Vesicoureteral Reflux

Prem Puri • Atsuyuki Yamataka
Editors

Vesicoureteral Reflux

Springer

Editors
Prem Puri
Beacon Consultants Clinic
University College Dublin
Dublin, Ireland

Atsuyuki Yamataka
Pediatric Surgery and Urogenital Surgery
Juntendo University School of Medicine
Tokyo, Japan

ISBN 978-3-031-95090-2 ISBN 978-3-031-95091-9 (eBook)
https://doi.org/10.1007/978-3-031-95091-9

This Springer imprint is published by the registered company Springer Nature Switzerland AG
The registered company address is: Gewerbestrasse 11, 6330 Cham, Switzerland

To Nina, Rumi, Hinata, Ichika, and Karen- bright young hearts who remind us daily why we care for children and strive to build a healthier future

Contents

About the Editors

Prem Puri MBBS, LRCP, LRCS(Ed), DCH, MS, FRCS, FRCS(Ed), FACS, FCS Paed Surg(SA)(Hon), FAAP(Hon), D.Sc(Hon), MEA, the Newman Clinical Research Professor at the University College Dublin, is a globally recognized leader in pediatric surgery. He is a Past President of the World Federation of Associations of Pediatric Surgeons (WOFAPS), the European Pediatric Surgeons Association (EUPSA), and the WOFAPS Foundation.

He served as the Editor-in-Chief of *Pediatric Surgery International* from 2001 to 2021, and is on the Editorial Board of several other journals. As Director of Research (1989–2009) and later President (2009–2016) of the National Children's Research Centre at Our Lady's Children's Hospital in Dublin, he led the largest pediatric research institute in Ireland.

Renowned for his pioneering research into the mechanisms and management of congenital disorders, his work has significantly advanced global clinical practices. His groundbreaking research on vesicoureteral reflux (VUR) led to the development of a minimally invasive 15-minute endoscopic procedure that replaced traditional open surgery and transformed patient care worldwide.

He is one of the most widely cited pediatric surgical researchers in the world. His research work has been cited over 28,000 times in peer-reviewed articles with h-index of 83 and i10-index of 540. He has published 11 books and monographs, 147 chapters in textbooks and over 700 articles in peer-reviewed journals.

He has been awarded many Honorary Memberships/Fellowships, including the American Surgical Association (ASA), German Society of Surgery, Association of Surgeons of India, American Academy of Pediatrics, American Pediatric Surgical Association, Canadian Association of Pediatric Surgeons, Japanese Society of Pediatric Surgeons, and Argentinean, Austrian, Canadian, Czech, Croatian, Cuban, Indian, and South African pediatric surgical associations.

He is a multi-award-winning researcher whose previous awards include People of the Year Award (Ireland), the prestigious Denis Browne Gold Medal by the British Association of Pediatric Surgeons, Rehbein Medal by the European Paediatric Surgeons Association, and Colles Medal by the Royal College of Surgeons in Ireland, for outstanding contribution to pediatric surgery. He has been a visiting professor to many leading universities all over the world and invited speaker at over 250 international scientific meetings.

Atsuyuki Yamataka MD, PhD, FAAP (Hon.), is a distinguished figure in pediatric surgery and currently holds the position of Special Professor at the Department of Pediatric General and Urogenital Surgery at Juntendo University School of Medicine in Tokyo. He also serves as a Visiting Professor in the Department of Gastrointestinal and Pediatric Surgery at Tokyo Medical University. From 2006 to 2024, he was Professor and Chief of Pediatric Surgery at Juntendo University.

A recognized leader in minimally invasive pediatric surgery, Professor Yamataka is Past President of the International Pediatric Endosurgery Group (IPEG), the Asian Association of Pediatric Surgeons, and the Pacific Association of Pediatric Surgeons. He is an Associate Editor of both the *Journal of Pediatric Surgery* and the *European Journal of Pediatric Surgery*, and serves on the Executive Editorial Board of *Pediatric Surgery International.*

His prolific academic contributions include over 500 peer-reviewed publications. His key research interests span the developmental biology of Hirschsprung's disease, pediatric hepatobiliary disorders, and emerging fields such as organoid research.

His excellence in academic mentorship and clinical innovation has earned him honorary memberships in premier organizations such as the American Academy of Pediatrics, the American Pediatric Surgical Association, and the European Paediatric Surgeons' Association.

He is a sought-after speaker, having been invited as guest lecturer at over 100 international scientific meetings, and has served as visiting professor at leading universities across the globe.

Contributors

Diana A. Aponte-Colon Department of Urology, Duke University School of Medicine, Durham, NC, USA

Angela M. Arlen Department of Urology, Yale School of Medicine, Yale University, New Haven, CT, USA

J. Christopher Austin Department of Urology, Division of Pediatric Urology, School of Medicine, Oregon Health and Sciences University, Portland, OR, USA

David L. Barquin Department of Urology, Duke University School of Medicine, Durham, NC, USA

Lorenzo Biassoni Department of Radiology, Great Ormond Street Hospital for Children, London, UK

Per Brandström Queen Silvia Children's Hospital, Sahlgrenska University Hospital, Gothenburg, Sweden
Department of Pediatrics, Institute of Clinical Science at Sahlgrenska Academy, University of Gothenburg, Gothenburg, Sweden
The Department of Pediatric Nephrology, Pediatric Uro-Nephrologic Center, Queen Silvia Children's Hospital, Sahlgrenska University Hospital, Gothenburg, Sweden
Inst of Clinical Science, Dept of Pediatrics, Sahlgrenska Academy, University of Gothenburg, Gothenburg, Sweden

Nicola Capozza Department of Surgery, Luigi Maria Monti Foundation, Rome, Italy

Salvatore Cascio School of Medicine, University College Dublin and Children's Health Ireland, Dublin, Ireland

Boris Chertin Departments of Urology & Pediatric Urology, Shaare Zedek Medical Center, Faculty of Medicine, Hebrew University, Jerusalem, Israel

Leon Chertin Department of Urology, Shamir Medical Center, Faculty of Medicine Tel Aviv University, Zerifin, Israel

Emily K. Clennon Department of Urology, Oregon Health & Science University, Portland, OR, USA

Christopher J. Corbett Division of Pediatric Urology, Children's National Medical Center, Washington, DC, USA

David Coyle Department of Pediatric Urology, Children's Health Ireland at Crumlin, Dublin, Ireland

John M. Darlow Formerly of Department of Genetics, Children's Health Ireland, Dublin, Ireland

Fulvia Del Conte Pediatric Surgery Unit, "Federico II" University of Naples, Naples, Italy

Amane Endo Department of Pediatrics, Faculty of Medicine, Juntendo University, Tokyo, Japan

Maria Escolino Pediatric Surgery Unit, "Federico II" University of Naples, Naples, Italy

Ciro Esposito Pediatric Surgery Unit, "Federico II" University of Naples, Naples, Italy

Marie-Klaire Farrugia Department of Paediatric Urology, Chelsea and Westminster Hospital and Imperial College (West London Children's Healthcare), London, UK

Sverker Hansson Queen Silvia Children's Hospital, Sahlgrenska University Hospital, Gothenburg, Sweden
Inst of Clinical Science, Dept of Pediatrics, Sahlgrenska Academy, University of Gothenburg, Gothenburg, Sweden

Gundela Holmdahl Division of Pediatric Urology, Astrid Lindgren's Children's Hospital, Karolinska University Hospital, Stockholm, Sweden
Department of Women's and Children's Health, Karolinska Institutet, Stockholm, Sweden

Manuela Hunziker University Hospital Zurich, Zurich, Switzerland

Laura Jackson Department of Paediatric Surgery and Urology, Bristol Royal Hospital for Children, Bristol, UK

Andrew J. Kirsch Department of Pediatric Urology, Emory University and Children's Healthcare of Atlanta, Atlanta, GA, USA

Martin A. Koyle Department of Urology, University of Minnesota Faculty of Medicine and Masonic Children's Hospital, Minneapolis, Minnesota, USA

Balazs Kutasy Division of Pediatric Urology, Astrid Lindgren's Children's Hospital, Karolinska University Hospital, Stockholm, Sweden

Magnus Lindén Department of Pediatrics, Halland Hospital, Halmstad, Sweden
Inst of Clinical Science, Dept of Pediatrics, Sahlgrenska Academy, University of Gothenburg, Gothenburg, Sweden

Armando Lorenzo Division of Urology, The Hospital for Sick Children, University of Toronto, Toronto, ON, Canada

Tej K. Mattoo Division of Pediatric Nephrology, Wayne Pediatrics, Departments of Pediatrics and Urology, Wayne State University School of Medicine, Detroit, MI, USA

Ermelinda Mele Department of Pediatric Urology, Bambino Gesù Children's Hospital, Rome, Italy

Dunya Mohammad Division of Pediatric Nephrology, Department of Pediatrics, University of South Alabama, Mobile, AL, USA

Mayu Nakagawa Department of Pediatrics, Faculty of Medicine, Juntendo University, Tokyo, Japan

Tryggve Nevéus Department of Women's and Children's Health, Uppsala University, Uppsala, Sweden

Josefin Nordenström Department of Pediatrics, Institute of Clinical Science at Sahlgrenska Academy, University of Gothenburg, Gothenburg, Sweden
The Department of Pediatric Surgery/Urology, Pediatric Uro-Nephrologic Center, Queen Silvia Children's Hospital, Sahlgrenska University Hospital, Gothenburg, Sweden

Benjamin H. Press Department of Pediatric Urology, Emory University and Children's Healthcare of Atlanta, Atlanta, GA, USA

Prem Puri Beacon Consultants Clinic, University College Dublin, Dublin, Ireland

G. Raisin Departments of Urology & Pediatric Urology, Shaare Zedek Medical Center, Faculty of Medicine, Hebrew University, Jerusalem, Israel

Jonathan C. Routh Department of Urology, Duke University School of Medicine, Durham, NC, USA

Mohamed Sameh Shalaby Department of Paediatric Surgery and Urology, Bristol Royal Hospital for Children, Bristol, UK

Soichi Shibuya Department of Pediatric General and Urogenital Surgery, Juntendo University School of Medicine, Tokyo, Japan

Yvonne Simrén Department of Radiology, Institute of Clinical Sciences at Sahlgrenska Academy, University of Gothenburg, Gothenburg, Sweden
The Department of Pediatric Radiology, Queen Silvia Children's Hospital, Sahlgrenska University Hospital, Gothenburg, Sweden

Yutaka Tanami Division of Radiology, Saitama Children's Medical Center, Saitama, Japan

Priyank Yadav Department of Urology and Renal Transplantation, Sanjay Gandhi Postgraduate Institute of Medical Sciences, Lucknow, India

Atsuyuki Yamataka Department of Pediatric General and Urogenital Surgery, Juntendo University School of Medicine, Tokyo, Japan

Historical Aspects of Vesicoureteral Reflux

Prem Puri

Abstract The management of vesicoureteral reflux (VUR), characterized by the retrograde flow of urine from the bladder into the ureters and kidneys has been controversial from the outset. The role of continuous antibiotic prophylaxis and surgical intervention is still debated. Understanding the historical context and current perspectives surrounding VUR is essential for a comprehensive grasp of the disease, especially given its significance in the evolution of pediatric urology as a subspecialty. The contributions of key leaders and the advancements in diagnostic and therapeutic approaches have significantly improved patient outcomes. Recognising the historical milestones and important contributions from key leaders in the field should allow clinicians to effectively address the complexities of this condition and provide the best possible care for their patients.

Keywords Vesicoureteral reflux · Historical aspects · Continuous antibiotic prophylaxis · Ureteral reimplantation · Endoscopic treatment · Renal parenchymal damage · Urinary tract infections

Introduction

Primary vesicoureteral reflux (VUR), a congenital anatomical defect of the ureterovesical junction, is one of the most prevalent urological abnormalities in infants and children. The association between VUR, urinary tract infections (UTIs), and renal parenchymal damage is well established. However, the management of VUR remains controversial. Research over the past two decades has enhanced our understanding of the natural history of VUR and identified patients at higher risk for both VUR and associated renal parenchymal damage. Despite this progress, debate persists over key management issues, such as the timing of diagnostic imaging and

P. Puri (✉)
Beacon Consultants Clinic, University College Dublin, Dublin, Ireland

P. Puri, A. Yamataka (eds.), *Vesicoureteral Reflux*,
https://doi.org/10.1007/978-3-031-95091-9_1

determining which pediatric patients benefit from continuous antibiotic prophylaxis or surgical intervention.

A comprehensive understanding of any disease requires a deep knowledge of historical developments and the insights of key leaders in the field, which have shaped current practices. This is especially true for Vesicoureteral Reflux (VUR), a condition that has been fundamental to the emergence of pediatric urology as a subspecialty [1]. This chapter provides a comprehensive summary of the historical aspects of primary VUR, covering various important aspects such as anatomical and functional basis of vesicoureteral reflux, VUR associated renal parenchymal damage, grading systems for VUR, and medical and surgical management of VUR.

Historical Aspects of Anatomical and Functional Basis of Vesicoureteral Reflux

Properly functioning ureterovesical junction (UVJ) permits urine to pass from the ureters into the bladder while preventing the backflow of urine into the ureters during both bladder filling and voiding. The anatomy of the ureterovesical junction has been studied for centuries. The earliest recognition of the antireflux mechanism of the normal ureterovesical junction dates to Galen (129–217 AD), whose influence on medical science including anatomy and physiology, remained unchallenged in Europe and the Middle East throughout the Middle Ages and Renaissance [2]. Galen proposed that the oblique passage of the ureter through the bladder wall results in the one directional flow of urine and thus provides protection against reflux. Leonardo da Vinci (1452–1519 AD) performed dissections and created anatomical illustrations, suggesting an antireflux mechanism to prevent urine from returning into upper urinary tracts [3]. His anatomical sketches illustrate the path of the ureter as it enters the bladder near the bladder neck, makes a U-turn, and then runs upward to the middle of the bladder lumen.

Our current understanding of the anatomical basis of vesicoureteral reflux is derived from the detailed research work on the musculature of the distal ureter and trigone, length of the intravesical ureter, and size and configuration of the ureteral orifice by a number of investigators [4–7]. In the normal urinary tract as the ureter approaches the bladder it loses its circular muscle fibres and within the bladder wall it is surrounded solely by longitudinal muscle fibres. These longitudinal fibres continue beyond the ureteral orifice into the trigone, fanning out and mingling with similar fibres from the opposite side and being firmly attached to the mucosa of the trigone. Thus the ureter has only one firm attachment to the bladder-that is, at its orifice by its longitudinal muscle fibres running into the trigone. During micturition or when the bladder contracts, the competent UVJ provides a predominantly passive one-way valve mechanism and closes. In this way, the UVJ is structurally and functionally adapted to allow the intermittent passage of urine into the bladder as well as prevent the retrograde flow of urine into the ureter or kidney. The main mechanism for an incompetent UVJ is believed to be the presence of a short intramural tunnel and the absence of adequate detrusor support for the intravesical ureter. Congenital deficiency or absence of the longitudinal muscle fibers of the intravesical ureter, as seen in primary VUR, results in upward and lateral displacement of the ureteral orifice, thereby reducing the length and obliquity of the intravesical ureter [6]. Paquin [5] was the first to describe the normal anatomical dimensions of the intravesical submucosal tunnel of the ureter, characterized by an oblique entry of the ureter into the bladder, resulting in a 5:1 ratio of submucosal tunnel length to ureteral diameter. In addition, the intramural ureter must be supported behind by a firm muscle and terminate low in the bladder base where it is firmly anchored.

VUR is classified as either primary or secondary VUR. Primary VUR is attributed to structural failed development or immaturity of the UVJ, which results in an abnormally short and inadequate intravesical submucosal tunnel length and an absence of adequate detrusor support behind the intravesical ureter. Secondary VUR is much less common and is usually due to abnormal bladder dynamics and/or elevated voiding pressures seen with lower urinary tract dysfunction stemming from bladder outlet obstruction, neurogenic bladder, or dysfunctional voiding [8].

VUR Associated Renal Parenchymal Damage

The association of UTI, VUR and renal parenchymal damage has been the subject of much discussion since 1952, when Hutch [9] first drew attention to the damaging effects of VUR with UTI on the renal parenchyma. In 1960 Hodson and Edwards [10] reported that focal scarring in VUR is due to UTIs. Rolleston et al. [11] reported that UTI plays an important role in producing renal parenchymal damage in the presence of VUR, but they also suggested that gross reflux can cause progressive damage in the absence of infection. They suggested that the hydrodynamic effect of VUR is an important factor in producing renal damage in the prenatal and neonatal period causing continuing insult to and atrophy of the sensitive developing renal tissue [11, 12]. Hodson et al. [13] demonstrated in their high pressure porcine model that linear cortical scars could develop at the location of the intrarenal reflux even though the urine was kept sterile throughout the experiment by means of chemoprophylaxis and asserted that a high intravesical pressure was the most important initiating event, bacteriuria playing a secondary role. Ransley and Risdon [14] observed renal scarring in a porcine model with the combination of VUR, UTI and elevated intravesical pressure. The investigators found that the intrarenal reflux of infected urine through compound papillae is central to the acquired scarring process. Therefore, permanent renal injury associated with VUR can result either from congenital renal dysplasia secondary to embryological alterations in bladder dynamics or from acquired postinfectious damage following an UTI due to pyelonephritis [15, 16]. The term reflux nephropathy (RN) was first introduced by Bailey [17] to emphasize the association between VUR and the coarse renal scarring. While congenital RN is more common in male infants with high-grade VUR, acquired renal scarring after a single or recurrent UTI is more common in girls [18, 19].

Grading of Vesicoureteral Reflux

Despite the concerns about ionizing radiation and its invasive nature, voiding cysto-urethrography (VCUG) remains the gold standard for diagnosing VUR (Fig. 1). However, until 1985, no common grading system for VUR existed. In 1974, Colodny and Lebowitz [20] made a plea for grading VUR, suggesting that both medical and surgical therapies could only be evaluated if results were discussed with an internationally acceptable standardized system. The lack of standardization hampered

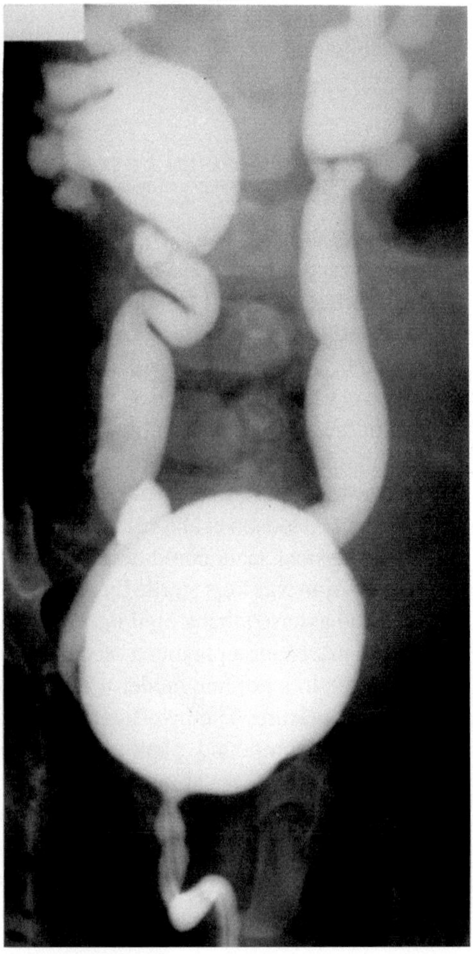

Fig. 1 VCUG showing bilateral high grade vesicoureteral reflux in a 10-month-old infant. Note normal urethra and bladder wall

communication not only between institutions, but also clinicians working in the same institution [21].

In 1962, Melick et al. [22] proposed the first system for grading VUR, based on the visualization that cine cystourethrography offered of the voiding mechanism:

Group1: No reflux on filling the bladder, reflux only on raised intravesical pressure.
Group2: Reflux at large volumes with low or normal intravesical pressure
Group 3: Reflux at normal volumes with an elevated intravesical pressure
Group 4: Reflux at an extremely low volume with low or normal intravesical pressure
Group 5: Reflux at an extremely low volume and markedly elevated intravesical pressure

Howerton and Lich [23] in 1963 proposed the first grading system based on degree of dilatation:

Group1: Opacification of the terminal ureter alone or of the entire ureter and kidney, but without dilatation.
Group 2: Moderate ureteral dilatation and calyceal fullness.
Group 3: Marked ureteral dilatation and gross calyceal damage
Group 4: Profound dilatation of the renal pelvis, calyces, and ureter associated with ureteral tortuosity.

During the next few years there were number of other grading systems for VUR reported ([24, 25]; In 1985, Lebowitz et al. [26] reported International Reflux Study grading system based upon the contrast VCUG. Currently, this is the most used grading system and has been used by the clinicians to predict resolution of VUR as well as guide medical and surgical therapy. The severity of VUR in the International Reflux Study grading system includes domains such as height of retrograde flow as well as degree of dilatation and tortuosity of the ureter on voiding cystourethrogram. This grading system includes five grades, ranging from grade I with reflux into a non-dilated ureter to grade V with reflux through a massively dilated and tortuous ureter into a severely dilated renal pelvis and blunt calyces (Fig. 2). Depending on the grade of VUR, the probability of spontaneous reflux resolution and risk of permanent renal injury has been estimated. In general, a lower reflux grade correlates with a higher chance of spontaneous resolution, whereas higher grades of VUR are associated with an increased occurrence of renal scarring.

Medical Management

The concept of continuous antibiotic prophylaxis (CAP) in the management of vesicoureteral reflux (VUR) emerged in response to the recognition of the link between VUR, urinary tract infections (UTIs), and renal scarring. Early studies in the mid-twentieth century established that recurrent UTIs in children with VUR could lead to significant renal damage, including scarring and potential long-term

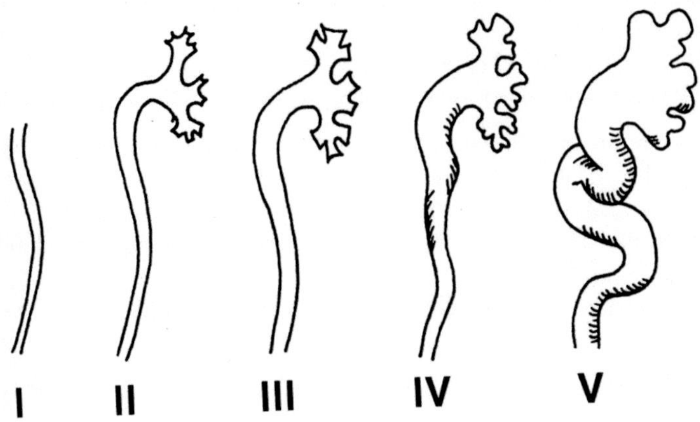

Fig. 2 International classification of vesicoureteral reflux (Grade I–V)

consequences such as hypertension and chronic kidney disease. The medical management is based on three important assumptions: (1) Sterile VUR in most cases is not harmful to the kidneys (2) Children can outgrow VUR, at least the lower grades (3) continuous low-dose antibiotic prophylaxis can prevent infection for years while VUR is still present.

One of the earliest studies advocating for the use of antibiotics to prevent recurrent UTIs in children with VUR was conducted by Normand and Smellie [27] and they demonstrated that continuous low-dose antibiotics could reduce the incidence of recurrent UTIs in children, thereby potentially preventing renal scarring. By the 1980s, CAP had become a widely accepted standard of care for managing children with VUR, particularly those with low to moderate grades of reflux. Several studies provided evidence that CAP was effective in reducing the frequency of UTIs in children with VUR [28–31]. It has also been reported that CAP is superior to watchful waiting or surveillance concerning prevention of UTIs in children with high grade VUR [28, 32, 33]. There is known concomitant relationship between VUR, UTIs, and bowel and bladder dysfunction (BBD), characterized by a high bladder capacity and incomplete bladder emptying associated with an increased post-void residual [34]. The Swedish reflux trial in children reported that 20% of patients enrolled with high grade reflux had BBD [35]. Dilating reflux directly correlated with bladder dysfunction and successful treatment of bladder dysfunction was associated with improvement of reflux grade. They recommended CAP for those with concomitant BBD and VUR due to an increased risk of UTI.

Mixed results have been reported in relation to the role of CAP in the prevention of renal scarring in VUR. The Swedish reflux study reported a significant higher risk of developing renal scarring without treatment [19]. However, the Randomized Intervention for Children with Vesicoureteral Reflux (RIVUR) trial showed that there was a 50% reduction in the risk of recurrence of UTI in children who were on CAP but the prophylaxis did not decrease the risk of renal scarring [36, 37]. Furthermore, A meta-analysis that included seven randomized controlled trials revealed that antimicrobial prophylaxis did not prevent UTI-related renal scarring in children with VUR [38].

In recent years various professional organizations like the National Institute for Health and Clinical Excellence [39], American Academy of Pediatrics (AAP) [40] and the European Association of Urology (EAU)/European Society of Pediatric Urology (ESPU) [41], have developed comprehensive guidelines for the diagnosis, management, and follow-up of patients with VUR. These guidelines provide practical considerations for the management of VUR in children based on risk analysis and selective indications for diagnostic tests, medical management including treatment of bladder and bowel dysfunction and surgical interventions. The AAP guidelines of 2011 recommended renal and bladder ultrasound in patients between 2 and 24 months of age with their first febrile UTI and no VCUG without ultrasound detectable abnormalities, thereby significantly reducing the use of VCUG.

More recently, artificial intelligence (AI) and machine learning is gaining increased popularity and credibility in pediatric urology for predicting the outcome of surgical procedures and demonstrating the severity of the condition based on imaging. Several AI and machine learning models have been developed for VUR [42]. Computer vision models using VCUG have been investigated. An optimal tree model to predict the recurrence of UTI associated with VUR from the RIVUR and Careful Urinary Tract Infection Evaluation (CUTIE) study patients was developed. This predictive model provided promising performance to facilitate individualized treatment in children with an initial UTI and identify those most likely to benefit from VCUG after the initial UTI [43]. Prediction models have also been developed to predict VUR by RBUS, spontaneous resolution of primary VUR, VUR grade using VCUG, predict VUR *vs.* UTI using clinical data, UTI following VUR and likely benefit from antimicrobial prophylaxis [44–46].

Surgical Management

Open Ureteral Reimplantation

The genesis of open ureteral reimplantation for the treatment of VUR began when Hutch [9] recognised a casual relationship between VUR and pyelonephritis in paraplegic patients. He performed antireflux surgery in 9 paraplegic patients, after which six patients were cured of their VUR. The principle behind antireflux operations was to lengthen the intravesical ureter against a solid detrusor support to allow its compression against the detrusor. The 1950s and 1960s saw a significant progress in the development of surgical techniques for ureteral reimplantation. Various intravesical, extravesical and combined intra and extravesical techniques for ureteral reimplantation were described for the surgical correction of VUR. In 1958, Politano and Leadbetter [47] introduced an intravesical reimplantation technique combined with extravesical dissection to create a neo-hiatus insertion site into the posterior bladder wall superior and medial to the original hiatus. This technique which created a submucosal tunnel for the ureter within the bladder wall, providing a valve like effect to prevent reflux became very popular. In 1959, Paquin reported a technique whereby the ureters were divided extravesically. The defunctionalized, distal ureter was left intact and the ureteral stumps were reimplanted, creating an intravesical nipple [48]. In 1960s, Lich and Gregoir simultaneously developed the extravesical technique of ureteral reimplantation [49, 50]. This technique involves extravesical dissection of the ureter towards the ureteral orifice, followed by an incision through the seromuscular layer but not through the mucosal layer to create a bed for the extravesical ureter, followed by a closure of the detrusor muscle defect upon the ureter [8]. This technique was not popular originally but in recent years it is gaining popularity for laparoscopic extravesical ureteral reimplantation or robot-assisted extravesical ureteral reimplantation.

Another notable contribution was the cross-trigonal technique introduced by Cohen in 1975. Cohen [51] reported some of the best success rates with low complication rates due to the preservation of the original ureteral hiatus into the bladder and maintaining completely intravesical dissection. Currently, Cohen's cross-trigonal and Politano Leadbetter techniques are considered gold standards for open ureteral reimplantation surgery.

Laparoscopic and Robot-Assisted Ureteral Reimplantation

Traditional open ureteral reimplantation, while effective, involved significant morbidity, including larger incisions and dissection, considerable postoperative pain, and prolonged recovery [52, 53]. The 1980s and 1990s saw the introduction of minimally invasive techniques in pediatric urology, including endoscopic, laparoscopic and robotic-assisted approaches to treat VUR. These methods aimed to reduce the surgical trauma and recovery time associated with open surgery.

The first laparoscopic ureteral reimplantation was performed by Ehrlich [54] in 1994. Over the following years, the laparoscopic approach was refined to improve outcomes and reduce operative times. Techniques such as the laparoscopic extravesical (LEVUR) and trans-vesicoscopic (TVUR) ureteral reimplantation were developed, mirroring the principles of open surgery but with the advantages of minimally invasive methods [55–58]. Babu and Chandrasekharam [59] in a meta-analysis compared outcomes of LEVUR versus TVUR and found that LEVUR had a shorter operating time, higher success rate, and shorter hospital stay compared to TVUR. They attributed this to higher number of unilateral VUR cases and lower number of grade V VUR cases in the LEVUR group. Although laparoscopic ureteral reimplantation has been reported as a safe and effective option, its widespread adoption has been limited because of the difficult intra-corporeal suturing [60].

The early 2000s saw the introduction of robotic surgical systems, such as the da Vinci Surgical System, which provided enhanced precision, dexterity, and three-dimensional imaging which were particularly useful for the visualization and handling of the delicate anatomical structures in infants and children. This technology quickly gained interest in the field of pediatric urology, allowing better suturing precision, reduced blood loss, and shorter hospital stays. In 2005, Peters and Woo [61] reported the first case of robotic-assisted ureteral reimplantation. Over the past decade, robot-assisted laparoscopic ureteral reimplantation (RALUR) has become a viable minimally invasive surgical option for vesicoureteral reflux (VUR), although there is evidence that the success rate with this method is lower and the incidence of postoperative urinary retention higher in patients undergoing bilateral procedures compared to open reimplantation [62, 63]. High cost of robotic systems, need for specialized training and the slow development of miniaturized robotic instruments have restricted accessibility to these approaches [60]. Future efforts should aim at reducing costs to make the robotic technology more accessible, better robotic instrumentation suited to pediatric population, and improved training programs for surgeons.

Endoscopic Treatment

The introduction of endoscopic treatment of VUR by Puri & O'Donnell was a radical change from the previously standard observational management and surgical intervention [12]. They induced VUR in 2- to 4-weeks-old piglets VUR by opening the bladder and slitting the anterior wall of both intravesical ureters and cured it by injecting polytetrafluoroethylene (PTFE) paste subureterically [64]. This novel approach, in addition to producing a solid support behind the refluxing intravesical ureter also provided a firm anchorage to the intravesical ureter, thereby preventing VUR. The authors called this new procedure "*The STING*", which stands for subureteric Teflon injection [65, 66]. This innovation brought about a revolution in the surgical management of VUR that has largely stood the test of time with only relatively minor modifications as advances in materials science and our understanding of VUR have progressed [12]. The various bulking agents that have been used endoscopically to treat VUR include PTFE, collagen, polydimethylsiloxane, dextranomer/hyaluronic acid and polyacrylate polyalcohol copolymer hydrogel [67].

The greatest paradigm shift in the endoscopic treatment of VUR occurred when the Food and Drug Administration (FDA) in 2001 approved dextranomer/hyaluronic acid (Deflux®) as an acceptable and biocompatible tissue augmenting substance for the endoscopic treatment of VUR in children. Another important milestone in the endoscopic treatment of VUR was in 2002. This year the Journal of Urology accorded "Classic Article Status" to important urological innovations published in the last century which had major impact on patient treatment worldwide. The STING article published in the British Medical Journal in 1984 was accorded "Classic Article in Pediatric Urology" status [68]. Since Deflux® was approved by the FDA for the endoscopic treatment of VUR in children in 2001, the procedure rapidly gained worldwide popularity and is today an integral part of the AUA guidelines [33] and the EAU/European Society of Pediatric Urology guidelines [41] for the management of primary VUR in children. Currently, Deflux® is considered the preferred choice and the most used tissue augmenting substance for the endoscopic injection. This 15-min outpatient procedure has several advantages. In contrast to long-term antimicrobial prophylaxis, it offers immediate cure of VUR, its success does not rely on patient or parent compliance and the procedure is virtually free of complications.

The indications for endoscopic treatment of VUR are basically the same as for open, laparoscopic and robotic-assisted anti-reflux procedures, including high-grade primary VUR, breakthrough UTIs on continuous antibiotic prophylaxis (CAP), non-compliance with CAP and new renal scarring [67]. Endoscopic injection therapy has also been used successfully to treat VUR in duplex renal systems, VUR secondary to neuropathic bladder or posterior urethral valves, VUR in failed reimplanted ureters, VUR following renal transplantation and VUR in refluxing ureteral stumps [12].

Several injection techniques for the endoscopic treatment of VUR have been described, including subureteric injection (STING) [65, 66], intraureteric hydrodistention implantation technique (HIT) [69], combined HIT/STING and double HIT (i.e., proximal and distal intraluminal submucosal injections) [70]. The STING procedure, introduced by Puri in 1984, is the most adopted technique for endoscopic correction of VUR worldwide, whereas double HIT is the most utilized technique in the United States [71]. Most multivariate analyses did not show any significant outcome differences between both techniques [72–74].

The 40 years' experience with endoscopic correction of VUR has demonstrated that this outpatient procedure is safe, effective, and has had a much less negative impact on patients than any other surgical technique to treat reflux [12]. Clinical data from several studies have confirmed the long-term safety and efficacy of endoscopic treatment [12, 71]. Endoscopic correction is currently the first line of treatment for children with grade III to V primary reflux and complex cases of VUR in many institutions worldwide because of the simplicity of the procedure [71, 75–79]. In contrast to CAP, this procedure offers immediate cure with resolution rates ranging from 77% to 83% after first injection [67] and is independent of patient or parent compliance. Parental preferences, opinion of the nephrologist/pediatric urologist and the treating hospital play a major role in the selection of endoscopic treatment over the traditional methods of CAP or ureteral reimplantation [80–84].

References

1. Penna FJ, Caldamone A, Koyle MA. Coming full circle with vesicoureteral reflux: from Hutch to bladder and bowel dysfunction. Pediatr Urol. 2017;13(2):189–91.
2. Bloom DA, Milen MT, Heininger JC. Claudius Galen: from a 20th century genitourinary perspective. J Urol. 1999;161:12–9.
3. Schultheisis D, Grunewald V, Jonas U. Urodynamics in the anatomical work of Leonardo da Vinci (1452–1519). World J Urol. 1999;17:137–14.
4. Hutch JA. Theory of maturation of the intravesical ureter. J Urol. 1961;86:534–8.
5. Paquin AJ. Ureterovesical anastomosis: the description and evaluation of a technique. J Urol. 1959;82:573–83.
6. Stephens FD, Lenaghan D. The anatomical basis and dynamics of vesicoureteral reflux. J Urol. 1962;87:669–80.
7. Tanagho EA, Pugh RC. The anatomy and function of the ureterovesical junction. Br J Urol. 1963;35:151–65.
8. Rensing A, Austin P. The diagnosis and treatment of vesicoureteral reflux: an update. Open Urol Nephrol J. 2015;8:96–103.
9. Hutch JA. Vesico-ureteral reflux in the paraplegic: cause and correction. J Urol. 1952;68(2):457–69.
10. Hodson CJ, Edwards D. Chronic pyelonephritis and vesico-ureteric reflex. Clin Radiol. 1960;11:219–31.
11. Rolleston GL, Shannon FT, Utley WL. Relationship of infantile vesicoureteric reflux to renal damage. Br Med J. 1970;1(5694):460–3.
12. Kutasy B, Coyle D. History of endoscopic treatment of vesicoureteral reflux. Pediatr Surg Int. 2023;39:187.
13. Hodson CJ, Mailing TMJ, McManamon PJ, Lewis MG. The pathogenesis of reflux nephropathy (chronic atrophic pyelonephritis). Brit J Radiol. 1975;Suppl 13:1–26.
14. Ransley PG, Risdon RA. Renal papillae and intra-renal reflux in the pig. Lancet. 1974;2:1114.
15. Peters C, Rushton HG. Vesicoureteral reflux associated renal damage: congenital reflux nephropathy and acquired renal scarring. J Urol. 2010;184:265–73.
16. Swerkersson S, Jodal U, Sixt R, Stokland E, Hansson S. Relationship among vesicoureteral reflux, urinary tract infection and renal damage in children. J Urol. 2007;178:647–51.
17. Bailey PR. The relationship of vesicoureteric reflux to urinary tract infection and chronic pyelonephritis- reflux nephropathy. Clin Nephrol. 1973;1:132–41.
18. Alsaywid BS, Saleh H, Deshpandey A, et al. High grade primary vesicoureteral reflux in boys: long-term results of a prospective cohort study. J Urol. 2010;184:1598–603.
19. Brandstrom P, Neveus T, Sixt R, et al. The Swedish reflux trial in children: IV. Renal damage. J Urol. 2010;184:292–7.
20. Colodny AH, Lebowitz RL. A plea for grading vesicoureteric reflux. Urology. 1974;4:357–8.
21. Duckett JW, Bellinger MF. Cystographic grading of primary reflux as an indicator of treatment. In: Johnston JH, editor. Management of vesicoureteric reflux. Baltimore/London: Williams & Wilkins; 1984. p. 97–109.
22. Melick WF, Brodeur A, Karellos D. A suggested classification of ureteral reflux and suggested treatment based on cineradiolographic findings and simultaneous pressure recordings by means of the strain gauge. J Urol. 1962;88:35–7.
23. Howerton LW, Lich R. The cause and correction of ureteral reflux. J Urol. 1963;89:672–5.
24. Heikel PE, Parkkulainen KV. Vesicoureteric reflux in children. A classification and results of conservative treatment. Ann Radiol. 1966;9:37–40.
25. Williams DI, Eckstein HB. Surgical treatment of reflux in children. Br J Urol. 1965;37:13–24.
26. Lebowitz RL, Olbing H, Parkkulainen KV, Smellie JM, Tamminen-Möbius TE. International system of radiographic grading of vesicoureteric reflux. International reflux study in children. Pediatr Radiol. 1985;15:105–9.

27. Normand ICS, Smellie JM. Prolonged maintenance chemotherapy in the management of urinary infection in childhood. Br Med J. 1965;1:1023–6.
28. Craig JC, et al. Antibiotic prophylaxis and recurrent urinary tract infection in children. N Engl J Med. 2009;361:1748–59.
29. Elder JS, Peters CA, Arant BS Jr, et al. Pediatric vesicoureteral reflux guidelines panel summary report on the management of primary vesicoureteral reflux I children. J Urol. 1997;157:1846–51.
30. Wheeler DM, Vimalachandra D, Hodson EM, et al. Interventions for primary vesicoureteral reflux. Cochrane Database Syst Rev. 2004;2:CD001532.
31. Williams GJ, Wei L, Lee A, Craig JC. Long-term antibiotics for preventing recurrent urinary tract infections in children. Cochrane Database Syst Rev. 2006;3:CD001534.
32. Brandstrom P, Esbjorner E, Herthelius M, et al. The Swedish reflux trial in children: III. Urinary tract infections pattern. J Urol. 2010;184:286–91.
33. Peters CA, et al. Summary of the AUA guideline on management of primary vesicoureteral reflux in children. J Urol. 2010;184:1134–44.
34. Koff SA, Lapides J, Piazza DH. Association of urinary tract infection and reflux with uninhibited bladder contractions and voluntary sphincteric obstruction. J Urol. 1979;122:373–6.
35. Sillén U, Brandström P, Jodal U, et al. The Swedish reflux trial in children: v. bladder dysfunction. J Urol. 2010;184:298–304.
36. Mathews R, Mattoo TK. The role of antimicrobial prophylaxis in the management of children with vesicoureteral reflux- the RIVUR study outcomes. Adv Chronic Kidney Dis. 2015;22:325–30.
37. Mattoo TK, et al. Renal scarring in the randomized intervention for children with vesicoureteral reflux (RIVUR) trial. Clin J Am Soc Nephrol. 2016;11:54–61.
38. Hewitt IK, Pennesi M, Morello W, Ronfani L, Montini G. Antibiotic prophylaxis for urinary tract infection-related renal scarring: a systematic review. Pediatrics. 2017;139:e20163145.
39. National Institute for health and clinical excellence: urinary tract infections in children. NICE; 2007. http://guidance.nice.org.uk/CG054.
40. Finnell SME, Carroll AE, et al. Diagnosis and management of an initial UTI in febrile infants and children. Pediatrics. 2011;128(3):e749–70. https://doi.org/10.1542/peds.2011-1332.
41. Gnech M, Hoen L, Zachou A, Bogaert G, Castagnetti, O'Kelly F, et al. Update and summary of the European Association of Urology/European Society of Pediatric Urology Paediatric guidelines on vesicoureteral reflux in children. Eur Urol. 2024;85:433–42.
42. Scott Wang HH, Vasdev R, Nelson CP. Artificial intelligence in pediatric urology. Urol Clin North Am. 2024;51:91–103.
43. Advanced Analytics Group of Pediatric Urology and ORC Personalized Medicine Group. Targeted workup after initial febrile urinary tract infection: using a novel machine learning model to identify children most likely to benefit from voiding cystourethrogram. J Urol. 2019;202:144–52.
44. Bertsimas D, Li M, Estrada C, Nelson C, Scott Wang HH. Selecting children with vesicoureteral reflux who are most likely to benefit from antibiotic prophylaxis: application of machine learning to RIVUR. J Urol. 2021;205:1170–9.
45. Eroglu Y, Yildirim K, Çinar A, Yildirim M. Diagnosis and grading of vesicoureteral reflux on voiding cystourethrography images in children using a deep hybrid model. Comput Methods Prog Biomed. 2021;210:106369.
46. Keskinoğlu A, Özgür S. The use of artificial neural networks for differential diagnosis between vesicoureteral reflux and urinary tract infection in children. J Pediatr Res. 2020;7:230–5.
47. Politano VA, Leadbetter WF. An operative technique for the correction of vesicoureteral reflux. J Urol. 1958;79(6):932–41.
48. Benway B, Slaughenhoupt B, Lich R Jr. Innovator in pediatric and adult urology. J Urol. 2007;177:845–8.
49. Gregoir W. Congenital vesico-ureteral reflux. Acta Urol Belg. 1962;30:286–300.
50. Lich R, Howerton LW, Davis LA. Recurrent urosepsis in children. J Urol. 1961;86:554–8.

51. Cohen SJ. Ureterozystonneostomie. Eine neue antirefluxtech-nik. Akt Urol. 1975;6:1.
52. Kurtz MP, Leow JJ, Varda BK, et al. Robotic versus open pediatric ureteral reimplantation: costs and complications from a nationwide sample. J Pediar Urol. 2016;12(408):e1–6.
53. Wang HH, Tejwani R, Cannon GM Jr, et al. Open versus minimally invasive ureteroneocystostomy; a population-level analysis. J Pediatr Urol. 2016;12(232):e1–6.
54. Ehrlich RM, Gershman A, Fuchs G. Laparoscopic vesicoureteroplasty in children: initial case reports. Urology. 1994;43:255–61.
55. Bayne AP, Shoss JM, Starke NR, et al. Single -center experience with pediatric laparoscopic extravesical reimlantation: safe and effective in simple and complex anatomy. J Laparoendosc Adv Surg Tech. 2012;22:102–6.
56. Bustangi N, Kailas Chemaly A, Scalabre A, et al. Extravesical ureteral reimplantation following Lich-Gregoir technique for the correction of vesicoureteral reflux: retrospective comparative study open versus laparoscopy. Front Pediatr. 2018;18:388.
57. Jayanthi VR. Vesicoscopic cross-trigonal ureteral reimplantation: high success rate for elimination of primary reflux. J Pediatr Urol. 2018;14:324.
58. Valla JS, Steyaert H, Griffin SJ, et al. Transvesicoscopic Cohen ureteric reimplantation for vesicoureteral reflux in children: a single- centre 5-year experience. J Pediatr Urol. 2009;5:466–71.
59. Babu R, Chandrasekharam VVS. A systematic review and meta-analysis comparing outcomes of laparoscopic extravesical versus vesicoscopic ureteric reimplantation. J Pediatr Urol. 2020;16:783–9.
60. Esposito C, Masieri L, Fourcade L, et al. Pediatric robot-assisted extravesical ureteral reimplantation (revur) in simple and complex anatomy: report of a multicenter experience. J Pediatr Urol. 2023;19:136–42.
61. Peters CA, Woo R. Intravesical robotically assisted bilateral ureteral reimplantation. J Endourol. 2005;19:618–21.
62. Boysen WR, Akhavan A, Ko J, et al. Prospective multicenter study on robot-assisted laparoscopic extravesical ureteral reimplantation(RALUR_EV): outcomes and complications. J Pediatr Urol. 2018;14:262.
63. Herz D, Fuchs M, Todd A, et al. Robot assisted-laparoscopic extravesical ureteral reimplant: a critical look at surgical outcomes. J Pediatr Urol. 2016;12:402.
64. Puri P, O'Donnell B. Correction of experimentally produced vesicoureteric reflux in the piglet by intravesical injection of Teflon. Br Med J (Clin Res Ed). 1984;289:5–7.
65. O'Donnell B, Puri P. Treatment of vesicoureteric reflux by endoscopic injection of Teflon. Br Med J (Clin Res Ed). 1984;289:7–9.
66. Puri P. Endoscopic correction of primary vesicoureteric reflux by subureteric injection of polytetrafluoroethylene. Lancet. 1990;335:1320–2.
67. Friedmacher F, Puri P. Endoscopic treatment of vesicoureteral reflux. In: Puri P, editor. Pediatric surgery. Berlin, Heidelberg: Springer; 2023. p. 59–61.
68. O'Donnell B, Puri P. Classic article in pediatric urology: treatment of vesicoureteric reflux by endoscopic injection of Teflon. J Urol. 2002;167:1808–9.
69. Kirsch AJ, Perez-Brayfield M, Smith EA, Scherz HC. The modified sting procedure to correct vesicoureteral reflux: improved results with submucosal implantation within the intramural ureter. J Urol. 2004;171(6 Pt 1):2413–6.
70. Kirsch AJ, Arlen AM. Evaluation of new Deflux administration techniques: intraureteric HIT and double HIT for the endoscopic correction of vesicoureteral reflux. Expert Rev Med Devices. 2014;11:439–46.
71. Escolino M, et al. Endoscopic injection of bulking agents in pediatric vesicoureteral reflux: a narrative review of literature. Pediatr Surg Int. 2023;39:133.
72. Routh JC, et al. Multivariate comparison of the efficacy of intraureteral versus subtrigonal techniques of dextranomer/hyaluronic acid injection. J Urol. 2007;178(4 Pt 2):1702–5.
73. Watters ST, Sung J, Skoog SJ. Endoscopic treatment for vesicoureteral reflux: how important is technique? J Pediatr Urol. 2013;9(6 Pt B):1192–7.

74. Yucel S, Gupta A, Snodgrass W. Multivariate analysis of factors predicting success with dextranomer/hyaluronic acid injection for vesicoureteral reflux. J Urol. 2007;177:1505–9.
75. Friedmacher F, Colhoun E, Puri P. Endoscopic injection of dextranomer/hyaluronic acid as first line treatment in 851 consecutive children with high grade vesicoureteral reflux: efficacy and long-term results. J Urol. 2018;200:650–5.
76. Hunziker M, Mohanan N, Puri P. Dextranomer/hyaluronic acid endoscopic injection is effective in the treatment of intermediate and high grade vesicoureteral reflux in patients with complete duplex systems. J Urol. 2013;189:1876–81.
77. Lackgren G, Cooper CS, Neveus T, Kirsch AJ. Management of vesicoureteral reflux: what have we learned over the last 20 years. Front Pediatr. 2021;9:650326.
78. Molitierno JA Jr, Scherz HC, Kirsch AJ. Endoscopic injection of dextranomer hyaluronic acid copolymer for the treatment of vesicoureteral reflux in duplex ureters. J Pediatr Urol. 2008;4:372–6.
79. Puri P, Kutasy B, Colhoun E, Hunziker M. Single center experience with endoscopic subureteral dextranomer/hyaluronic acid injection as first line treatment in 1,551 children with intermediate and high grade vesicoureteral reflux. J Urol. 2012;188(4 Suppl):1485–9.
80. Capozza N, et al. Treatment of vesico-ureteric reflux: a new algorithm based on parental preference. BJU Int. 2003;92:285–8.
81. Hsieh MH, et al. Cross-sectional evaluation of parental decision making factors for vesicoureteral reflux management in children. J Urol. 2010;184(4 Suppl):1589–93.
82. Ogan K, Pohl HG, Carlson D, Belman AB, Rushton HG. Parental preferences in the management of vesicoureteral reflux. J Urol. 2001;166:240–3.
83. Routh JC, Nelson CP, Graham DA, Lieu TA. Variation in surgical management of vesicoureteral reflux: influence of hospital and patient factors. Pediatrics. 2010;125:e446–51.
84. Puri P, Friedmacher F, Farrugia MK, Sharma S, Esposito C, Mattoo TK. Primary vesicoureteral reflux. Nat Rev Dis Primers 2024;10:75.

Anatomical and Functional Basis of Primary Vesicoureteral Reflux

Emily K. Clennon and J. Christopher Austin

Abstract Vesicoureteral reflux is due to abnormalities of the ureterovesical junction. Reflux is prevented by an adequate submucosa ureter within the bladder, which acts as a passive one-way flap valve. Primary vesicoureteral reflux is due to a short submucosal tunnel and enlarged ureteral orifice. The normal and abnormal anatomy and histological findings associated with VUR are reviewed. Bladder dysfunction is associated with VUR and is a negative predictor for spontaneous resolution and a risk factor for urinary tract infections. The normal development of bladder function and the types of bladder dysfunction associated with VUR are reviewed. The importance of recognition and treatment of bladder and bowel dysfunction is reviewed.

Keywords Vesicoureteral reflux · Anatomical basis · Ureterovesical junction · Histological findings · Bladder function

Anatomic and Functional Basis of Vesicoureteral Reflux

Vesicoureteral reflux (VUR) is the retrograde flow of urine from the bladder into the ureter. It is present in a high percentage of children with pyelonephritis and is associated with renal scarring. It has been a controversial subject in pediatric urology. The number of children being seen for VUR has decreased due to organizations which have released guidelines that have discouraged the practice of evaluating children after their first urinary tract infection with a voiding cystourethrogram [7, 22, 29, 36]. While the controversy will continue about the benefits of treatment of

E. K. Clennon
Department of Urology, Oregon Health & Science University, Portland, OR, USA
e-mail: clennon@ohsu.edu

J. C. Austin (✉)
Department of Urology, Division of Pediatric Urology, School of Medicine, Oregon Health and Sciences University, Portland, OR, USA
e-mail: austin@ohsu.edu

P. Puri, A. Yamataka (eds.), *Vesicoureteral Reflux*,
https://doi.org/10.1007/978-3-031-95091-9_2

VUR, its existence due to anatomical and functional abnormalities of the ureterovesical junction is well documented and still seen in children who undergo surgical correction of VUR.

Some of the earliest descriptions of surgical repair of VUR were in adult paraplegics with hydronephrosis, pyelonephritis, and VUR [13]. VUR was also noted to be associated with pyelonephritis and renal scaring in children. While initially all children with VUR were thought to have an anatomical defect at the ureterovesical junction as the etiology of the reflux, it has become clear that bladder physiology plays an additional role in this disorder. The classic concept of a dichotomous classification of VUR into a primary (congenital anatomical defect of the ureterovesical junction) and secondary (VUR due to abnormal bladder function or obstruction) is likely an oversimplification of a continuous spectrum with those children with VUR and dysfunctional elimination syndrome (or bladder/bowel dysfunction) bridging the ends of the spectrum. Recent evaluations of gender dichotomies in VUR have supported the notion that primary VUR may itself be a spectrum ranging from physiologic delay in urinary tract development to syndromic and non-syndromic pathology [1]. In this chapter, the anatomical defects of the ureterovesical junction and bladder physiology that results in VUR will be reviewed.

The normal function of the ureterovesical junction is to allow urine to be propelled by the peristaltic muscular contractions from the kidney unimpeded into the bladder. As the bladder nears capacity or the pressure within the bladder rises, it must also prevent the retrograde flow of urine back up the ureter. There has been much speculation and study regarding the precise mechanisms by which this occurs. Features such as the length of the intravesical ureter, size and configuration of the ureteral orifice, and the importance of the trigone and distal ureteral musculature have all been investigated [10, 13, 33, 47, 48]. The prevention of VUR has been shown to be independent of active muscular contractions by its absence in postmortem specimens, although the anatomic structure of these muscles still leads to some speculation that they may play a partial or small role in the overall competency of the ureterovesical junction [49]. Collectively, these findings favor the competency of ureterovesical junction to be due to a passive flap valve mechanism. The length of the submucosal ureter allows the distal ureter, which is supported by the detrusor muscle, to be compressed when the pressure increases with the bladder. The compression of the distal ureter prevents urine from refluxing up the ureter toward the kidney. Figures 1 and 2 illustrate this principle in the normal and refluxing ureterovesical junctions.

Normal Anatomy of the Ureterovesical Junction and Trigone

The normal anatomy of the ureterovesical junction has been studied for well over a century, with a resurgence of interest following the discovery of the clinical importance of VUR. This has consisted of both gross and microscopic studies, often combined. The ureter has two distinct muscle layers—an outer circular which is the bulk

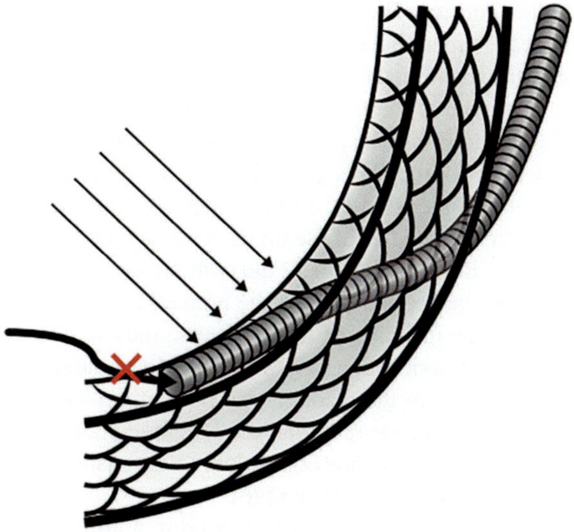

Fig. 1 Diagram of the normal ureterovesical junction illustrating how a normal submucosal tunnel can act as a one way flap valve. The detrusor muscle supporting the distal ureter will compress the submucosal ureter when the intravesical pressure rises (denoted by the long arrows). This will create enough resistance in the distal ureter to prevent urine from refluxing

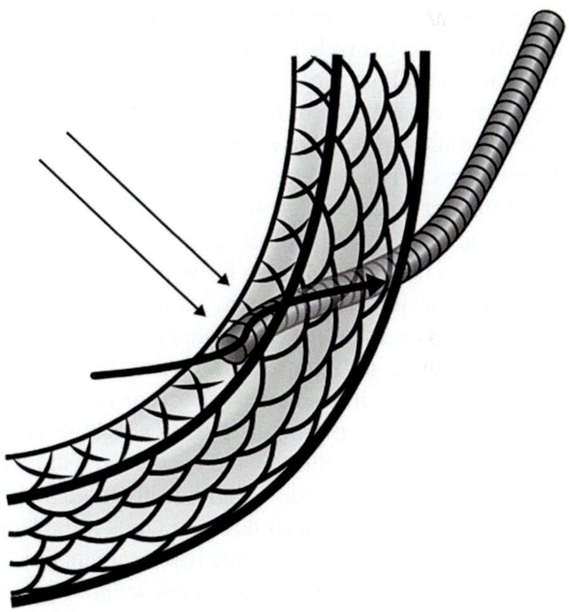

Fig. 2 Diagram of refluxing ureterovesical junction. A short submucosal ureter is illustrated here. With a small segment of ureter to compress when the intravesical pressure rises there is not enough resistance to prevent urine refluxing up the ureter

of the musculature and an inner longitudinal layer. As the distal ureter approaches the ureterovesical junction and enters the bladder, the two layers coalesce into a single longitudinal layer [57]. These fibers then continued into the trigone, anchoring the ureter to the bladder. The intravesical ureter can be divided into an intramural and a subepithelial part. After entering the bladder, the muscular fibers of the roof of the ureter spread laterally and medially, to coalesce at the inferior wall of the ureteral orifice. These muscle fibers on gross dissections seemed to be in continuity with the superficial trigonal musculature [48]. The trigonal musculature crosses the midline to meet the fibers from the contralateral ureter forming the interureteric ridge. Some of these fibers fan downward toward the bladder neck and traverse the bladder neck into the prostatic urethra in males and the posterior urethra in females. The origin of the fibers was originally thought to be ureteric based on these findings, but histologic studies favor a detrusor origin of the trigonal muscle fibers. Microscopic studies of the ureterovesical junction in both human and porcine models have failed to document the continuation of the longitudinal fibers of the ureter into the bladder and support the ureteral muscle fibers terminating at the distal ureter near the insertion of the transverse muscle fibers of the trigone, which traverse the interureteric ridge [17, 32, 50]. Morphologic studies have demonstrated that muscle mass in the bladder wall and intramural ureteral tunnel increase with age though at a slower rate than the length and angle of the tunnel, implying that the muscular structure contributes less to the maturation of the ureterovesical junction than other structural factors [26].

The juxtavesical ureter is encased in a fibromuscular attachment to the bladder. This tissue is often referred to as "Waldeyer's Sheath." Originally described as an injectable space between the intravesical ureter and bladder wall, this structure has been the subject of much debate. The true existence of an actual "sheath" around the ureter has been both reported and refuted over the years [17, 37, 48, 50, 57]. It is clear that there are little or no direct attachments of the intravesical ureter along its course through the detrusor and submucosally. The origin of the extravesical attachments seems to be an extension of detrusor muscle fibers. It becomes more fibrous in nature as it reaches its proximal extent, usually a short distance (2–3 cm) proximal to the bladder wall. Histologic studies have supported the bladder rather than the ureter as the origin of these fibers [35, 50]. This space provides a looseness and freedom of the intravesical ureter, but most histologic studies fail to demonstrate an actual sheath encasing the ureter along its course. Clinically, this space is encountered during ureteral reimplantation after the trigonal and detrusor muscle attachments have been divided from the distal ureter. At this point, a short length of intravesical ureter is essentially free of attachments until the fibromuscular attachments of "Waldeyer's Sheath" are encountered more proximally. Once these fibers are fully divided, the ureter is significantly more mobilized, and suitable length can be advanced into the bladder during ureteral reimplantation surgery.

Anatomical studies of the ureterovesical junction highlight that the passive flap which prevents VUR requires a suitable length of subepithelial ureter to be competent (see Figs. 1 and 2). For a normal, competent ureterovesical junction the ratio of the length of this ureteral submucosal tunnel to the diameter of ureteral orifice is 5:1. The importance of a 5:1 tunnel length to diameter ratio has been passed down over the past half century as dogma for successful ureteral reimplantation to correct VUR. The basis for these findings is shown in Figs. 3 and 4, which shows the anatomical findings of Paquin's study of postmortem bladders in adults and children [33]. His original series only included five children ages 2 days to 14 years. The average length of the intravesical ureter was 7 mm (range 197 3.5–10 mm), and the average maximal diameter of the ureteral orifice was 1.5 mm (range 0.5–3 mm). This has led to the recommendation that during surgical repair of reflux, the ureter should be reimplanted with submucosal tunnel of at least 5: 1 length to diameter ratio.

Mechanical simulations have evaluated the relative importance of submucosal tunnel length versus ureteral diameter in ureteral coaptation. Villanueva et al. [54] found that the ureteral diameter played a larger role in coaptation than tunnel length but that no one structural variable explained the initiation of reflux. In simulations, a dynamic interaction between tunnel length, ureteral diameter, ureteral thickness, and shape of the ureteral orifice was necessary to explain observed reflux mechanics [54, 55]. These findings call into question the necessity of a predetermined length to diameter ratio during reimplantation.

Innervation of the Ureterovesical Junction

The innervation of the bladder from the pelvic plexus and branches along the ureter has been studied. Fetal studies have mapped the nerves running superficial to the adventitia along the medial border of the distal ureter [61]. Upon reaching the bladder, the nerves form a complex network of branches over the outer surface of the bladder. The nerves course over Waldeyer's sheath and innervate the trigone and

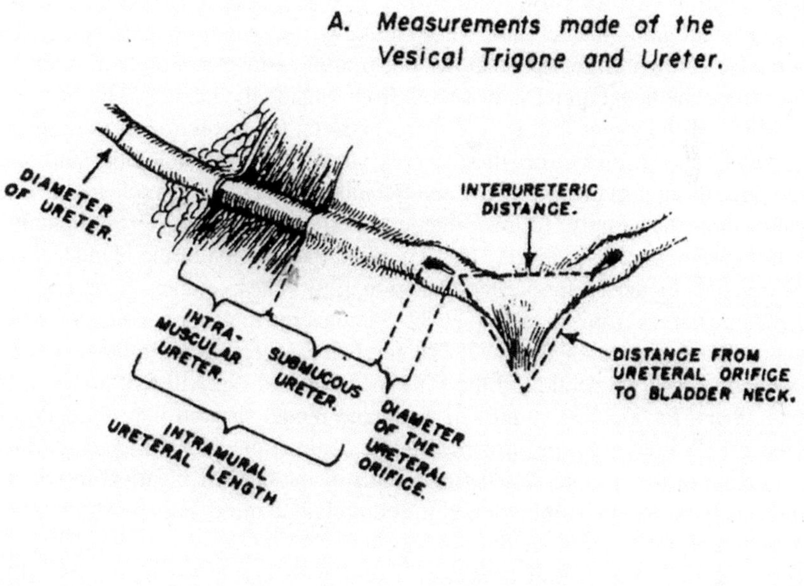

Fig. 3 Diagram of the trigone and intravesical ureter. Defines the measurements that were taken to evaluate normal and refluxing bladders. (Reproduced with permission from [33])

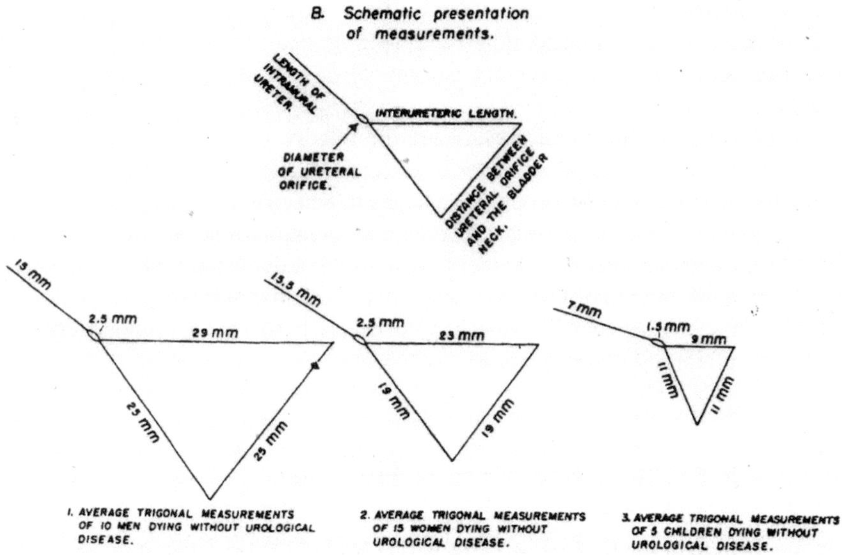

Fig. 4 Summary of the measurements of the intravesical ureter, diameter of the ureteral orifice, and trigone in post mortem bladders dying without urological disease. (Reproduced with permission from [33])

caudal areas of detrusor muscle. Immunohistochemical staining of these nerves shows them to express nitric oxide synthase, which is characteristic of the motor neurons innervating the detrusor. These findings are hypothesized to be a potential source for voiding difficulties that can occur after extravesical ureteral reimplantation, where the distal ureter is dissected from outside the bladder. The intravesical dissection of the ureter follows the plane between the adventitia of the ureter and Waldeyer's sheath, away from these nerves. However, no physiological studies have been done to support the role of the ureteral innervation playing a role in the voiding dysfunction that rarely follows bilateral extravesical ureteral reimplantation. Anatomical studies of cadavers have described the location of the bladder innervation relative to the ureterovesical junction [23]. These studies have shown the splanchnic nerves from sacral nerves S2–S4 converge to the pelvic plexus, which is located dorsal and medial the UVJ. The nerve fibers then branch to the region of the UVJ and trigone. Dissection of the UVJ medial and distal will risk injury to these nerve fibers. Physiologic studies in a porcine model showed that dissection of a unilateral UVJ led to lower pressure bladder contractions [27]. There was a lack of contraction of the ipsilateral detrusor muscle of the bladder identical to when that produced by unilateral stimulation of the contralateral motor nerves. More proximal dissection of the ureter alone did not have an effect on the contraction. These findings suggested that even unilateral extravesical dissection of the ureterovesical junction could disrupt the innervation of the ipsilateral detrusor muscle. Pirker et al. [35] analyzed the development of smooth muscle components of the ureterovesical junction and their nerve supply in the fetal, newborn, and adolescent pig. They demonstrated that the smooth muscle components and innervation of the ureterovesical junction continue to mature during the postnatal period.

Anatomical Findings in VUR

Animal models have shown the importance of an abnormal ureteral bud in the development of VUR and renal development [14], and studies in children with ureteral duplication provide direct evidence for the embryological mechanism for VUR. Mackie et al. postulated that an abnormally located ureteral bud led to abnormal insertion within the bladder causing reflux and renal dysmorphia. Patients with duplicated systems were carefully evaluated to note the location of the ureteral orifices along with the presence and absence of VUR in the lower pole ureter or ureteral ectopia of the upper pole ureter. Renal moieties with normally located ureteral orifices were typically normal whereas ectopic ureteral orifices were associated with renal abnormalities, and VUR was found primarily in ureters with more lateral and superior orifices [25].

The location of the ureteral orifice has the potential to dictate other mechanics of the submucosal tunnel and ureterovesical junction. More lateral ureteral orifices have less steep angles of insertion which increase the cross-sectional diameter of the ureter, decrease tunnel length and flow resistance, and increase the likelihood of reflux [19]. These findings are all in alignment with Paquin's descriptions of tunnel length to diameter ratio. With his original measurements of the trigone and intravesical ureters, he reported unpublished data that the average ratio was 1.4:1 in patients with VUR [33]. In addition to the location and angle of the ureteral orifice, the actual configuration of the ureteral orifice has been shown to correlate with the presence of VUR. The classic description of the ureteral orifice configurations was in the shape of a cone, stadium, horseshoe, or golf hole as shown in Fig. 5 [24]. These observations were based on the review of the cystoscopic findings of 671 ureteral orifices. The appearance of the orifice combined with relative location along the trigone was associated with different rates of VUR. They showed that orifices in the horseshoe configuration were refluxing 83% of the time, and 100% of golf hole orifices had VUR. Figure 6 shows the cystoscopic appearance of a golf hole orifice. Additionally, all configurations of the orifices when located farther lateral on the trigone were more likely refluxing (75%–100%) versus those that were in the normal position (2–50%). VUR resolution during follow-up was more common in those with cone and stadium orifices and if the ureteral orifice was located more medially along the trigone. Other authors have confirmed these findings [4], and simulation models suggest that orifice configuration may be more important than tunnel length [55]. Within models of the UVJ with varied tunnel lengths and either golf hole or cone orifice configurations, bladder pressure required to induce ureteral closure was compared. With the same orifice configuration, increasing tunnel length to diameter ratio from 3:1 to 5:1 reduced closing pressures by only 7%

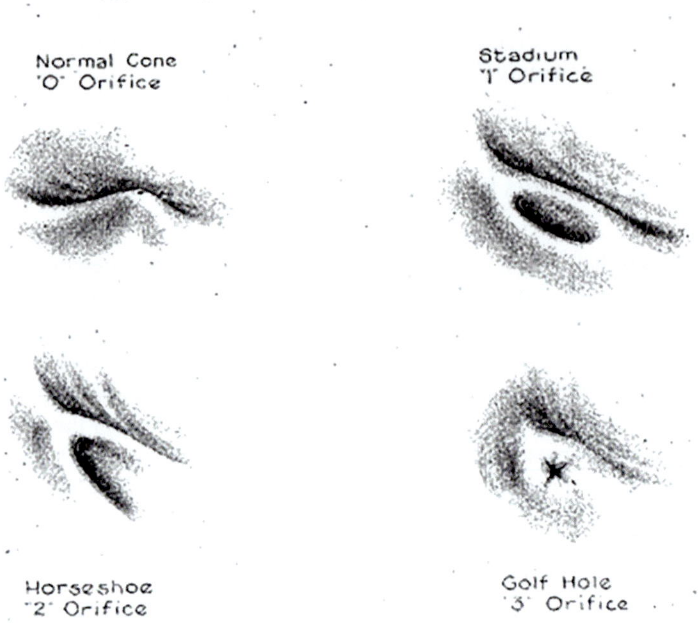

Fig. 5 The 4 types ureteral orifices. Findings were based on the cystoscopic appearances of the ureteral orifices. Note the differences in the size of orifice and direction of the effluxing urine bolus progressing from the cone shaped with the urine entering at nearly 90 degrees to the surface of the bladder to the horseshoe and cone which run parallel to the bladder wall. (Reproduced with permission from [24])

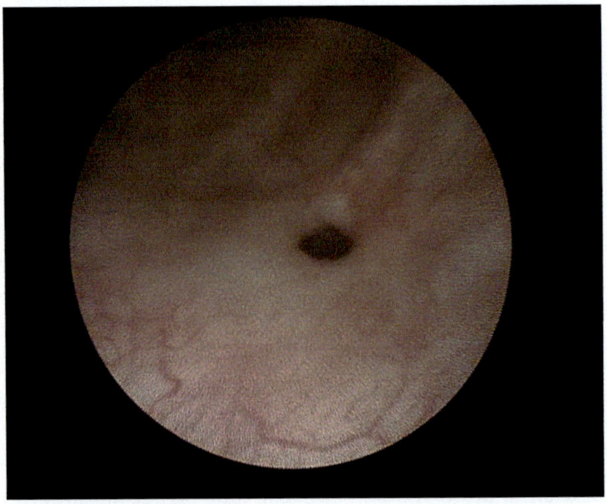

Fig. 6 Cystoscopic appearance of the left ureteral orifice in a female with high grade VUR. The orifice is gaping open at rest in a golf hole configuration. The ureteral is located far lateral along the trigone at the lateral wall of the bladder

whereas maintaining tunnel length but changing configuration from golf hole to volcano reduced closing pressures by 78%. For golf hole configurations, closing pressures were consistently >20 cm H_2O compared to 4-5 cm H_2O for volcano configurations.

With the increase in the use of endoscopic injection therapy for VUR in the past two decades, there has been resurgence in interest in the association of the degree of competency of the ureteral orifice and VUR. Dynamic hydrodistention during cystoscopy has been described as a way to assess the competency of the ureteral orifice during these procedures [2]. To hydrodistend the orifice, the flow from the cystoscope is directed at the ureteral orifice to open it. The degree of hydrodistention has been graded H0 through H3. If there is no opening of the orifice, it is grade H0. For H1, the orifice opens minimally, but the intramural ureter is not visible. Grade H2 hydrodistention is when the orifice opens and the intramural ureter is visible. When the orifice opens widely and the extravesical ureter is visible, it is grade H3. A cystoscopic appearance of grade H3 is shown in Fig. 7. In patients with grade H3, a small (7–8 Fr) cystoscope may be able to be passed into the distal ureter. In patients with no history of VUR or urinary tract infections, hydrodistention is rare and low grade (69% H0 and 31% H1). Hydrodistention grades H2 and H3 are considered abnormal and associated with VUR and pyelonephritis. In patents with grade V VUR, dynamic hydrodistention was grade H3 in 77% and H2 in 23%. Hydrodistention has also been shown to be predictive of new onset contralateral VUR after treatment, which was seen more commonly in "non-refluxing" contralateral ureters with hydrodistention grades H2 or H3. This did not occur in ureters with lower grades of hydrodistention. In a small series of patients with unilateral VUR, the prophylactic treatment of contralateral ureters with hydrodistention grades H2–3 eliminated new onset contralateral VUR [3]. This classification doesn't consider the orifice location along the trigone, but it is reproducible and simple to perform during cystoscopy.

Histological Findings in VUR

The histological findings in refluxing ureters have been studied examining the distal ureters excised during ureteral reimplantation surgery. Early studies reported no differences based on routine histological staining of the longitudinal muscle [5]. More recent studies using immunohistochemical staining for alpha-actin, myosin, desmin, and collagen subtypes have shown decreased smooth muscle and increased connective tissue in distal most aspect of the refluxing ureters compared to control ureters obtained from postmortem specimens [31, 51]. The proximal portions of the refluxing ureters were identical to the normal control. Additional studies on these specimens have revealed lower microvessel density (relative marker of ischemia), a decrease in the number of interstitial cells of Cajal (loss of which is associated with dysmotility problems), and decreased staining for connexin 43 (a transmembrane protein that is part of the gap junctions that permit communication from cell to cell [38, 39]. Genetic studies have implicated mutations in uroplakin genes, but their pathogenic role and importance remain unclear [15]. Collectively, these histologic findings confirm that there are microscopic changes affecting the distal ureter; however, it is not clear if these findings are related to the cause or a consequence of VUR. Given the gross appearance of refluxing orifices and the findings of a short

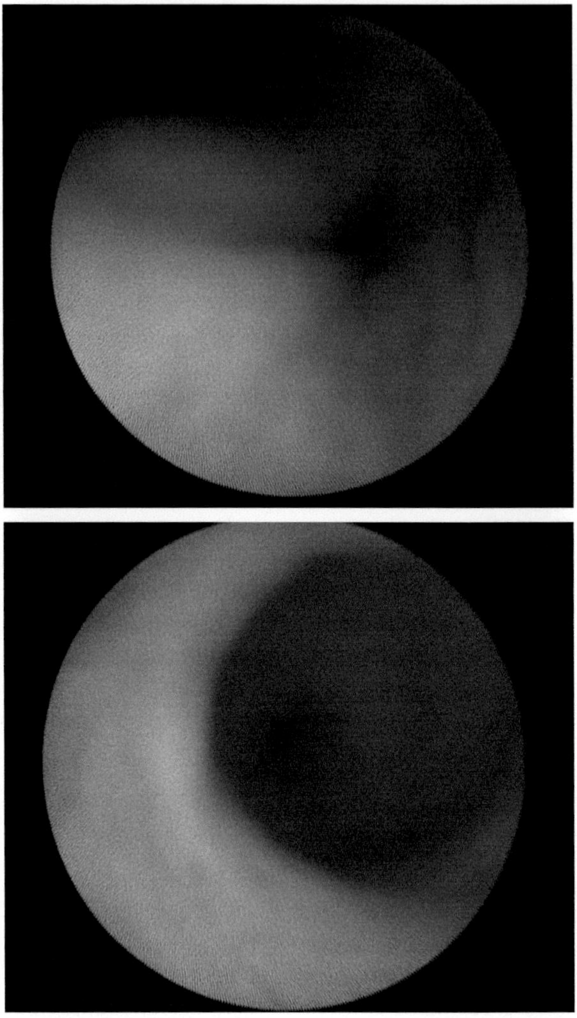

Fig. 7 Cystoscopic appearance of the L ureteral orifice before and after hydrodistention during cystoscopy in a male with high grade VUR. The ureter opens such that the extravesical ureter is visible-hydrodistention grade H3

submucosal tunnel and the lateral attachment to the trigone, these findings are not unexpected.

Bladder Function and VUR

Bladder dysfunction has long been known to be associated with VUR. It is associated with increased risk for urinary tract infection and renal scarring [34]. There have been multiple studies examining the role of bladder dysfunction on VUR. This has primarily focused on two distinct groups of children, the first being infants and toddlers and the second being older children who often present with symptoms of bladder and bowel dysfunction after the age of toilet training.

Infants and Toddlers

Bladder function changes as children mature from birth through childhood. Natural fill cystometry studies in normal children have revealed that normal bladder voiding pressures are quite high in male infants and less so in female infants [58]. Observational studies have given insight into the normal voiding pattern and relative frequency of incomplete voiding in this population. Infants void nearly every hour, voiding is associated with some degree of arousal, and voiding is incomplete nearly 1/3 of the time [16]. The findings of high voiding pressures, with mean voiding pressures near 150 cmH20 for males and 100 cmH20 for females, have helped to define what is normal versus abnormal bladder function for these patients in this age group [58, 59].

Studies in infants with high grade VUR have demonstrated worsening bladder dysfunction as the children age, most notably in males [45]. In this study of 114 infants with high-grade VUR, there were three urodynamic patterns found in males—low bladder capacity with high-pressure voiding +/− overactivity, normal bladder capacity, and increased bladder capacity and elevated postvoid residual. In females, only the later pattern (increased capacity) is found. At 20 months of age, 42% of the patients had voiding dysfunction. The early pattern of low bladder capacity with high pressures disappears after 1 year of age (and may be a normal finding except for the presence of unstable contractions in a minority of these). These patients with bladder dysfunction beyond 1 year of age were described as having dilated bladder dysfunction (bladder capacity >200% predicted capacity and postvoid residual greater than 25% of bladder capacity) and overactive bladder). Only 10% had isolated overactive bladder with a normal capacity. The majority had dilated bladder dysfunction with a small subset having both patterns present. Predictors of bladder dysfunction at presentation during infancy were an elevated postvoid residual and grade V VUR [42]. These difference in bladder mechanics between male and female infants may explain gendered differences in the natural course of VUR. Capozza et al. evaluated 464 cases of primary reflux at a single center and found a strong male predominance in the first year of life with a high rate of spontaneous resolution and a steady prevalence among females creating equal disease prevalence at 5 years [1].

There were similar findings regarding bladder dysfunction reported from Swedish Reflux Trial (randomized study in children ages 1–2 years with Gr III and IV VUR). Patients were evaluated prospectively for voiding problems at entry and 2 years. At entry, 20% of patients had lower urinary tract dysfunction characterized by increased bladder capacity and elevated postvoid residual urine. At 2 years, there was an increase to 34%. In children that were toilet trained, symptoms of overactive bladder (frequency, urgency, urge incontinence) were present in nearly all with bladder dysfunction. Voiding phase problems were defined at dysfunctional voiding (interrupted voiding pattern, straining, or hesitancy), dysfunctional elimination (bowel dysfunction with dysfunctional voiding), and dilated bladder dysfunction (VCUG capacity >200% age predicted volume or maximum voided volume > 150% age predicted volume). Lower urinary tract dysfunction was more common in grade IV VUR than grade III [44].

An additional series of patients with dilated bladder dysfunction and VUR were treated with intermittent catheterization to facilitate emptying, but this failed to improve the resolution of VUR in these patients [43]. A follow up of patients from the Swedish Reflux Trial found that a majority of patients had persistent bladder/bowel dysfunction at age 7 despite resolution of VUR and infections after surgical intervention [41]. These findings indicate bladder dysfunction in VUR patients may be either inherent or secondary to the pathophysiology of VUR. Furthermore, the presence of abnormal bladder function is a negative predictor for VUR resolution [30, 46, 60]. Multiple classification strategies have been proposed to categorize urinary dysfunction to predict resolution after endoscopic treatment [28, 53].

Older Children

Studies in older children with VUR have documented that VUR usually occurs as a low-pressure phenomenon [10, 56]. A study of 36 children with unilateral VUR, the mean detrusor pressure at VUR onset was 24 cm H2O and did not differ by reflux grade [8]. Among these children, those who developed renal scarring outside the context of infection had mean onset pressures of 34 cm H_2O compared to 9 cm H_2O in those without scarring. High pressure phenotypes may be more damaging, but lower pressure at onset of VUR had been shown to be a negative predictor for reflux resolution over time independent of grade of reflux [52]. Though high pressures overwhelming the ureterovesical junction do not appear to explain new reflux in older children, voiding dysfunction among these patients is common and increases risk of infections and renal scarring [21, 34]. Urodynamic patterns in these children include most commonly detrusor overactivity, followed by dysfunctional voiding (incomplete or intermittent pelvic floor relaxation), and primary bladder neck dysfunction was the least common [12, 18, 20, 53]. Sharifi-Rad et al. also found that 2/3 of neurologically normal children diagnosed with VUR after toilet training had abnormal uroflowmetry and half had active pelvic floor contraction during voiding [40]. Unlike in infants, recognition and treatment of bladder dysfunction in this group of patients (with biofeedback to treat pelvic floor dysfunction, anticholinergics to treat overactive bladder, or alpha-blockers for primary bladder neck dysfunction) have been shown to increase rates of VUR resolution and decrease need for surgical repair [9, 11, 18]. Conversely, untreated bladder and bowel dysfunction has been associated with lower success rates of endoscopic injection [6, 28, 34]. These findings are strong indicators that bladder dysfunction in older patients after toilet training plays a significant role in the VUR. Because of this, it has been stressed that identification and management of bladder and bowel dysfunction are important factors in treating patients with VUR.

References

1. Capozza N, Gulia C, Bateni ZH, Zangari A, Gigli S, Briganti V, Tursini S, Koh CJ, Gaffi M, Baldassarra S, Signore F, Porrello A, Piergentili R. Vesicoureteral reflux in infants: what do we know about the gender prevalence by age? Eur Rev Med Pharmacol Sci. 2017;21:5321–9.
2. Cerwinka W, Scherz H, Kirsch A. Dynamic hydrodistention classification of the ureter and the double hit method to correct vesicoureteral reflux. Arch Esp Urol. 2008;61(8):882–7.
3. Cerwinka WH, Kaye JD, Leong TL, Elmore JM, Scherz HC, Kirsch AJ. Selective endoscopic treatment of the non-refluxing contralateral ureter prevents new contralateral vesicoureteral reflux. J Pediatr Urol. 2013;9(1):51–5.
4. Dikshit M, Acharya V, Shikare S, Merchant S, Pardanani D. Comparison of direct radionuclide cystography with micturating cystourethrography for the diagnosis of vesicoureteral reflux, and its correlation with cystoscopic appearances of the ureteric orifices. Nephrol Dial Transplant. 1993;8:600–2.
5. Dixon J, Jen P, Yeung C, Chow L, Mathews R, Gearhart J, Gosling J. The structure and automomic innervation of the vesico-ureteral junction in cases of primary reflux. Br J Urol. 1998;81(1):146–51.
6. Elder J, Diaz M, Caldemone A, Cendron M, Greenfield S, Hurwitz R, Kirsch A, Koyle M, Pope J, Shapiro E. Endoscopic therapy for vesicoureteral reflux: a meta-analysis. I. Reflux resolution and urinary tract infection. J Urol. 2006;10(6):716–22.
7. Garcia-Roig M, Travers C, McCracken CE, Kirsch AJ. National Trends in the Management of Primary Vesicoureteral Reflux in children. J Urol. 2018;199(1):287–93.
8. Goren MR, Ceyhan E, Ozer C, Kilinc F, Ozkardes H. The impact of reflux pressure on renal scarring in children with sterile vesicoureteral reflux. J Pediatr Urol. 2023;19:130e1-e5.
9. Herndon C, DeCambre M, McKenna P. Changing concepts concerning the management of vesicoureteral reflux. J Urol. 2001;166(4):1439–43.
10. Hinman F, Miller E, Hutch J, Gainey M, Cox C, Goodfriend R, Marshall S. Low pressure reflux: relation of vesicoureteral reflux to intravesical pressure. J Urol. 2002;167:1063–8.
11. Homsy Y, Nsouli I, Hamburger B, Laberge I, Schick E. Effects of oxybutynin on vesicoureteral reflux in children. J Urol. 1985;134(6):1168–71.
12. Hong Y, Altobelli E, Borer J, Bauer S, Nguyen H. Urodynamic abnormalities in toilet trained children with primary vesicoureteral reflux. J Urol. 2011;185(5):1863–8.
13. Hutch J. Vesic-ureteral reflux in the paraplegic: cause and correction. J Urol. 2002;167:1410–4.
14. Ichikawa I, Kuwayama F, Pope J, Stephens F, Miyazaki Y. Paradigm shift from classic anatomic theories to contemporary cell biological views of CAKUT. Kidney Int. 2002;61(3):889–98.
15. Jackson AR, Ching CB, McHugh KM, Backnell B. Roles for urothelium in normal and aberrant urinary tract development. Nat Rev Urol. 2020;17(8):459–68.
16. Jannson U, Hanson M, Hanson E, Hellstrom A, Sillen U. Voiding pattern in healthy children 0-3 years old: a longitudinal study. J Urol. 2000;164(6):2050–4.
17. Juskiewenski S, Vaysse P, Moscovici J, de Graeve P, Guitard J. The ureterovesical junction. Anat Clin. 1984;5:251–9.
18. Kajbafzadeh A, Baradaran N, Sedeghi Z, Tourchi A, Saeedi P, Madani A, Ataei N, Taghavinejad A, Mohsseni M. Vesicoureteral reflux and primary bladder neck dysfunction in children: urodynamic evaluation and randomized, double blind, clinical trial on the effect of alpha-blocker therapy. J Urol. 2010;184:2128–33.
19. Kalayeh K, Fowlkes JB, Schultz WW, Sack BS. Ureterovesical junction deformation during urine storage in the bladder and the effect on vesicoureteral reflux. J Biomech. 2020;113:1–12.
20. Karami H, Razi A, Mazloomfard M, Javanmard B. Is there a role for urodynamic study in children with high-grade vesicoureteral reflux. Urology. 2012;79(4):888–91.

21. Koff S, Wagner T, Jayanthi R. The relationship among dysfunctional elimination syndromes, primary vesicoureteral reflux and urinary tract infections in children. J Urol. 1998;160(3 pt 2):1019–22.
22. Lee T, Ellimoottil C, Marchetti KA, Banerjee T, Ivančić V, Kraft KH, Bloom DA, Park JM, Wan J. Impact of clinical guidelines on voiding Cystourethrogram use and vesicoureteral reflux incidence. J Urol. 2018;199(3):831–6.
23. Leissner J, Allhoff E, Wolff W, Feja C, Hochel M, Black P, Hohenfellner R. The pelvic plexus and antireflux surgery: topographical findings and clinical consequences. J Urol. 2001;165:2652–5.
24. Lyon R, Marshall S, Tanagho E. The ureteral orifice: its configuration and competency. J Urol. 1969;102:504–9.
25. Mackie G, Awang H, Stephens F. The ureteric orifice: the embryologic key to radiologic status of duplex kidneys. J Pediatric Surg. 1975;10(4):473–81.
26. Makosiej R, Orkisz S, Czkwianianc E. Morphologic study of the ureterovesical junction in children. J Anat. 2018;232:449–56.
27. Martinez Portillo F, Seif C, Braun P, Bohler G, Osmonov D, Leissner J, Hohenfeller R, Aleken P, Juenemann K. Risk of detrusor denervation in antireflux surgery demonstrated in a neurophysiological animal model. J Urol. 2003;170:570–4.
28. Marzullo-Zucchet L, March-Villalba JA, Hinarejos CD, Rodrigo AP, Serrano-Durba A, Tormo FB. Usefulness of the classification of urinary dysfunction for the prognosis of the first endoscopic treatment of vesicoureteral reflux in children over the age of 3. Actas Urol Esp. 2019;43(4):212–9.
29. NICE (National Institute for Clinical Excellence) Guidelines (CG54). Urinary tract infection in under 16s: diagnosis and management. www.nice.org.uk 2007.
30. Nordenstrom J, Sillen U, Holmdahl G, Linner T, Stokland E, Sjostrom S. The Swedish infant high-grade reflux trial – bladder function. J Pediatr Urol. 2017;13:139–45.
31. Oswald J, Brenner E, Schwentner C, Deibl M, Bartsch G, Fritsch H, Radmayr C. The intravesical ureter in children with vesicoureteral reflux: a morphological and immunohistochemical characterization. J Urol. 2003;598(170):2423–7.
32. Oswald J, Schwentner C, Lunacek A, Fritsch H, Longato S, Sergi C, Bartsch G, Radmayr C. Reevaluation of the fetal muscle development of the vesical trigone. J Urol. 2006;176:1166–70.
33. Paquin A. Ureterovesical anastomosis: description and evaluation of a technique. J Urol. 1959;82(5):573–83.
34. Peters C, Skoog S, Arant B, Copp H, Elder J, Hudson R, Khoury A, Lorenzo A, Pohl H, Shapiro E, Snodgrass W, Diaz M. Summary of the AUA guideline on management of primary vesicoureteral reflux in children. J Urol. 2010;184(3):1134–44.
35. Pirker M, Rolle U, Shinkai T, Shinkai M, Puri P. Prenatal and postnatal neuromuscular development of the ureterovesical junction. J Urol. 2007;177:1546–51.
36. Roberts K, Downs S, Finnell S, Hellerstein S, Shortliffe L, Wald E, Zerin J, Davidson C. Urinary tract infection: clinical practice guideline for the diagnosis and management of the initial UTI in febrile infants and children 2-14 months. Pediatrics. 2011;128(3):595–610.
37. Rusu MC, Pop F, Petre N, Dobra MA. The sheath of Waldeyer is not a specific anatomical trait of the ureterovesicaljunction. Morphologie. 2018;102(336):6–11.
38. Schwentner C, Oswald J, Lunacek A, Fritsch H, Deibl M, Bartsch G, Radmayr C. Loss of interstitial cells of Cajal and gap junction protein connexin 43 at the vesicoureteral junction in children with vesicoureteral reflux. J Urol. 2005;174:1981–6.
39. Schwentner C, Oswald J, Lunacek A, Schlenck B, Berger A, Deibl M, Fritsch H, Bartsch G, Radmayr C. Structural changes of the intravesical ureter in children with vesicoureteral reflux-does ischemia have a role? J Urol. 2006;176:2212–8.
40. Sharifi-Rad L, Ladi-Seyedian S, Amirzargar H, Kajbafzadeh A. Pelvic floor electromyography and urine flow patterns in children with vesicoureteral reflux and lower urinary tract symptoms. IBJU. 2018;44(6):1207–14.

41. Sjostrom S, Ekdahl H, Abrahamsson K, Sillen U. Bladder/bowel dysfunction at school age is seen in children with high-grade vesicoureteral reflux and lower urinary tract dysfunction in infancy. Acta Paediatr. 2019;109:388–95.
42. Sillen U, Hellstrom A, Hermanson G, Abrahmson K. Comparison of urodynamic and free voiding pattern in infants with dilating reflux. J Urol. 1999;161:1928–33.
43. Sillen U, Holmdahl G, Hellstrom A, Sjostrom S, Solsnes E. Treatment of bladder dysfunction and high-grade vesicoureteral reflux does not influence the spontaneous resolution rate. J Urol. 2007;177:325–30.
44. Sillen U, Brandstrom P, Jodal U, Holmdahl G, Sandin A, Sjoberg I, Hansson S. The Swedish reflux trial in children: V. Bladder dysfunction. J Urol. 2010;184:298–304.
45. Sjostrom S, Bacherlard M, Sixt R, Sillen U. Change in urodynamic patterns in infants with dilating vesicoureteral reflux: 3-year followup. J Urol. 2009;182:2446–54.
46. Sjostrom S, Sillen U, Jodal U, Sameby L, Sixt R, Stokland E. Predictive factors for resolution of congenital high grade vesicoureteral reflux in infants: results of univariant and multivariate analysis. J Urol. 2010;183:1177–84.
47. Stephens F, Lenaghan D. The anatomical basis and dynamics of vesicoureteral reflux. J Urol. 1962;87(5):669–80.
48. Tanagho E, Pugh R. The anatomy and function of the ureterovesical junction. Br J Urol. 1963;35:151–65.
49. Tanagho E, Meyers F, Smith D. The trigone: anatomical and physiological considerations in relation to the ureterovesical junction. J Urol. 1968;100:623–32.
50. Thomson A, Dabhoiwala N, Verbeek F, Lamers W. The functional anatomy of the ureterovesical junction. Br J Urol. 1994;73(3):284–91.
51. Tokhmafshan F, Brophy PD, Gbadegesin RA, Gupta IR. Vesicoureteral reflux and the extracellular matrix connection. Pediatr Nephrol. 2017;32(4):565–76.
52. Van Arondonk K, Austin J, Hawtrey C, Graham M, Cooper C. Nuclear cystometrogram-determined bladder pressure at the onset of vesicoureteral reflux predicts spontaneous resolution. Urology. 2007;69(4):862–5.
53. Van Batavia J, Ahn J, Fast A, Combs A, Glassberg K. Prevalence of urinary tract infection and vesicoureteral reflux in children with lower urinary tract dysfunction. J Urol. 2013;190:1495–500.
54. Villanueva CA, Nelson CA, Stolle C. Intravesical tunnel length to ureteral diameter ratio insufficiently explains ureterovesical junction competence: a parametric simulation study. J Pediatr Urol. 2015;11(3):144.e1–5.
55. Villanueva CA, Tong J, Nelson C, Gu L. Ureteral tunnel length versus ureteral orifice configuration in the determination of ureterovesical junction competence: a computer simulation model. J Pediatr Urol. 2018;14(3):258.e1–6.
56. Weiss R, Biancani P. Characteristics of normal and refluxing ureterovesical junctions. J Urol. 1983;129:858–61.
57. Woodburne R. The ureter, ureterovesical junction, and vesical trigone. Anat Rec. 1965;151:243–50.
58. Yeung C, Godley M, Duffy P, Ransley P. Natural filling cystometery in infants and children. Br J Urol. 1995;75(4):531–7.
59. Yeung C, Godley M, Dhillon H, Duffy P, Ransley P. Urodynamic patterns in infancts with normal lower urinary tracts or primary vesico-ureteric reflux. Br J Urol. 1998;81(3):461–7.
60. Yeung C, Sreedhar B, Sihoe J, Sit F. Renal and bladder functional status at diagnosis as predictive factors for the outcome of primary vesicoureteral reflux in children. J Urol. 2006;176:1152–7.
61. Yulcek S, Baskin L. Neuroanatomy of the ureterovesical junction: clinical implications. J Urol. 2003;170:945–8.

Familial Vesicoureteral Reflux

Prem Puri and Manuela Hunziker

Abstract Primary vesicoureteral reflux (VUR) is the most common disease of the urinary tract in children, occurring in 1–2% of the pediatric population and in 30–50% of those who present with urinary tract infection (UTI). It is caused by the maldevelopment and malfunction of the ureterovesical junction, which causes the urine to flow retrogradely from the bladder to the kidneys. The association of VUR, urinary tract infection and renal damage is well known, and reflux nephropathy is a major cause of childhood hypertension and chronic renal failure. The hereditary and familial nature of VUR is well recognized. Several studies have shown that siblings of index patients with VUR have a much higher incidence of VUR than the general population with a reported incidence of 26–50%. The transmission of VUR from parent to child has been reported at a rate up to 66%. The screening of asymptomatic siblings and offspring is controversial. The aim in the management of childhood VUR is prevention of permanent renal damage by minimizing the risk of recurrent febrile UTIs. It is reported that there is increased risk of renal cortical abnormalities in siblings with a previous urinary tract infection, siblings with high-grade VUR and siblings older than 1 year of age. It is recommended that the families of children with VUR should be informed that siblings and offspring have a higher chance of VUR and be counseled regarding prompt treatment of acute UTI and subsequent voiding cystourethrography especially if there is evidence of renal cortical abnormalities or renal size asymmetry on ultrasound.

Keywords Vesicoureteral reflux · Familial vesicoureteral reflux · Siblings · Offspring · Genetics · Urinary tract infections · Renal damage · Screening siblings

---

P. Puri (✉)
Beacon Consultants Clinic, University College Dublin, Dublin, Ireland

M. Hunziker
University Hospital Zurich, Zurich, Switzerland
e-mail: Manuela.hunziker@usz.ch

P. Puri, A. Yamataka (eds.), *Vesicoureteral Reflux*,
https://doi.org/10.1007/978-3-031-95091-9_3

Introduction

Primary vesicoureteral reflux (VUR), the retrograde flow of urine from the bladder into the upper urinary tract, is caused by maldevelopment and malfunction of the vesicoureteral junction. The defect usually involves a shortening of the submucosal ureteral segment due to congenital lateral ectopia of the ureteral orifice. It is the most common urological anomaly in children. VUR occurs in 1–2% of the pediatric population and in 30–50% of children who present with urinary tract infection (UTI) [1, 2]. Among infants in whom hydronephrosis is prenatally identified on ultra- sound (US) and who are screened for VUR, the VUR prevalence is reported to be 16.2% (7–35%) [3]. The association of VUR, urinary tract infection and renal damage is well known, and reflux nephropathy is a major cause of childhood hypertension and chronic renal failure.

The hereditary and familial nature of VUR is well recognized. Several studies have shown that siblings of index patients with VUR have a much higher incidence of VUR than the general population with a reported incidence of 26–50% [4–8]. The transmission of VUR from parent to child has been reported at a rate up to 66% [9–11]. As primary VUR is often asymptomatic and can resolve spontaneously with age, it is difficult to determine the exact prevalence of VUR in family members [12, 13].

The familial clustering of VUR, syndromes associated with VUR, and demonstration of VUR in transgenic or knock-out mouse models imply that genetic factors play an important role in the pathogenesis of this condition. A study by Kaefer et al. of 46 twin pairs provides strong evidence for a genetic origin, in that there was 80–100% concordance for VUR in monozygotic twins compared with 35–50% concordance in dizygotic twins [14]. The high transmission rate and sibling risk suggests that VUR is inherited in an autosomal dominant manner in most families, though autosomal recessive inheritance and X-linked inheritance has been demonstrated in some families.

Understanding the familial nature of VUR is crucial when counseling parents about the increased likelihood of another family member having VUR.

Transmission of VUR from Parent to Child

Primary VUR is known to occur in families. There is a risk of transmitting VUR from parent to child, but the inheritance pattern is complex and still not completely understood. Miller and Caspari, in a pedigree analysis of 10 affected families, were the first to propose an autosomal dominant mode of transmission in 1972 [15]. Noe et al. studied a total of 36 offspring of 23 parents with radiologically proven primary vesicoureteral reflux [10]. Reflux was identified in 24 of the 36 offspring (66%), and all had grade II or higher grade of VUR. Scott et al. performed a 3-year prospective collaborative study in three maternity hospitals to estimate the incidence of VUR transmission to a child from parent or close relative with a documented history of VUR [11]. Of the 186 infants who met study inclusion criteria and underwent voiding cystourethrography after birth, VUR was detected in 38 (20.4%). The predominant relationship was through the mother. The high transmission rate suggests that VUR is inherited in an autosomal dominant manner in most families.

Prevalence of VUR in Siblings

As VUR can resolve spontaneously as the child grows older, it is difficult to accurately determine the exact prevalence in siblings. Several prospective and retrospective studies have investigated the prevalence of VUR and the extent of renal damage in siblings of index patients with vesicoureteral reflux. Prevalence rates of 27–51% in siblings of children with VUR have been reported [4–8]. In 1992, Noe reported the results of long-term follow up siblings of index patients with VUR [4]. Of the 354 screened siblings 119 (34%) had VUR. Most siblings discovered to have VUR were asymptomatic and 61% had grade III-IV reflux. There was no difference in the incidence of VUR in female and male siblings. Wan et al. reported results of a dual center retrospective study of sibling reflux [16]. A total of 422 families comprising 622 siblings were identified. VUR was identified in 144 siblings (27%) with a male to female ratio of 1:1.7. High grade VUR (grade III- V) was identified in 25% of all refluxing ureters, while 57% showed grade II VUR. Parekh et al. reported 40 (51%) screened siblings of the 78 index patients showed evidence of VUR, with 31% having grade III-V reflux. Hunziker et al. investigated the prevalence of VUR and renal cortical abnormalities in the siblings less than 6 years of age of index patients with grade III-V VUR in a large cohort of families with VUR [8]. There were 275 families with a total of 593 children with VUR, including 239 (40%) boys and 354 (60%) girls. Four hundred twenty-four siblings were screened, and 190 (45%) siblings were found to have VUR. In addition, 128 siblings were diagnosed with VUR following a UTI. The number of families with 2, 3, 4, and 5 siblings was 237, 34, 3, and 1 respectively. This study showed that most siblings, whether symptomatic or asymptomatic, had intermediate or high grade VUR. A striking finding in this study was that the prevalence of renal parenchymal damage in screened siblings without previous UTI was 15%, whereas it was 34% in siblings with a previous UTI. The study showed increased risk of renal cortical abnormalities in siblings with a previous history of UTI, siblings with high grade VUR, and siblings older than 1 year of age. Other studies have also reported that the most important risk factors for the development of renal parenchymal damage in familial VUR include history of urinary tract infection, reflux grade and age at diagnosis [17–19]. Another study reported that the incidence of sibling VUR is maximal in patients who are younger than 3 years and the VUR in symptomatic siblings in this age group is usually intermediate or high grade and associated with a higher incidence of renal scarring [20]. A major goal of screening siblings is to identify children who may be at higher risk for reflux nephropathy, because with early detection the incidence of renal damage in siblings may be decreased compared with that in index patients.

Impact of Age and Gender on Familial Reflux

Age at diagnosis plays an important role in familial VUR. Studies have shown that mostly young children are discovered to have VUR if they have been screened. Especially in younger children, VUR may resolve spontaneously. Therefore, the age at which VUR is diagnosed is important in understanding the likelihood of spontaneous resolution. While some studies show that siblings younger than 18 months have a significantly higher rate of VUR than older children [4], others have shown that the rate of VUR is maximal in siblings who are younger than 3 years of age [10].

The main goal of treating patients with VUR is prevention of recurring febrile UTIs and minimizing the risk of renal damage and long-term renal impairment. Renal parenchymal damage can be congenital (hypoplasia or dysplasia) or acquired scarring resulting from pyelonephritis induced renal injury. Exposure to UTIs in patients with congenital renal dysplasia can lead to progression of renal damage. A number of prospective and retrospective studies have investigated the extent of renal scarring in the siblings of patients with VUR [8, 16, 17, 20, 21]. Overall, it has been shown that 20% of siblings of index cases of VUR had renal scars [22]. While some investigators have shown that younger siblings (<18 months) have a higher rate of renal scarring [4], others have shown that the risk of renal cortical abnormalities is increased in siblings over the age of 1 year [8].

Gender differences have been noted in patients with VUR. Those with prenatally diagnosed hydronephrosis, male infants dominate clearly over female infants, show higher grades of VUR and a higher percentage of renal damage [23, 24]. On the contrary, when VUR is diagnosed after symptomatic urinary tract infection, prevalence is higher in females. Pirker et al. investigated influence of gender on the prevalence and expression of familial VUR [25]. They subdivided families into siblings' groups with only male affected, only female affected and mixed affected siblings [25]. They found that sisters of female index patients were significantly more likely to have reflux than brothers (68% vs 45%). Boys in families with exclusively boys affected had a significantly higher grade of reflux than boys in families with mixed affected siblings and girls in all family groups. Another striking finding was the high (15.3%) rate of duplex renal systems in families with only boys affected compared to 5.7% in the group of siblings with only girls affected. It is possible that the underlying genetic defect in families with only boys affected is different than the defect dominating in the families with mixed affected siblings and only females affected siblings.

Reflux Related Morbidity in Relatives of Index Patients with Vesicoureteral Reflux

There is little information available regarding reflux related morbidity in relatives of index patients with VUR. Noe et al. studied a total of 36 offspring of 23 parents with radiologically proven primary vesicoureteral reflux [10]. Reflux was identified in 24 of the 36 offspring (66%). They also found a high incidence of reflux related morbidity in the parents. Four of the 23 parents underwent nephrectomy due to nonfunctioning kidneys and 3 were known to have renal scars and hypertension. Hunziker and Puri determined the prevalence of VUR and reflux related morbidity in first, second and third-degree relatives of index patients with high grade VUR [26]. A total of 300 siblings of the 259 index patients were found to have vesicoureteral reflux on voiding cystourethrography. In terms of the other relatives of the 259 index patients, 127 relatives also had radiologically proven vesicoureteral reflux. Reflux related morbidity among the first, second and third-degree relatives included end stage renal disease in 21, nephrectomy in 12 and hypertension in 4. Fifty-nine relatives continued to suffer from recurrent urinary tract infections for many years. In 73% of the relatives, vesicoureteral reflux was seen on the mother's side.

Screening of Asymptomatic Siblings and Offspring of Refluxing Parents

Screening of siblings of index patients with VUR and offspring of refluxing parents has been proposed to detect a population at risk, potentially allowing treatment to prevent acute illness and decrease adverse outcomes associated with VUR, including UTIs, pyelonephritis, and renal injury. However, screening of asymptomatic siblings and offspring of parents with VUR is controversial. There is no evidence-based consensus on the indications for screening siblings This is due to the lack of randomized clinical trials for screened patients to assess clinical benefits of screening siblings. Furthermore, the lack of a sensitive, noninvasive screening method has limited the acceptance of screening asymptomatic siblings as a routine.

The main goal of screening siblings is to identify children who may be at higher risk for reflux nephropathy, because with early detection the incidence of renal damage in siblings may be decreased compared with that in index patients. Data from sibling screening program in Dublin from a large cohort of families with VUR has provided useful information [8, 17–20, 25, 26]. The unique features of this screening program were that it included both symptomatic and asymptomatic siblings of index patients and 55% of siblings were less than 1 year of age. It showed that the prevalence of sibling VUR was maximal in children under the age of 3 years and most siblings, whether symptomatic or asymptomatic had intermediate to high-grade VUR. Furthermore, the incidence of renal scarring in symptomatic siblings was identical to that in index patients and significantly higher than in asymptomatic siblings. It was also observed that the risk of VUR and the severity of VUR in siblings is dependent upon the gender of the child affected, boys having a significantly higher grade of VUR and significantly higher prevalence of severe renal scarring than girls. It has been recommended to consider screening siblings under 3 years of age, particularly male siblings of index patients. Current knowledge indicates that male siblings of patients with VUR should get particular attention in screening programs. Although a certain proportion of siblings with moderate to severe kidney damage seems to have congenital renal damage, which cannot be influenced by early screening. However, in these patients it is mandatory to discover VUR at early stages to prevent exposure to UTIs and avoid possible progression of renal parenchymal damage [27].

Conclusions

Given the hereditary nature of the condition, children with a family history of VUR are at an increased risk, and screening may be warranted, especially in male siblings of index patients who have higher grades of VUR and predisposition to severe renal scarring. Early detection can contribute to timely intervention, reducing the risk of complications such as recurrent UTIs and renal scarring, and thus minimizing the risk of reflux-related morbidities such as hypertension and end-stage renal disease. However, the decision to screen should be individualized, considering various factors such as age, gender, clinical presentation, and the presence of other risk factors. It is important at least to counsel parents regarding prompt treatment of acute UTI and subsequent voiding cystourethrography in siblings of index patients with VUR, especially if there is evidence of renal cortical abnormalities or renal size asymmetry on ultrasound [28].

References

1. Smellie JM, Barratt TM, Chantler C, et al. Medical versus surgical treatment in children with severe bilateral vesicoureteric reflux and bilateral nephropathy: a randomised trial. Lancet. 2001;357(9265):1329–33.
2. Hoberman A, Charon M, Hickey RW, et al. Imaging studies after a first febrile urinary tract infection in young children. N Engl J Med. 2003;348(3):195–202.
3. Gnech M, Hoen L, Zachou A, Bogaert G, Castagnetti, O'Kelly F, et al. Update and summary of the European Association of Urology/ European Society of Pediatric Urology Paediatric guidelines on vesicoureteral reflux in children. Eur Urol. 2024;85:433–42.
4. Noe HN. The long-term results of prospective sibling reflux screening. J Urol. 1992;148(5 Pt 2):1739–42.
5. Aggarwal VK, Verrier Jones K. Vesicoureteric reflux: screening of first degree relatives. Arch Dis Child. 1989;64(11):1538–41.
6. Parekh DJ, Pope JCIV, Adams MC, et al. Outcome of sibling vesicoureteral reflux. J Urol. 2002;167(1):283–4.

7. Chertin B, Puri P. Familial vesicoureteral reflux. J Urol. 2003;169:1804–8.
8. Hunziker M, Colhoun E, Puri P. Renal cortical abnormalities in siblings of index patients with vesicoureteral reflux. Pediatrics. 2014;133(4):e933–7.
9. Eccles MR, Bailey RR, Abbott GD, et al. Unravelling the genetics of vesicoureteric reflux: a common familial disorder. Hum Mol Genet. 1996;5 spec no:1425–9.
10. Noe HN, Wyatt RJ, Peeden JN, et al. The transmission of vesicoureteral reflux from parent to child. J Urol. 1992;148(6):1869–71.
11. Scott JE, Swallow V, Coulthard MG, et al. Screening of newborn babies for familial ureteric reflux. Lancet. 1997;350(9075):396–400.
12. Scoog SJ, Peters CA, Arant BS Jr, et al. Pediatric vesicouretral reflux guidelines panel summary report: clinical practice guidelines for screening siblingsof children with vesicoureteral reflux and neonates/infants with prenatal hydronephrosis. J Urol. 2010;184:1145–51.
13. Tekgul S, Riedmiller H, Hoebeke P, et al. EAU guidelines on vesicoureteral reflux in children. Eur Urol. 2012;62(3):534–42.
14. Kaefer M, Curran M, Treves ST, et al. Sibling vesicoureteral reflux in multiple gestation births. Pediatrics. 2000;105:800–4.
15. Miller HC, Caspari EW. Ureteral reflux as a genetic trait. JAMA. 1972;220:842–3.
16. Wan J, Greenfield SP, Ng M, et al. Sibling reflux: a dual center retrospective study. J Urol. 1996;156(2 Pt 2):677–9.
17. Pirker ME, Colhoun E, Puri P. Renal scarring in familial vesicoureteral reflux: is prevention possible? J Urol. 2006;176(4 Pt 2):1842–6. discussion 1846.
18. Cascio S, Yoneda A, Chetin B, Colhoun E, Puri P. Renal parenchymal damage in sibling vesicoureteric reflux. Acta Paediatr. 2003;92:17–20.
19. Yoneda A, Cascio S, Oue T, Chertin B, Puri P. Risk factors for the deveopment of renal parenchymal damage in familial reflux. J Urol. 2002;168:1704–7.
20. Menezes M, Puri P. Familial vesicoureteral reflux—is screening beneficial? J Urol. 2009;182(4 Suppl):1673–7.
21. Connolly LP, Treves ST, Connolly SA, et al. Vesicoureteral reflux in children: incidence and severity in siblings. J Urol. 1997;157(6):2287–90.
22. Hari P, Meena J, Kumar M, et al. Evidence-based clinical practice guideline for management of urinary tract infection and primary vesicoureteric reflux. Pediatr Nephrol. 2023;39:1639–68.
23. Yeung CK, et al. The characteristics of primary vesico-ureteric reflux in male and female infants with pre-natal hydronephrosis. Br J Urol. 1997;80(2):319–27.
24. Marra G, Barbieri G, Dell'Agnola CA, et al. Severe vesicoureteral reflux and chronic renal failure: a condition peculiar to male gender? Data from the ItalKid project. J Pediatr. 2004;144(5):677–81.
25. Pirker ME, Mohanan N, Colhoun E, Barton D, Green A, Puri P, et al. Familial vesicoureteral reflux: influence of sex on prevalence and expression. J Urol. 2006;176(4 Pt 2):1776–80.
26. Hunziker M, Puri P. Familial vesicoureteral reflux and reflux related morbidity in relatives of index patients with high grade vesicoureteral reflux. J Urol. 2012;188(4 Suppl):1463–6.
27. Houle AM, Cheikhelard A, Barrieras D, et al. Impact of early screening for reflux in siblings on the detection of renal damage. BJU Int. 2004;94(1):123–5.
28. Puri P, Friedmacher F, Farrugia MK, Sharma S, Esposito C, Mattoo TK. Primary vesicoureteral reflux. Nat Rev Dis Primers 2024;10:75.

Genetics of Vesicoureteral Reflux

John M. Darlow

Abstract A genetic cause for nonsyndromic primary VUR has been sought for about seven decades and we are still only part of the way there, though much has been done. This chapter begins with an explanation of why the study of VUR genetics is difficult. This is followed by descriptions of the different methods of searching for the answers, what we can learn from each, and some of the results that each has brought. It covers observations of inheritance patterns in families, genetic linkage and association, studies of optically visible chromosomal defects and methods of detecting chromosomal defects or rearrangements too small to see with the light microscope, and mention of haplotypes. We have learnt that there are many genes in which some variants can cause nonsyndromic VUR, and that they can be dominant or recessive, and autosomal or X-linked, but the majority autosomal dominant. There are millions of genomic differences between individuals throughout the genome. Brief descriptions are given of some of the databases and prediction methods used to determine whether a particular gene might be relevant and whether any particular genetic variant might be pathogenic, and accounts are given of some of the DNA sequencing studies and their yields.

Keywords VUR genetics · Modes of inheritance · Genetic linkage · Genetic association · Chromosome anomalies · Copy-number variation · Gene sequencing · Exome sequencing · Whole genome sequencing · miRNAs

J. M. Darlow (✉)
Formerly of Department of Genetics, Children's Health Ireland, Dublin, Ireland
e-mail: john.darlow@ucd.ie

P. Puri, A. Yamataka (eds.), *Vesicoureteral Reflux*,
https://doi.org/10.1007/978-3-031-95091-9_4

Introduction–The Problems of Investigating VUR Genetics

The first report of the familial incidence of vesicoureteric reflux was at least as long ago as 1955 [78], at which time the structure of DNA had only just been elucidated [31, 89, 94], the genetic code had not yet been deciphered, and genetics was primarily a bio-mathematical subject. The exact normal number of human chromosomes was not even established until a few months later, and was published in April 1956 [80]. Since that time, the technology for elucidating human genetics has advanced enormously, and the genetics of many human disorders have been established, but discovering the genetic causes of non-syndromic primary VUR has only started gaining momentum in recent years. There are good reasons for this.

There are several methods for searching for the variants in the genome that cause any inherited disorder, some requiring the study of whole families, and some just comparing patients with controls, who do not have the disorder, but whatever means is tried, it is of course necessary to establish who has the disorder, and extremely helpful to establish who has not. So, the first problem is that, though some patients with VUR develop renal scarring, and some of those progress to renal failure, VUR itself is asymptomatic, and the only reliable way of diagnosing it till now involves an invasive investigation using a radiological contrast medium, a micturating cystourethrogram (MCUG, known as a VCUG, voiding cystourethrogram in the USA) or a radionuclide cystogram, so screening has not been a practical or ethical possibility. Because of this, children are generally only investigated if they develop recurrent urinary tract infections (UTIs, see chapter "Vesicoureteral Reflux and Urinary Tract Infection"), or if prenatal ultrasound of the mother picks up possible hydronephrosis of the fetus (see chapter "Prenatally Detected Vesicoureteral Reflux"), or if the parents of a child diagnosed with VUR consent to screening of their other (asymptomatic) children—so collecting families in which two or more people are known to have VUR is difficult.

Furthermore in many, but not all children, the condition resolves spontaneously as the child grows, and the prevalence drops quite rapidly with age [13, 17, 27, 60]. The result of this is that if older siblings of an affected small child are screened, VUR may not be detected even though they did have it when younger and have got the genetic variant that caused the condition. It also follows that any collection of controls is liable to contain individuals who have or used to have VUR.

There have been several attempts to develop a reliable non-invasive diagnostic method, and when one of these is proved successful, and universally adopted, it will make the investigation of the genetics of VUR very much easier. Taking a family history is useful. The parents usually do not know whether either of them had VUR, and as the doctor diagnosing the children is a paediatric physician or surgeon, he or she cannot investigate the parents. However, sometimes enquiries elicit a history of VUR in cousins of the affected children, or occasionally other relatives, and this allows one to identify obligate carriers (relatives intermediate in the family tree, who must have transmitted the pathogenic variant, and therefore must have the variant themselves, even if never diagnosed with VUR).

The above information poses several questions: Why does VUR resolve in some children but not in others? Why do some children with VUR develop kidney damage and others do not? Why do some individuals who develop renal scarring progress to renal failure while others do not, and how much of the answer to this is genetic and how much possibly due to other factors? But that is not the end of the complexity with which the geneticist has to grapple. Most VUR is caused by a congenital anomaly of the development of the urinary tract—a deviation of the vesicoureteric junction from its normal anatomical construction so as to produce incompetence of the combined sphincteric and valvular mechanism that prevents urinary reflux—and VUR can occur as a feature of any of a number of different multiple developmental anomaly syndromes. This of course indicates that there must be a number of different genes that can cause VUR as part of a syndrome, and these have mainly been identified. It also tells us that each of these genes is involved in the development of several different organs, so when mutated, usually several organs fail to develop normally. However, most children with VUR do not have any anomaly of any other organ system, and that has been the question that has been taking so long to answer: where and what are the mutations that cause VUR without producing a syndrome?

What we do observe, though, is that children with VUR commonly have other anomalies of the genitourinary tracts, and that these may be different between siblings in the same family [26]. The same is also observed in mice. Also, though in our own observation, the grade of VUR is usually similar in siblings, it is sometimes widely different between siblings, and between them and other members of the same family. So here is another question: is the variation between individuals carrying the same genetic mutation due to chance (chaotic, butterfly-effect) perturbations in the intricate and complicated course of embryological development, or different environmental effects on the same mother in different pregnancies, or genetic background—the fact that each sibling has a different random selection of the other variants of their two parents? We can also deduce that the mutations causing non-syndromic VUR are either different mutations from the ones that cause syndromes with VUR, but in the same genes, or in genes other than the ones identified in connection with syndromes, genes that somehow continue to evade detection despite the huge advances in genomic exploration, or they are not in genes at all, but instead are in non-coding sequences that regulate the expression of the already-known genes specifically within differentiated urinary tract cells. A lot of work has been done in recent years to explore and understand the functions of the more than 98% of the human genome that is non-coding, but there is more to be done. However, it is already well established that a gene expressed in several tissues may have several different regulators, and some of these may be specific to a particular tissue or set of tissues [47], so it is logical to propose that mutations in regulatory sequences that only operate in the urinary tract could cause VUR and other urinary tract anomalies while leaving the expression of the same genes unimpaired in their co-operation in the construction of other organs.

The other anomalies that may be observed in individuals with VUR include duplex kidneys (the most common, unilateral or bilateral, partial or complete, and within this variation, two separate complete ureters on the same side or ureters connecting into one from separate hila) unilateral renal agenesis, horseshoe kidney, renal dysplasia, renal cysts, multicystic dysplastic kidney, ureterocele, posterior urethral valve, bladder diverticulae, hypospadias, imperforate hymen, labial synechia, hydroceles and ovarian cysts. Readers might here remark that posterior urethral valve and ureterocele are causes of secondary, rather than primary VUR, but as they are part of the spectrum of developmental anomalies of the urinary tract, it is not logical to consider them separately from a genetical point of view. Besides, in our own cohort, we had a sibship in which one child with VUR had a posterior urethral valve and another did not, yet it is unlikely that the two children did not have the same genetic variant causing their VUR. The same goes for another family in which only one of the children with VUR had a ureterocele.

The commonly used overall term for the many and various urinary (and occasionally also genital) tract anomalies that can occur when genes involved in embryonic development of the urinary tract are mutated or deleted or fail to function normally is 'CAKUT', standing for Congenital Anomalies of the Kidneys and Urinary Tract. This is a clumsy invention, since the urinary tract surely runs from the glomeruli to the external opening of the urethra, and so includes the kidneys, which therefore do not need to be mentioned separately. It has been suggested [95] that the term has outlived its usefulness and should be dropped. An alternative acronym, UTM, standing for Urinary Tract Malformations was suggested, with the additional benefit of not using the word 'anomaly' which can include functional defects with normal anatomy, but the proposer was not keen on the use of any collective term.

However, as to usefulness, an overall term like 'CAKUT' was never useful for some people, particularly those treating patients with particular malformations, but it is still useful for others, in particular geneticists and developmental biologists trying to complete the picture of all the genetic causes of malformations of the urinary tract. It will be seen in the proceeding account that many genes can be the cause of a range of different malformations when mutated, and quite often more than one in the same patient, the ranges differing a little depending on which stage, or usually several stages, in the developmental process the particular gene plays a role. UTM will be used as much as possible in this chapter (though in the case of some genes, UGTM might be even better), and a little more will be said about the use of these collective terms in the next section, on how we look for causes.

The inclusion of renal dysplasia in the above list brings us on to one more complexity not yet mentioned, concerning the main reason for investigating the genetics of VUR, 'reflux nephropathy'. This term covers three different pathologies, congenital renal dysplasia, a part of the spectrum of urinary-tract malformation due to genetic perturbation of the embryological development of the kidney, mechanical damage due to hydronephrosis, and acquired renal scarring due to inflammatory reaction to infection. Patients who have urinary tract infections do not all develop renal scarring. Apart from the grade of VUR, the reasons for this might include the type and virulence of the infecting microbe, and environmental and other factors affecting the patient's immune system, but also genetic differences in the immune systems of patients, difference specified by another large set of genes, which may not overlap at all with the set involved in the development of the urinary tract. Work on this set of genes has largely been carried out by a different set of investigators.

Many genes have so far been found to be involved in the embryonic development of the urinary tract. Until relatively recently, these have all been identified by often long investigations of the genetics of human syndromes that include VUR, and by developmental genetic work on animals, particularly mice. However, the development and rapidly falling price of 'next-generation' DNA sequencing, applied to cohorts of patients with all kinds of urinary tract malformations (UTMs), with or without any accompanying syndromic phenotype, has been bringing in new discoveries at a rapid rate, but sequencing alone cannot provide all the answers.

There is so much to relate about the genetics of VUR that it has been decided to divide the information into two chapters. In this chapter a description is given of the different methods of searching for the genes and mutations that are involved in VUR, and the different information that these methods can uncover, and have revealed so far. Search for genes involved in non-syndromic VUR has proceeded simultaneously with investigation of syndromes that include VUR and work on mice, and has constantly been informed by, and related to, information from these other investigations, and in chapter "Embryological Development of the Lower Urinary Tract and the Genes Involved" the embryological development of the urinary tract and interconnected parts of the genital tracts will be described, because familiarity with this is essential to understanding how the genes have their effects. Then, what is known about genes so far identified as being involved in the relevant embryological processes will be described along with the evidence from animal work and the mutations discovered in patients. There is so much to recount about these genes that unfortunately there is not room in these chapters to go into the work on the genetic factors affecting acquired renal scarring as well.

The Different Types of Genetic Investigation of Patients with Nonsyndromic VUR, and What Each Has Told Us So Far

Genetics has gone through a series of revolutions that have dramatically changed what we are able to discover, and the speed at which we can do things. It is only in the past few years that we have had the technology to sequence a whole human genome rapidly and cheaply, and the computing power and storage to process the massive amounts of data that this produces, in order to search for potentially pathogenic mutations. It should be remembered that until the first human genomes were sequenced around the beginning of this century, we only had maps of the chromosomes created tediously over many decades and sparsely-populated with genes. And even after we had our first very imperfect reference human genome sequence, populated with genes that were mostly predicted from clues in the sequence, and had genome browser software allowing us to scroll or search through the genome, we had no idea what most of the predicted genes did, and that was only 20 years ago and less. In the meantime our sequencing methods had improved from the early days, when we used to label DNA bases with radioactivity and read our sequences from X-ray films, and was now partially mechanised and radioactivity-free, but it was still labour-intensive, and expensive to sequence even small bits of the genome. So, if we wanted to find a gene whose mutation might be the cause of a particular condition of interest, such as VUR, we still had to use the mathematical techniques of classical genetics to identify exactly what part of the genome to start sequencing to look for variations from the reference sequence. This reliance on mathematical techniques to determine where to look for relevant genes has applied throughout most of the time for which the genetics of VUR have been investigated, from before we could sequence the DNA at all until very recently. Now, massive computing power is used to search and sort the massive amounts of data in many different ways. This section describes what we have been able to discover about the genetics of VUR at each stage, as technology has advanced.

Establishing Whether the Disorder Is Inherited and, If So, What the Mode of Inheritance Is

A standard investigation to determine whether a disorder might be inherited is to carry out a twin study. There were lots of reports of VUR in twins from 1955 onwards, but there appears to be only one report in which the appropriate genetic investigation was done, i.e. collect all pairs of twins in which at least one is affected, and then see whether monozygous twins are more often 'concordant' (*i.e.* both have the condition) than 'discordant' (one has it and the other hasn't) compared with dizygous twins. As they did not know anything about the genetic aetiology of VUR, the investigators [41] played safe and excluded all pairs in which there was any additional UTM, such as posterior urethral valve, duplex collecting system or a bladder diverticulum, and were left with 46 pairs (i.e. 46 index cases with VUR and 46 twin siblings) collected over a ten-year period. Their finding was that 12/15 of the identical twin siblings (80%) had VUR compared with only 11/31 (35%) of the fraternal twin siblings. When only the youngest individuals in each group were considered, to reduce the possibility of spontaneous resolution, the results were 100% (7/7) of the monozygotics and 50% (5/10) of the dizygotics. (They did not specify what their cut-off age was). This showed that VUR was definitely inherited, and that probably it was autosomal dominant, if they assumed that there was only one gene, though the number of young pairs was too small to be certain of that.

In the meantime (i.e. from long before this was published in 2000) others had been considering possibilities. One of these that was considered early on was that there are many genes, whose variations can each affect the chance of developing VUR, and that these effects can add together to make a continuous scale of risk, and that beyond a certain critical risk point, VUR occurs. It was put forward that this continuous variable might be the length of the intravesical ureter, VUR only occurring when the length was below a critical one [9]. The authors of a study of 186 families of index cases with established primary VUR (which found very small proportions of siblings affected compared with most other reports) considered that this mode of inheritance, known as polygenic, or multifactorial, inheritance was the most likely [25]. This view was held by some until very recently, on the grounds that VUR is so common (like, say, hypertension) that this must be the mode.

Others had been collecting family pedigrees to determine the mode of inheritance on the assumption that only a single gene was involved in any one family, if indeed there was more than one gene. No doubt many of these studies will have been described in chapter "Familial Vesicoureteral Reflux". Here, let us just go over the details of the three simplest and most likely familial patterns that might be seen in any inherited condition, to illustrate why studying VUR genetics was so difficult. (1) The family has an autosomal dominant pattern with no homozygotes. One of the parents is affected, and each child has a 50% chance of being affected (i.e. having the condition), and girls and boys have an equal chance of being affected. (2) The family has an autosomal recessive pattern, in which neither parent is affected and each child has a 25% chance of being affected. If the condition is rare, the parents in most families will be related, whereas if it is a common condition (like VUR), most couples having affected children will not be related. (3) The family will show an X-linked recessive pattern. The parents will not be affected. The mother has the mutation, but she is not affected, so the observer does not know that she has it. Each son has a 50% chance of being affected. The daughters are not affected, but each of them also has a 50% chance of carrying the mutation, and if those daughters have children, each of their sons has a 50% chance of being affected. The problems of assessing which of these possibilities might be the answer are that the parents hardly ever know whether they had reflux as a child, and most families these days are small, and of course, that spontaneous resolution can affect the proportions affected.

A 1985 study of 88 families [14] concluded that a single major genetic locus was the most important cause of non-syndromic VUR, with dominant inheritance, and there were others that came to the same conclusion. We now know that there are many genes whose disturbance can result in nonsyndromic VUR and, as will be seen, most of those found so far do have their effects in an autosomal dominant manner.

Earlier, a family appearing to show X-linked recessive inheritance was described in which all 3 brothers and the maternal grandfather had VUR, whereas the father, mother and 3 daughters were urologically normal [61]. At that time, finding the relevant mutation would have been very difficult, and there does not appear to be anything in the literature to say that the mutation has ever been found subsequently. It may well be interesting if it is found, because so far only one X-linked gene with recessive mutations has been identified as being involved in urinary tract development, *AGTR2*, which will be described later and produces angiotensin II receptor type 2, and no mutations in it have yet been published in a nonsyndromic VUR case.

Later, a few reports of families showing an autosomal recessive inheritance pattern appeared, the first being [67]. Several genes will be described later that show autosomal recessive inheritance, but the mutation in this Somali family has not been identified yet. Further work which has come closer to the solution will be mentioned later.

Lastly, a fourth pattern of VUR inheritance was published [62]. This paper (from Iran) has been cited several times as showing X-linked inheritance (which is mentioned in its title) without any appreciation by the citers that this paper does not show the well-known X-linked recessive inheritance pattern, as seen for instance in Duchenne muscular dystrophy. It suggests X-linked *dominant* inheritance. In this, the pattern is completely different. One of the parents will always be affected, and the pattern depends upon which one it is. The mother of course has two X-chromosomes, and if she is the affected one, every child has a 50% chance of being affected, girls as well as boys. However, the father only has one X-chromosome and one Y-chromosome, so if he is the affected one, *all* his daughters will be affected, and *none* of his sons, and that was the pattern seen in this family (but not mentioned in the title of the paper).

The index case was a girl with end-stage renal failure due to reflux nephropathy. The parents and siblings (three female and two male) were screened for VUR although they had not presented episodes of urinary tract infection, and VUR was identified in the father, who also had renal scarring, and in all the three sisters, aged up to 18 years, two of whom also had renal scarring, while the two brothers (aged 5 years and 8 years) had normal renal ultrasonograms and cystograms. No mutated gene has yet been identified in this family so far in the literature. This pattern could of course be produced by chance by autosomal dominant inheritance, but if it is indeed X-linked dominant, then one candidate for the gene is *OFD1*, in which mutations can cause the X-linked dominant Orofacial-Digital Syndrome, but in which mutations have been found in two families in patients with nonsyndromic VUR [81]. However, Orofacial Digital syndrome is usually lethal in males in intrauterine or early neonatal life. Perhaps the milder reported mutations of this gene reported in VUR cases are compatible with life to adulthood, but unfortunately the sexes of these two children are not reported. Another possible candidate gene might be *PRKX*, of which more later.

Identification of Where in the Genome the Mutations Lie

Linkage and Association Studies

Having decided that a condition is inherited, the next step is to identify where causative mutations are in the genome. There are two methods of doing this by applying mathematics to observations, linkage and association studies. They each use 'markers'—observable or testable places of difference between genomes at known positions—but the ways in which these methods work, and what they tell us, are completely different.

Linkage studies came long before association. The principle is simple: if a common characteristic that you can easily observe or test for is possessed by every member of a large family who has a particular disorder, then you may assume that the genes responsible for the characteristic and the disorder are on the same chromosome, because at every meiosis producing every egg and sperm, the chromosomes are assorted, so if the two are not on the same chromosome, they will frequently be separated. Chromosomes of course are subject to recombination (crossing over) at each meiosis too, so even if the gene variants responsible for the characteristic and for the disorder are on the same chromosome, they can be separated by crossing over. The closer the disease gene and the marker are, the less likely it is that they will be separated, i.e. the more likely that every family member with the disorder will also have the marker. SO, if you have lots of markers all along every chromosome, and you observe them in family members, you can work out where the disease gene is by a probability calculation. It's called a LOD score, for 'Logarithm of the odds'. We don't need to go into the mathematics of how it is calculated here, but the score, which is a statistical estimate of the relative probability that the marker and the mutation are located near each other on a chromosome, and therefore likely to be inherited together, is $-\text{Log}_{10}\text{p}$, where p is the well-known p value, so if $p = 0.001$, i.e. 10^{-3}, then the LOD score is 3, which is generally considered to be the minimum score worthy of interest.

The first markers used for linkage studies in humans were blood groups, which are produced by genes, but there aren't very many of them compared with the later markers, VNTRs and SNPs, which are DNA variations that are not genes. SNPs are 'single nucleotide polymorphisms' so called, though they are nearly all dimorphisms (one or other of two bases at a particular position) and they are not all single-nucleotide variants. There are two very important points to note about these markers. Suppose a marker is an SNP that can be either a T or a C on a particular member of a chromosome pair. The marker will only be useful in a family member with the inherited disorder that you want to study if the genotype is T/C (or C/T) so that you can see which one is passed on with the disorder, and if the frequencies of T and C are exactly equal, only 50% of people will be heterozygous (and 25% C/C and 25% T/T), and if the frequencies are not equal, heterozygotes will be less than 50%, so, at best, a particular SNP is only useful half the time. (The first method of detecting SNPs relied on the fact that bacterial restriction enzymes, of which there are very many, each recognize a particular exact short DNA sequence, and will cut the DNA only at an exact position in each strand only in the exact sequence. Therefore if a DNA variant occurs in a restriction-enzyme recognition-sequence, the DNA with the variant will not be cut at that position. The technique was called RFLP, restriction fragment length polymorphism, and came into use for genetic linkage studies in human samples in about 1973.)

The other type of marker, a VNTR, is a variable number tandem repeat. This is a set of multiple copies of a particular sequence in a row. VNTRs are named as two categories, minisatellites, in which the repeating sequence is typically around 10–100 bp in length, and microsatellites, in which the repeating sequence is typically 1 to 6 bp in length, and it is the latter that are used as markers, and are used as the basis for DNA fingerprinting, originated by Alec Jeffreys in 1984. The number of copies of the little sequence varies within a range, of typically 5 to 50 between different copies of the same chromosome. The huge advantage of this type of marker is that nearly every person is a heterozygote for nearly every VNTR across the genome. The disadvantages are that there is more work involved in determining the genotype of each VNTR, and that there are fewer of them compared with SNPs. Now that the human genome has been sequenced, we know a lot more of each, and there are over 600,000 microsatellites, but there are millions of SNPs, so one can refine the genomic position of a mutant gene much more precisely with the latter, even though only SNPs in which the (usually just two) alleles are of similar frequencies are useful.

The other important point is that a different allele of the same SNP will be linked to the disorder in different families. The main reason for this is that unrelated families with the same inherited disorder, caused by mutation of the same gene, will nearly always have a different mutation in the same gene. Any mutation occurs first in a particular individual on a particular chromosome before it is spread through generations to other family members and later to the wider population, and if there is a nearby SNP, that again say is C or T, some mutations will occur on a chromosome that happens to have a C, and other mutations in the same gene in other families, will occur on a chromosome bearing a T at the SNP position. Of, course, if the SNP is not very close to the mutation, there can sometimes be a cross-over between the two, so this is another reason why the other allele may be on the chromosome carrying the mutation. The marker is just a marker; it does not cause the disorder.

An association study is completely different. This does not use families. It involves comparing a cohort of thousands, or preferably hundreds of thousands, of unrelated patients with a particular disorder with matched control subjects. The genotypes of as many SNPs as possible are determined all across the genome of each participant. Then the frequency of each allele of each SNP is determined and compared between the two groups by a computer program that searches for SNPs for which one allele is much more common in the patients than in the controls with a highly significant p value.

Thus, in a linkage study, either allele of a marker can pass with the disorder through generations, whereas in an association study, it is the same allele. Some of these polymorphisms have been around for tens of thousands, or even hundreds of thousands, of years, and have spread throughout the population concerned over many generations. This means that either the genetic variant causing the disorder is so close to the SNP that there is hardly ever a cross-over between them, or the SNP allele itself is the cause of the increased risk. Association studies are used to study common disorders that are expected to be multifactorial, whereas linkage is used for disorders in which the expectation is that the disorder will be caused by a variant in, or relating to, a single gene in any particular family. It is because VUR is common that some investigators, or (in our case) their grant-application reviewers, believed that VUR must be multifactorial, that association studies were done.

One of the frustrations that investigators have had with the results of these enormously expensive studies is that each SNP, found to be highly significantly associated with the disorder in question, only contributes a very small amount to the overall risk. But this is only to be expected. Any variant that causes a large risk that its bearer will develop the disorder, and thereby be less likely to survive to pass the variant on to the next generation, will be swiftly brought to rarity by natural selection, so variants that have been common for thousands of years are necessarily ones that only make a small difference, and are usually balanced (prevented from dying out) by giving their bearer an advantage in some other way.

The other frustration is that almost all SNPs found to be highly significantly associated with any disorder, are 'in the middle of nowhere', i.e. in non-coding DNA, often far from any gene. Since we have had the first human reference genome (now revised many times and still being revised) we have been able to see that genes occur in clusters—sections of the genome where there are many genes—with gene deserts in between. These are regions of a megabase or more in width with no genes at all, but hundreds of predicted transcription-factor binding-sites. These regions harbour enhancers and other types of regulatory sequence that are each composed of several or many recognition sites for various DNA-binding proteins. Each of these proteins binds best to a particular consensus DNA sequence, and variations in that sequence may increase or decrease its binding, and thereby cause a particular gene or several genes to be up-regulated or down-regulated. Thus SNPs contribute to phenotypic variation necessary to the survival of any species as the basis of adaptation to different conditions. However, to prove that a particular alteration in non-coding DNA has a measurable effect, and to find out which gene it affects, requires a lot of laboratory work. Regulatory sequences can be upstream or downstream of the gene that they control, and up to a megabase or more away, and even inside another gene [45].

Because of expense and labour-intensity of techniques at the time, early linkage and association studies to look for genes involved in nonsyndromic VUR were not genome-wide investigations but used small numbers of markers around and within individual candidate genes suggested by mouse work, or involvement in human syndromes that include VUR, and sequencing studies of individual genes carried out without prior checking for linkage or association. Some of these studies proved negative of course, but the first four discoveries of mutations in one or a very few patients with nonsyndromic VUR were made in patient cohorts not selected on the basis of VUR, in the following genes, more details of which will be given in chapter

"Embryological Development of the Lower Urinary Tract and the Genes Involved" (section "Genes Involved in the Formation of a Functioning One-Way Urine Flow System"). ***PAX2*:** Having read a report that renal hypoplasia can occur as part of renal-coloboma syndrome, which is caused by dominant mutations in *PAX2*, a team [65] sequenced the gene in a group of 20 patients with renal hypoplasia without obvious evidence of the syndrome, and found mutations in two of them. One was then found to have mild features of the syndrome, but the other patient, who had bilateral small kidneys and grade III VUR, and subsequently developed renal failure, had normal visual acuity and a normal optic nerve, normal growth, intelligence, and hearing. His mother also had the mutation and was awaiting a second renal transplant. She also had no signs of the syndrome, and was not investigated for VUR. DNA of her family was examined, and it was found that the mutation had occurred *de novo* in this mother, so this was not a mutation that had been circulating in the population Only one other patient with nonsyndromic VUR has since been found to have a mutation in this gene, 20 years later (see section "Genes Involved in the Formation of a Functioning One-Way Urine Flow System"). ***UPK3A*:** This gene, suggested as a candidate by mouse work, was sequenced in 17 children with renal failure caused by adysplasia, of whom four had mutations, all *de novo*, and two of these children had VUR [38]. ***UPK2*:** This gene, also suggested by mouse work, was sequenced in 42 children with various UTM, and a mutation was found in just one, who had VUR, bilateral nephropathy and renal failure [39]. ***HNF1B***, in which mutations can cause a syndrome of cystic kidneys and diabetes, but can also cause various other anomalies, was sequenced in 99 unrelated patients with renal hypodysplasia, and mutations were found in eight patients, two of whom also had VUR [90].

Commercial companies sprung up that could do large amounts of genotyping of markers, or DNA sequencing, using robots to handle the samples, and prices came down, and it became possible, and affordable to carry out genome-wide linkage and association studies of cohorts of VUR patients and their families, and then sequence in regions showing high probabilities of containing relevant genetic variants. 'Targeting' of sequencing to regions indicated by these studies reduced the cost, but as the price of sequencing came down, it became affordable for some to sequence the whole 'exomes', i.e. all the coding exons of all the known genes, or whole genomes of their patients, and then search them all for potentially pathogenic mutations, such as deletions of all or parts of genes, or mutations causing frame-shifts, or that introduce stop codons by substitution, or that change amino acids predicted to be important for function of the encoded protein and not found in healthy control subjects, and occur in all affected members of the family concerned, if DNA from family members is available.

If you have a large family with numerous affected members, you may well be able to get a high enough LOD score in a narrow enough genomic region that you can confine your search to one or a few genes, and a search for any information on those genes may further help you to refine your choice of which to try sequencing first to look for mutations. But large families with multiple members with nonsyndromic VUR are not common, and if your families are mainly small, you have to add the genotyping results from a group of families together and hope that they all have mutations in the same gene. The trouble, as became increasingly obvious, is that there are many genes of which disturbance in their expression or function can cause VUR, so in any cohort of families recruited, there will inevitably be mutations relating to several or many different genes, and when the LOD score was plotted out, marker by marker along the genome, a confusing picture appeared of several or many peaks of different sizes, and every linkage study from different cohorts gave different results, though there were some correspondences. Small false peaks of apparent linkage can also occur by chance sharing, between affected members of small families, of identical parts of the genome inherited from the same parent but in which the relevant mutation does not lie.

The first genome-wide linkage 'scan' for nonsyndromic VUR was conducted in the U.K. with a group of seven quite large European families that appeared to exhibit autosomal dominant inheritance, with three to seven affected members per family, and genotyped in-house for 387 microsatellite markers [30]. The next scan used a cohort of 133 mostly small Irish families genotyped commercially with a set of 4753 SNP markers, reducing to 129 families and 4710 markers after results revealed some aberrant results [43]. The third linkage scan used 382 microsatellite markers in 16 Italian families [18], and the fourth, on 12 large 'Caucasian' American families (including Hasidic Jewish and Italian families) used 393 microsatellite markers, followed by 10,204 SNP markers [92], and the fifth was performed by a group in Boston on 98 mainly small 'Caucasian' American families, and used approximately 6000 SNP markers [8]. Then the UK group published a second scan, using 262,264 SNP markers on a total of 189 families from the UK and Slovenia [20]. A family-based association analysis was also carried out in this study, using data from 2938 previously-genotyped control subjects from the Wellcome Trust Case Control Consortium, but it brought no significant results. Then the Boston group published another analysis [58], on the same group of 98 families analysed earlier, this time sorting families to give results supposedly to show linkage to different autosomal loci depending upon gender, but it is not clear how they did this.

All of these studies used additional markers after analysis of the initial results, to try to refine the position of the highest scoring linkage peak or peaks, except that no more lab work was done after the repeat analysis by the Boston group. Most groups also tried analysis on the bases of autosomal dominant and of autosomal recessive inheritance, and looking for sharing of genomic segments between siblings without any assumption of the mode of inheritance (non-parametric linkage analysis), and in some studies, some families were removed from the group after the first analysis if their results pointed to a different part of the genome from the rest, so as to try again to get more focussed results. All of them found some genomic regions achieving quite high linkage scores in one or more of the different analyses, and in some cases peaks of linkage corresponded with genomic regions indicated as harbouring urinary tract development genes from other evidence, including cytogentically-detected deletions, but none of them resulted in identifying a gene.

Two targeted linkage studies, in seven [71] and four [82] large extended VUR families respectively, used markers covering the positions of previously reported peaks of linkage with VUR and of genes known to be involved in urinary tract development, and found no significant linkage of any of these to their families, even though some of them were already known to harbour mutations in a few VUR cases, and others have been found to do so subsequently. The authors rightly concluded that VUR is very heterogeneous.

The second UK/Slovenian study specifically looked for linkage to six genes previously identified as being involved in lower urinary tract development by mouse and or human studies, *AGTR2*, *HNF1B*, *PAX2*, *RET*, *ROBO2* and *UPK3A*, but did not find linkage to any of them. This does not mean that none of the families had mutations in any of these genes; any linkage in a small number of small families would be swamped by signals from many different parts of the genome from all the other families whose pathogenic mutations were in other parts of the genome, and the small families on their own would be insufficient for linkage to be detected.

This does not mean that linkage analysis cannot find genes whose mutation can cause VUR; it just taught us that VUR can be caused by mutation of so many different genes that lumping lots of small families together is likely to fail. Analysis of single very large families can find even genes mutated in VUR. There were some results from analysis of large groups of VUR families, though.

The Irish group recruited more families and genotyped them and the original families with a set of 900,000 SNP markers, and used 592 blood-donor controls from the Trinity-College-Dublin-Irish-Blood-Transfusion-Service Biobank that had previously been genotyped by another group with the same markers [22]. This resulted in establishing the true identities of some samples that had evidently been mislabelled, enabling families that had been rejected before to be used. It also revealed that some of the nuclear families were related, enabling them to be assembled into larger extended families. After this, and again sifting out samples and markers that did not give satisfactory results, there were 118 'old' families, some now extended, and 81 new families that were not part of previously recruited families, and 643,691 usable markers. Some samples that could not be used for linkage analysis because only one affected family member's sample had genotyped successfully, could still be used for association, and there were a total of 900 samples, 500 from affected members, that could be used for one or more of analysis of linkage and two different association methods.

The two groups of families, when analysed by linkage separately, gave linkage peaks in different regions, emphasising the heterogeneity of VUR, and adding them together did not make linkage peaks from the first scan a great deal larger. However, four of the linkage peaks were in the same genomic regions indicated by a different kind of study, a 'copy-number variation' study, to which we shall come below. The association results were not of very high significance, and also did not identify specific genes. However there were two interesting findings from the study. The first relates to the Somali family mentioned in section "Establishing Whether the Disorder Is Inherited and, If So, What the Mode of Inheritance Is" in which an autosomal recessive inheritance pattern had been noted [67]. The unaffected parents were first cousins who had fifteen children, of whom seven had at that time been noted to have UTM, consisting of VUR and/or pelviureteric junction obstruction and/

or unilateral renal agenesis. Subsequently, the investigators found that another child was also affected, obtained blood for DNA extraction from the parents and all eight affected children and four of the seven unaffected, and genotyped them at 50,000 SNPs [3]. Analysis then showed that the only part of the genome in which all eight affected children had inherited part of the same chromosome (of a pair), known as a haplotype, from their father, and the same haplotype from their mother, was a region on chromosome 8q24 only 2·5 Mb wide, which contained a single gene, *KHDRBS3*, very close to the centromeric side of the region. They sequenced all the exons of the gene and found no mutations.

The new linkage scan of Irish VUR families [22] also showed a recessive linkage peak at the same position. Just three of the 199 families contributed to this linkage peak. They were all in the 'old' group of families, but the smaller number of markers in the previous set were too far apart to detect it. One of the families had six children, all affected, five of whom had been genotyped, and the other two families each had three children, all affected. As the families were smaller than the Somali one, it was not surprising that the region that the affected children all shared was a bit wider, 5 Mb, but it covered the whole of the previously-reported region, and *KHDRBS3* was in the very centre. Ashraf et al. did not examine the promoter of the gene in their family, so we examined 1000 bp upstream of the gene and the 5′ untranslated region in our three linked families, and found no new variants that segregated with VUR there either.

KHDRBS3, 'KH RNA-binding-domain containing, signal transduction associated 3', does not seem to be a very likely candidate to be involved in urinary tract development. It codes for a protein that forms part of a complex that is predicted to be involved in regulation of alternative mRNA splicing, and since there were no mutations in the gene, we must presume that somewhere in the linkage region there is a non-coding sequence involved in the regulation (at a distance) of a gene that is involved in urinary tract development. None of the nearby genes seem likely candidates either, and none of the genes so far proven to take part in developing a functional ureterovesical junction are anywhere near 8q24, so at the moment, it is still a mystery.

The other interesting finding that came out of the second Irish VUR genome scan was that there was one family with a boy and a girl, both with VUR, in which the genotyping indicated that the boy had two X-chromosomes and no Y. Cytogenetic study then showed that he had a Yp;Xp translocation. This can occur by recombination in regions of homology between the X and Y chromosomes, and one of these is close to a pair of highly homologous genes on the X and Y chromosomes, *PRKX*, 'Protein kinase cAMP-dependent X-linked catalytic subunit', and *PRKY*, and recombination within or near to these genes is a frequent cause of sex reversal disorder in XX males and XY females [46, 74]. *PRKY* is thought to be non-functional, but *PRKX* is developmentally regulated and, in the developing urinary tract is restricted to the ureteric bud epithelium [53], and it has been shown that increased expression of the gene in ureteric bud epithelium in a mouse embryonic kidney organ culture system that recapitulates early kidney development *in vitro*, stimulates branching morphogenesis and results in increase in glomerular number [54].

It is thus perhaps possible that a mutation in this region of Xp caused some dysregulation of *PRKX* and caused VUR in both children, as well as making the DNA wore susceptible to a translocation event that occurred in one of them. It would have to be a dominant mutation, and on the father's X chromosome, if it also increased the liability to translocation in the generation of a gamete. There was a small dominant linkage peak near the tip of Xp (though too small to be statistically significant), and, as mentioned before, X-linked dominant VUR has been reported [62]. Also, VUR has previously been reported in an XX male [50]. The instability region is not inside *PRKX* but adjacent to it on the centromeric side [70], so the gene would be lost in the translocated chromosome of the boy. However, it is possible that the same mutation that increased the instability of the region might have inactivated the adjacent copy of the gene in his sister.

Linkage and association analyses were then carried out on the combined UK, Slovenian and Irish cohorts of VUR families [23]. Family-based association analysis of 1098 parent-affected-child trios and case/control association analysis of 1147 cases and 3789 controls did not reveal any compelling associations, but parametric linkage analysis of 460 families with 1,062 affected individuals, under a dominant model identified a single region, on 10q26, that showed strong linkage (HLOD = 4.90; ZLRLOD = 4.39) to VUR (where HLOD is a Heterogeneity LOD, which takes account of the fact that only some of the families in the cohort will have linkage to any particular part of the genome, and ZLRLOD is another type of calculation that does not assume any particular mode of inheritance). However, the linkage region was about 9 Mb wide and contained 69 genes. Sequencing their exons in the members of the eight largest families in the combined cohort did not identify any gene in which all the affected members of any family had a rare variant.

Sequencing was then carried out across the whole linkage region (including all the non-coding DNA) in one affected member of each of the 32 families showing highest linkage to the region, and a search was made for short sequences, that might potentially be regulatory elements, such as enhancers, in which affected individuals from several families all had novel or very rare variants. No such sequences were found except that right in the middle of the linkage region, at the position of highest LOD score, was a sequence nearly 42·5 kb long, in which there were apparently hundreds of variants. This sequence included the first exon of a gene called *FANK1*, Fibronectin type III and ankyrin repeat domains 1, and sequence up- and downstream of the exon, containing the promoter and a potential enhancer. The trouble was that it turned out that this region was what is known as a 'segmental duplication'; meaning that there were multiple, non-functional and slightly different, copies of it in other parts of the genome. It was clear that a lot of the sequence reads came from these other copies, and it was impossible to determine which of the sequence reads were from the true *FANK1* sequence on 10q. The only way to resolve this would be to get long-range sequences right across the whole 42·5 kb between unique 10q sequences on either side, but at the time, neither of the two long-range sequencing companies were able to carry out targeted sequencing of such a long distance, so the regulatory element and mutations, if there, are still not found.

A homozygous nonsynonymous (i.e. amino-acid-changing) mutation, predicted to be deleterious, has subsequently been found in *FANK1* in one patient in a large whole-exome sequencing survey of families with all sorts of UTM, but unfortunately the phenotype of the patient was not given [81] (in their Supplementary Table 4, red section). The gene codes for an extracellular matrix protein, and other extracellular matrix proteins have been found to be mutated in a few VUR cases (see section "Genes Involved in the Formation of a Functioning One-Way Urine Flow System" in chapter "Embryological Development of the Lower Urinary Tract and the Genes Involved").

Cytogenetic and Copy-Number Variation Studies

Chromosome deletions large enough to see on light microscopy are rather large, and usually contain many genes and result in many congenital anomalies, but if these anomalies happen to include the phenotype in which one is interested, it alerts one to the fact that at least one of the genes within the deletion must be related to the condition. Comparing cases with deletions in the same region whose phenotypes include the phenotype of interest and overlapping them can narrow the search for the relevant gene.

Overlapping the 10q26 terminal deletions of a collection of ten patients with urinogenital malformations (including VUR) or genital malformations or both, defined a region for genital malformations within a larger one that included the urinary tract malformations [66]. Already at least four of the genes on 10q were known to be involved in urinary tract development from mouse work or human syndromes, and the authors noted that *PAX2*, *GFRA1* and *EMX2* were all present in both copies in all of their patients, and therefore were outside the deletions. (*RET* is also on 10q but much further away.) The linkage region on 10q in the first Irish linkage scan mentioned above [43], was much wider than the deletions, and stretched from 10q25.2–q26.3, but the highest-scoring SNP for non-parametric linkage within the region was on 10q26.3, and was within the deletion region for the patients with UTMs. The much larger linkage peak obtained later from the combined UK, Slovenian and Irish cohorts [23] was a little to the centromeric side of that, in 10q26.2. Another study [85] reports three patients with 10q terminal deletions, two with UTM as part of their multiple anomaly phenotypes (one of them having VUR) and one without UTM, and aligns the deletions with those of Ogata et al. and of six other reports that had been published subsequently, some patients having UTM and some not. This shows a rather confusing picture, but suggests that the true position of the genetic element, whatever it is that is responsible for UTM, is even further towards the centromere, in 10q26.13. This is still within the linkage region and still does not include any of the genes excluded by Ogata et al.

Another study [84] presented three children with congenital anomalies, including UTMs, with deletions of 13q33–q34. One of the linkage regions found in the first linkage study by the UK group [30], with a non-parametric linkage score of 2·34, was on 13q. It was much wider than the deletion region but covered the whole of it. The Irish group's first scan had a very small linkage peak, scoring only 1·55, on 13q33.3, completely within the deletion region. A gene involved in urinary tract development, some mutations of which have been found in a few cases of nonsyndromic VUR, has subsequently been identified within the deletion region. It is *COL4A1*, the collagen type IV alpha 1 chain gene. It is on 13q34, so the tiny Irish linkage peak just missed it, probably because evidently there were very few families in the Irish cohort with mutations at that locus and the position of the peak was skewed by interference from chance signals from other families whose mutations lay in other parts of the genome.

The same authors [83] also presented patients with overlapping deletions in another part of the same chromosome, 13q12–q22, whose urinary tract manifestations included hydronephrosis, ureterocele, renal dysplasia, and mesangioproliferative steroid-resistant nephrotic syndrome. This was outside the UK linkage region for VUR, the boundary of which on that side was in 13q32.1. The responsible gene has also been found in this region of deletion overlaps. It is *FREM2*, standing for FRAS1 related extracellular matrix 2. Recessive mutations of both genes, *FREM2* and *FRAS1*, amongst others, have been found to cause Fraser syndrome, but less severe recessive mutations of each have been found in a few cases of nonsyndromic VUR. Details and references will be given in chapter "Embryological Development of the Lower Urinary Tract and the Genes Involved".

The above were examples. It is not intended to describe every deletion region or genetic linkage region in which genes related to VUR have subsequently been found. Another cytogenetic event by which genes related to many disorders have been found is chromosomal translocation. Translocations can occur without causing any abnormality of phenotype if no chromosome section is lost and the breaks are in places that are neither within genes nor place the promoter of one gene next to a different gene on the chromosome to which it is joined, but if one or both of the chromosomal breaks is/are within a gene, a syndrome will result. At least one gene of which mutations can cause nonsyndromic VUR was found as a result of cytogenetic examination of a patient with multiple congenital anomalies which included VUR. The patient was found to have a Yp;3p translocation. The breaks in both chromosomes went through genes, and the one on chromosome 3, which was then found to carry genetic variants in a few VUR patients, was *ROBO2*.

The markers described as being used in genetic linkage and association investigations can also be used to define the limits of optically visible chromosomal rearrangements and of ones that are too small to be seen in stained chromosomes under light microscopy. The margins of some of the deletions described in the papers cited above were defined by the use of arrays of DNA markers. SNP arrays are 'chips' bearing arrays of oligonucleotides, each designed to detect a particular SNP or the number of copies of a short invariant stretch of the genome. Such arrays were used to genotype participants in some of the genetic linkage and association studies cited above, but they can also be used to detect a class of variation below the level of conventional cytogenetic detection, CNVs.

CNVs, or Copy-Number Variations, may be simple deletions, duplications, insertions, or inversions of DNA segments, or may be more complex combinations of two or more of these. The sequences involved can be up to several megabases in length and contain several genes. This means that a person with a normal karyotype, who might be expected to have two copies of any autosomal gene, might only have one, or have three or even four or none at all. We all have many CNVs in our chromosomes, and frequently when genomes of members of a population somewhere in the world, not previously sequenced are sequenced, quite large stretches of genome never seen before are found. It has become apparent that there is no single standard human genome. Some CNVs appear not to be detrimental and can be quite common and are part of normal variation. Others are pathogenic.

Copy number variations in the genome can be of any length, but the official lower limit is 50 base-pairs, and common variations below and up to about that length appear in the SNP database, dbSNP. SNP arrays can be used to detect large CNVs but are unreliable for detecting small ones. Until very recently, the best arrays available have had a little over one million SNPs so, considering that our genome is over 3000 million bp in length, that means that the average distance between them was about 3 kb, and several SNPs in a row, all present at half or one-and-a-half times the detection intensity of those on either side, will be needed to be sure that a deletion or duplication respectively is probably real. Some genome-wide studies of cohorts of patients have therefore limited themselves to searching for CNVs upwards of 100 kb in length. Smaller CNVs may be detected in sequencing studies by comparison of the number of 'reads' generated between different sections of the genome, but this is not very reliable. Very recently, a new cytogentics array has become available that has two million invariant markers and 750,000 SNP markers, and this will allow smaller CNVs to be detected, as well as closer definition of larger ones.

Before going on to describe results of CNV search with SNP arrays, it should be noted that there is another technique, used principally by cytogeneticists, to detect micro-imbalances in chromosomes, comparative genomic hybridization (CGH), which was then adapted to arrays, 'array-CGH', giving higher resolution, and has been used in search for genes involved in UTMs. These techniques and the SNP arrays are all descended from Southern blotting, a technique invented by Ed(win) Southern in 1973, and published in 1975 [77], a technique which we all used to use back in the day but needn't go into here. The principal, however, which is relevant here, is that mixed single strands of DNA of different sequences will find their exact matches amongst all the other sequences, and bind back together into double-stranded DNA. So, if you bind pieces of single-stranded DNA to a substrate and you label your test DNA (originally with a radioactive isotope but nowadays with a fluorescent dye) and you melt the strands apart (by heating to 96 °C or above) and then pour it onto the substrate, you will be able to see where it binds.

Arrays used for array-CGH have arrays of clusters of multiple copies of short bits of genomic sequence chosen at intervals across the genome (not designed to detect SNPs). Then the genomic DNA of a control subject is cut up and labelled with a dye of one colour and the genomic DNA of the patient with another colour, and then the two are mixed together and melted and then applied to the array, and they compete for binding. Then you can detect any region of imbalance, where one binds more than the other—because your patient has a deletion or a duplication in that region. Obviously the resolution depends upon how far apart your markers are. Arrays used for array-CGH detect genomic imbalances below the resolution of light microscopy of banded chromosomes, but generally do not have as high a resolution as current SNP arrays. An array-CGH study of 30 patients with syndromic UMTs (having at least one 'extra-renal' manifestation was an entry criterion) [91] discovered three patients with chromosomal imbalances, and though none of these patients was nonsyndromic, they are still of interest. One patient had two imbalances, a duplication of 2q37.1–q37.3 and a deletion of 7q36.2–q36.3 in an unbalanced translocation. These were both regions of genetic linkage found in a genome scan for nonsyndromic VUR [43]. Of the other two patients with detected genomic imbalances, one had a duplication in 1q21.1, a region in which deletions were found in nonsyndromic VUR patients in a CNV study described below. The remaining patient had deletion in 3q23–q25.1. This region includes the gene for the Angiotensin II receptor type 1, *AGTR1* (which is in 3q24), in which a mutation was later found in a patient with nonsyndromic VUR in a big sequencing study to be mentioned later [64].

Several genome-wide searches for CNVs using SNP arrays in groups of patients, fetuses, or families with UTMs have been used to find the genes whose deletions cause the UTMs [2, 10–12, 72, 76, 86, 87, 93, 96, 97]. Also, CNV analyses within chromosomal deletion regions associated with syndromes that can sometimes include UTMs have been carried out, finding *CRKL* in the 22q11.2 deletion region of DiGeorge Syndrome [56] and *TBX6* in 16p11.2 microdeletion syndrome [98]. However, so far there has just been one large study specifically to look for CNVs as a cause of nonsyndromic VUR [88].

This collaboration of teams from eight countries sought pathogenic CNVs and carried out GWAS in pooled cohorts of VUR patients genotyped with genome-wide SNP arrays. Both types of analysis were association studies, comparing patients with controls. CNVs $\geq$100 Kb were sought in 1737 multiethnic patients, and 24,765 controls, and GWAS in 1395 unrelated patients of European ancestry and 5366 matched controls.

In the CNV analysis, a significant excess of large, rare, gene-intersecting CNVs was found in VUR patients compared with controls, principally due to CNVs over 500 kb in length, and was considered to be the aetiology of the VUR in 2.23% of patients. Then CNVs were checked for known pathogenicity against a list of 148 CNVs already noted to be pathogenic in some condition (not necessarily previously associated with VUR). 18 such CNVs were found in 35 of the 1737 patients (2.02%) and 162 out of the 24,765 controls (0.65%) giving an odds ratio of 3.12, $p = 6.35 \times 10^{-8}$. Patients with these known pathogenic CNVs were found in all of the contributed cohorts, including ones for which chromosomal anomalies had been specifically excluded as entry an entry criterion.

As with the results of the linkage and association studies described in the previous section, there is not time and space to describe all the details here, but the three most prominent of the 18 were 16p11.2 deletion, in which, as noted above *TBX6* had been noted to be the contributor to UTMs (4 patients, as compared with 5 in the

14.26 times as many controls), 22q11.21 duplication, in which *CRKL* had previously been implicated in UTMs (5 against 7 amongst the controls), and trisomy of the X-chromosome (3 *vs.* 1 control). These CNVs, all including many genes, had previously been found in patients with autism, schizophrenia, developmental delay, congenital cardiac defects, and vertebral defects. One of the other known pathogenic CNVs, present in one patient, was a homozygous deletion in 2q13. This region contains *NPHP1*, in which mutations can cause Senior-Loken Syndrome type 1, also known as juvenile nephronophthisis with Leber amaurosis, or Joubert syndrome type 4, characterized by cerebellar ataxia, oculomotor apraxia, psychomotor delay and neonatal breathing abnormalities, but sometimes including retinal dystrophy and renal disease. A homozygous deletion of the first 20 of 23 exons has also been reported in a patient who, in addition to short stature and a ventriculoseptal defect had grade I VUR and bilateral renal hypodysplasia [55]. However, homozygous or compound heterozygous mutations of *NPHP1* have also been found in patients with nonsyndromic nephronophthisis [79]. Another patient had a deletion in 7q36, which was one of the loci of weak genetic linkage (nonparametric score 2.19) in a previous genome scan for nonsyndromic VUR [43] and a deletion in the array-CGH study of syndromic UMT patients [91].

Apart from the 18 CNVs previously known to be pathogenic, CNVs previously unseen but likely to be pathogenic were found in 16 patients (0.92% of the 1737). Among these were heterozygous deletions in chr 2q31.1, which includes *BBS5* and *ITGA6;* 10q24.2, including *HPSE2*; 10q26.11–10q26.3, which includes *FGFR2*; 12p13.33, including *CACNA1C*; 12q21.31–12q21.33, encompassing *NPHP6*; and two female patients with heterozygous deletions of *COL4A5* on chromosome X, insertions and duplications in 6q14.3, including *TBX18*; 16q24.1, encompassing *FOXC2 and FOXF1*; and 17q25.1–17q25.3, including *ITGB4*. These named genes are all ones known to be involved in urinary tract development or in the same gene family as, genes that are so known.

Genome-wide association analyses were carried out separately for dominant, recessive and additive risk (two copies of the variant giving more risk than one), and all of these on the whole cohort and on males and females separately. Three significant associations ($p < 7.58 \times 10^{-9}$) and five suggestive ones ($p < 1.52 \times 10^{-7}$) were found. The most significant SNP was in an intron of *WDPCP* on Chromosome 2p15. 3.3% of the patients were homozygous for the risk allele, compared with 1.2% of controls. Mutations in the coding sequence of this gene cause Bardet-Biedl Syndrome, of which VUR is included in the features, and mutant mice exhibit, amongst many other malformations, failure of septation of the cloaca, failure of the ureters to reach the urogenital sinus, and duplex kidneys [21]. However, which gene is actually affected in the region of the significant SNP association is unknown; it could be one of the other genes nearby, and *OTX1*, which has high expression levels in the urinogenital system, is another candidate.

The other highly significant SNP associations were in the 3′-untranslated region of *BMP5* in females, and in a noncoding RNA, *LOC101928570*, 203 kb upstream of the nearest coding gene, *HTRB1*. The latter codes for Hydroxytryptamine receptor 1b, which binds serotonin, and might be involved in the control of smooth muscle in the ureter, as serotonergic mechanisms have been found to influence the urine flow rate in male rats [29].

One of the five suggestive loci was on 3p14.13 downstream of *WNT5A*, which had already been implicated in kidney and ureteric development in mice and, following up the discovery of this association, in this same CNV and association study [88], *Wnt5a* knockout mice were examined. Fused kidneys and renal hypoplasia or renal agenesis were observed as previously reported, but also persistence of the cloaca, rudimentary bladder and urethra in 13 out of 18 embryos, and absence of the bladder or defective urethral differentiation in the other five. The patients, of course, only had nonsyndromic VUR, so clearly whatever genetic element the association was indicating was, it was one that did not have such a severe effect when mutated.

There is one more study to relate that takes yet another approach to searching for regions of the genome containing genetic variation causing VUR, and does not fit neatly into either this or the previous subsection, though perhaps better into the latter, but is easier to explain here after covering these other topics. It is a search for shared haplotypes between affected members of families within a particular population. The word 'haplotype' was introduced in section "Linkage and Association Studies". It means a recognizable stretch of a part of the genome—recognizable as having a particular combination of variations on it that distinguishes it from other copies of the same DNA sequence, and here it is worth describing what this means.

Think of making 100 copies of a long sentence (say written in small writing on a large piece of paper so that each can occupy a single line and you can line them up one below the other). Then make spelling mistakes in every sentence. Some mistakes you make (in the same letter or letters of the same word) in a lot of the 100 copies, some in smaller numbers of copies, and some in only one copy each, resulting in 100 slightly different copies of the same sentence. That is what haplotypes of the genome are like, with the spelling-mistakes corresponding to all the many different types of genetic variation. We all have haplotypes on our chromosomes that have been handed down to us through countless generations of our families, though cut and modified through time.

In the first division of every meiosis making an egg or a sperm, crossing-over occurs between chromatids of members of each chromosome pair, making a new combination of the genetic variants on the recombined chromatids of each member of the pair (and leaving the other chromatids untouched). The copy of Chromosome 3 that you received from your father may thus have pieces from both of his parents, and from their parents, and from their parents, and so on (but not from all ancestors on his side of the family; chance will determine that you have no part from some particular ancestor several generations back on that chromosome, and that for some ancestors further back, no part on any chromosome). The longest human chromosome, Chromosome 1, is over 248.9 million base-pairs long, and will usually have three or four cross-overs, dividing it into four or five bits, and the shortest, Chromosome 21 (which turned out to be a little smaller than chromosome 22 when it was sequenced), is about 46.7 million bp, and will always have at least one cross-over.

So, after a single meiosis, the chromosome sections are tens of millions of base-pairs long, but at every generation, some of these pieces, haplotypes, are cut in to smaller sections. However, there are many millions of genetic variations all along the chromosomes, and the shorter a haplotype becomes, the less likely it is that a cut will occur within it again, so even after thousands of years, it is still possible to recognize particular haplotypes. This is how we can study the relationships between different races, and study and map migrations and mixtures and replacements of populations over thousands of years. It is how we know that all non-African modern humans have small pieces of Neanderthal and Denisovan chromosomes, and have recently learnt that the more recent Neanderthals had stretches of sequence from modern humans in their genomes [35].

Now we can come to this other VUR study. It was a study of fourteen families in south-western Sweden, each having at least three members with mainly high-grade VUR with renal hypodysplasia to look for shared ancestral haplotypes [4] in case there might be one containing a variant causing VUR. They used an array containing about 262,000 SNP markers. The search revealed that there was no single haplotype shared by all the families that might have suggested a 'founder mutation' from a single ancestor. This is no surprise, since we know that VUR is very common and there are many variants that can cause it. However, there was one haplotype shared by the affected members of thirteen families, and there were 18 haplotypes shared by as many as seven families when only one affected members of each family was investigated. The investigators then started comparing the haplotypes with unaffected controls, one at a time, and found that by the time they had compared with just four control individuals, there was only one haplotype left that was present in as many as seven of the affected families and not in any control, and they reckoned that this was enough controls to exclude haplotypes that were very common in the local population of the region but not too many to exclude less common haplotypes on which a copy might have a VUR-causing variant, though not in the controls.

Varying numbers of shared haplotypes were counted depending upon how many affected families shared the haplotype and how many of the controls did not have that haplotype. The investigators looked at the contents of the 32 haplotypes that they found to be shared between seven or more families when all affected members of all 14 families were included and after excluding only haplotypes that were present in all four of the controls. These haplotypes varied in length between 200,000 kb and 1·93 mb, long enough to contain many SNPs in each, but relatively quite short in terms of the length of the whole genome, and only covering 0.76% of the genome when all 32 were added together. Some of them contained no coding sequences and others contained genes that the investigators could not relate to the developing urinary tract, but in nine of them they found a total of thirteen coding genes (and two non-coding RNAs that are no longer recognized in the latest genome builds) that they could relate in some way to the developing urinary tract, and there were a few more such genes in some of the haplotypes shared between smaller numbers of families. However, they are not listed here because, as will be revealed in section "Mutation-Detection and Sequencing Studies", when sequencing was carried out later [5], genes in which mutations were found were not any of those previously identified.

In this first study, the same SNP results in these families were also used to detect CNVs. Many CNVs were found, but there was only one that was present in all the affected members of any family, and this in just one family. This CNV was a deletion of about 109 kb within the gene *FSTL4*, Folistatin-like 4, which had been detected in mouse embryos to be expressed during renal tubule development, but not in the ureteric bud or metanephric mesenchyme during the earlier stages of development vital to functional ureterovesical junction formation.

Resources for Identifying Genes and Genetic Variants Involved in VUR and Other UTMs

Many animal models of urinary tract malformations have been created, particularly in mice, some of which will be mentioned in the rest of this chapter, but an extremely valuable database has also been created of gene expression studies of every tissue in the urinary tract at every stage of development, mainly but not exclusively in the mouse. This is called GUDMAP, The GenitoUrinary Development Molecular Anatomy Project [34, 59]. This is a huge resource, continually updated, showing every gene expressed in each tissue at each stage of genitourinary development, and including histological images of gene and protein expression by *in situ* hybridisation and immunohistochemistry. Of course, not every gene expressed in any particular structure at any particular time in development is involved in the developmental process itself, but GUDMAP will show where and when your gene of interest is or is not expressed. The database has recently been incorporated into a larger one, ATLAS-D2K (Analysis, Technology, Leadership, Administration, and Science—Data to Knowledge) with data from another consortium, RBK (ReBuilding a Kidney).

Another type of resource needed is one to help pick out the likely pathogenic variants from the vast number of harmless variants to be found in any genome by predicting pathogenicity. There are many of these, and most genetic studies use several of them. They include, amongst others, the following: **SIFT** (Sorting Intolerant From Tolerant), which uses protein sequence homology across species to give a score of the likelihood that a particular amino-acid replacement might be damaging [63]; **PolyPhen-2** (Polymorphism Phenotyping v2) predicts possible impact of an amino acid substitution on the structure and function of a human protein using physical and comparative considerations [1]; **GERP** (Genomic Evolutionary Rate Profiling), which uses genome-wide DNA sequence homology across species [19, 24]. This has the apparent advantage of being able to predict the pathogenicity of variants in noncoding sequences. However, this has limitations because though humans have most of the same genes as other mammals, and many of them require to be regulated in similar ways, we humans have also evolved a lot of differences, and have an estimated 80 Mb of noncoding DNA unlikely to have high GERP scores because of its rate of change [36]; **CADD** (Combined Annotation

Dependent Depletion) scores the deleteriousness of insertion/deletion variants in the human genome as well as single nucleotide variants by integrating multiple annotations into one metric by contrasting variants that survived natural selection with simulated mutations. CADD scores strongly correlate with allelic diversity, pathogenicity of both coding and non-coding variants, and experimentally measured regulatory effects, and also highly rank causal variants within individual genome sequences [44, 69].

In addition to genes encoding proteins and all of the many types of non-coding RNAs, the genome browsers are annotated with sequences matching to binding sites for transcription factors, the SNPs in the SNP database, dbSNP referred to earlier, and many other details. In particular, relevant to the possible effect of a mutation at any particular position is the ENCODE Project. Quoting directly from its website 'The Encyclopedia of DNA Elements (ENCODE) Consortium is an ongoing international collaboration of research groups funded by the National Human Genome Research Institute (NHGRI). The goal of ENCODE is to build a comprehensive parts list of functional elements in the human genome, including elements that act at the protein and RNA levels, and regulatory elements that control cells and circumstances in which a gene is active.' The regulatory elements include enhancers and the project includes a range of different assays to identify parts of the genome likely to be regulatory regions, and these are also marked on the genome in genome browsers.

Finally, there is the empirical method: how common is this variant? If it is very common then it cannot be very dangerous. If it is very rare, or has never been seen before, it may well be harmful. All human ancestry groups have variants that developed in their own populations, often adapting them to their particular environments and ways of life, so a variant common in one population may be rare in another, so it is important for predicting pathogenicity to make sure that a variant under consideration is rare in all populations. What is needed is a database in which one can check any position at all in the best reference human genome sequence (constructed from many genome sequences) available, and find out whether any variant has been found there in any population, and if so, how often. The first database came out of the 1000 Genomes Project, the goal of which was to find common genetic variants with frequencies of at least 1% in the populations studied, and was planned during a meeting at The Welcome Genome Campus, Hinxton, U.K., in September 2007, and has now expanded to the International Genome Sample Resource (IGSR) [7, 28]. However, the largest and most used resource for checking the frequencies of variants at any human genome position started with the ExAC Database, of variants found in exome sequencing, which has since been incorporated into '**gnomAD**', the Genome Aggregation Database, which covers noncoding as well as coding sequence and includes data from over 125,000 exome sequences and many tens of thousands of whole genome sequences [33]. For CNVs there is DGV, the Database of Genomic Variants [57], which catalogues all the structural variations larger than 50 bp in healthy control subjects but does not give frequencies in vast population collections.

These resources have been and continue to be essential for identifying mutations found in the sequencing studies of which some descriptions and their findings are below. However, one that can only come from the investigations themselves when families containing several affected members are recruited, is checking whether any variant presumed to be the causative one is present in all other affected family members.

Mutation-Detection and Sequencing Studies

When the invention of the polymerase chain reaction (PCR) became widely known and started to be used in research laboratories in the second half of the 1980s, DNA sequencing was still laborious and hazardous, and only enabled short stretches of DNA to be read, and even when sequencing could be done by capillary electrophoresis on computer-controlled machines using different coloured fluorescent dyes to detect the four different nucleotides, in the mid 1990s, it was still quite time-consuming and expensive.

As a result, techniques were used to screen DNA samples from different individuals to detect which ones had mutations in the sequence under study, so that only those samples need be sequenced. There were several different methods but the principle was the same. PCR amplification of short stretches (150–400 bp) of the gene under study was carried out on all the samples to be screened. Then the DNA was melted (by heating to 96 °C) and then cooled extremely rapidly (such as by plunging the tubes into iced water) so that in samples in which there was a heterozygous variant, complementary single strands that did not quite match but had started to pair, could not melt apart again to find a perfect match. Then the samples could either be run on a gel by electrophoresis, when double-stranded DNA containing a mismatch would run a different rate to perfectly-matched samples, and/or samples could be melted again by very slow heating, whereupon mismatched samples would melt earlier than perfectly-matched ones, and with a differently shaped melting-curve (high-resolution melting-curve analysis, HRM).

Whether searching candidate genes by mutation-detection first or by directly sequencing all samples, searches were often negative even when the gene was relevant to VUR, because it was not realized how tremendously heterogeneous is the genetic aetiology of VUR, meaning that even in a large cohort of patients or families, only a few, or one, or even none at all in that cohort, will have a causative mutation in any one particular gene. A compounding problem was that in the first decade of this (21st) century many common polymorphisms in the human genome had not been discovered, so variants that were found more often turned out to be common polymorphisms than pathogenic mutations. For instance, a search of the exons and surrounding intronic splicing sequences of all four uroplakin genes in 76 nonsyndromic VUR patients discovered 18 SNPs, seven of which change amino-acids coded, but which also occurred in unaffected controls, and no pathogenic variants were found [40]. Another study failed to find any mutations in the gene for Uroplakin

IIIA, *UPK3A*, in 25 VUR patients [32] and a targeted linkage and association study of the same gene in 126 sibling pairs with VUR found no linkage or association with it [42]. However, very soon afterwards, a report published the finding of pathogenic mutations in *UPK3A* in four out of 17 children with renal failure caused by renal adysplasia, two of whom also had severe VUR [38].

These and many other small studies of candidate genes for VUR and other UTMs led to the strategies of (a) searching very large cohorts of patients by international collaborations, (b) including as many patients with more severe phenotypes as possible, and (c) screening for mutations in several or many candidate genes at the same time. Once gene sequencing technology had advanced to the stage of being able to read vast amounts of DNA sequence with very small samples (carefully purified) at relatively low cost compared with former times, the latter (c) could be achieved by sequencing a 'panel' of genes, selected by evidence from animal studies and/or human syndromes, or by sequencing whole 'exomes' (all the coding exons of all the known genes, WES = whole exome sequencing), or by sequencing whole genomes (WGS = whole genome sequencing).

These strategies have only been practical within not much more than the past decade, and have become easier and cheaper to do as time has gone on, resulting in a flood of results in very recent times. (The lab-work is less, but the effort of co-ordinating the collaborations and collecting the cohorts can be huge.) The problem with all of these strategies is selection. If you use a panel of genes, there will inevitably be some patients in the cohort who have mutations in genes not included in the panel, and if you sequence whole exomes or whole genomes, you find tens of thousands of sequence variants, which you have to sort to try to decide which are relevant, and however hard you try, inevitably you will reject some that actually are the relevant ones, because your knowledge or ability to predict the effect of every possible variant is never complete. Most of these studies have quite modest yields, leaving the majority of patients or families in the cohort with no discovered genetic cause, yet frequently adding several more genes to the list of ones that can be found mutated in UMT cases.

Some of these studies are carried out on patients with a particular type of UTM, while others include all types, and often mix syndromic and nonsyndromic patients in the same cohort, and one has to search through often many tables of results from any one study (often hidden in supplementary material online because the results far exceed the word-limits of the journal) to find cases of nonsyndromic VUR. Much of the information that one needs is inevitably not in the abstracts. It is not possible even to list, let alone to go through the results of all these studies here, but here follow brief descriptions of some of the studies that the author hopes include all of the large ones, giving some details of the yields, and a few of the many smaller ones.

Chatterjee at al [15]. sequenced three genes, *RET*, *GDNF* and *SPRY1* in 122 patients with UMTs and found mutations in six patients, with *RET* or *GDNF* variants. *RET* mutation is recessive and two patients had the same *RET* variant but, though one was homozygous, the other patient only had the variant heterozygously. This patient was then investigated further and found to have a heterozygous mutation in *GFRA1*, of which the protein product is the co-receptor with RET.

Hwang et al. [37] carried out WES of the only 17 genes they knew at the time to cause UTMs in a dominant inheritance pattern when mutated, in a cohort of 749 individuals from 650 families with UTMs. The most common phenotypes in the cohort were VUR in 288 patients, renal hypodysplasia in 120, and unilateral renal agenesis in 90 patients. They identified 37 different heterozygous mutations (33 novel) in 12 of the 17 genes in 47 patients from 41 of the 650 families (just 6·3%). The genes and number of families with mutations in each were: *BMP7* (1), *CDC5L* (1), *CHD1L* (5), *EYA1* (3), *GATA3* (2), *HNF1B* (6), *PAX2* (5), *RET* (3), *ROBO2* (4), *SALL1* (9), *SIX2* (1), and *SIX5* (1). Of the individuals with these mutations, 13 had nonsyndromic VUR with mutations in six of the genes, and can be found in Table 1, chapter "Embryological Development of the Lower Urinary Tract and the Genes Involved". The investigators also judged, from the evidence on variant pathogenicity, that several genetic variants previously reported to be pathogenic were likely to be benign.

In the same year, Kohl et al. [48] knew of 23 genes reported to be mutated and dominant in human UTM families, and in search of more, they reckoned that genes mutated in recessive mouse models with the specific UTM phenotype of unilateral renal agenesis might also be mutated in humans with nonsyndromic UTMs. They used targeted exon sequencing of 12 recessive murine candidate genes in 574 individuals with nonsyndromic UTMs from 590 families, and found recessive mutations in six of the genes in a total of 15 families (2½%). The investigators observed that biallelic (i.e. recessive) mis-sense (i.e. nonsynonymous) mutations in these genes cause nonsyndromic UTMs, whereas recessive truncating mutations cause Fraser syndrome, which involves many organs. The genes were *FRAS1*, *FREM1*, *FREM2*, *GREM1*, *GRIP1* and *ITGA8*, and are all described in section "Genes Involved in the Formation of a Functioning One-Way Urine Flow System".

Nicolaou et al. [64] carried out targeted exon sequencing of 208 of the genes by then known to be involved in urinary tract development in 453 patients with UTMs. Previously reported pathogenic mutations were detected, but only five were considered fully-penetrant causal mutations that improved diagnosis. They also found 148 variants in 82 genes in 151 patients that had high likelihood of being pathogenic (including being predicted pathogenic and absent from or very rare in controls), which they prioritised for follow-up studies, and those in nonsyndromic VUR will be mentioned in chapter "Embryological Development of the Lower Urinary Tract and the Genes Involved", section "Genes Involved in the Formation of a Functioning One-Way Urine Flow System" and/or in Table 1.

Bekheirnia et al. [6] carried out WES on 62 families with UTMs and found a total of six pathogenic variants in the 35 genes that they knew to have been reported to have mutations in UTM patients, 1 in *PAX2*, 2 in *HNF1B* and 3 in *EYA1*. They also found a *de novo* mutation in a new candidate, *FOXP1*, and so searched the ExAC database and found seven more individuals with *de novo* pathogenic single nucleotide variants in this gene, and six of them had syndromic genitourinary tract malformations. They also searched their families for CNVs and found a known pathogenic one (at triplication in 22q11.1–q11.21) and in six other families CNVs which were of uncertain significance at the time, but these included four in CNV regions later recognised to be pathogenic, a duplication and a deletion in 16p11.2, in which a deletion was later also found in the nonsyndromic VUR CNV study mentioned above [88] and a duplication in 16p13.11 where there was also found a duplication and a deletion in that VUR study, and a duplication in 3p29, which is within the deletion of 3pter-p25 found in the VUR study. So, if the *FOXP1* variant and all the CNVs were pathogenic, that is a yield of 14 out of 62 families (22·6%).

Sanna-Cherchi et al. [73] carried out whole exome sequencing on 202 patients with renal hypodysplasia, RHD (some of them with other anomalies) who had already been found not to have pathogenic CNVs in four earlier studies, and found mutations in six genes previously known to be mutated in RHDs (two in *PAX2* and one each in *EYA1*, *GATA3*, *SIX5*, *HNF1B*, and *UMOD*) in a total of just seven patients, of whom two had VUR, one with an *HNF1B* mutation, who had multicystic dysplastic kidneys and epispadias, and the other in the patient with a UMOD mutation, who had renal hypoplasia and hydronephrosis along with the VUR, but also had hyperuricaemia. They also found 28 rare variants in 18 other genes that were candidates for causing RHD when mutated, on evidence from human syndromes or mouse mutants, in another 26 patients. They then carried out an exome-wide association study with 6905 control subjects and identified at least 11 more candidate genes, of which the top one was *GREB1L*. They identified 9 patients with likely causative variants in this gene and then carried out targeted 'next-generation' sequencing on that one gene in a further 410 RHD patients and found mutations in a further 8. None of the 17 patients had VUR, but relatives of two of them did have VUR and may have had the same variants, though they were not tested. They then carried out work on zebrafish which will be mentioned in chapter "Embryological Development of the Lower Urinary Tract and the Genes Involved".

Van der Ven et al. [81] carried out analysis of WES data of members of 232 families with 329 members with UTMs (79 of whom had other phenotypic features beyond the urinary tract) for mutations in the 40 genes known at the time in which mutations caused nonsyndromic UTMs, 179 genes of which mutations were known to cause syndromic UTMs, and 185 other genes mutated in murine UTMs, a total of 404 genes. They found a causative mutation in a known gene for isolated or syndromic UTMs that sufficiently explained the patient's UTM phenotype in 29 families and, in three families, a mutation in a gene in which previous mutations had been reported to cause UMT phenotypes earlier ascribed to other genes (a total of 14%). They also detected deleterious mutations in 15 of the 155 families with nonsyndromic UTMs, in genes in which mutations had previously been reported to cause UTMs as part of syndromes (making 9·7% of the nonsyndromic familes and a further 6·4% of the total number). They also searched for novel monogenic causes of UTMs in consanguineous and multiplex families and found a potential single, novel monogenic UTM gene in 19 of the 232 families (another 8%), making a total yield of 66/232 families (28·4%).

Liu et al. [55] carried out WES of 379 unrelated children with primary VUR of whom 165 (43·5%) showed the coexistence of other UTMs and a total of 64 (16·9%) had extrarenal manifestations. They found a genetic variant in a gene associated with UTMs in just 28 patients (7·4%), and a look at their results shows that in 17 of these patients the variant was of uncertain significance. In another one of the 28, two variants were found in a recessive gene, one of which was predicted pathogenic and the other of uncertain significance, but which it seems likely was sufficient to cause the phenotype in the presence of the other variant.

Following up the finding of a homozygous mis-sense mutation in *ETV4* in a Kuwati patient with grade II VUR [16], a search of exome sequencing data of 731 families revealed just one patient, an American of Nigerian origin, who also had a homozygous variant in *ETV4*, a nonsense variant, making a stop codon at a very early position, the 6th codon [51]. The authors of this report called this a truncating variant but this is surely incorrect. A truncating variant causes the production of a truncated protein as the result of a stop codon, but many mutations that result in stop codons do not lead to the production of protein. This is because of a process called nonsense-mediated decay, by which RNAs that are too short are degraded. It can occur during splicing of the primary transcript to make mRNA or during attempted translation of a very short mRNA. This mutation is so early in the coding sequence that it is inconceivable that any protein would be produced, as the investigators admit. The patient had a posterior urethral valve and renal dysplasia. His parents were not related, which was proven by the finding of very little homozygosity in the patient's genome. The mother was heterozygous for the variant but the father was not tested. The variants of both patients had never been seen before.

Occasionally a surprising yield can result from a small study [5]. This was a sequencing study of 13 of the 14 families previously investigated for shared haplotypes and CNVs [4], and in this second paper, it was stated that these, 13 families that each had at least three members with VUR that was confirmed by MCUG and who were able to give samples for DNA extraction, were selected from 1054 non-syndromic VUR patients from western Sweden seen in a 15-year period. As previously mentioned, these selected families were ones in which most affected members had high-grade VUR and renal hypodysplasia, on the assumption that these families would be more likely to have a recognisable genetic aetiology. Whole exome sequencing of initially one member of each family found a total of 68,770 variants, of which 5718 were rare and predicted deleterious in addition to being reliably real variants in the sequencing data, and of them, 40 were in genes or pathways associated with urinary tract development or found in animal models of UTMs or were expressed in relevant tissues. Of those 40, only three segregated with VUR, each in one family, when the DNA samples of other members were sequenced. None of these three genes had ever been found mutated in VUR before. The genes were *LAMC1*, in which there was a frameshift variant, and *KIF26B* and *LIFR*, in which there were mis-sense variants. The index case of the family with the *KIF26B* mutation had scoliosis, mitral insufficiency and juvenile idiopathic arthritis, and was thought possibly to have Marfan Syndrome, but the other family members with VUR and the same mutation had no syndromic features. In the family with the *LIFR* mutation, one of the affected members, a child of the index case, had a ventriculoseptal defect, but again, none of the other affected family members had this or any other anomaly outside the urinary tract. Though not mentioned in this paper, a check of the family identification numbers shows that this family is the same one in which the CNV deleting part of the gene *FSTL4* was found in the previous study [4]. No members of the family with the *LAMC1* variant had any syndromic features. This gene, which is on 1q25.3, is within a previous wide VUR linkage region, 1q23.3–q32.2 [43] and a wider one found by an earlier study using fewer markers [30]. Also, heterozygous variants in this gene, predicted to be deleterious, had been reported in one case each of ureteropelvic junction obstruction and duplex collecting system [64]. Several other sequencing studies, each identifying one more gene in single families will be mentioned in the next chapter.

Finally, there is a sequencing study to report that investigated one of the sources of gene regulation. Micro RNAs, miRNAs, are small noncoding RNAs that each have a target mRNA to whose 3′-untranslated region they bind, and restrain the production of the protein that the mRNA codes for by affecting its stability and/or down-regulating its translation [75]. The genomic DNA sequences that specify the miRNAs sequences occur in intergenic DNA and within gene introns, singly or in clusters. The initially single-stranded RNA is processed in a series of steps which include folding into a double-stranded hairpin by co-operation of the proteins DROSHA and DGCR8 and held together by complementary base-pairing, and then cut by another called DICER. These proteins process many different miRNAs (and DICER processes other types of RNA too and is a strong anti-viral agent against RNA viruses, including the Zika virus and SARS-CoV-2), so one would expect mutation of the genes of any of these proteins to have dire consequences not restricted to a single organ system; indeed general knock-out causes failure of gastrulation. Mouse experiments have shown that knocking out the genes for any one of them specifically in ureteric bud or other cells of the developing urinary tract leads to UTMs, demonstrating that miRNAs are involved in urinary tract development.

In the light of this knowledge, Kohl et al. [49] carried out 'next-generation' sequencing of 96 stem-loop sequences of 73 miRNA genes (some coding for clusters of several miRNAs) with conserved expression in the urinary tract in 1213 individuals with nonsyndromic UTMs from 980 families. They identified in 31 individuals from 26 families with 17 different single nucleotide variants. Two variants did not segregate with the disease in the families, and so could not be causative, and thirteen variants they presumed to be benign because they occurred in control populations and/or they affected nucleotides of weak evolutionary conservation, but two unrelated individuals had potentially pathogenic variants with unknown biological relevance. These affected miRNAs MIR19B1 and MIR99A. The patient with the former mutation had right renal agenesis, but the one with the mutation in MIR99A had VUR and right renal ptosis.

The authors concluded that mutations affecting mature microRNAs in individuals with UTMs are rare and therefore probably not a common cause of human UTMs, but this conclusion may not be correct. The investigators sequenced the stem-loop sequences of the miRNA genes because they are evolutionarily highly conserved, whereas the recognition sequences are not conserved [68]. But regulatory sequences in DNA are the fastest evolving sequences. They make major differences between species precisely because they regulate developmental genes differently [52], therefore surely the recognition sequences are a highly likely place to find mutations affecting development. Each recognition sequence of an miRNA has to match a specific sequence in the 3′-untranslated region of the mRNA of the target gene or genes, so a mutation in either of these two complementary sequences could cause a failure of normal regulation. So, there may be more work to be done on this subject before we have a certain answer.

Concluding Remarks

This chapter has covered the difficulties and changing methods of searching for the genetic aetiology of nonsyndromic VUR over the past 70 years or so during which the technologies both of studying genes and of computing have repeatedly made enormous advances that probably could not even have been imagined at the beginning, yet we are still a long way from being able to account for the cause of VUR in the majority of cases, let alone all of them. We have discovered that VUR is not a simple Mendelian disorder caused by mutation of a single gene, but instead that different cases can be caused by mutation of any one of many different genes, autosomal and X-linked, dominant and recessive. It is also clear that the coding sequences of genes do not contain as much as half of the answer, and that we may have to understand all the many layers of gene regulation which include non-coding DNA sequences, where presumably many relevant mutations lie, alternative transcription initiation sites and alternative splicing of mRNAs, the many different kinds of non-coding RNAs, DNA and RNA base modifications, histone modifications and modifications of the protein products of some of the genes relevant to VUR, and of course exactly how all of the genes have their effects on controlling the differentiation and co-operation of cells to build the urinary tract, before we have the whole picture of how the normal anatomy is formed and the different ways in which this process can be disturbed. New developments in refined genomic scan techniques could assist in predicting the occurrence of VUR and in understanding its pathogenesis and could lead to improvements in accurate molecular genetic diagnosis and prognosis [99].

The enormous amount of work carried out by developmental biologists on mice to explore the embryological construction of the urinary tract has not been described here, where the concentration has been upon investigation of human patients, but work on mice has frequently been referred to in this chapter and will also be in the next. In chapter "Embryological Development of the Lower Urinary Tract and the Genes Involved", what we have learnt so far of how the genes interact and have their effects will be described.

References

1. Adzhubei IA, Schmidt S, Peshkin L, Ramensky VE, Gerasimova A, Bork P, Kondrashov AS, Sunyaev SR. A method and server for predicting damaging missense mutations. Nat Methods. 2010;7:248–9.
2. Ahram DF, Lim TY, Ke J, Jin G, Verbitsky M, Bodria M, Kil BH, Chatterjee D, Piva SE, Marasa M, Zhang JY, Cocchi E, Caridi G, Gucev Z, Lozanovski VJ, Pisani I, Izzi C, Savoldi G, Gnutti B, Capone VP, Morello W, Guarino S, Esposito P, Lambert S, Radhakrishnan J, Appel GB, Uy NS, Rao MK, Canetta PA, Bomback AS, Nestor JG, Hays T, Cohen DJ, Finale C, Wijk J, La Scola C, Baraldi O, Tondolo F, Di Renzo D, Jamry-Dziurla A, Pezzutto A, Manca V, Mitrotti A, Santoro D, Conti G, Martino M, Giordano M, Gesualdo L, Zibar L, Masnata G, Bonomini M, Alberti D, La Manna G, Caliskan Y, Ranghino A, Marzuillo P, Kiryluk K, Krzemien G, Miklaszewska M, Lin F, Montini G, Scolari F, Fiaccadori E, Arapovic A, Saraga M, McKiernan J, Alam S, Zaniew M, Szczepanska M, Szmigielska A, Sikora P, Drozdz D, Mizerska-Wasiak M, Mane S, Lifton RP, Tasic V, Latos-Bielenska A, Gharavi AG, Ghiggeri GM, Materna-Kiryluk A, Westland R, Sanna-Cherchi S. Rare single nucleotide and copy number variants and the etiology of congenital obstructive uropathy: implications for genetic diagnosis. J Am Soc Nephrol. 2023;34:1105–19.
3. Ashraf S, Hoskins BE, Chaib H, Hoefele J, Pasch A, Saisawat P, Trefz F, Hacker HW, Nuernberg G, Nuernberg P, Otto EA, Hildebrandt F. Mapping of a new locus for congenital anomalies of the kidney and urinary tract on chromosome 8q24. Nephrol Dial Transplant. 2010;25:1496–501.
4. Bartik Z, Sillen U, Ostensson M, Fransson S, Djos A, Sjoberg R, Martinsson T. A genome-wide scan to locate regions associated with familial vesicoureteral reflux. Exp Ther Med. 2022;23:92.
5. Bartik ZI, Sillen U, Djos A, Lindholm A, Fransson S. Whole exome sequencing identifies KIF26B, LIFR and LAMC1 mutations in familial vesicoureteral reflux. PLoS One. 2022;17:e0277524.
6. Bekheirnia MR, Bekheirnia N, Bainbridge MN, Gu S, Coban Akdemir ZH, Gambin T, Janzen NK, Jhangiani SN, Muzny DM, Michael M, Brewer ED, Elenberg E, Kale AS, Riley AA, Swartz SJ, Scott DA, Yang Y, Srivaths PR, Wenderfer SE, Bodurtha J, Applegate CD, Velinov M, Myers A, Borovik L, Craigen WJ, Hanchard NA, Rosenfeld JA, Lewis RA, Gonzales ET, Gibbs RA, Belmont JW, Roth DR, Eng C, Braun MC, Lupski JR, Lamb DJ. Whole-exome sequencing in the molecular diagnosis of individuals with congenital anomalies of the kidney and urinary tract and identification of a new causative gene. Genet Med. 2017;19:412–20.
7. Birney E, Soranzo N. Human genomics: the end of the start for population sequencing. Nature. 2015;526:52–3.
8. Briggs CE, Guo CY, Schoettler C, Rosoklija I, Silva A, Bauer SB, Retik AB, Kunkel L, Nguyen HT. A genome scan in affected sib-pairs with familial vesicoureteral reflux identifies a locus on chromosome 5. Eur J Hum Genet. 2010;18:245–50.
9. Burger RH. A theory on the nature of transmission of congenital vesicoureteral reflux. J Urol. 1972;108:249–54.
10. Cai M, Lin N, Su L, Wu X, Xie X, Li Y, Chen X, Dai Y, Lin Y, Huang H, Xu L. Detection of copy number disorders associated with congenital anomalies of the kidney and urinary tract in fetuses via single nucleotide polymorphism arrays. J Clin Lab Anal. 2020;34:e23025.
11. Cai M, Lin N, Su L, Wu X, Xie X, Li Y, Chen X, Lin Y, Huang H, Xu L. Copy number variations associated with fetal congenital kidney malformations. Mol Cytogenet. 2020;13:11.
12. Caruana G, Wong MN, Walker A, Heloury Y, Webb N, Johnstone L, James PA, Burgess T, Bertram JF. Copy-number variation associated with congenital anomalies of the kidney and urinary tract. Pediatr Nephrol. 2015;30:487–95.
13. Chand DH, Rhoades T, Poe SA, Kraus S, Strife CF. Incidence and severity of vesicoureteral reflux in children related to age, gender, race and diagnosis. J Urol. 2003;170:1548–50.

14. Chapman CJ, Bailey RR, Janus ED, Abbott GD, Lynn KL. Vesicoureteric reflux: segregation analysis. Am J Med Genet. 1985;20:577–84.
15. Chatterjee R, Ramos E, Hoffman M, VanWinkle J, Martin DR, Davis TK, Hoshi M, Hmiel SP, Beck A, Hruska K, Coplen D, Liapis H, Mitra R, Druley T, Austin P, Jain S. Traditional and targeted exome sequencing reveals common, rare and novel functional deleterious variants in RET-signaling complex in a cohort of living US patients with urinary tract malformations. Hum Genet. 2012;131:1725–38.
16. Chen J, Van Der Ven AT, Newman JA, Vivante A, Mann N, Aitkenhead H, Shril S, Ityel H, Schulz J, Schmidt JM, Widmeier E, Gileadi O, Costantini F, Thowfeequ S, Wenger RH, Bauer SB, Lee RS, Lu W, Getwan M, Kaminski MM, Lienkamp SS, Lifton RP, Tasic V, Kehinde EO, FH. ETV4 mutation in a patient with congenital anomalies of the kidney and urinary tract. Int J Pediatr Child Health. 2016;4:61–71.
17. Connolly LP, Treves ST, Connolly SA, Zurakowski D, Share JC, Bar-Sever Z, Mitchell KD, Bauer SB. Vesicoureteral reflux in children: incidence and severity in siblings. J Urol. 1997;157:2287–90.
18. Conte ML, Bertoli-Avella AM, de Graaf BM, Punzo F, Lama G, La Manna A, Grassia C, Rambaldi PF, Oostra BA, Perrotta S. A genome search for primary vesicoureteral reflux shows further evidence for genetic heterogeneity. Pediatr Nephrol. 2008;23:587–95.
19. Cooper GM, Stone EA, Asimenos G, Green ED, Batzoglou S, Sidow A. Distribution and intensity of constraint in mammalian genomic sequence. Genome Res. 2005;15:901–13.
20. Cordell HJ, Darlay R, Charoen P, Stewart A, Gullett AM, Lambert HJ, Malcolm S, Feather SA, Goodship TH, Woolf AS, Kenda RB, Goodship JA. Whole-genome linkage and association scan in primary, nonsyndromic vesicoureteric reflux. J Am Soc Nephrol. 2010;21:113–23.
21. Cui C, Chatterjee B, Lozito TP, Zhang Z, Francis RJ, Yagi H, Swanhart LM, Sanker S, Francis D, Yu Q, San Agustin JT, Puligilla C, Chatterjee T, Tansey T, Liu X, Kelley MW, Spiliotis ET, Kwiatkowski AV, Tuan R, Pazour GJ, Hukriede NA, Lo CW. Wdpcp, a PCP protein required for ciliogenesis, regulates directional cell migration and cell polarity by direct modulation of the actin cytoskeleton. PLoS Biol. 2013;11:e1001720.
22. Darlow JM, Dobson MG, Darlay R, Molony CM, Hunziker M, Green AJ, Cordell HJ, Puri P, Barton DE. A new genome scan for primary nonsyndromic vesicoureteric reflux emphasizes high genetic heterogeneity and shows linkage and association with various genes already implicated in urinary tract development. Mol Genet Genomic Med. 2014;2:7–29.
23. Darlow JM, Darlay R, Dobson MG, Stewart A, Charoen P, Southgate J, Baker SC, Xu Y, Hunziker M, Lambert HJ, Green AJ, Santibanez-Koref M, Sayer JA, Goodship THJ, Puri P, Woolf AS, Kenda RB, Barton DE, Cordell HJ. Genome-wide linkage and association study implicates the 10q26 region as a major genetic contributor to primary nonsyndromic vesicoureteric reflux. Sci Rep. 2017;7:14595.
24. Davydov EV, Goode DL, Sirota M, Cooper GM, Sidow A, Batzoglou S. Identifying a high fraction of the human genome to be under selective constraint using GERP++. PLoS Comput Biol. 2010;6:e1001025.
25. de Vargas A, Evans K, Ransley P, Rosenberg AR, Rothwell D, Sherwood T, Williams DI, Barratt TM, Carter CO. A family study of vesicoureteric reflux. J Med Genet. 1978;15:85–96.
26. Devriendt K, Groenen P, Van Esch H, van Dijck M, Van de Ven W, Fryns JP, Proesmans W. Vesico-ureteral reflux: a genetic condition? Eur J Pediatr. 1998;157:265–71.
27. Edwards D, Normand IC, Prescod N, Smellie JM. Disappearance of vesicoureteric reflux during long-term prophylaxis of urinary tract infection in children. Br Med J. 1977;2:285–8.
28. Fairley S, Lowy-Gallego E, Perry E, Flicek P. The International Genome Sample Resource (IGSR) collection of open human genomic variation resources. Nucleic Acids Res. 2020;48:D941–7.
29. Fan WJ, Chen SC, Hsieh TH, Lai CH, Lin YS, Peng CW, Kou YR. Influence of serotonergic mechanisms on the urine flow rate in male rats. Am J Physiol Regul Integr Comp Physiol. 2014;307:R1239–50.

30. Feather SA, Malcolm S, Woolf AS, Wright V, Blaydon D, Reid CJ, Flinter FA, Proesmans W, Devriendt K, Carter J, Warwicker P, Goodship TH, Goodship JA. Primary, nonsyndromic vesicoureteric reflux and its nephropathy is genetically heterogeneous, with a locus on chromosome 1. Am J Hum Genet. 2000;66:1420–5.
31. Franklin RE, Gosling RG. Evidence for 2-chain helix in crystalline structure of sodium deoxyribonucleate. Nature. 1953;172:156–7.
32. Giltay JC, van de Meerakker J, van Amstel HK, de Jong TP. No pathogenic mutations in the uroplakin III gene of 25 patients with primary vesicoureteral reflux. J Urol. 2004;171:931–2.
33. Gudmundsson S, Singer-Berk M, Watts NA, Phu W, Goodrich JK, Solomonson M, Rehm HL, MacArthur DG, O'Donnell-Luria A. Variant interpretation using population databases: lessons from gnomAD. Hum Mutat. 2022;43:1012–30.
34. Harding SD, Armit C, Armstrong J, Brennan J, Cheng Y, Haggarty B, Houghton D, Lloyd-MacGilp S, Pi X, Roochun Y, Sharghi M, Tindal C, McMahon AP, Gottesman B, Little MH, Georgas K, Aronow BJ, Potter SS, Brunskill EW, Southard-Smith EM, Mendelsohn C, Baldock RA, Davies JA, Davidson D. The GUDMAP database - an online resource for genitourinary research. Development. 2011;138:2845–53.
35. Harris DN, Platt A, Hansen MEB, Fan S, McQuillan MA, Nyambo T, Mpoloka SW, Mokone GG, Belay G, Fokunang C, Njamnshi AK, Tishkoff SA. Diverse African genomes reveal selection on ancient modern human introgressions in Neanderthals. Curr Biol. 2023;33:4905–4916.e5.
36. Huber CD, Kim BY, Lohmueller KE. Population genetic models of GERP scores suggest pervasive turnover of constrained sites across mammalian evolution. PLoS Genet. 2020;16:e1008827.
37. Hwang DY, Dworschak GC, Kohl S, Saisawat P, Vivante A, Hilger AC, Reutter HM, Soliman NA, Bogdanovic R, Kehinde EO, Tasic V, Hildebrandt F. Mutations in 12 known dominant disease-causing genes clarify many congenital anomalies of the kidney and urinary tract. Kidney Int. 2014;85:1429–33.
38. Jenkins D, Bitner-Glindzicz M, Malcolm S, Hu CC, Allison J, Winyard PJ, Gullett AM, Thomas DF, Belk RA, Feather SA, Sun TT, Woolf AS. De novo Uroplakin IIIa heterozygous mutations cause human renal adysplasia leading to severe kidney failure. J Am Soc Nephrol. 2005;16:2141–9.
39. Jenkins D, Bitner-Glindzicz M, Malcolm S, Allison J, de Bruyn R, Flanagan S, Thomas DF, Belk RA, Feather SA, Bingham C, Southgate J, Woolf AS. Mutation analyses of Uroplakin II in children with renal tract malformations. Nephrol Dial Transplant. 2006;21:3415–21.
40. Jiang S, Gitlin J, Deng FM, Liang FX, Lee A, Atala A, Bauer SB, Ehrlich GD, Feather SA, Goldberg JD, Goodship JA, Goodship TH, Hermanns M, Hu FZ, Jones KE, Malcolm S, Mendelsohn C, Preston RA, Retik AB, Schneck FX, Wright V, Ye XY, Woolf AS, Wu XR, Ostrer H, Shapiro E, Yu J, Sun TT. Lack of major involvement of human uroplakin genes in vesicoureteral reflux: implications for disease heterogeneity. Kidney Int. 2004;66:10–9.
41. Kaefer M, Curran M, Treves ST, Bauer S, Hendren WH, Peters CA, Atala A, Diamond D, Retik A. Sibling vesicoureteral reflux in multiple gestation births. Pediatrics. 2000;105:800–4.
42. Kelly H, Ennis S, Yoneda A, Bermingham C, Shields DC, Molony C, Green AJ, Puri P, Barton DE. Uroplakin III is not a major candidate gene for primary vesicoureteral reflux. Eur J Hum Genet. 2005;13:500–2.
43. Kelly H, Molony CM, Darlow JM, Pirker ME, Yoneda A, Green AJ, Puri P, Barton DE. A genome-wide scan for genes involved in primary vesicoureteric reflux. J Med Genet. 2007;44:710–7.
44. Kircher M, Witten DM, Jain P, O'Roak BJ, Cooper GM, Shendure J. A general framework for estimating the relative pathogenicity of human genetic variants. Nat Genet. 2014;46:310–5.
45. Kleinjan DA, van Heyningen V. Long-range control of gene expression: emerging mechanisms and disruption in disease. Am J Hum Genet. 2005;76:8–32.
46. Klink A, Schiebel K, Winkelmann M, Rao E, Horsthemke B, Ludecke HJ, Claussen U, Scherer G, Rappold G. The human protein kinase gene PKX1 on Xp22.3 displays Xp/Yp homology and is a site of chromosomal instability. Hum Mol Genet. 1995;4:869–78.

47. Ko JY, Oh S, Yoo KH. Functional enhancers as master regulators of tissue-specific gene regulation and cancer development. Mol Cells. 2017;40:169–77.
48. Kohl S, Hwang DY, Dworschak GC, Hilger AC, Saisawat P, Vivante A, Stajic N, Bogdanovic R, Reutter HM, Kehinde EO, Tasic V, Hildebrandt F. Mild recessive mutations in six Fraser syndrome-related genes cause isolated congenital anomalies of the kidney and urinary tract. J Am Soc Nephrol. 2014;25:1917–22.
49. Kohl S, Chen J, Vivante A, Hwang DY, Shril S, Dworschak GC, Van Der Ven A, Sanna-Cherchi S, Bauer SB, Lee RS, Soliman NA, Kehinde EO, Reutter HM, Tasic V, Hildebrandt F. Targeted sequencing of 96 renal developmental microRNAs in 1213 individuals from 980 families with congenital anomalies of the kidney and urinary tract. Nephrol Dial Transplant. 2016;31:1280–3.
50. Kolon TF, Ferrer FA, McKenna PH. Clinical and molecular analysis of XX sex reversed patients. J Urol. 1998;160:1169–72. discussion 1178
51. Kolvenbach CM, Zheng B, Merz LM, Mertens ND, Mansour B, Wang C, Seltzsam S, Schneider S, Schierbaum L, Pantel D, Chen J, van der Ven AT, Bello JO, Shril S, Hildebrandt F. A homozygous truncating ETV4 variant in a Nigerian family with congenital anomalies of the kidney and urinary tract. Am J Med Genet A. 2023;191:1355–9.
52. Kuderna LFK, Ulirsch JC, Rashid S, Ameen M, Sundaram L, Hickey G, Cox AJ, Gao H, Kumar A, Aguet F, Christmas MJ, Clawson H, Haeussler M, Janiak MC, Kuhlwilm M, Orkin JD, Bataillon T, Manu S, Valenzuela A, Bergman J, Rouselle M, Silva FE, Agueda L, Blanc J, Gut M, de Vries D, Goodhead I, Harris RA, Raveendran M, Jensen A, Chuma IS, Horvath JE, Hvilsom C, Juan D, Frandsen P, Schraiber JG, de Melo FR, Bertuol F, Byrne H, Sampaio I, Farias I, Valsecchi J, Messias M, da Silva MNF, Trivedi M, Rossi R, Hrbek T, Andriaholinirina N, Rabarivola CJ, Zaramody A, Jolly CJ, Phillips-Conroy J, Wilkerson G, Abee C, Simmons JH, Fernandez-Duque E, Kanthaswamy S, Shiferaw F, Wu D, Zhou L, Shao Y, Zhang G, Keyyu JD, Knauf S, Le MD, Lizano E, Merker S, Navarro A, Nadler T, Khor CC, Lee J, Tan P, Lim WK, Kitchener AC, Zinner D, Gut I, Melin AD, Guschanski K, Schierup MH, Beck RMD, Karakikes I, Wang KC, Umapathy G, Roos C, Boubli JP, Siepel A, Kundaje A, Paten B, Lindblad-Toh K, Rogers J, Marques Bonet T, Farh KK. Identification of constrained sequence elements across 239 primate genomes. Nature. 2023;625:735–42.
53. Li X, Li HP, Amsler K, Hyink D, Wilson PD, Burrow CR. PRKX, a phylogenetically and functionally distinct cAMP-dependent protein kinase, activates renal epithelial cell migration and morphogenesis. Proc Natl Acad Sci USA. 2002;99:9260–5.
54. Li X, Hyink DP, Polgar K, Gusella GL, Wilson PD, Burrow CR. Protein kinase X activates ureteric bud branching morphogenesis in developing mouse metanephric kidney. J Am Soc Nephrol. 2005;16:3543–52.
55. Liu JL, Shen Q, Wu MY, Zhu GH, Li YF, Wang XW, Tang XS, Bi YL, Gong YN, Chen J, Fang XY, Zhai YH, Wu BB, Li GM, Sun YB, Gao XJ, Liu CH, Jiang XY, Hao S, Kang YL, Gong YL, Rong LP, Li D, Wang S, Ma D, Rao J, Xu H. Responsible genes in children with primary vesicoureteral reflux: findings from the Chinese Children Genetic Kidney Disease Database. World J Pediatr. 2021;17:409–18.
56. Lopez-Rivera E, Liu YP, Verbitsky M, Anderson BR, Capone VP, Otto EA, Yan Z, Mitrotti A, Martino J, Steers NJ, Fasel DA, Vukojevic K, Deng R, Racedo SE, Liu Q, Werth M, Westland R, Vivante A, Makar GS, Bodria M, Sampson MG, Gillies CE, Vega-Warner V, Maiorana M, Petrey DS, Honig B, Lozanovski VJ, Salomon R, Heidet L, Carpentier W, Gaillard D, Carrea A, Gesualdo L, Cusi D, Izzi C, Scolari F, van Wijk JA, Arapovic A, Saraga-Babic M, Saraga M, Kunac N, Samii A, McDonald-McGinn DM, Crowley TB, Zackai EH, Drozdz D, Miklaszewska M, Tkaczyk M, Sikora P, Szczepanska M, Mizerska-Wasiak M, Krzemien G, Szmigielska A, Zaniew M, Darlow JM, Puri P, Barton D, Casolari E, Furth SL, Warady BA, Gucev Z, Hakonarson H, Flogelova H, Tasic V, Latos-Bielenska A, Materna-Kiryluk A, Allegri L, Wong CS, Drummond IA, D'Agati V, Imamoto A, Barasch JM, Hildebrandt F, Kiryluk K, Lifton RP, Morrow BE, Jeanpierre C, Papaioannou VE, Ghiggeri GM, Gharavi AG, Katsanis

N, Sanna-Cherchi S. Genetic drivers of kidney defects in the DiGeorge syndrome. N Engl J Med. 2017;376:742–54.

57. MacDonald JR, Ziman R, Yuen RK, Feuk L, Scherer SW. The Database of Genomic Variants: a curated collection of structural variation in the human genome. Nucleic Acids Res. 2014;42:D986–92.
58. Marchini GS, Onal B, Guo CY, Rowe CK, Kunkel L, Bauer SB, Retik AB, Nguyen HT. Genome gender diversity in affected sib-pairs with familial vesico-ureteric reflux identified by single nucleotide polymorphism linkage analysis. BJU Int. 2012;109:1709–14.
59. McMahon AP, Aronow BJ, Davidson DR, Davies JA, Gaido KW, Grimmond S, Lessard JL, Little MH, Potter SS, Wilder EL, Zhang P. GUDMAP: the genitourinary developmental molecular anatomy project. J Am Soc Nephrol. 2008;19:667–71.
60. Menezes M, Puri P. Familial vesicoureteral reflux--is screening beneficial? J Urol. 2009;182:1673–7.
61. Middleton GW, Howards SS, Gillenwater JY. Sex-linked familial reflux. J Urol. 1975;114:36–9.
62. Naseri M, Ghiggeri GM, Caridi G, Abbaszadegan MR. Five cases of severe vesico-ureteric reflux in a family with an X-linked compatible trait. Pediatr Nephrol. 2010;25:349–52.
63. Ng PC, Henikoff S. SIFT: predicting amino acid changes that affect protein function. Nucleic Acids Res. 2003;31:3812–4.
64. Nicolaou N, Pulit SL, Nijman IJ, Monroe GR, Feitz WF, Schreuder MF, van Eerde AM, de Jong TP, Giltay JC, van der Zwaag B, Havenith MR, Zwakenberg S, van der Zanden LF, Poelmans G, Cornelissen EA, Lilien MR, Franke B, Roeleveld N, van Rooij IA, Cuppen E, Bongers EM, Giles RH, Knoers NV, Renkema KY. Prioritization and burden analysis of rare variants in 208 candidate genes suggest they do not play a major role in CAKUT. Kidney Int. 2016;89:476–86.
65. Nishimoto K, Iijima K, Shirakawa T, Kitagawa K, Satomura K, Nakamura H, Yoshikawa N. PAX2 gene mutation in a family with isolated renal hypoplasia. J Am Soc Nephrol. 2001;12:1769–72.
66. Ogata T, Muroya K, Sasagawa I, Kosho T, Wakui K, Sakazume S, Ito K, Matsuo N, Ohashi H, Nagai T. Genetic evidence for a novel gene(s) involved in urogenital development on 10q26. Kidney Int. 2000;58:2281–90.
67. Pasch A, Hoefele J, Grimminger H, Hacker HW, Hildebrandt F. Multiple urinary tract malformations with likely recessive inheritance in a large Somalian kindred. Nephrol Dial Transplant. 2004;19:3172–5.
68. Praher D, Zimmermann B, Dnyansagar R, Miller DJ, Moya A, Modepalli V, Fridrich A, Sher D, Friis-Moller L, Sundberg P, Foret S, Ashby R, Moran Y, Technau U. Conservation and turnover of miRNAs and their highly complementary targets in early branching animals. Proc Biol Sci. 2021;288:20203169.
69. Rentzsch P, Witten D, Cooper GM, Shendure J, Kircher M. CADD: predicting the deleteriousness of variants throughout the human genome. Nucleic Acids Res. 2019;47:D886–94.
70. Rosser ZH, Balaresque P, Jobling MA. Gene conversion between the X chromosome and the male-specific region of the Y chromosome at a translocation hotspot. Am J Hum Genet. 2009;85:130–4.
71. Sanna-Cherchi S, Reese A, Hensle T, Caridi G, Izzi C, Kim YY, Konka A, Murer L, Scolari F, Ravazzolo R, Ghiggeri GM, Gharavi AG. Familial vesicoureteral reflux: testing replication of linkage in seven new multigenerational kindreds. J Am Soc Nephrol. 2005;16:1781–7.
72. Sanna-Cherchi S, Kiryluk K, Burgess KE, Bodria M, Sampson MG, Hadley D, Nees SN, Verbitsky M, Perry BJ, Sterken R, Lozanovski VJ, Materna-Kiryluk A, Barlassina C, Kini A, Corbani V, Carrea A, Somenzi D, Murtas C, Ristoska-Bojkovska N, Izzi C, Bianco B, Zaniew M, Flogelova H, Weng PL, Kacak N, Giberti S, Gigante M, Arapovic A, Drnasin K, Caridi G, Curioni S, Allegri F, Ammenti A, Ferretti S, Goj V, Bernardo L, Jobanputra V, Chung WK, Lifton RP, Sanders S, State M, Clark LN, Saraga M, Padmanabhan S, Dominiczak AF, Foroud T, Gesualdo L, Gucev Z, Allegri L, Latos-Bielenska A, Cusi D, Scolari F, Tasic V, Hakonarson

H, Ghiggeri GM, Gharavi AG. Copy-number disorders are a common cause of congenital kidney malformations. Am J Hum Genet. 2012;91:987–97.

73. Sanna-Cherchi S, Khan K, Westland R, Krithivasan P, Fievet L, Rasouly HM, Ionita-Laza I, Capone VP, Fasel DA, Kiryluk K, Kamalakaran S, Bodria M, Otto EA, Sampson MG, Gillies CE, Vega-Warner V, Vukojevic K, Pediaditakis I, Makar GS, Mitrotti A, Verbitsky M, Martino J, Liu Q, Na YJ, Goj V, Ardissino G, Gigante M, Gesualdo L, Janezcko M, Zaniew M, Mendelsohn CL, Shril S, Hildebrandt F, van Wijk JAE, Arapovic A, Saraga M, Allegri L, Izzi C, Scolari F, Tasic V, Ghiggeri GM, Latos-Bielenska A, Materna-Kiryluk A, Mane S, Goldstein DB, Lifton RP, Katsanis N, Davis EE, Gharavi AG. Exome-wide Association Study identifies GREB1L mutations in congenital kidney malformations. Am J Hum Genet. 2017;101:789–802.
74. Schiebel K, Winkelmann M, Mertz A, Xu X, Page DC, Weil D, Petit C, Rappold GA. Abnormal XY interchange between a novel isolated protein kinase gene, PRKY, and its homologue, PRKX, accounts for one third of all (Y+)XX males and (Y-)XY females. Hum Mol Genet. 1997;6:1985–9.
75. Shukla GC, Singh J, Barik S. MicroRNAs: processing, maturation, target recognition and regulatory functions. Mol Cell Pharmacol. 2011;3:83–92.
76. Siomou E, Mitsioni AG, Giapros V, Bouba I, Noutsopoulos D, Georgiou I. Copy-number variation analysis in familial nonsyndromic congenital anomalies of the kidney and urinary tract: evidence for the causative role of a transposable element-associated genomic rearrangement. Mol Med Rep. 2017;15:3631–6.
77. Southern EM. Detection of specific sequences among DNA fragments separated by gel electrophoresis. J Mol Biol. 1975;98:503–17.
78. Stephens FD, Joske RA, Simmons RT. Megaureter with vesico-ureteric reflux in twins. Aust N Z J Surg. 1955;24:192–4.
79. Stokman MF, van der Zwaag B, van de Kar N, van Haelst MM, van Eerde AM, van der Heijden JW, Kroes HY, Ippel E, Schulp AJA, van Gassen KL, van Rooij I, Giles RH, Beales PL, Roepman R, Arts HH, Bongers E, Renkema KY, Knoers N, van Reeuwijk J, Lilien MR. Clinical and genetic analyses of a Dutch cohort of 40 patients with a nephronophthisis-related ciliopathy. Pediatr Nephrol. 2018;33:1701–12.
80. Tjio J-H, Levan A. The chromosome number in man. Hereditas. 1956;42:1–6.
81. van der Ven AT, Connaughton DM, Ityel H, Mann N, Nakayama M, Chen J, Vivante A, Hwang DY, Schulz J, Braun DA, Schmidt JM, Schapiro D, Schneider R, Warejko JK, Daga A, Majmundar AJ, Tan W, Jobst-Schwan T, Hermle T, Widmeier E, Ashraf S, Amar A, Hoogstraaten CA, Hugo H, Kitzler TM, Kause F, Kolvenbach CM, Dai R, Spaneas L, Amann K, Stein DR, Baum MA, Somers MJG, Rodig NM, Ferguson MA, Traum AZ, Daouk GH, Bogdanovic R, Stajic N, Soliman NA, Kari JA, El Desoky S, Fathy HM, Milosevic D, Al-Saffar M, Awad HS, Eid LA, Selvin A, Senguttuvan P, Sanna-Cherchi S, Rehm HL, MacArthur DG, Lek M, Laricchia KM, Wilson MW, Mane SM, Lifton RP, Lee RS, Bauer SB, Lu W, Reutter HM, Tasic V, Shril S, Hildebrandt F. Whole-exome sequencing identifies causative mutations in families with congenital anomalies of the kidney and urinary tract. J Am Soc Nephrol. 2018;29:2348–61.
82. van Eerde AM, Koeleman BP, van de Kamp JM, de Jong TP, Wijmenga C, Giltay JC. Linkage study of 14 candidate genes and loci in four large Dutch families with vesico-ureteral reflux. Pediatr Nephrol. 2007;22:1129–33.
83. Vats AN, Ishwad C, Vats KR, Moritz M, Ellis D, Mueller C, Surti U, Parizhskaya MZ, Meza MP, Burke L, Schneck FX, Saxena M, Ferrell R. Steroid-resistant nephrotic syndrome and congenital anomalies of kidneys: evidence of locus on chromosome 13q. Kidney Int. 2003;64:17–24.
84. Vats KR, Ishwad C, Singla I, Vats A, Ferrell R, Ellis D, Moritz M, Surti U, Jayakar P, Frederick DR, Vats AN. A locus for renal malformations including vesico-ureteric reflux on chromosome 13q33-34. J Am Soc Nephrol. 2006;17:1158–67.

85. Vera-Carbonell A, Lopez-Gonzalez V, Bafalliu JA, Ballesta-Martinez MJ, Fernandez A, Guillen-Navarro E, Lopez-Exposito I. Clinical comparison of 10q26 overlapping deletions: delineating the critical region for urogenital anomalies. Am J Med Genet A. 2015;167A:786–90.
86. Verbitsky M, Westland R, Perez A, Kiryluk K, Liu Q, Krithivasan P, Mitrotti A, Fasel DA, Batourina E, Sampson MG, Bodria M, Werth M, Kao C, Martino J, Capone VP, Vivante A, Shril S, Kil BH, Marasa M, Zhang JY, Na YJ, Lim TY, Ahram D, Weng PL, Heinzen EL, Carrea A, Piaggio G, Gesualdo L, Manca V, Masnata G, Gigante M, Cusi D, Izzi C, Scolari F, van Wijk JAE, Saraga M, Santoro D, Conti G, Zamboli P, White H, Drozdz D, Zachwieja K, Miklaszewska M, Tkaczyk M, Tomczyk D, Krakowska A, Sikora P, Jarmolinski T, Borszewska-Kornacka MK, Pawluch R, Szczepanska M, Adamczyk P, Mizerska-Wasiak M, Krzemien G, Szmigielska A, Zaniew M, Dobson MG, Darlow JM, Puri P, Barton DE, Furth SL, Warady BA, Gucev Z, Lozanovski VJ, Tasic V, Pisani I, Allegri L, Rodas LM, Campistol JM, Jeanpierre C, Alam S, Casale P, Wong CS, Lin F, Miranda DM, Oliveira EA, Simoes ESAC, Barasch JM, Levy B, Wu N, Hildebrandt F, Ghiggeri GM, Latos-Bielenska A, Materna-Kiryluk A, Zhang F, Hakonarson H, Papaioannou VE, Mendelsohn CL, Gharavi AG, Sanna-Cherchi S. The copy number variation landscape of congenital anomalies of the kidney and urinary tract. Nat Genet. 2019;51:117–27.
87. Verbitsky M, Westland R, Perez A, Kiryluk K, Liu Q, Krithivasan P, Mitrotti A, Fasel DA, Batourina E, Sampson MG, Bodria M, Werth M, Kao C, Martino J, Capone VP, Vivante A, Shril S, Kil BH, Marasa M, Zhang JY, Na YJ, Lim TY, Ahram D, Weng PL, Heinzen EL, Carrea A, Piaggio G, Gesualdo L, Manca V, Masnata G, Gigante M, Cusi D, Izzi C, Scolari F, van Wijk JAE, Saraga M, Santoro D, Conti G, Zamboli P, White H, Drozdz D, Zachwieja K, Miklaszewska M, Tkaczyk M, Tomczyk D, Krakowska A, Sikora P, Jarmolinski T, Borszewska-Kornacka MK, Pawluch R, Szczepanska M, Adamczyk P, Mizerska-Wasiak M, Krzemien G, Szmigielska A, Zaniew M, Dobson MG, Darlow JM, Puri P, Barton DE, Furth SL, Warady BA, Gucev Z, Lozanovski VJ, Tasic V, Pisani I, Allegri L, Rodas LM, Campistol JM, Jeanpierre C, Alam S, Casale P, Wong CS, Lin F, Miranda DM, Oliveira EA, Simoes ESAC, Barasch JM, Levy B, Wu N, Hildebrandt F, Ghiggeri GM, Latos-Bielenska A, Materna-Kiryluk A, Zhang F, Hakonarson H, Papaioannou VE, Mendelsohn CL, Gharavi AG, Sanna-Cherchi S. Author correction: the copy number variation landscape of congenital anomalies of the kidney and urinary tract. Nat Genet. 2019;51:764.
88. Verbitsky M, Krithivasan P, Batourina E, Khan A, Graham SE, Marasa M, Kim H, Lim TY, Weng PL, Sanchez-Rodriguez E, Mitrotti A, Ahram DF, Zanoni F, Fasel DA, Westland R, Sampson MG, Zhang JY, Bodria M, Kil BH, Shril S, Gesualdo L, Torri F, Scolari F, Izzi C, van Wijk JAE, Saraga M, Santoro D, Conti G, Barton DE, Dobson MG, Puri P, Furth SL, Warady BA, Pisani I, Fiaccadori E, Allegri L, Degl'Innocenti ML, Piaggio G, Alam S, Gigante M, Zaza G, Esposito P, Lin F, Simoes ESAC, Brodkiewicz A, Drozdz D, Zachwieja K, Miklaszewska M, Szczepanska M, Adamczyk P, Tkaczyk M, Tomczyk D, Sikora P, Mizerska-Wasiak M, Krzemien G, Szmigielska A, Zaniew M, Lozanovski VJ, Gucev Z, Ionita-Laza I, Stanaway IB, Crosslin DR, Wong CS, Hildebrandt F, Barasch J, Kenny EE, Loos RJF, Levy B, Ghiggeri GM, Hakonarson H, Latos-Bielenska A, Materna-Kiryluk A, Darlow JM, Tasic V, Willer C, Kiryluk K, Sanna-Cherchi S, Mendelsohn CL, Gharavi AG. Copy number variant analysis and Genome-wide Association Study identify loci with large effect for vesicoureteral reflux. J Am Soc Nephrol. 2021;32:805–20.
89. Watson JD, Crick FH. Molecular structure of nucleic acids; a structure for deoxyribose nucleic acid. Nature. 1953;171:737–8.
90. Weber S, Moriniere V, Knuppel T, Charbit M, Dusek J, Ghiggeri GM, Jankauskiene A, Mir S, Montini G, Peco-Antic A, Wuhl E, Zurowska AM, Mehls O, Antignac C, Schaefer F, Salomon R. Prevalence of mutations in renal developmental genes in children with renal hypodysplasia: results of the ESCAPE study. J Am Soc Nephrol. 2006;17:2864–70.
91. Weber S, Landwehr C, Renkert M, Hoischen A, Wuhl E, Denecke J, Radlwimmer B, Haffner D, Schaefer F, Weber RG. Mapping candidate regions and genes for congenital anomalies of

the kidneys and urinary tract (CAKUT) by array-based comparative genomic hybridization. Nephrol Dial Transplant. 2011;26:136–43.
92. Weng PL, Sanna-Cherchi S, Hensle T, Shapiro E, Werzberger A, Caridi G, Izzi C, Konka A, Reese AC, Cheng R, Werzberger S, Schlussel RN, Burk RD, Lee JH, Ravazzolo R, Scolari F, Ghiggeri GM, Glassberg K, Gharavi AG. A recessive gene for primary vesicoureteral reflux maps to chromosome 12p11-q13. J Am Soc Nephrol. 2009;20:1633–40.
93. Westland R, Verbitsky M, Vukojevic K, Perry BJ, Fasel DA, Zwijnenburg PJ, Bokenkamp A, Gille JJ, Saraga-Babic M, Ghiggeri GM, D'Agati VD, Schreuder MF, Gharavi AG, van Wijk JA, Sanna-Cherchi S. Copy number variation analysis identifies novel CAKUT candidate genes in children with a solitary functioning kidney. Kidney Int. 2015;88:1402–10.
94. Wilkins MH, Stokes AR, Wilson HR. Molecular structure of deoxypentose nucleic acids. Nature. 1953;171:738–40.
95. Woolf AS. The term CAKUT has outlived its usefulness: the case for the prosecution. Pediatr Nephrol. 2022;37:2785–91.
96. Wu CW, Lim TY, Wang C, Seltzsam S, Zheng B, Schierbaum L, Schneider S, Mann N, Connaughton DM, Nakayama M, van der Ven AT, Dai R, Kolvenbach CM, Kause F, Ottlewski I, Stajic N, Soliman NA, Kari JA, El Desoky S, Fathy HM, Milosevic D, Turudic D, Al Saffar M, Awad HS, Eid LA, Ramanathan A, Senguttuvan P, Mane SM, Lee RS, Bauer SB, Lu W, Hilger AC, Tasic V, Shril S, Sanna-Cherchi S, Hildebrandt F. Copy number variation analysis facilitates identification of genetic causation in patients with congenital anomalies of the kidney and urinary tract. Eur Urol Open Sci. 2022;44:106–12.
97. Xi Q, Zhu X, Wang Y, Ru T, Dai C, Wang Z, Li J, Hu Y. Copy number variations in multicystic dysplastic kidney: update for prenatal diagnosis and genetic counseling. Prenat Diagn. 2016;36:463–8.
98. Yang N, Wu N, Dong S, Zhang L, Zhao Y, Chen W, Du R, Song C, Ren X, Liu J, Pehlivan D, Liu Z, Rao J, Wang C, Zhao S, Breman AM, Xue H, Sun H, Shen J, Zhang S, Posey JE, Xu H, Jin L, Zhang J, Liu P, Sanna-Cherchi S, Qiu G, Wu Z, Lupski JR, Zhang F. Human and mouse studies establish TBX6 in Mendelian CAKUT and as a potential driver of kidney defects associated with the 16p11.2 microdeletion syndrome. Kidney Int. 2020;98:1020–30.
99. Puri P, Friedmacher F, Farrugia MK, Sharma S, Esposito C, Mattoo TK. Primary vesicoureteral reflux. Nat Rev Dis Primers 2024;10:75

Embryological Development of the Lower Urinary Tract and the Genes Involved

John M. Darlow

Abstract This chapter begins with a description of the embryological development of the lower urinary tract, because it is during this development that the genes have their effect, and it is only by understanding this that we can appreciate how they do so. This is followed by description of genes and their protein products identified to be involved in various processes in the development, and how they interact. This involves cell signalling and gene regulation, and the effects on development if the genes are mutated. Different types of mutations are explained and the differences between mutations found so far in non-syndomic compared with syndromic VUR are described.

Keywords VUR genetics · Lower urinary tract embryology · Gene function · Gene interactions · Cell signalling · Transcription factors · Types of mutation

Introduction

In order to understand how the disturbance of function of any gene can result in vesicoureteric reflux, it is necessary to understand the function of the gene in normal development. In this chapter, a description is first given of the embryological development of the urinary tract and interconnected parts of the genital tracts. Then, what is known about the genes and their protein products so far identified as being involved in the relevant embryological processes and how they have their effects will be described, along with the evidence from animal work and the mutations discovered in patients.

J. M. Darlow (✉)
Formerly of Department of Genetics, Children's Health Ireland, Dublin, Ireland
e-mail: john.darlow@ucd.ie

P. Puri, A. Yamataka (eds.), *Vesicoureteral Reflux*,
https://doi.org/10.1007/978-3-031-95091-9_5

Embryological Development of the Lower Urinary Tract

The anatomical and functional basis of VUR has already been described (Chapter "Anatomical and Functional Basis of Primary Vesicoureteral Reflux"). To understand the genetics, we need to understand the normal developmental processes that construct the bladder, the ureter and the ureterovesical junction, and the consequences of mutations affecting the many different genes involved in producing the valvular and sphincteric closure mechanism.

All metazoa more than a few cells thick require an excretory system, and this has evolved increasing complexity and functional ability throughout evolution. Its stages are known as the protonephridium and nephridium, the pronephros, mesonephros and metanephros, which all have characteristic micro-anatomical features that distinguish between them. It is worth mentioning this because the genes involved are the same throughout, but more have been added through the course of evolution. One of the major innovations that enabled the transition from amphibians, which have to remain moist, and reptiles, which can walk far away from water and inhabit dry places, was the loop of Henle, present in the nephrons of the metanephros but not those of the mesonephros possessed by adult teleost fish and amphibia. It conferred much increased ability to concentrate urine and retain water.

Very early embryos of many species are extremely similar, and differences appear as development proceeds, so early embryos tend to display, transitorily and often incompletely, features of earlier stages of evolution. *Amphioxus*, the living representative of our chordate ancestor, has protonephridia in its gills, and a larger version, the nephridium (of Hatchek), in the pharynx, and it is commonly claimed that the embryos of mammals first develop (bilaterally) a pronephros, followed by a mesonephos and finally a metanephros, in rostral to caudal and in temporal order. A detailed histological examination of human embryos has now concluded that no structure classifiable as a pronephros ever develops [44]. However, the work finds that, at its fullest extent, at 42–44 days, the cranial limit of the mesonephros is at the level of the fifth cervical vertebra.

The mesonephroi lie beside and lateral to the indeterminate gonads on either side of the vertebral column dorsally and aorta ventrally, and the mesonephric (Wolffian) ducts open into a part of the cloaca, which becomes the urogenital sinus, and later the bladder and urethra. During human embryonic days 31–35 [44] a bulge, which becomes a protrusion, the ureteric bud, emerges from the mesonephric duct caudally to the mesonephros. The ureteric bud secretes signalling molecules that stimulate the adjacent cells, known as the metanephric mesenchyme, to start organizing to form a kidney, and the metanephric mesenchyme in turn secretes signals that stimulate the ureteric bud to branch and to extend. (References to the details will be given in section "Genes Involved in the Formation of a Functioning One-Way Urine Flow System"). The ureteric bud tissue forms the ureter, renal pelvis, and collecting ducts, and the metanephric mesenchyme forms the nephroi proper—the glomeruli, the convoluted tubules and the loop of Henle. It is commonly stated that the extension of the ureteric bud to form the ureter, causes the kidney to migrate cranially in the embryo, but it has been shown that the kidney actually develops in roughly its adult position relative to the vertebrae, and the impression of migration is given by the relative rates of growth of other structures [43, 44], so it might be better to say that the body extends caudally, and the ureter with it.

Post mortem examination of infants with duplex kidneys [113], observing the relationship of the position of the ureteric orifice to the condition of the kidney, led the investigators to propose the now well-known Ureteric Bud 'Theory' (hypothesis), which proposes that the precise position of emergence of the ureteric bud from the mesonephric duct is of supreme importance to the development of the whole metanephric urinary tract. It was suggested that if the ureteric bud arose more cranially to its optimum position, the ureter would connect into the urethra, and if it emerged more caudally than the optimum position, then it would be inserted into the bladder laterally to the trigone, and that in either case, the kidney would be dysplastic because the cells towards which the emerging bud grew, were less capable of forming normal kidney tissue. Years later, after many advances in developmental genetics, this story was modified in the light of discoveries that the same genes that are involved in regulating the precise position of emergence of the ureteric bud are also involved in later stages of development, leading to the new understanding that mutations that cause the bud to emerge atopically and the ureter to be inserted anomalously, also cause the kidney to develop dysplasticly [18, 73]. However, it is certainly true that if two ureteric buds emerge, duplex kidneys will inevitably form.

By the fourth week of development, a cloaca, an endodermal structure, has formed, into which the alimentary canal and mesonephric ducts run. Soon afterwards, septation occurs, dividing the cloaca into dorsal rectum and ventral urogenital sinus [61]. Subsequently, the urogenital sinus divides. The most anterior part, the anterior ureterovesical canal, becomes the bladder, which initially drains through an outflow tract, the urachus, to the allantois, running through the umbilical cord. The posterior ureterovesical canal becomes the entire urethra in the female, and the pelvic portion of the urethra in the male, further divided into pre-prostatic, prostatic and post-prostatic parts, and the most posterior part of the urogenital sinus becomes penile urethra in the male and the lower portion of the vagina and the vulva in the female. (The allantois regresses, and the bladder separates from the umbilicus at about 15 weeks, the remains of the urachus becoming the umbilical ligament.)

The part of the mesonephric duct between the point of ureteric budding and the urogenital sinus, is called the common nephric duct. After the formation of the ureteric bud, and its elongation to form the ureter, the mesonephric duct, the ureter and the common nephric duct form a Y shape, but the common nephric duct broadens and shortens, becoming a connection between the distal ends of the metanephric duct and the ureter, and spreads out over the surface of the urogenital sinus, and merges into it, its cells disappearing by apoptosis, leaving the two ducts entering the sinus at separate positions. This process is brought about by vitamin A-induced signalling from the urogenital sinus [18, 19]. Rapid growth of the bladder then considerably widens the distance between them, and the distal end of the ureter, which is initially blind, forms an opening into the bladder, also by apoptosis [117]. In normal development, the final positions of the ureteric orifices, along with the urethral orifice, form the trigone of the bladder. In the female, the mesonephric duct degenerates along with the mesonephros, by apoptosis, but in the male, though the mesonephros also disappears likewise, the mesonephric duct, which from the start lay parallel with the then indeterminate gonad, becomes the epididymis, vas deferens and seminal vesicles, and is connected with the urethra via the prostate gland.

In the meantime, the structure of the ureter develops from a simple beginning of inner epithelial and outer mesenchymal cell layers. The epithelium starts as simple cuboidal cells and develops into a multilayered mucosa known as the urothelium, covered by a lamina propria. The bladder and urethra also have urothelium but in them it develops from endoderm, whereas the urothelium of the ureter, renal pelvis and collecting ducts is derived from intermediate mesoderm. The urothelium has a basal layer of regenerative cells, several layers of intermediate cells and a luminal surface layer of fully differentiated specialized cells known as umbrella cells or facet cells. The umbrella cells present a surface layer of hexagonal 'plaques', composed of proteins called uroplakins, which protect the urothelium from the caustic effects of urine while allowing flexibility and dilatation [78, 188]. The urothelium is covered by mesenchymal cells which differentiate into stromal cells, smooth muscle with inner circular and outer longitudinal layers, and adventitial cells, which form the outer fibrous serosa [11]. In the lower third of the ureter, there is a third muscle layer, another longitudinal layer, on the luminal side of the circular layer.

Differentiation of the muscle layers proceeds from the ureterovesical junction towards the pelviureteric junction. Then pacemaker cells, that form between the calyces and the pelviureteric junction, initiate waves of peristalsis from kidney to bladder [103]. These cells are similar, if not identical, to the interstitial cells of Cajal, seen in the gut [12]. The musculature of the ureter does not end at the vesicoureteric junction but is continuous with the trigone, as is an adventitial fibromuscular sheath, Waldeyer's sheath, which covers the distal ureter, but traces of which are also seen further up the ureter [151, 170].

The kidneys are thought to start producing urine between the end of the second month and 11 weeks [3, 66]. At this time, the developing bladder is still connected with the allantois. Smooth muscle starts to appear in the wall at about the 12th week, but the urothelium does not appear to be fully developed till 21 weeks, by which time the muscle coat is also fully developed [131]. During this development, the collagen content decreases and the elastin content increases [90]. The passive valve mechanism of the ureterovesical junction results from the long intramural course of the distal ureter through the bladder wall that results as the ureteric orifice is displaced laterally during normal development, and a low ratio of diameter to length, but of course this is not the whole story. There is also an active closure mechanism effected by the muscle layers surrounding the junction and their innervation.

We are not aware of our ureterovesical junctions, and cannot close them by conscious control, but their closure and relaxation are tied by a reflex to the operation of a urethral sphincter, over which we do have conscious control. In females, having no prostate gland, there is a single urethral sphincter 'complex', composed of both smooth muscle (lithosphincter) and striated muscle (rhabdosphincter) components. Examination of female fetuses showed that it first appears on the anterior wall of the urogenital sinus at 9 weeks gestation before the formation of the urethra. By 15 weeks, the lithosphincter and rhabdosphincter could be clearly distinguished, and by 20 weeks the lower third had formed a cross-section like a capital omega, closed by a narrow posterior connective tissue raphe, attached to the ventral wall of the vagina, which by that time has formed [159]. In the upper third there is only smooth muscle, in the middle third, circular layers of inner smooth and outer striated muscle, and in the lower third the lithosphincter remains circular but the rhabdosphincter forms the omega shape described above [87]. In males, there are two sphincters, the internal sphincter, which lies at the bladder outflow proximal to the prostate gland and is composed of smooth muscle confluent with the bladder muscle, and the external sphincter, immediately distal to the prostate gland, which is composed of an inner layer of smooth muscle under autonomic control, and an outer layer of striated muscle, under conscious control [86].

The muscle layers that surround the outlet of the ureter act as a sphincter, which contracts during bladder contraction during micturition, and relaxes when the (external) urethral sphincter closes, the 'sphinctero-ureterovesical reflex' [161]. The importance of the augmentation of the passive flap-valve mechanism by the active closure mechanism is emphasised by the finding in ureterovesical junctions of children with VUR that the muscle layers in the distal ureter are dysplastic, with disordered fibre arrangement and increased extracellular matrix collagen, and the intramural nerve supply is absent, rendering the active mechanism impossible [8, 138, 144].

Genes Involved in the Formation of a Functioning One-Way Urine Flow System

Embryonic development is controlled by an immense network of genes controlling other genes controlling yet other genes, and including many instances of collaboration between gene products, and many of processes that are required in a variety of different organs. For instance, branching occurs of course not only in the ureteric bud, forming the calyces and collecting ducts of the kidney, but in the lungs, and the exocrine glands, and the blood and lymphatic vessels (though these do not all happen in exactly the same way), so the same genes are often used at different stages in many different organs. The number of genes so far known to be involved in urinary tract development from the earliest stages of the mesonephros to the fully developed kidney, ureter, etc., is very large, including many feedback loops of genes maintaining the expression of genes that activated them [114]. Here the aim is to concentrate on just those genes that have a direct bearing on VUR.

For those unfamiliar with gene and protein terminology, each gene has an official full name and an official short name consisting of a few letters and often a number too. The gene names are in italics and short names for the proteins are the same but in regular text. For human genes, the whole short name is in capitals, for other mammals, only the first letter is capital, and for invertebrates, such as *Drosophila* species, the gene or protein name is entirely without capitals.

It is also worth here remarking about the nature of mutations. 'Dominant' and 'recessive' are relative terms. The normal state of affairs is of course to have two fully-functioning copies of an autosomal gene, but while some genes are sufficient in only one copy, others show 'dosage effects'. A mutation may be classified as recessive because the described phenotype is only seen if both copies of the gene have the same mutation, or different mutations that have very similar effects on the gene or its product(s), but a heterozygous individual (in whom only one copy of the gene is mutant) may have unobserved differences in phenotype, and may be liable to have all or part of the phenotype if there is a variant in another, interacting gene, or in the presence of a particular environmental factor. Also, 'dominant' mutations are of two types. The phenotypes caused by most dominant mutations are due to a dosage effect, 'haploinsufficiency', meaning that the amount of product from one unmutated copy of the gene is not sufficient for normality. In this case, loss of function of both copies of the gene may be lethal, or there may be a more severe phenotype, compatible with survival because the loss may be partially compensated for by other genes. However, some mutations are known as 'dominant negative'. This means that the product of the mutated gene interferes with the function of the product of the unmutated gene. For instance, a mutant ligand protein may bind to a receptor but fail to cause it to transmit its message to the inside of the cell, thereby blocking the normal ligand from the other gene copy from stimulating that receptor, or the mutant ligand may bind so firmly that it will not come off, so that the effect cannot be switched off without the cell removing and destroying the receptor. Furthermore, different mutations in the same gene can have different consequences (see *SALL1* below). This variation in the effects of different mutations is one of the possible ways in which some mutations could cause nonsyndromic VUR while other mutations in the same gene cause a syndrome. In the following account, readers can take it that genes described are autosomal, and that mutations are dominant haploinsufficient unless otherwise stated.

From the description in section "Embryological Development of the Lower Urinary Tract", one would expect to find that in patients with VUR there might be disordered function of one or more genes involved in any of the processes necessary to producing a functioning one-way urine flow system: precise positioning of the emergence of the ureteric bud from the mesonephric duct, vitamin A metabolism, development of smooth muscle on the ureters and bladder, the nerve-supply of the latter, and connective tissue. To clarify what is coming below, it is worth mentioning that sequencing of the *Amphioxus* genome has shown that since the common ancestor of *Amphioxus* and vertebrates, the whole genome was duplicated twice [53, 69, 172], and before and since that time, over 500 thousand years ago, there have been other gene duplications and some losses of some copies, making families of genes, and selected mutations that have modified the copies so that through evolution they have developed different related and sometimes overlapping roles, and many genes involved in urinary tract development are replicates of single genes seen in *Drosophila*, the model organism from which the gene names are often derived.

In order to co-operate to build structures during embryonic development, cells need to send signals to one-another, and these signals are often to upregulate some genes and to downregulate others, so a lot of the relevant genes are those for receptors, the ligands that bind to them, and transcription factors that regulate the expression of genes by binding to specific sites in DNA.

Emergence of the Ureteric Bud

Many genes have been shown to be involved in this, but a key is signalling between RET (whose gene is also known as 'ret proto-oncogene'), a transmembrane receptor which is a member of the tyrosine protein kinase family of proteins, with the co-receptor, GFRA1 (GDNF family receptor alpha 1) and the ligand, GDNF (Glial cell derived neurotrophic factor). Inactivation of any of the genes encoding these three proteins in mice can cause failure of emergence of a ureteric bud, resulting in renal agenesis [39, 164].

The name 'RET' comes from 'Rearranged during Transfection', a historical left-over from the accidental way that its gene was found. The primary RNA transcript of *RET*, in common with those of many other genes, is spliced into numerous different mRNA 'isoforms' containing different numbers and different combinations of exons. According to the latest information on the NCBI Gene website (https://www.ncbi.nlm.nih.gov/gene), there are 41 different isoforms, coding for proteins with different numbers of amino-acids. Of these, three are well recognized, which differ in their N-terminal domains, which are the extracellular domains, and vary in length between 29 and 635 amino-acids. There is a family of four co-receptor proteins that can each form a heterodimer with RET, GFRA1-4, and the combination of RET with each of these binds a different signalling ligand [23]. In the urinary tract, RET forms a heterodimer with GFRA1 and they bind the ligand GDNF.

The gene *GFRA1* encodes a preprotein that is processed proteolytically to produce the mature co-receptor. The gene *GDNF* also encodes a preprotein, and it is proteolytically processed to produce a peptide of which two copies form a homodimer. RET and GFRA1 are expressed on the surface of the mesonephric duct, and GDNF is secreted by the metanephric (metanephrogenic) mesenchyme all along the side of the duct, so multiple ureteric buds will grow out from the duct if its expression is not suppressed everywhere except the optimum position. A complex network of gene products upregulating and suppressing GDNF and ureteric bud outgrowth exists to confine the outgrowth to a single exact position.

As the full name for GDNF (above) suggests, this signalling is also involved in nerve growth, so one would not *expect* mutation of any of these genes themselves to cause non-syndromic VUR. Indeed, though mice with *Ret* gene knock-out have impaired distal ureter maturation and impaired calyceal branching or renal agenesis [18, 158], mutation in humans of either *RET* or *GFRA1* or *GDNF* can cause Hirschsprung Disease [189] as well as other neurological disorders. Various heterozygous nonsynonymous *RET* variants have been found in fetuses with bilateral renal agenesis or other urinary tract malformations [80, 164], and homozygous mutations of *GFRA1* have been found it six cases of non-syndromic bilateral renal agenesis [5, 9]. However, two mis-sense (nonsynonymous) mutations have been found in RET in nonsyndromic VUR patients. One of them was in a patient with unilateral VUR accompanying a duplex collecting system and hydroureter [71]. The mutation having this mild effect compared with most other reported mutations, was towards the end of the gene, changing a leucine to a valine at position 1,027 in the 1,114-amino-acid polypeptide chain of the longest isoform. As mentioned earlier, like many other genes, *RET* has numerous different transcripts (40 at the latest count) using different start sites and/or different combinations of exons, many but not all transcripts, coding and producing proteins of different lengths, whose individual functions have yet to be determined. The amino-acid that is No. 1027 in the longest protein isoform, is the very last amino-acid of one of the other isoforms. The other variant, found in a patient with bilateral grade III VUR and no other anomaly, was at position 427 in the protein, which is not within any of the important domains [111].

One common polymorphic mis-sense variant of *RET* (p.Gly691Ser) was reported to be associated with VUR [191], but this association was proven to be false [42]. However, in a later study, this variant was found in combination with a nonsynonymous *GDNF* variant (p.Arg93Trp) in a patient with bilateral VUR and no other anomalies [34]. This *GDNF* variant, which is registered as an SNP (rs36119840) but was not found in any of the 363 unrelated controls used in the study, was found in two more of the 122 patients with UTMs investigated, neither of whom had the common RET variant. One of these also had VUR, unilaterally, with an ectopic hydronephrotic kidney on the other side, and the other did not have VUR but had unilateral renal agenesis and an ectopic kidney on the other side. In the same study, a child with right cystic-dysplasia, left dysplasia, bilateral megaureter, and cryptorchidism was found to have two nonsynonymous *RET* variants inherited from his unaffected father and a nonsynonymous *GFRA1* variant inherited from his unaffected mother. The child did not have VUR, but this is mentioned to make the point that a combination of otherwise silent ('hypomorphic') variants can have phenotypic effect.

Now we turn to genes that regulate GDNF/RET-GFRA1 signalling in the urinary tract. Multiple factors positively and negatively regulate this signalling system. Positive regulation occurs both through activating the expression of GDNF and of RET.

Activators of GDNF Expression

These proteins are the transcription factors PAX2, EYA1, SIX1, SIX5, HOX11 paralogues, DACH and SALL1, and the receptor-ligand pairs ITGA8/ITGB1 with NPNT, and a TGFβ family receptor with GDF11.

PAX2 is one of a family of nine 'Paired Box' proteins. These are all involved in embryonic development and have a 'paired box' domain of approximately 126 amino-acids, that is divided into three sub-domains, the ones at each end binding DNA, with the one in the middle acting as a linker, hence the name. However, the linker can also bind in the minor groove of DNA. The PAX genes also have a homeobox domain (or homeodomain) of about 60 amino-acids that also binds DNA, and occurs also in other groups of embryonic organizer proteins, the homeobox protiens, which include the HOX proteins, and are major regulators of many other genes.

Along with PAX8, PAX2 is one of the earliest indicators of urinary tract cell lineage, and if both copies of the gene are inactivated, the mesonephric duct never fully develops and degenerates by apoptosis, and metanephric kidneys never form [162]. In the normal course of events, expression of PAX2 protein activates expression of *GDNF* in the mesenchyme by binding to regulatory elements upstream of the gene in combination with EYA1, SIX1 and HOX11 [30, 57, 152]. After the ureteric bud has invaded the metanephric mesenchyme, it undergoes about ten rounds of branching, and a series of reciprocal signalling interactions, between the tip of each branch and the metanephric mesenchyme, induces the development of a nephron at the end of each branch. Mesenchyme cells divide into ones that express PAX2 and SIX2 and form nephrons and ones that express another transcription factor, FOXD1, which become stromal cells [40].

In the light of this, it is not surprising that if one copy of *PAX2* is mutated, there might be VUR and renal hypo-dysplasia, but PAX2 is also involved in the development of the nervous system, eye and ear, and heterozygous mutation of *PAX2* in humans can result in Renal-Coloboma Syndrome, also known as Papillorenal Syndrome [154]. As in all syndromes, the phenotype is variable, depending upon the type of mutation and position in the coded protein, as well as the genetic background of variants in other genes in the individual. The core features are optic nerve dysplasia, coloboma, and renal hypodysplasia, or oligomeganephronia, but patients may also have hearing loss, malformations of the central nervous system, and joint and skin anomalies, and about 25% have VUR [129]. However, two patients have been described with nonsyndromic VUR. One had bilateral small kidneys and bilateral grade III VUR, and was found to have no eye or external ear anomalies or hearing loss, and normal intelligence. The mutation was a base-substitiution, a C-to-A transversion at position 1566 in exon 9 (out of 12), creating a stop codon [133]. This would have resulted in a protein truncated towards the end of the transactivation domain (a domain that binds to other proteins), but with a normal paired-box domain and homeodomain (see Fig. 1 in [129] for a diagram of the gene structure). The other patient had right grade I VUR, left hydronephrosis, and bilateral hypodysplasia [111]. This patient also had a heterozygous base-substitution creating a stop codon, but at cDNA coding position 906 in exon 7, replacing amino-acid 302. This truncation is in the homeodomain and is rather more surprising.

As already mentioned, **EYA1, SIX1, and 'HOX11'** are required in addition to PAX2 to activate GDNF expression in the metanephric mesenchyme. *EYA1* is one of the four human homologues of the *Drosophila* 'Eyes absent' (*eya*) gene. *SIX1* is one of six homologues in humans, and other mammals, of the Drosophila *sine oculis* (without eyes) gene (*so*) and *optix* gene. pax, so/six and eya genes have been co-operating in the development of the eyes and other organs since the common ancestor of all bilaterians over 550 million years ago [88]. Human HOX genes are present in four clusters, A – D, on different chromosomes, with thirteen different patterns, numbered 1–13 in order of temporal and physical expression, rostrally to caudally in the embryo, that have similar paralogues on the other chromosomes. However, in each cluster, some genes have been lost over evolutionary time since the two genomic duplications mentioned earlier, so that birds and mammals have a total of 39 HOX genes rather than the potential of $4 \times 13 = 52$, and only sets 4 and 13 have a copy in all four clusters [105]. As also occurs in some other sets of paralogous genes, there is a degree of redundancy, i.e., if mutation inactivates both copies of a particular gene, its paralogues can compensate or partially compensate for its loss. It's a useful evolutionary survival mechanism. In the HOX11 group there are three paralogs, *HOXA11*, *HOXC11* and *HOXD11*, and in mice it has been shown [187] that if both copies of either *Hoxa11* or *Hoxd11* are rendered non-functional, there is no discernible kidney abnormality. If both genes are knocked out, there is renal dysplasia, but if *Hoxc11* is then also knocked out, the metanephric blastema condenses, GDNF is not expressed, and no ureteric bud forms. HOX genes are involved in so many early embryonic processes that it is not surprising that no mutations of any of the *HOX11* paralogues have been found in a living child.

Whereas in the mesonephros and mesonephric duct, *PAX2* is expressed independently of *EYA1* and *SIX1*, in the metanephric mesenchyme, EYA1 activates *SIX1* and *PAX2*, and SIX1 also upregulates *PAX2* [114, 152]. The EYA proteins have a 271-amino-acid 'EYA domain' or 'EyaHR', Eyes absent homologous region, which is essential for protein-protein interactions, but have no DNA-binding domain [32], so it appears that they activate genes by binding to other proteins that do bind DNA. Different mutations of one copy of *EYA1* have been found as causes of branchio-oto-renal syndrome [1, 2, 101] and of branchio-otic syndrome [180], as well as of sporadic cases of congenital cataracts and ocular anterior segment anomalies [10]. The range of clinical features of branchio-oto-renal syndrome includes a variety of malformations of the outer, middle, and inner ear associated with conductive, sensorineural, or mixed hearing impairment, branchial fistulae and cysts, and urinary tract anomalies ranging from mild renal hypoplasia to bilateral renal agenesis, and including pelviureteric junction obstruction and VUR, as well as palate anomalies, euthyroid goitre and facial palsy [165, 176]. They can also include congenital cataracts [10].

The appearance of ear and branchial cleft remnants along with urinary tract anomalies relates to the evolutionary origin, mentioned earlier, of the proximity of the excretory organs to the gills. Homozygous mouse mutants of *Eya1* have no ears and no kidneys. In these mice, GDNF is not expressed in the metanephric mesenchyme, and the ureteric bud does not appear, whereas heterozygous mutants have conductive hearing loss and renal anomalies similar to those in human branchio-oto-renal syndrome [190]. So far only one patient with non-syndromic VUR has been found to have an *EYA1* mutation, a base substitution replacing a glycine with an aspartic acid residue at position 66 in the protein, and is currently of uncertain significance [111] so may not actually be the cause of the patient's VUR. This patient had bilateral grade V VUR and left hypodysplasia.

Some cases of Branchio-oto-renal Syndrome have been in found to have mutations of *SIX1* [150, 176], as might be expected from knowledge of the co-operation of the EYA1 and SIX1 proteins, as mentioned above, but other cases have been found to have mutations in *SIX5* [65], *SALL1*, or a partial tetrasomy of chromosome 22q [150, 176].

The SIX proteins all have two DNA-binding domains, a 60-amino-acid homeodomain, and a 110–115-amino-acid Six domain. All six *SIX* genes and their protein products have slight differences in both domains, and the family can be divided into three sub-families SIX1/2, 3/6 and 4/5, by their overall lengths and structures, and by the similarities of their DNA-binding domains [88] and by their closest homologies to the Drosophila *so*, *optix* and *DSix4* genes respectively [100] (Yes, that *Drosophila* gene has, atypically, some capital letters in its name). The discovery that some cases of Branchio-oto-renal Syndrome were caused by mutations in *SIX5* [65] was made by a deliberate search for such mutations in 95 patients, following the discovery that in the nematode worm *Caenorhabditis elegans*, unc-39—the homologue of human SIX5—interacts with eya-1, and the speculation that this protein-protein interaction might have been conserved over the course of over 600 million years. Four different mutations were found in 5 of the 95 patients, and functional analyses of these mutations showed that two of them affect EYA1-SIX5 binding and the ability of SIX5 or the EYA1-SIX5 complex to activate gene transcription.

No cases of nonsyndromic VUR have yet been found to have a *SIX1* mutation, but cases have been found with mutations in *SIX5* [71] or *SIX2* [186] which has not been reported to be mutated in any branchio-oto-renal syndrome patient. The patient with the *SIX5* mutation had a duplex kidney with VUR on that side, and ureterovesical junction obstruction on the other side, and the mutation was in a part of the protein well beyond the two DNA-binding domains. Functional inactivation of *Six2* in mice was found to result in premature and ectopic differentiation of metanephric mesenchymal cells into epithelia, and depletion of the progenitor cell population, and failure to renew the mesenchymal cells resulted in severe renal hypoplasia [160]. This led Weber et al. [186] to screen 250 children with renal hypodysplasia and impaired renal function for *SIX2* mutations. They specifically excluded patients who had VUR but normal kidneys on ultrasound, but some of the selected children did have VUR in addition to renal anomalies. They found three different mutations, one of which was within the region coding for the SIX domain of the protein, and the other two in the *SIX2*-specific C-termianal domain. Two of the mutations were each found in a single patient, and one of these had VUR on the opposite side from a dysplastic kidney. The third mutation was found in three children, two of whom had VUR, one having bilateral cystic dysplasia and bilateral VUR, and the other unilateral hypoplasia with VUR on the same side.

DACH1 (Dachshund family transcription factor 1) is one of two homologues of the *Drosophila dachshund* gene, *dac*, so called because mutations cause the flies to have very short legs in relation to their body length, and is yet another transcription factor that regulates gene expression and cell fate determination during development. DACH1 protein contains two domains that are highly conserved since our common ancestor with *Drosophila*, DD1 near the N-terminal, which binds DNA, and DD2 near the C-terminal, which binds to other proteins. In *Drosophila*, *dac* (DACH) was found to interact with the SIX and EYA homologues in eye development, and has been shown to do also in kidney development in the mouse [108]. It interacts directly with SIX proteins but only indirectly with EYA proteins, through another transcription factor, CREBBP (CREB binding protein) which binds both to EYA1 and to DACH1 [74]. DACH1 can act both as a suppressor and as an activator of gene expression. When bound to DNA upstream of a gene combined with a SIX protein and other factors, it suppresses transcription, but when an EYA protein is attached to the complex through CREBBP, the gene is activated [108]. Exon sequencing of 208 genes known to be involved in urinary tract development in 453 patients with UTMs [132] found a *DACH1* mutation as the likely cause in a single case. The patient had unilateral renal dysplasia, VUR and megaureter and no anomalies of the eyes or other organs.

SALL proteins are zinc-finger proteins. A zinc finger is a protein fold that is stabilized by one or more zinc (Zn^{2+}) ions, and zinc-finger proteins have many functions, including recognizing specific DNA sequences, and assisting in folding of other proteins, and the SALL proteins bind DNA as transcription factors. The proteins also have a glutamine-rich domain with which they interact with other proteins. There are three human *SALL* genes, and heterozygous mutation of *SALL1* was found to be the cause of Townes-Brocks Syndrome [94], defined by the triad of dysplastic ears (often accompanied by sensorineural deafness), thumb abnormalities (and often foot anomalies too) and imperforate anus. 42% have renal insufficiency with or without a wide variety of urinogenital tract malformations, including VUR. 25% have heart anomalies, 10% intellectual impairement, and rare cases can include eye defects (congenital cataracts, micro-ophthalmia or iris coloboma), Duane anomaly, Arnold-Chiari malformation Type 1, or growth retardation [95].

Subsequent to the discovery that *SALL1* mutation was the culprit in Townes-Brocks Syndrome, *Sall1* gene-knock-out mice were created [135]. Two types were made, one in which no Sall1 protein was produced, the other producing only a part of the protein, and both types were homozygous. Mice with the partial protein expression had renal agenesis or severe dysgenesis and died in the perinatal period, whereas in those with no protein expression mesonephros development was normal and metanephric mesenchyme was formed but small, and the ureteric bud formed but either it failed to invade the metanephric mesenchyme, which then failed to differentiate and bud branching did not occur, or the bud invaded partially but mesenchymal condensation and ureteric branching were poor.

Further understanding of the effects of mutation *SALL1* mutations has been revealed as more human mutations have been reported. Most mutations causing Townes-Brocks Syndrome have been found in a hot-spot region located between the coding region for the glutamine-rich domain and 65 bp 3′ of the coding region for the first double zinc finger domain [25], and can produce a truncated protein that is able to bind to its interacting proteins but unable to bind to DNA to regulate its target genes because it lacks the zinc-finger domain. These mutations are demonstrably dominant negative mutations because complete deletion of one copy of *SALL1* results in a milder (haploinsufficient) phenotype [15, 24, 76, 121]. In the sequencing study of the coding exons of 17 dominant genes, known to be involved in congenital UTMs, in a cohort of 749 individuals from 650 families mentioned in section "Mutation-Detection and Sequencing Studies" in chapter "Genetics of Vesicoureteric Reflux" [71], seven different genetic variants in *SALL1* were found in ten individuals. Of these, five patients had VUR, four of whom were nonsyndromic, with three different variants, all of which changed highly evolutionarily conserved amino-acids and were predicted to be deleterious.

ITGA8 codes for Integrin subunit α8. Integrins form heterodimers of α and β subunits and are receptors which mediate many cellular processes including cell adhesion, cytoskeletal rearrangement, and activation of signalling pathways. ITGA8 forms a heterodimer with ITGB1 (Integrin subunit β1). These heterodimers serve as receptors for various different ligands in different tissues, and in urinary tract development, the ligand has been identified and named Nephronectin (NPNT) [28], though it is now known to be expressed in a number of other tissues too. ITGA8 is expressed in many tissues and is involved in neurite outgrowth and vestibular hair-cell growth amongst other processes. It is expressed in the mesenchyme adjacent to the mesonephric (Wolffian) duct and in the metanephric mesenchyme, and is induced by contact with the ureteric bud in the cells surrounding it. In mouse *Itgα8* mutant homozygotes, growth and branching of the ureteric bud and recruitment of mesenchymal cells into epithelial structures are defective, and result in renal dysgenesis or agenesis [127] and, in humans also, homozygous mutations can cause bilateral renal agenesis [70].

It has been pointed out that the homozygous or compound heterozygous mutations in ITGA8 (and several other genes to be mentioned later) that cause renal agenesis are truncating mutations, and shown that less-damaging biallelic mutations can cause nonsyndromic UTM phenotypes [93]. So far, two nonsyndromic VUR patients have been reported to have mutations in *ITGA8*, both biallelic. One of these, with unilateral duplex kidney and grade III VUR, had a homozygous intronic mutation predicted to affect the splice-site upstream of Exon 28 of a total of 31 exons [93]. The other, with unilateral grade III VUR and no other anomaly, had a stop codon in Exon 27 of one allele and a nonsynonymous substitution in Exon 20 in the other [111]. A heterozygous nonsynonymous ***ITGB1*** mutation has also been reported in one patient with VUR and a duplex collecting system, but this patient also had heterozygous mutations in two other urinary tract development genes—one in *SIX2* and one in *WNT5A*, both also amino-acid substitution mutations [132]. The mutation in *SIX2* was in the homeobox domain rather than in either of the domains in which Weber et al. (mentioned above) found mutations.

Homozygous null mutations of ***NPNT*** have been found in several cases of bilateral renal agenesis in three consanguineous families [4, 41]. However, in one of the families there was one individual homozygous for the family mutation, who only had unilateral renal aplasia [4], and lived to have ten children, all heterozygotes of course. No urinary tract anomalies were reported in any of the heterozygous individuals in any of the families, which would suggest that in the case of this gene, *NPNT* one functioning copy is sufficient, and the finding of the exceptional homozygote with one normal kidney demonstrates that in some, as yet unknown circumstance, renal development is possible in the absence of any nephronectin. It was not reported whether any of the heterozygous individuals in any of the families was investigated for VUR. This is a pity, because the investigators were perhaps unaware that two individuals with UTM phenotypes had already been reported to have (different) heterozygous nonsynonymous mutations in *NPNT* [132]. One of these patients had pelviureteric junction obstruction and was not found to have a second mutation in any of the other 207 urinary tract development genes investigated at the same time. The other patient had VUR and had a heterozygous *ROBO2* mutation in addition to the *NPNT* mutation. *ROBO2* is described later below.

GDF11 (Growth differentiation factor 11) encodes a ligand of the TGFβ (transforming growth factor-beta) superfamily of proteins. Ligands of this family bind various TGFβ receptors, leading to recruitment and activation of SMAD family transcription factors. The gene encodes a preproprotein that is proteolytically processed to generate each subunit of the disulfide-linked homodimer, GDF11, which plays a role in the development of the nervous and other organ systems, and has been shown to control anterior/posterior patterning in the axial skeleton. In mice, deletion of the gene caused a spectrum of renal abnormalities, with the majority of mutant animals lacking both kidneys, and further investigation showed that GDNF was not secreted and ureteric buds did not form, and that if GDF11 was added to urogenital tracts taken from *Gdf11* null embryos, induced ectopic ureteric bud formation occurred along the mesonephric duct [49]. GDF11 is therefore essential for ureteric bud outgrowth. However, a group of six probands, four with nonsense or frameshift mutations and two with mis-sense mutations in *GDF11*, presented with neurological, craniofacial, vertebral, visual, cardiac, auditory, and connective tissue abnormalities [147], but there have been no reports of *GDF11* mutations in patients with urinary tract anomalies. The specific receptor of GDF11 in the mesenchyme of the urinary tract seems not to have been identified yet.

Activators of RET Expression

These are PAX2, CTNNB1, GATA3, and retinoic acid and receptors RARA/RXRA and RARB/RXRB, modulated by their co-activator GREB1L and repressor NRIP1, and subsequently EMX2 is required to sustain RET expression.

CTNNB1, Catenin β1, better known as β-catenin, anchors the actin cytoskeleton in epithelial cells. It is an intracellular protein and, with two other related intracellular proteins, CTNNA1 and CTNND1, and a transmembrane protein, CDH1 (Cadherin 1), forms a complex called an adherens junction. These junctions are necessary for the creation and maintenance of epithelial cell layers by regulating cell growth and adhesion between cells. In the mouse it has been shown that CTNNB1 is necessary to keep the cells of the mesonephric duct, and of the ureteric bud when it emerges, in an undifferentiated state so that the bud can continue to grow and branch within the metanephric mesenchyme. If the gene *CTNNB1* is deleted in the mesonephric duct, the cells of the ureteric bud soon begin to differentiate, causing growth and branching to slow and cease, resulting in renal aplasia or hypoplasia [115].

GATA3, GATA binding protein 3, is one of a family of six genes (without homologues in most invertebrates) that encode zinc finger transcription factors that recognize the nucleotide sequence GATA in the promoters of target genes that they activate or repress. They play an important role in the regulation of cellular differentiation and organogenesis during development. GATA3 has two GATA-type zinc fingers. PAX2 (described earlier) takes part in activating *GATA3* [27, 59], which in turn takes part in turning on *RET* expression in the mesonephric duct [60]. CTNNB1 is also required to activate *GATA3*, as deletion of *Ctnnb1* in mice causes almost complete extinction of Gata3 and Ret expression, but does not affect Pax2 expression [60, 115]. Counterintuitively, inactivation of *Gata3* specifically in the nephric duct of mice leads to massive ectopic ureter budding. This is due to ectopic budding of interspersed cells along the mesonephric duct still expressing the Ret receptor, but Ret expression soon ceases, and this results in a spectrum of urogenital malformations including renal adysplasia, duplex systems, and hydroureter, as well as vas deferens hyperplasia and uterine agenesis [60].

Four patients with nonsyndromic VUR have been reported to have mutations in *GATA3*, all of them heterozygous and causing amino-acid substitutions, and all of them different. Two of the substitutions, both in patients with bilateral VUR and no other anomalies, were of highly evolutionarily-conserved amino-acids and predicted to be deleterious [71]. The other two, one in a patient with bilateral grade III VUR and the other in one with unilateral hypodysplasia and grade III VUR, were of uncertain significance [111], while another patient in the same study, who had a heterozygous frame-shift mutation in the gene had short stature grade V VUR on one side and a multicystic dysplastic kidney on the other.

ALDH1A2 (previously known as *RALDH2*), which encodes the enzyme Aldehyde dehydrogenase 1family member A2, is one of a subfamily of three genes, *ALDH1A1-3*, which form part of a larger family with 19 functional members which encode enzymes which carry out detoxification or biotransformation of different endogenous and exogenous aldehyde substrates. A study of all the polymorphic variants in all of the 19 genes reported in gnomAD (see section "Resources for Identifying Genes and Genetic Variants Involved in VUR and Other UTMs") has found that this small subfamily of three genes appear to have a much lower tolerance of loss-of-function mutations than the other ALDH genes, and concluded that these three enzymes may serve more essential functions than the others [35]. Alternatively, it may be that their specificities do not overlap much with those of the rest of the family, so their losses can less easily be compensated for. ALDH1A2 catalyzes the synthesis of retinoic acid (the active ingredient of Vitamin A, chemical name retinol) from retinaldehyde.

The retinoic acid receptors (RARα, β, and γ) are multi-domain polypeptides that heterodimerize with retinoid X receptors (RXRα, β, and γ) to form functional transcription factors [146]. All six proteins have DNA-binding domains. Their genes are

RARA, *B* & *G*, and *RXRA*, *B* & *G*. Retinoic acid signalling has been shown to be necessary for RET expression because in the mouse either deletion of *Raldh2* (*ALDH1A2*) or a dominant negative retinoic acid receptor mutation cause loss of Ret expression and Ret-dependent functions including ureteric bud formation and branching morphogenesis [148]. The picture thus emerges that both PAX2 and CTNNB1 are necessary for GATA3 expression, and both GATA3 and retinoic acid signalling are necessary for RET expression. In addition to emergence and growth of of the ureteric bud, the retinoic acid-GATA3-RET pathway has also been shown to be necessary for insertion of the mesonephric duct into the cloaca [37].

Heterozygous mutation of *CTNNB1* can cause Neurodevelopmental Disorder with Spastic Diplegia and Visual Defects (NEDSDV) [99], which can include cardiovascular, facial, and skeletal defects [89, 163] and is also one of the causes of Familial Exudative Vitreo-Retinopathy (FEVR) [38], and homozygous mutation can cause a severe syndromic form of FEVR including microphthalmia and persistent fetal vasculature [171], but strangely there have been no reports of any urinary tract anomalies in any of these cases, let alone of nonsyndromic VUR. Mutations of *GATA3* can cause Barakat Syndrome, also known as HDR Syndrome, whose core components are hypoparathyroidism, sensorineural deafness and renal dysplasia, but has a very variable phenotype and can include VUR [13, 14].

A homozygous duplication of a 752,216 bp region on 15q21.3 containing five genes, which included *ALDH1A2* was found in a search for CNVs in Hirschsprung Disease [104], and two heterozygous mutations in *ALDH1A2* have been found in two cases of Fallot's tetralogy [140], but no *ALDH1A2* mutations have so far been found in patients with urinary tract anomalies. One patient has been reported with a mutation of *RARA*. She was referred for congenital chorioretinal coloboma but also had facial, skeletal and other anomalies, amongst which was an ectopic kidney [79]. There have been more reports of heterozygous *RARB* mutations, including cases of microphthalmia and dystonia [174], pulmonary hypoplasia, diaphragmatic eventration, microphthalmia, and cardiac defect [7], colonic agangliosis [52], and intellectual disability with progressive motor impairment [168], amongst others, and biallelic mutation has been found in autism spectrum disorder [45], but no reports of *RARB* mutation have included urinary tract anomalies. The RXR proteins, in addition to forming heterodimers with the RAR proteins, also form heterodimers with the thyroid hormone receptors and with the Vitamin D receptors, so mutation of any of them would be even more devastating and not confined simply to urinary tract anomalies.

Transcriptional activation initiated by the binding of retinoic acid to the RAR/RXR receptors may be activated by GREB1L and is repressed by NRIP1. **GREB1L** is GREB1 like retinoic acid receptor coactivator, where GREB1 is a similar protein, 'Growth regulation by estrogen in breast cancer 1'. In 2017, two studies found *GREB1L* mutations in human subjects, one was a study of renal hypodysplasia patients [153], mentioned in section "Mutation-Detection and Sequencing Studies", and the other was a study of two large extended families in which there had been fetuses with renal agenesis [31]. The first mentioned, which was a large study identifying many genes, carried out zebrafish studies which established that *greb1l* is necessary for genesis of the proximal convoluted tubule of the pronephros, and that injection of mutant embryos with mRNA of human *GREB1L* with either of two different genetic variants found in control subjects prevented the renal tubule loss phenotype from happening, but injection of mRNA with any of four of the variants found in the 17 human renal hypodysplasia patients did not rescue the embryos. They were able to conclude that the damaging mutations caused loss of function and were dominant due to haploinsufficiency. The 17 patients had either unilateral renal aplasia, or renal hypoplasia, or multicystic dysplastic kidneys. None of them had VUR, but the sister of one of them and two cousins of another had VUR, but none of them was checked for the family mutation. The other team [31] also carried out work on zebrafish, and on mice. GREB1L is expressed in the metanephric mesenchyme and at a low level in the ureteric bud. It is still unclear exactly how it acts but the authors concluded from their own animal work and that of various others that retinoic acid may activate GREB1L, which then combines with the retinoic acid receptors to promote kidney formation. None of the members of their families was reported to have VUR. A patient with VUR and congenital vaginal atresia (and no kidney malformation) was found to have a variant in *GREB1L* which was a nonsynonymous variant in exon 31out of 35, but was of uncertain significance [111].

Exome sequencing of members of a four generation family with various UTM found a frame-shift truncating mutation in ***NRIP1***, Nuclear receptor interacting protein 1, in all seven sequenced affected members, four of whom had VUR in addition to other UTMs (listed in Table 1) [182]. mRNA, transcribed from the genome in the nucleus, has to be taken out into the cytoplasm to be translated by the ribosomes, and then nuclear proteins have to be transported back into the nucleus. Using human embryonic kidney cells (HEK293 cells) the investigators found that the mutated protein of this family was not transported into the nucleus, failed to bind RARA, and failed to inhibit retinoic acid–dependent transcriptional activity, and further experiments with mice and the frog, *Xenopus laevis*, confirmed that NRIP1 regulation of retinoic acid signalling is required for normal urinary tract development.

EMX2, empty spiracles homeobox 2, encodes yet another transcription factor with a name derived from earlier *Drosophila* work, and, like *GATA3*, its expression is also activated by PAX2 and CTNNB1 [26, 29]. In mice with both copies of *Emx2* inactivated, the ureteric bud fails to branch after invading the mesenchyme and soon degenerates [123]. This is recessive, as mice with heterozygous knock-out of *Emx2* do not show any defects unless *Pax2* is also heterozygously mutated, in which case duplex systems associated with urinary tract obstruction, bifid ureter and a high penetrance of VUR are found [26] and so far no mutations of *EMX2* have been found in human patients.

Table 1 Genes in which variants have been found in cases of nonsyndromic VUR

Developmental process	Gene	Location	Additional UT anomalies (ALL reported patients have VUR)	References
UB outgrowth	*RET*	10q11.21	Lt Duplex kidney, ureterocele	[71]
			None—nonsynonymous VUS in Exon 7	[111]
UB outgrowth	*GDNF*	5p13.2	Lt VUR with Rt ectopic hydronephrotic kidney; bilat none in presence of common RET nonsynonymous variant	[34]
Related to FGF10 which has been shown to act like GDNF	*FGF8*	10q24.32	None	[132]
Receptor for FGFs	*FGFR1*	8p11.23	Lt renal agenesis, Rt VUR & hypospadia s with bladder extrophy	[177]
Activator of GDNF expression	*PAX2*	10q24.31	Bilateral small kidneys	[133]
			Rt grade I, Lt hydronephrosis, and bilateral hypodysplasia	[111]
As above	*EYA1*	8q13.3	Bilateral grade V and left hypodysplasia—VUS	[111]
As above	*SIX2*	2p21	Lt Dys, Rt VUR; bilat multi-cystic dysplasia; unilat hypoplasia	[186]
As above	*SIX5*	19q13.32	Rt duplex with VUR, Lt UVJO	[71]
As above	*SALL1*	16q12.1	None × 2; RA; Rt duplex but bilat VUR; MCDK	[71]
As above	*DACH1*	13q21.33	Unilat RD and megaureter	[132]
As above	*ITGA8*	10p13	Unilateral duplex with VUR (homozygous mutation)	[93]
			None (biallelic mutations)	[111]
As above	*ITGB1*	10p11.22	Duplex collecting system, also had mutations in *SIX2* & *WNT5A*	[132]
As above	*NPNT*	4q24	None, patient also had a mutation in *ROBO2* (see below)	[132]

(continued)

Table 1 (continued)

Developmental process	Gene	Location	Additional UT anomalies (ALL reported patients have VUR)	References
Activator of RET expression	*GATA3*	10p14	None—2 cases, different mutations	[71]
			None—2 cases, other different mutations both VUS (another patient, who had a frame-shift mutation had short stature in addition to VUR and MCDK)	[111]
Regulator of retinoic acid transcriptional activity required in RET expression	*NRIP1*	21q11.2–q21.1	4/7 patients with UMT in one family had VUR as follows: Lt MCDK + Rt VUR dilated ureter & dysplasia, unilateral VUR & renal dysplasia, Bilat Gr 2, Lt Gr 5 & renal dysplasia, Rt Gr 2.	[182]
Retinoic acid receptor co-activator involved in RET expression for UB outgrowth	*GREB1L*	18q11.1–q11.2	Suggestive evidence only in both reports below	
			Congenital vaginal atresia—but heterozygous nonsynonymous variant in Exon 31 of uncertain significance.	[111]
			Sister of one of 17 renal a/hypo/dysplasia patients reported with *GREB1L* mutations had VUR, but the sister was not tested for the variant (which was also a heterozygous nonsynonymous one but predicted damaging)	[153]
Signalling; mutations can cause syndromic nephrono-phthysis	*NPHP1*	2q13	This gene is within a homozygous deletion reported in one case of nonsyndromic VUR. The deletion of this particular gene is likely to be the cause but not yet proven.	[179]
Suppressor of ectopic ureteric bud emergence	*BMP4*	14q22.2	2 cases, unilat. renal dysplasia or hypoplasia and contralat. VUR	[186]
Interacts with BMPs	*CRIM1*	2p22.2	None	[132]
Probable overlap with ROBO2 function	*ROBO1*	3p12.3	None (another patient with the same variant had a duplex collecting system but no VUR)	[132]

(continued)

Table 1 (continued)

Developmental process	Gene	Location	Additional UT anomalies (ALL reported patients have VUR)	References
Suppression of ectopic ureteric bud emergence	*ROBO2*	3p12.3	None, renal hypoplasia & nephropathy; duplex kidney and collecting system—one of these variants predicted benign but not found in controls	[112]
			None × 2, and RN, and Rt PUJO + Lt dysplastic kidney but no VUR; none × 2; none × 2; none × 2, one of whom developed ESRD	[22]
			None × 2	[46]
			None	[71]
			None × at least 4; none × at least 2	[48]
			None, also had *FAT1* mutation; none, also had *NPNT* mutation	[132]
			None; bilateral renal hypodysplasia—VUS in both patients	[111]
Suppression of ectopic ureteric bud emergence	*SLIT2*	4p15.2	None; none; Duplex kidney—all 3 VUS	[111]
As above	*AGT*	1q42.2	None	[132]
As above	*AGTR1*	3q24	Duplex collecting system and phymosis	[132]
Transcription factor related to SPRY1 which suppresses ectopic ureteric bud emergence	*SOX17*	8q11.23	6 patients with the same mutation, 4 nonsyndromic = a mother & son (son also has unilat PUJO) and 2 sporadic cases, one of whom had PUJO but no VUR. (Other two in another family were syndromic.); 2 more sporadic cases with different mutations.	[56]
Acts downstream of GDNF/RET signalling to promote UB growth	*ETV4*	17q21.31	None—homozygous mis-sense mutation	[36]

(continued)

Table 1 (continued)

Developmental process	Gene	Location	Additional UT anomalies (ALL reported patients have VUR)	References
Required for ureteric bud invasion into metanephric mesenchyme	*KIF26B*	1q44	One family with high-grade VUR and renal hypodysplasia: none × 2. (Another family member with VUR and the genetic variant had a Marfan-like syndrome.) Two further family members with the variant had strong history of VUR but no radiological examinations.	[16]
Transcriptional repressor regulating differentiation of ureteric mesenchyme and smooth muscle cells	*TBX18*	6q14.3	Bilat renal dysplasia with unilat VUR (6 other family members with same variant had other UMT but not VUR)	[181]
			Rt RHD – VUS	[111]
Cell adhesion, growth and tissue-patterning	*DCHS1*	11p15.4	None	[132]
As above	*DCHS2*	4q31.3	None	[132]
As above	*FAT1*	4q35.2	None, patient also had a *ROBO2* mutation (see above)	[132]
Regulates cell growth and tissue patterning but exact role in VUR not yet determined	*SEMA3A*	7q21.11	None; PUV; DCS	[132]
A type I cytokine receptor regulating cell pluripotency	*LIFR*	5p13.1	One family with high-grade VUR and renal hypodysplasia: none × 2, bladder diverticula (one other affected individual had a VSD)	[16]
Extracellular matrix	*FRAS1*	4q21.21	None (homozygous mutation)	[93]
As above	*FREM1*	9p22.3	Bilat grade III; unilat grade V + ipsilat renal hypodysplasia (homozygous mutations in both patients)	[93]
			None	[132]
As above	*FREM2*	13q13.3	Bilat VUR with CKD (homozygous mutation); Rt VUR with Lt PUJO, PUV and CKD (compound heterozygous mutations)	[93]
			None; none	[132]

(continued)

Table 1 (continued)

Developmental process	Gene	Location	Additional UT anomalies (ALL reported patients have VUR)	References
As above	*TNXB*	6p21.33-p21.32	None × 4 + 1 with DCS (at least 2 with nephropathy, +4 with DCS but no VUR); none except nephropathy.	[54]
			None except nephropathy (this patient had 2 variants in the same copy of the gene); none × 2; none × 2; none; none.	[48]
			7/49 children with VUR, no indication of other UTM.	[173]
			None, VUS; bilat VUR Gr V, unilat RHD, VUS; unilat VUR Gr IV, ipsilat RHD, FS; none, FS; none, VUS.	[111]
As above	*COL4A1*	13q34	None × 3; none; PUV; PUV and single kidney	[91]
			None VUS	[111]
As above	*LAMC1*	1q25.3	None × 3	[16]
Luminal lining of ureter	*UPK2*	11q23.3	RN and renal failure	[83]
As above	*UPK3A*	22q13.31	Unilateral renal aplasia, contralateral severe dysplasia, and persistent cloaca; bilateral severe cystic dysplasia unrelated but same de novo mutation	[82]
			Unilateral multicystic dysplasia	[157]
Unknown mechanism	*HNF1B*	17q12	2 unrelated patients with same mutation, one with bilateral cystic dysplasia, ectopy and horseshoe fusion but carrier father with normal kidneys, the other with bilateral renal hypoplasia	[185]
			3 cases with cystic kidneys and different deletion or frame-shift mutations	[64]
			None; neurogenic bladder; PUV.	[71]
			Bilateral MCDK and epispadius	[153]
			bilat VUR with unilat hypodysplasia	[111]
Cilliary function	*INVS*	9q31.1	Unliat duplex collecting system with VUR	[132]

(continued)

Table 1 (continued)

Developmental process	Gene	Location	Additional UT anomalies (ALL reported patients have VUR)	References
Cilliary function; mutations can cause orofacial-digital syndrome	*OFD1*	Xp22.2	Right MCDK, left complete duplex and left grade III VUR with ureterocoele; Bilateral VUR with right hydronephrosis	[177]
Not yet determined	*UMOD*	16p12.3	PUV & meatal stenosis	[132]
			Renal hypoplasia, hydronephrosis (& hyperuricaemia)	[153]
			bilat VUR with unilat hypodysplasia	[111]
Role in glucose homeostasis & cell growth & differentiation	*TBC1D1*	4p14	2 patients with different heterozygous mutations, both with the same phenotype: bilateral grade IV VUR, renal hypodysplasia, hydronephrosis, megaureters, and ESRD	[98]

All variants are heterozygous unless otherwise stated. All variants are predicted pathogenic unless otherwise stated—*VUS* variant of uncertain significance, *FS* frame-shift variant, *CKD* chronic kidney disease, *DCS* duplex collecting system, *ESRD* end-stage renal disease, *MCDK* multicystic dysplastic kidney, *PUV* posterior urethral valve, *PUJO* pelviureteric junction obstruction, *RD* renal dysplasia, *RHD* renal hypodysplasia, *RN* reflux nephropathy, *UTM* urinary tract malformation, semicolons (;) separate unrelated patients with variants in the same gene, × N number of patients in same family (with same variant)

Suppressors of Ureteric Bud Outgrowth

These proteins, which limit ureteric bud outgrowth to a precise position, include the transcription factors FOXC1 and FOXC2 and the receptor-ligand pairs, BMPR1A/BMPR2 & BMP4, ROBO2 & SLIT2 and AGTR2 & Angiotensin II, and the receptor tyrosine kinase agonist Sprouty 1.

FOXC1 and ***FOXC2***, Forkhead box C1 and C2, are members of a larger family of forkhead box genes that produce transcription factors that can act both as activators and repressors in different circumstances. Each can act in combination with other transcription factors, and in urinary tract development, they are both required. Mice with deletion of both copies of *Foxc1*, have congenital hydrocephalus, but most also have abnormalities of the metanephric kidney, including duplex kidneys and double ureters, one of which is a hydroureter, and analysis of embryos reveals that *Foxc1* homozygotes have ectopic mesonephric tubules and rostrally ectopic ureteric buds. Along with this, Gdnf expression in the intermediate mesoderm surrounding the mesonephric duct is extended rostrally too compared with that in wild type embryos. Mice with heterozygous mutations of *Foxc1* are normal, as are those with heterozygous mutations of *Foxc2*, but most compound heterozygotes (mice heterozygous for mutations in both genes) have hypoplastic kidneys and a single hydroureter [96, 102].

In addition to taking part in controlling the position of ureteric bud emergence, *FOXC1* and *FOXC2* are also essential to maintaining the nephron and stromal progenitor cell populations in the developing kidney by regulating other genes [126], hence the hypoplasia when they are mutated in mice. However, they are also involved in maintaining chondral progenitor cells [6] and those of Schlemm's canal [175], and cytoskeletal activity during lymphatic valve maturation [136], and neural crest cells during heart development [75, 136], and mutation of these genes does not cause VUR. In humans, duplication of a segment of chromosome 6p including *FOXC1* can cause renal hypoplasia or hydronephrosis with proteinuria/hematuria, and focal segmental glomerular sclerosis, and can result in chronic end-stage renal failure [193]. A frameshift mutation of *FOXC2* was found in a family with hereditary lymphoedema-distichiasis syndrome associated with renal disease and diabetes mellitus [192]. Subsequently, other cases have had ectopic kidney, complete duplex kidney, partial duplex and malrotation with duplex collecting system, or bilateral hydronephrosis, and in some fetuses, bilateral renal agenesis, and other associated features that have been reported in living cases include varicose veins, cleft palate, congenital heart defects, and ptosis [84, 118].

The BMPs (Bone morphogenic proteins) are a family of ten ligands of the TGFB (Transforming growth factor β) family, and bind to BMP receptors. BMP4 and BMP7 are involved in urinary tract development. ***BMP4*** encodes a preproprotein that is proteolytically processed to generate each subunit of the disulfide-linked homodimer, BMP4. It is expressed in the mesenchyme adjacent to the mesonephric duct, and is another factor that suppresses ureteric bud outgrowth [30], but mouse models also show that in the metanephric mesenchyme it promotes ureteric branching and promotes growth of the mesenchyme and, in the mesenchyme surrounding the ureter, promotes differentiation into smooth muscle cells. Heterozygous knockout of the gene in the mouse can result variously in ectopic vesicouretric junctions due to ectopic ureteric budding from the mesonephric duct, double collecting systems due to ectopic budding from the ureter, dysplastic kidneys due to reduced ureteric branching and apoptosis of PAX2-positive metanephric mesencyme cells and expansion of FOXD1-positive stromal cells, and megaureter due to reduced smooth muscle actin in the ureter [124, 125].

The same screen mentioned earlier of 250 children with renal hypodysplasia and impaired renal function (excluding patients with VUR but normal kidneys) for *SIX2* mutations, finding three different ones in five children [186], also looked for *BMP4* mutations, and also found 3 different mutations in five children. All of the patients were unrelated, and all of the mutations were mis-sense mutations, and all in the prodomain of *BMP4*, and were not found in 300 control chromosomes (*i.e.* 150 control people). The prodomain of the protein is necessary for forming the active dimer molecules [130]. Two of the children, with different heterozygous mutations, had VUR, both having VUR on one side and renal hypoplasia or dysplasia on the other side. One of the mutations was a *de novo* mutation (not present in either parent), and the other was inherited from the father, who was found to have a normal renal ultrasound. Two of the other patients also had heterozygous mutations, one having unilateral renal aplasia and the other unilateral renal dysplasia (but no VUR).

The fifth child came from a consanguineous family, and had a homozygous mutation and had bilateral cystic dysplasia. The parents of that child were both heterozygous carriers of the mutation but had no urinary tract investigations. In a separate report of another consanguineous family, a child with bilateral cystic renal dysplasia and end-stage renal disease at the age of five, whose parents were double first cousins, was found to have homozygous mutations of both *BMP4* and *DACH1* [156].

BMP7 is expressed in many developing organs, but mutations in the mouse result only in anomalies of the kidneys, eyes and skeleton [81], and it is thought that this may be because compensation by overlapping functions of other members of the BMP family in other sites, such as the notochord, gut and heart [47]. BMP7 is involved in regulation of ureteric bud branching, and maintains the nephron progenitor cell population by inhibiting differentiation [67, 107, 139]. Two related individuals with nonsyndromic urinary tract anomalies were found to have a mis-sense variant in *BMP7*, changing a glutamic acid to a lysine in the protein [71]. One had unilateral hypodysplasia, and the other had unilateral ureterovesical junction obstruction, but so far no mutations of *BMP7* have been found in VUR.

The BMP receptors are a family of transmembrane serine/threonine kinases that include the type I receptors BMPR1A (previously known as ALK3) and BMPR1B and the type II receptor BMPR2. BMPR2 can bind ligand (any of the BMP family) but not pass the signal on into the cell, whereas the type I receptors can signal but not bind ligand, so a combination of either BMPR1A or BMPR1B with BMPR2 is required for function. Whereas BMP4 is expressed in the mesenchyme along beside the mesonephric duct, the receptors are expressed on the surface of the duct, to receive the signal to prevent ectopic budding. Mice homozygous for knock-out of *BMPR1A* show abnormal ureteric bud branching, resulting in dysplastic kidneys [63]. BMP receptors occur in many tissues. Mutations in them have been found in disorder of small pulmonary arteries and in juvenile polyposis coli, but have not been reported in patients with urinary tract anomalies.

GREM1 is an antagonist of BMP4. It was found that *Grem1* knock-out mouse embryos had had no kidneys as well as lung septation defects [119], and the investigators concluded that Grem1-mediated BMP antagonism is essential to induce metanephric kidney development, as initiation of ureter growth, branching, and establishment of RET/GDNF signalling were disrupted in Grem1-deficient embryos. A mathematical model was proposed, suggesting the importance of the opposite effects of BMP and GREM 1on GDNF/RET-GFRA1 signalling in regulating the emergence of the ureteric bud to a single point [106]. Kohl et al. [93] listed *GREM1* amongst six genes in which homozygous truncating mutations cause multi-organ defects including renal agenesis but homozygous nonsynonymous mutations can cause nonsyndromic UTMs, and found such mutation in *GREM1* in a single case of nonsyndromic unilateral renal agenesis, but no nonsyndromic VUR patient has yet been found with *GREM1* mutations, though the gene was included amongst the 208 genes sequenced in 453 UTM cases [132].

The human four *ROBO* receptor and three *SLIT* ligand genes are homologues of single genes in *Drosphila* involved in axon and dendrite guidance in the nervous system, and have evolved various signalling functions in mammals. In the urinary tract, ***ROBO2***, *Roundabout axon guidance receptor 2*, is the receptor for ***SLIT2***, *Slit guidance ligand 2*, in confining the position of ureteric bud emergence, and in the mouse it was shown that inactivation of both copies of either *Slit2* or *Robo2* leads to the emergence of multiple buds [58].

Investigation of a young man who had numerous congenital anomalies, which included grade IV VUR, bilateral ureterovesical junction defects, unilateral megaureter, and had a Y;3 chromosomal translocation, revealed that the translocation had created a fusion between the *ROBO2* gene on Chromosome 3, and the gene *PCDH11Y, protocadherin 11 Y-linked*, whose protein product is thought to play a role in cell-cell recognition during development of the central nervous system [112]. This translocation left a normal copy of *ROBO2* on the other copy of Chromosome 3, but of course no other copy of *PCDH11Y* (there being only one Y chromosome, which was broken). Annotation of the human genome is constantly being revised and updated, and *ROBO2* is currently credited with 34 exons and numerous different transcripts, but at that time, human *ROBO2* was only shown in the genome browsers to have the 26 exons of a transcript now known as *ROBO2b*, (or more completely, 'Roundabout homolog 2, isoform ROBO2b precursor' because the 21 N-terminal amino-acids are later cleaved off proteolytically). Sequencing of all of those exons in 124 British and Dutch families with nonsyndromic VUR with potential autosomal dominant inheritance, reported in the same paper, discovered two different nonsynonymous variants in different families, that were not present in 276 controls, as well as another nonsynonymous variant that was present in three of the control subjects and therefore presumed to be a harmless polymorphism. The investigators also constructed mice with random levels of reduced expression of full-length ROBO2 protein, and the results suggested that reduced gene dosage can cause UTM.

Subsequently other groups have sequenced the exons of the same transcript in cohorts of patients or families with non-syndromic VUR, or cohorts or UTM cases including syndromic ones, and most have found more variants present heterozygously in nonsyndromic VUR patients and absent from controls: (1) four out of 95 patients with nonsyndromic VUR from a small region of Italy (and the polymorphic variant in others) [22]; (2) none in a Swedish study of 54 VUR families (not even the polymorphic one) [195]; (3) Four more new variants in 250 Irish families, but only two segregated with VUR, and one of those was present in one out of 592 controls (who could of course have had VUR as a child without ever knowing it) and the previously-reported polymorphic one [46]; (4) One out of 749 individuals from 650 families with UTMs, in a patient who had bilateral VUR, and three other new variants in patients who did not have VUR but respectively unilateral pelviureteric junction obstruction, posterior ureteric valve, and unilateral multicystic renal dysplasia, and were also nonsyndromic [71]; (5) two more different ones from 134 American families (nearly all white) [48]; (6) None in 103 Greek patients with VUR with or without renal hypodysplasia [122]; (7) Four more different ones (all in single patients in a study of 453 UTM patients) of which two were in patients with unilateral VUR, another with a duplex collecting system and the remaining one in a patient with a multicystic dysplastic kidney [132]; (8) two more different ones in 379 unrelated Chinese VUR patients [111] (see Table 1 for phenotypic details).

Further mouse work was also carried out. Hydronephrosis in Robo2-deficient mice (*i.e.* mice with reduced levels of normal Robo2 protein) was found to be progressive, with no sign of resolution, and was shown to be caused by high-grade VUR resulting from a dilated and incompetent ureterovesical junction rather than ureteric obstruction. The dilation occurred early, and Robo2 was concluded to be essential to the formation of a competent anti-reflux mechanism [184]. *ROBO2* has many different transcripts, encoding a variety of slightly different proteins, and in these transgenic mice, all transcripts would have been equally deficient. Another study used a different method to produce mice with 50% normal expression of the *Robo2* gene (a transposon called 'piggyBac'). The investigators found that the mice had VUR and pelviureteric junction obstruction, and microscopy showed disorganization of the smooth muscle fibres in the ureters, and they comment that this would have little chance of spontaneous resolution [110]. Another mouse study suggested that the mechanism of action of SLIT2-ROBO2 signalling is not to attenuate GDNF expression or activity, but to limit epithelial/mesenchymal interactions in the nascent metanephros and restrict the extent of the nephrogenic field [183].

When we sequenced the Irish cohort referred to above, we found that to that date (in 2013) there were 35 variants reported in *ROBO2* that caused different amino-acid substitutions, some of them common in some populations, and that the predicted pathogenicity of those that had so far been found exclusively in VUR patients did not differ from that predicted for those variants also found in controls. We therefore suggested that though this did not rule out the possibility that some variants might be the sole cause of VUR, it was clear from the overall frequency that most of them could not be, but that it was possible that some of the variants might cause VUR in combination with a mutation in another gene [46]. The continuing discoveries listed above bring the numbers up to at least 49 different nonsynonymous variants, of which 21 have been found exclusively in patients with VUR or other UTMs, and along with the mouse work, it seems certain that some variants can be the sole cause of VUR, but it still may well be that some of the other variants may result in VUR only if present with another mutation in another gene involved in the same developmental process. Indeed of the two mutations found with *ROBO2* variants in VUR patients in one of the studies mentioned above, both patients also had heterozygous variants of other genes, one having a variant in *FAT1* and the other in *NPNT* [132]. So if all the rest of us who sequenced *ROBO2* in patients with VUR or other UTMs had had the money or facility to sequence 207 other renal development genes in the same patients, perhaps we should also have found mutations in other genes in some of those patients. Nicolaou et al. also include a Supplementary Table 5 in which they list particular variants in a number of genes, previously reported in several papers as pathogenic which, on review, they had decided there was insufficient evidence to conclude that they actually are pathogenic. One of the variants listed is one of those reported in a VUR patient in the original paper by Lu et al. mentioned above, though Nicolaou et al. have clearly used the cDNA base and amino-acid numbering from a different transcript of the gene rather than the ROBO2b transcript.

NPNT was described earlier. ***FAT1***, Fat atypical cadherin 1, is the homologue of the *Drosophila* gene *fat*, which encodes a membrane protein which is essential for controlling cell proliferation during *Drosophila* development, and is a vital tumour suppressor in humans. It is expressed at high levels in a number of fetal epithelia and is thought to be involved in cell adhesion or signalling. Its precise role in urinary tract development has yet to be established but it certainly seems to have a role, because in the same series of patients [132], nine others were found to have *FAT1* mutations. Four of them had duplex collecting systems, two renal dysplasia, two pelviureteric junction obstruction, and one with megaureter. All of the mutations were heterozygous, and all were nonsynonymous substitutions except for one, which was a frame-shift mutation very near the end of the gene, where it would be likely to cause less damage. None of these other nine had recorded VUR but two of them also had a mutation in another urinary tract development gene, one in *HGF*, the other in *VANGL2*.

ROBO1 is adjacent to *ROBO2* but in the opposite direction on human chromosome 3p, the result of an ancient inverted duplication. In the sequencing of a panel of 208 genes mentioned earlier, the investigators [132] included *ROBO1*, giving as their reason a 2011 conference report of severe ureteric bud branching and reduced glomerular numbers in mice with double knock-out of *Robo1* and *Robo2*, and in their series of 453 UTM patients, they found three with candidate pathogenic variants in *ROBO1*. All of these were heterozygous and in-frame, one causing an amino-acid deletion, one an amino-acid duplication, and one a substitution. The one with the duplication had a duplex collecting system with VUR, and the others renal dysplasia and a posterior urethral valve respectively.

Subsequently, a study of 56 families in which there had been fetuses with bilateral kidney anomalies, found one family with *ROBO1* mutations [145]. Two pregnancies were terminated because of bilateral renal agenesis and both fetuses were found to have inherited mutations from both parents, one a nonsense mutation near the end of the gene, and the other a nonsynonymous substitution. Examination of the fetuses revealed that they also had genital hypoplasia, hypoplasia of halluces, intestinal malrotation, and anteriorly displaced anus, and one also had agenesis of the corpus callosum. Renal ultrasound of the heterozygous parents was normal and they were not examined further. Prenatal ultrasound of the two live children of the same parents also showed normal kidneys, but sequencing found that one of them also had both mutations, and the other was heterozygous for the nonsense mutation. Review of the young child with both mutations revealed frontal bossing, curled ears, and curled retinal arteries, chronic constipation requiring medication, nocturnal and diurnal enuresis, and delayed motor, social and emotional development, and growth retardation, but the elder child with the heterozygous mutation had no syndromic features and his urinary tract was not examined radiologically, so this family provided no confirmation that heterozygous *ROBO1* mutations could cause less severe, nonsyndromic UTM.

A more recent study in which deliberate search of databases for subjects with mutations of both copies of *ROBO1*, after the finding of two mutations in a syndromic UTM patient [128] has published a total of eight syndromic cases, but also did not look at or for nonsyndromic UTM patients with single heterozygous mutations in the gene. More animal work is also required to determine the exact role that *ROBO1* plays in urinary tract development.

Three different nonsynonymous coding variants in *SLIT2* have been found heterozygously each in one nonsyndromic patient in the same study of 379 unrelated Chinese VUR patients mentioned above [111] and three other mutations were previously found in patients with other nonsyndromic UTMs (bilateral subcortical cysts, unilateral multicystic renal dysplasia, and unilateral renal agenesis, respectively) who did not have VUR [72]. Two other genes whose products have also been found to act with ROBO2 and SLIT2 in regulating ureteric bud emergence are *SRGAP1*, whose product is SLIT-ROBO Rho GTPase activating protein 1, in which mutations have been found in patients with UTM but not so far in a VUR patient [72] and *Gen1*, investigated in the mouse [109] and again not so far found mutated in human VUR patients.

The renin-angiotensin-aldosterone system is well known for blood-pressure control, hence the name 'angiotensin', but signalling between angiotensin and its receptors is not only a trigger for secretion of aldosterone by the adrenal cortex, but is also involved in other processes, including urinary tract development. The product of the gene ***AGT***, is Angiotensinogen. (It is also absurdly known as pre-angiotensinogen, and as angiotensinogen precursor, but as its proper name, angiotensinogen implies, it is the precursor of angiotensin). It is produced in the liver, and is cleaved by the renal enzyme Renin (of which the gene is *REN*) to produce Angiotensin I, which is then further cleaved, by, Angiotensin Converting Enzyme (ACE), to produce the physiologically-active 'hormone'/signalling ligand Angiotensin II, which is only an octapeptide after these two cleavages. It has two receptors, types 1 and 2, of which the genes are *AGTR1* and *AGTR2*. The type 1 receptor occurs in many cell types, including those of the cardiovascular system, kidney, adrenal glands, pituitary, and central nervous system, whereas the type 2 receptor is mainly expressed in fetal tissues and neonates, and falls to much lower levels in adulthood, except in the brain, the adrenal medulla, and the atretic ovary.

Because it was known that a surge of renin-angiotensin release occurs when there is a mechanical hindrance to urine outflow, the effects of complete knock-out of either of the two angiotensin II receptors was investigated in mice, and it was found that both strains of mice displayed varying degrees of urinary tract obstruction [143]. In *Agtr2*-negative mice, obstructions developed early in embryonic urinary tract development, and in *Agtr1*-negative mice, during late development after birth. The conclusions of investigations were that signalling via a functioning Agtr2 acts to prevent obstruction of the growing ureter by causing removal (by apoptosis) of undifferentiated mesenchymal cells surrounding the ureteric bud and growing ureter, and that signalling via Agtr1 acts to promote the development of the renal pelvis when urine flow increases after birth.

The gene for the Angiotensin II receptor type 2 (***AGTR2***) is on the X-chromosome in both mice and humans, so the effect of its inactivation or mutation was studied mainly in males because of random X-inactivation in females. Targeted inactivation of the gene in the mouse was found to result in nonsyndromic VUR in a high proportion of offspring, and a range of other non-syndromic UTM phenotypes in a smaller proportion [134]. It was also found that Agtr2 is expressed in the undifferentiated mesenchymal cells surrounding the mesonephric duct and ureteric bud but not, initially, in the metanephric mesenchyme, and that in wild-type mice,

Angiotensin II causes apoptosis of undifferentiated mesenchymal cells that surround the mesonephric duct and ureteric bud, but that in the Agtr2 negative mice—that would go on to develop UTMs—this apoptosis was much reduced. Study of two small groups of human patients with UTM phenotypes, published in the same paper, found that a very common polymorphism in Intron 1 of the gene, that tends to cause Exon 2 to be spliced out of the mRNA, was much more common in the UTM patients than in controls.

Subsequently, 23 out of 470 mice with complete knock-out of *Agtr2* (3.1%) were found to have urinary tract malformations, of which the most common finding was duplex systems with hydronephrosis of the upper pole, and the investigators concluded that although not the sole regulator, angiotensin II type 2 receptor (which the investigators [137] mistakenly call 'angiotensin type II receptor') expression may have a role in the embryological development of the urinary tract by inhibiting aberrant ureteric budding. Presumably the reason for the low penetrance of the effect of *Agtr2* knock-out is that usually the other inhibitory mechanisms (two of which have already been discussed above) are sufficient, and anomalies perhaps only occur if one or more of these other mechanisms also has a defect. Redundancy—the existence of multiple back-up systems—is the principal reason that living organisms manage to survive. After the ureteric bud has entered the metanephric mesenchyme, AGTR2 is expressed by the mesenchyme cells and is involved in regulation of ureteric branching within the developing kidney [167].

In humans, mutations of *AGTR2* have been found several times in nonnsyndromic mental deficiency, but as far as the urinary tract is concerned, only one mutation, a heterozygous nonsynonymous substitution predicted as probably damaging, in a single patient with a unilateral duplex collecting system, has ever been reported [132]. Mutations have been found in *AGT* and in *AGTR1* in one case each of non-syndromic VUR, and in *AGT* in single cases of ureteropelvic junction obstruction, duplex collecting system, renal dysplasia, and renal aplasia, all unilateral, and in *AGTR1* of a single case of unilateral renal aplasia [132]. These mutations were all heterozygous nonsynonymous mutations. Bi-allelic mutations (homozygous or compound heterozygous) in either of these genes, or of the genes of the cleavage enzymes, *REN* or *ACE*, cause renal tubular dysgenesis [51]. *AGT* and *AGTR1* were each found to be mutated in one out of 100 fetuses with severe renal disorders [85]. Both pregnancies had had anhydramnios and the fetuses had dysplastic or small kidneys, and the one with *AGT* mutation also had hypocalvarium, and the other had a large fontanelle and died of lung hypoplasia. In these cases, the mutations were truncation mutations in both copies of the respective gene.

Sprouty1 (**SPRY1**) is one of a family of four receptor tyrosine kinase antagonists. Tyrosine kinases are enzymes that phosphorylate tyrosine amino acids within proteins, and this phosphorylation activates the receptor proteins, which otherwise do not signal. By being tyrosine kinase antagonists, sprouty proteins curb the exuberance of processes initiated and stimulated by such signalling by the interaction of growth factors with the receptors. However, the sprouty proteins also are only active if they too are phosphorylated, and in the case of SPRY1, it is a tyrosine at position 53 that has to be phosphorylated [62].

In mice, Spry1 it has been found not only to be involved in regulating ureteric bud outgrowth and branching, but branching of the blood vessels, the bronchi, and the mammary gland ducts, and to be involved in erythropoesis and development of external genitalia, the skull, the temporo-mandibular joint, eyelid closure, and epibranchial ganglia. Relevant to the urinary tract story, mouse embryos with homozygous knock-out of *Spry1* were found to have supernumerary ureteric buds, resulting in the development of multiple ureters and multiplex kidneys [17]. These defects were found to be due to increased sensitivity of the mesonephric duct to GDNF/RET signalling because reducing *Gdnf* gene dosage—by making *Gdnf* heterozygous negative—in *Spry1*-null embryos, saved this effect from occurring in about 75% of the mice. The authors therefore concluded that Spry1 down-regulates GDNF/RET signalling in the mesonephric duct, ensuring that kidney induction is restricted to a single site. It also regulates the amount of bud branching within the developing kidney [194]. No human VUR or other UTM patients have been found to have SPRY1 mutations so far. However, this is not the end of the story.

FGF10, *Fibroblast growth factor 10*, is one of a large family of genes. Numbers vary considerably in metazoa. Humans have 22, numbered 1-23 except 15. Most of their products are ligands for a family of four receptors FGFR1-4. Human FGF10 does not actually stimulate replication of fibroblasts, but is required for embryonic epidermal morphogenesis (and is also involved in wound healing). It has been revealed that FGF10 can initiate normal urinary tract development in the absence of GDNF/RET+GFRA1 signalling as long as ureteric bud outgrowth is not inhibited by SPRY1.

Tyrosine 1062 of mouse Ret is a binding site for several adaptor and effector proteins involved in signalling, and mice lacking Ret tyrosine 1062 nearly mimic the phenotype of Ret-knockout mice, which includes renal agenesis. However, knock-out of Sprouty1 in these mice was found to 'rescue' the renal agenesis and early postnatal lethality caused by lack of Ret tyrosine 1062. The kidneys and lower urinary tracts of the double-mutant mice developed normally [149]. This indicates that Gdnf/Ret+Gfra1 signalling is not the only final common path to ureteric bud outgrowth and thereby to the whole of metanephric urinary tract development. The renal agenesis that results from lack of Gdnf/Ret+Gfra1 signalling is seen actually to be caused by unopposed inhibition of ureteric bud outgrowth by Sprouty1, which means that in the absence of this inhibition, something else is stimulating ureteric bud outgrowth. This effect was specific to the urinary system, because loss of Sprouty1 did not rescue the Hirschsprung aspect of the phenotype, and the mice died within a week of birth [149].

Mice with homozygous knock-out of *Gdnf* and *Spry1* were found to develop normal metanephric urinary systems just like mice with homozygous knock-out of *Ret* and *Spry1*, and the signal taking over from the missing Gdnf/Ret+Gfra1 signalling was shown to be Fgf10 (which normally plays a minor role), as removal of even one copy of *Fgf10* in *Gdnf−/−;Spry*1−/− mutants caused complete failure of ureter and kidney development [120]. One would not expect to find *FGF10* mutations in human patients with VUR or other UTMs, because normally ureteric bud outgrowth is induced by GDNF/RET+GFRA1 signalling, but a mutation in ***FGF8*** has been found in a patient with nonsyndromic bilateral VUR [132], suggesting that this molecule can be yet another substitute. Mutation of *FGF8* had previously been reported in deficiency of gonadotropin-releasing hormone [50]. In the same study mentioned above [132], a mutation was also found in *FGF1* in a patient with a unilateral duplex collecting system without recorded VUR, and mutations were found in the genes of two of the FGF receptors: one in *FGFR1* in a patient with unilateral pelviureteric junction obstruction and one in *FGFR2* in a patient with unilateral multicystic renal dysplasia. In another study, a heterozygous nonsynonymous variant in ***FGFR1*** has also been found in one patient with nonsyndromic VUR [177], though other mutations in this gene can cause Kallmann Syndrome. This is not the last mention of *SPRY1* nor of *FGF10*; they will be mentioned again in relation to other genes.

Extracellular Matrix Genes

The three proteins FRAS1 (Fraser extracellular matrix complex subunit 1), FREM1 (once known as QBRICK) and FREM 2 (FRAS1 related extracellular matrix 1 and 2), produced by genes of the same names, form a protein complex lining the extracellular epithelial-mesenchymal interface, and function in the regulation of epidermal-basement membrane adhesion and organogenesis during development [92, 141]. GRIP1 (Glutamate receptor-interacting protein 1) is a scaffold protein that interacts with FRAS1 and is required for its localization to the basal side of cells [169]. Homozygous truncating mutations of any of the four genes, *FRAS1*, *FREM1*, *FREM2* or *GRIP1* cause Fraser Syndrome [77, 92, 116, 166, 169], whose most common features include subepidermal heamorrhagic blisters, cryptophthalmos, syndactyly, renal agenesis (unilateral or bilateral), genital anomalies and respiratory tract anomalies, but a wide range of other features may occur in smaller proportions of cases. Specific bi-allelic truncating or deletion mutations of *FREM1* can also cause Bifid Nose with or without Anorectal and Renal anomalies (BNAR) Syndrome, Manitoba oculotrichoanal (MOTA) Syndrome, or congenital diaphragmatic hernia [20]. However, homozygous *mis-sense* mutations of any of the same four genes can cause isolated (*i.e.* nonsyndromic) UTM of various types [93, 132], and so far these have included nonsyndromic VUR in all but *GRIP1* mutations.

Experiments with mice have shown that the reason for the urinary tract anomalies in Fraser and related syndromes caused by lack of the FRAS1-FREM1-FREM2 extracellular matrix complex, is that without this complex, the metanephric mesenchyme fails to receive enough stimulation to secrete sufficient GDNF to induce normal ureteric bud outgrowth and branching. 'Blebbed' is a mouse model of Fraser syndrome, in which the mice have a lack of function of *Fras1* due to a premature stop codon. It was found that reduction of Spry1 protein (that opposes the action of Gdnf) by introducing a null mutation into one copy of the *Spry1* gene in blebbed mice abolished renal agenesis, and null mutation of both copies of Spry1 resulted in duplex kidneys due to lack of opposition to the Gdnf that was produced. Also, application of Fgf10 (which substitutes for Gdnf) to blebbed mouse tissue with normal

Spry1 expression in culture induced kidney formation. However, these interventions to alleviate the failure of normal Gdnf/Ret signalling between the ureteric bud and metanephric mesenchyme due to lack of the extracellular matrix complex did not, of course, abolish the other phenotypic consequences of the missing extracellular matrix [142].

A heterozygous nonsynonymous mutation of another gene, ***TNXB***, encoding an extracellular matrix protein, Tenascin XB, was identified as the cause of nonsyndromic VUR and/or duplex collecting systems in a 97-member family with cases going back at least five generations [54], and the investigators then found other variants in this gene in six other VUR families [48, 54]. Mutations in *TNXB* were first found in some patients with a recessive form of Ehlers-Danlos Syndrome [33, 155], a group of 13 disorders, some showing dominant and some recessive inheritance, in which there is skin hyperextensibility and fragility, joint hypermobility, with proneness to dislocation of large joints, degenerative joint disease, and many other possible features including mitral valve prolapse, and rectal and uterine prolapse, and subsequently about half of heterozygous family members had been found to have isolated joint hypermobility [196].

VUR was first reported in Ehlers-Danlos Syndrome in 1995 [55]. As we now know, mutation of more than nineteen different genes can cause forms of Ehlers-Danlos Syndrome, and the causative gene was not identified in that patient, but the authors suggested that laxity of connective tissue had resulted in incompetence of the vesicoureteric junction. Gbadegesin and colleagues formed the same conclusion after finding that TNXB is normally expressed in the ureterovesical junction, and that fibroblast cell lines isolated from one of their affected individuals displayed reduced cell motility in response to platelet-derived growth factor and reduced expression of phosphorylated focal adhesion kinase [54]. However, they neglected to mention that this couldn't possibly explain the duplex collecting systems in five out of the nine members of their index family with the mutation whom they examined. Clearly TNXB must play a role in restricting the position of emergence of the ureteric bud, presumably by taking part in negative signalling.

It had previously been found that joint hypermobility is significantly more common in VUR patients than in the general population [178] and was subsequently found that VUR is very common (60%) in children with benign joint hypermobility 'syndrome' [21]. More recently, it was found that only 2/27 children with VUR and joint hypermobility had mutations in *TNXB*, while the other 5 out of the 49 DNA-tested children in the VUR cohort examined who also had *TNXB* mutations did not have joint hypermobility [173]. The investigators concluded that the association between VUR and joint hypermobility might be due to mutations in other extracellular matrix genes. However, joint hypermobility does not seem to have been reported in Fraser Syndrome, caused, as related above, by homozygous mutations in any of a group of genes producing extracellular matrix proteins, and the first cohort examined for *TNXB* mutations was also screened for mutations in the gene of another tenascin, Tenascin C (TNC), and no mutations were found [48].

The *TNXB* mutations in the first two VUR families reported to have them [54] had never been found before, in population surveys nor in Ehlers-Danlos Syndrome.

In one of the next five families or non-familial cases [48] two variants were found in the same *TNXB* allele. One was novel, but the other was present in the polymorphism database, dbSNP, as were the four variants found in *TNXB* in the other two families and two non-familial cases. However, none of these variants was present in the at least 200 ethnicity-matched controls, and all had low or fairly low allele frequencies in dbSNP and were predicted to be damaging by at least one *in silico* prediction program. All eight variants found were heterozygous and nonsynonymous. All of the seven *TNXB* variants judged to be potentially pathogenic in the other cohort mentioned above [173] were different from these, and two of them were intronic variants predicted to have an effect on mRNA splicing. Five further variants were found in the previously mentioned survey of 379 unrelated Chinese VUR patients [111], and two of them were frame-shift mutations, one a 17-base-pair insertion and the other a ten-base-pair deletion, both in exon 3 out of 44 exons. It is a great pity that TNXB was not included amongst the 208 genes sequenced in 453 UTM patients by Nicolaou et al., referred to many times above in relation to other genes.

The Lining of the Urothelium

The plaques which form a layer known as the asymmetric unit membrane on the luminal surface of the umbrella cells of the urothelium are composed of four types of uroplakins, UPK1A, 1B, 2 and 3A (previously known as Ia, Ib, II and IIIa) [78, 82]. There is another, UPK3B, which appears early on in development, but does not appear to play a major role in the fully-developed urothelium. The uroplakins are transmembrane proteins that pass through the lipid bilayer of the cell membrane once in the case of UPK2, UPK3A, and UPK3B, or four times in the case of UPK1A and UPK1B. All have large extracellular domains, but only UPK3A and UPK3B have significant cytoplasmic portions in their C-termini. The proteins form heterodimers, 1A with 2, and 1B with 3A or 3B, and the proteins cannot reach the cell surface unless the dimers form. In the absence of the appropriate partner, UPK1A, 2 and 3A cannot escape the endoplasmic reticulum, and UPK1B is mistargeted to the basolateral membrane of the cells. The heterodimers 'crystalize' to form plaques composed of an inner ring of 1A/2 and an outer ring of 1B/3A dimers. It might perhaps not be expected that disorder of the specialised lining of the urinary tract would cause mechanical failure of the vesicoureteric junction, but deletion in mice of either *Upk2* [97] or *Upk3a* or both [68] was found to result in severe VUR, hydronephrosis and impaired renal function. Mutations in the same two human uroplakin genes have been found in a few patients with VUR.

A heterozygous frameshift mutation in *UPK2* which, if expressed, would generate a truncated protein, was found in a child and mother [83]. The child presented with VUR, nephropathy and renal failure. The mother had not been investigated for

VUR in her own childhood, and had a normal renal ultrasound result, but the genetic variant was not found in 150 controls of the same ethnicity. The authors concluded that their study offered no definitive support for *UPK2* mutations causing human urinary tract malformations, but that in rare patients, such variants might be implicated in pathogenesis when acting in conjunction with other yet-to-be-defined, genetic or environmental modifying factors.

The same investigators found mutations in *UPK3A* in four out of 17 children with renal dysplasia and/or unilateral aplasia and renal failure without overt evidence of urinary obstruction, two of whom, from unrelated families, had VUR [82]. In all four children, the mutations were *de novo* (not present in the parents). The two with VUR, a boy and a girl (who also had persistent cloaca), had the same coding mutation at a CpG site (this means a cytosine followed by a guanine on the same DNA strand, not a C·G pair; CpG sites are prone to mutation) in the cytoplasmic domain, replacing a hydrophilic proline with a highly hydrophobic leucine in the protein, whereas the other two, without VUR, had different non-coding mutations in the 3′-untranslated region of the gene.

De novo mutations are rare events—we each have on average about 70 such mutations in the over 6000 million bases of our two copies of the genome—so nearly all cases of common inherited diseases (and VUR is very common on that scale) are caused by genetic variants passed on from one or both parents. The variant in these two children therefore represents a very rare cause of VUR. Dominant mutations causing conditions in which children seldom reach adulthood, or are seldom able to procreate if they do reach adulthood, are necessarily nearly all *de novo* mutations, which is why such conditions are rare. Renal failure in early childhood falls at least into the edge of this category, which is why it is not a surprise to find these mutations in this group, and one would not expect to find the one mutation that caused VUR, in familial VUR cases.

Another research group [157], investigating a cohort of 170 children with severe bilateral or unilateral renal hypodysplasia, found one with unilateral multicystic dysplasia and VUR who had another mis-sense mutation in *UPK3A*, which was also *de novo*. Nicolaou et al. [132] included all five uroplakin genes in their screening of 453 UTM patients. They found a heterozygous splice-site mutation in *UPK2* (which probably resulted in a lack of protein from that copy of the gene) in one patient with a duplex collecting system, and mutations in *UPK3A* in three patients. One of these patients had unilateral renal dysplasia and a heterozygous nonsense mutation. The other two patients had the same variant, a 5 bp deletion, causing a frame-shift of course, but the deletion began in codon 235 and the change of reading frame did not cause a stop codon till 41 new codons further on, and the normal length of the protein is 278 amino acids, so the mutant protein was almost the same length as the normal protein, but the last 41 amino-acids were different. One of the patients had pelviureteric junction obstruction and the variant was heterozygous, but in the other patient, who had a duplex collecting system, the variant was homozygous.

Other Genes

HNF1B (Hepatocyte nuclear factor homeobox 1B), which has numerous previous names including *TCF2* and *MODY5*, encodes a transcription factor that forms a homodimer and can also form a heterodimer with HNF1A. *HNF1B* is involved in the development of a number of organs including the kidneys and the pancreas, and mutations can cause a wide variety of phenotypic features of which a syndrome of cystic kidneys plus diabetes is best known. Though the gene's exact involvement in the development of the lower urinary tract does not seem to have been investigated, cases of VUR with *HNF1B* mutations have been reported by a number of teams: (1) In a cohort of 99 unrelated patients with renal hypodysplasia, eight were found to have *HNF1B* mutations, of whom two had nonsyndromic VUR [185]. Though unrelated, they both had the same nonsynonymous mutation in the activation domain. One had bilateral cystic dysplasia, ectopy and horseshoe fusion, but the carrier father had normal kidneys. The other had bilateral renal hypoplasia and the parents' DNA was not sequenced. (2) Three cases of VUR were reported amongst 75 patients with heterozygous *HNF1B* mutations, one with a complete deletion of the gene and bilateral hyperechogenic kidneys but no diabetes or other anomalies, and two with frame-shift mutations, one of whom had unilateral multicystic dysplastic kidney and chronic renal failure at 4 years of age but no other anomalies and no diabetes at the time, and the other having renal cysts and a normal GFR and no diabetes at 6 years old, while the mother, with the same mutation, had unilateral renal cysts and a normal GFR at 30 years, and no VUR, but gestational diabetes [64]. (3) In the study of 749 patients with UTM phenotypes from 650 families mentioned earlier [71], six were found to have *HNF1B* mutations, three of whom had nonsyndromic VUR, one with no other anomaly, one with a neurogenic bladder, and one with a posterior urethral valve. All of them had heterozygous nonsynonymous mutations. (4) one patient with bilateral VUR and unilateral renal hypodysplasia out of the 379 unrelated Chinese VUR patients of a study also referred to in relation to other genes [111].

Some other genes in which rare variants have been found in at least one patient with VUR but which there has not been time to explore in this account are included in Table 1, but probably there have been more published which there has not been time to find, in papers not seen or in supplementary data online that there has not been time to comb.

Concluding Remarks

The quest for the genetic causes of nonsyndromic VUR has been, and continues to be, a long and complicated one. What we have learnt so far, is that, of all the genes that are involved in development of the urinary tract, a list that is already well over 200 genes and still climbing, there are many in which some mutations can cause nonsyndromic VUR, though other mutations have more severe effects. We have also seen that the same mutation that causes VUR alone in one patient may cause a different UTM or both in another family member. We have also seen that the mutations that cause VUR are in general less damaging than ones that cause more severe phenotypes. Most of them are either nonsynonymous variants that result in a slightly altered but full-length protein, or are truncating mutations that only shorten the protein a little and do not interfere with any essential domain.

Most genes contain some polymorphic variants in their coding sequences, and some of these alter amino-acids without apparent ill effect, but it is quite possible that some of these, and other rare variants that are predicted not to be damaging, because the amino-acid substituted is similar, may have hypomorphic effects that become pathogenic when combined with another hypomorphic variant in an interacting protein. For instance, a variant in a receptor protein might alter its shape very slightly, yet it can still bind its ligand sufficiently to transmit an effective signal, but perhaps if there is also a hypomorphic variant in the ligand, that changes it just a little, but still allows it to bind to a normal receptor, the slightly altered ligand might not bind the slightly altered receptor, or not sufficiently to transmit a signal. The same might apply to variants in the protein-protein interaction domains of two different proteins, transcription factors perhaps, that have to form a heterodimer with one-another in order to bind to their target DNA sequence.

However, what we have also found is that we have accounted for a small proportion of nonsyndromic VUR cases so far, and though we shall no doubt find more variants in the same genes and in other genes in a few more VUR patients, it still seems likely to this author, as it has done for years, that the answers are not all in the genes. People go on investigating genes, because it's easy to spot a pathogenic variant in a coding sequence, and after that in a splice site, and at least a variant in a 5′ or 3′ untranslated region of the mRNA sequence can be recognised, and its effect can be investigated in the lab with a bit of effort. However, out in the great ocean of noncoding DNA there are millions of variants, and it is much harder to spot potentially pathogenic ones, and harder to prove that they *are* pathogenic if you can identify them, but probably that is what we are going to have to achieve before we eventually have an almost complete picture of the aetiology of nonsyndromic VUR. And of course there may be all sorts of environmental effects, such as a slight vitamin A deficiency perhaps, that might cause VUR without having any more serious effect. There is still a lot to learn—but science is fun!

What we need is a large cohort of nonsyndromic VUR patients, or preferably families with two or more members so affected, and to sequence their whole genomes, preferably with long-read sequencing technology, and to assemble their genomes *de novo* from overlapping the reads, rather than matching them to a reference sequence, and then to find in a first analysis how many can be found with reliable diagnostic variants—probably quite a small proportion—and then to keep the genome sequences as a resource for constant referral, as knowledge grows and more regulatory sequences and hypomorphic variants are investigated, until at last most of the cases are solved.

I apologise for all the information that I have undoubtedly left out, and to the authors of papers who might reasonably have expected to have been quoted but have not been. The literature is massive and goes on growing.

References

1. Abdelhak S, Kalatzis V, Heilig R, Compain S, Samson D, Vincent C, Levi-Acobas F, Cruaud C, Le Merrer M, Mathieu M, Konig R, Vigneron J, Weissenbach J, Petit C, Weil D. Clustering of mutations responsible for branchio-oto-renal (BOR) syndrome in the eyes absent homologous region (eyaHR) of EYA1. Hum Mol Genet. 1997;6:2247–55.
2. Abdelhak S, Kalatzis V, Heilig R, Compain S, Samson D, Vincent C, Weil D, Cruaud C, Sahly I, Leibovici M, Bitner-Glindzicz M, Francis M, Lacombe D, Vigneron J, Charachon R, Boven K, Bedbeder P, Van Regemorter N, Weissenbach J, Petit C. A human homologue of the Drosophila eyes absent gene underlies branchio-oto-renal (BOR) syndrome and identifies a novel gene family. Nat Genet. 1997;15:157–64.
3. Abramovich DR. The volume of amniotic fluid in early pregnancy. J Obstet Gynaecol Br Commonw. 1968;75:728–31.
4. Al-Hamed MH, Altuwaijri N, Alsahan N, Ali W, Abdulwahab F, Alzahrani F, Majrashi N, Alkuraya FS. A null founder variant in NPNT, encoding nephronectin, causes autosomal recessive renal agenesis. Clin Genet. 2022;102:61–5.
5. Al-Shamsi B, Al-Kasbi G, Al-Kindi A, Bruwer Z, Al-Kharusi K, Al-Maawali A. Biallelic loss-of-function variants of GFRA1 cause lethal bilateral renal agenesis. Eur J Med Genet. 2022;65:104376.
6. Almubarak A, Lavy R, Srnic N, Hu Y, Maripuri DP, Kume T, Berry FB. Loss of Foxc1 and Foxc2 function in chondroprogenitor cells disrupts endochondral ossification. J Biol Chem. 2021;297:101020.
7. Andijani AA, Shajira ES, Abushaheen A, Al-Matary A. Microphthalmia Syndrome 9: case report of a newborn baby with pulmonary hypoplasia, diaphragmatic Eventration, Microphthalmia, cardiac defect and severe primary pulmonary hypertension. Am J Case Rep. 2019;20:354–60.
8. Arena S, Fazzari C, Arena F, Scuderi MG, Romeo C, Nicotina PA, Di Benedetto V. Altered 'active' antireflux mechanism in primary vesico-ureteric reflux: a morphological and manometric study. BJU Int. 2007;100:407–12.
9. Arora V, Khan S, A WE-H, Dua Puri R, Rocha ME, Merdzanic R, Paknia O, Beetz C, Rolfs A, Bertoli-Avella AM, Bauer P, Verma IC. Biallelic pathogenic GFRA1 variants cause autosomal recessive bilateral renal agenesis. J Am Soc Nephrol. 2021;32:223–8.
10. Azuma N, Hirakiyama A, Inoue T, Asaka A, Yamada M. Mutations of a human homologue of the Drosophila eyes absent gene (EYA1) detected in patients with congenital cataracts and ocular anterior segment anomalies. Hum Mol Genet. 2000;9:363–6.
11. Baker LA, Gomez RA. Embryonic development of the ureter and bladder: acquisition of smooth muscle. J Urol. 1998;160:545–50.
12. Balikci Ö, Turunc T, Bal N, Celik H, Ozkardes H. Comparison of Cajal-like cells in pelvis and proximal ureter of kidney with and without hydronephrosis. Int Braz J Urol. 2015;41:1178–84.
13. Barakat AJ, Raygada M, Rennert OM. Barakat syndrome revisited. Am J Med Genet A. 2018;176:1341–8.
14. Barakat AY, D'Albora JB, Martin MM, Jose PA. Familial nephrosis, nerve deafness, and hypoparathyroidism. J Pediatr. 1977;91:61–4.

15. Bardakjian TM, Schneider AS, Ng D, Johnston JJ, Biesecker LG. Association of a de novo 16q copy number variant with a phenotype that overlaps with Lenz microphthalmia and Townes-Brocks syndromes. BMC Med Genet. 2009;10:137.
16. Bartik ZI, Sillen U, Djos A, Lindholm A, Fransson S. Whole exome sequencing identifies KIF26B, LIFR and LAMC1 mutations in familial vesicoureteral reflux. PLoS One. 2022;17:e0277524.
17. Basson MA, Akbulut S, Watson-Johnson J, Simon R, Carroll TJ, Shakya R, Gross I, Martin GR, Lufkin T, McMahon AP, Wilson PD, Costantini FD, Mason IJ, Licht JD. Sprouty1 is a critical regulator of GDNF/RET-mediated kidney induction. Dev Cell. 2005;8:229–39.
18. Batourina E, Choi C, Paragas N, Bello N, Hensle T, Costantini FD, Schuchardt A, Bacallao RL, Mendelsohn CL. Distal ureter morphogenesis depends on epithelial cell remodeling mediated by vitamin A and Ret. Nat Genet. 2002;32:109–15.
19. Batourina E, Tsai S, Lambert S, Sprenkle P, Viana R, Dutta S, Hensle T, Wang F, Niederreither K, McMahon AP, Carroll TJ, Mendelsohn CL. Apoptosis induced by vitamin A signaling is crucial for connecting the ureters to the bladder. Nat Genet. 2005;37:1082–9.
20. Beck TF, Veenma D, Shchelochkov OA, Yu Z, Kim BJ, Zaveri HP, van Bever Y, Choi S, Douben H, Bertin TK, Patel PI, Lee B, Tibboel D, de Klein A, Stockton DW, Justice MJ, Scott DA. Deficiency of FRAS1-related extracellular matrix 1 (FREM1) causes congenital diaphragmatic hernia in humans and mice. Hum Mol Genet. 2013;22:1026–38.
21. Beiraghdar F, Rostami Z, Panahi Y, Einollahi B, Teimoori M. Vesicourethral reflux in pediatrics with hypermobility syndrome. Nephrourol Mon. 2013;5:924–7.
22. Bertoli-Avella AM, Conte ML, Punzo F, de Graaf BM, Lama G, La Manna A, Polito C, Grassia C, Nobili B, Rambaldi PF, Oostra BA, Perrotta S. ROBO2 gene variants are associated with familial vesicoureteral reflux. J Am Soc Nephrol. 2008;19:825–31.
23. Bhattarai C, Poudel PP, Ghosh A, Kalthur SG. The RET gene encodes RET protein, which triggers intracellular signaling pathways for enteric neurogenesis, and RET mutation results in Hirschsprung's disease. AIMS Neurosci. 2022;9:128–49.
24. Borozdin W, Steinmann K, Albrecht B, Bottani A, Devriendt K, Leipoldt M, Kohlhase J. Detection of heterozygous SALL1 deletions by quantitative real time PCR proves the contribution of a SALL1 dosage effect in the pathogenesis of Townes-Brocks syndrome. Hum Mutat. 2006;27:211–2.
25. Botzenhart EM, Bartalini G, Blair E, Brady AF, Elmslie F, Chong KL, Christy K, Torres-Martinez W, Danesino C, Deardorff MA, Fryns JP, Marlin S, Garcia-Minaur S, Hellenbroich Y, Hay BN, Penttinen M, Shashi V, Terhal P, Van Maldergem L, Whiteford ML, Zackai E, Kohlhase J. Townes-Brocks syndrome: twenty novel SALL1 mutations in sporadic and familial cases and refinement of the SALL1 hot spot region. Hum Mutat. 2007;28:204–5.
26. Boualia SK, Gaitan Y, Murawski I, Nadon R, Gupta IR, Bouchard M. Vesicoureteral reflux and other urinary tract malformations in mice compound heterozygous for Pax2 and Emx2. PLoS One. 2011;6:e21529.
27. Boualia SK, Gaitan Y, Tremblay M, Sharma R, Cardin J, Kania A, Bouchard M. A core transcriptional network composed of Pax2/8, Gata3 and Lim1 regulates key players of pro/mesonephros morphogenesis. Dev Biol. 2013;382:555–66.
28. Brandenberger R, Schmidt A, Linton J, Wang D, Backus C, Denda S, Muller U, Reichardt LF. Identification and characterization of a novel extracellular matrix protein nephronectin that is associated with integrin alpha8beta1 in the embryonic kidney. J Cell Biol. 2001;154:447–58.
29. Bridgewater D, Cox B, Cain J, Lau A, Athaide V, Gill PS, Kuure S, Sainio K, Rosenblum ND. Canonical WNT/beta-catenin signaling is required for ureteric branching. Dev Biol. 2008;317:83–94.
30. Brophy PD, Ostrom L, Lang KM, Dressler GR. Regulation of ureteric bud outgrowth by Pax2-dependent activation of the glial derived neurotrophic factor gene. Development. 2001;128:4747–56.

31. Brophy PD, Rasmussen M, Parida M, Bonde G, Darbro BW, Hong X, Clarke JC, Peterson KA, Denegre J, Schneider M, Sussman CR, Sunde L, Lildballe DL, Hertz JM, Cornell RA, Murray SA, Manak JR. A gene implicated in activation of retinoic acid receptor targets is a novel renal agenesis gene in humans. Genetics. 2017;207:215–28.
32. Buller C, Xu X, Marquis V, Schwanke R, Xu PX. Molecular effects of Eya1 domain mutations causing organ defects in BOR syndrome. Hum Mol Genet. 2001;10:2775–81.
33. Burch GH, Gong Y, Liu W, Dettman RW, Curry CJ, Smith L, Miller WL, Bristow J. Tenascin-X deficiency is associated with Ehlers-Danlos syndrome. Nat Genet. 1997;17:104–8.
34. Chatterjee R, Ramos E, Hoffman M, VanWinkle J, Martin DR, Davis TK, Hoshi M, Hmiel SP, Beck A, Hruska K, Coplen D, Liapis H, Mitra R, Druley T, Austin P, Jain S. Traditional and targeted exome sequencing reveals common, rare and novel functional deleterious variants in RET-signaling complex in a cohort of living US patients with urinary tract malformations. Hum Genet. 2012;131:1725–38.
35. Chen CH, Kraemer BR, Lee L, Mochly-Rosen D. Annotation of 1350 common genetic variants of the 19 ALDH multigene family from global human genome aggregation database (gnomAD). Biomolecules. 2021;11:1423.
36. Chen J, Van Der Ven AT, Newman JA, Vivante A, Mann N, Aitkenhead H, Shril S, Ityel H, Schulz J, Schmidt JM, Widmeier E, Gileadi O, Costantini F, Thowfeequ S, Wenger RH, Bauer SB, Lee RS, Lu W, Getwan M, Kaminski MM, Lienkamp SS, Lifton RP, Tasic V, Kehinde EO, FH. ETV4 mutation in a patient with congenital anomalies of the kidney and urinary tract. Int J Pediatr Child Health. 2016;4:61–71.
37. Chia I, Grote D, Marcotte M, Batourina E, Mendelsohn C, Bouchard M. Nephric duct insertion is a crucial step in urinary tract maturation that is regulated by a Gata3-Raldh2-Ret molecular network in mice. Development. 2011;138:2089–97.
38. Cicerone AP, Dailey W, Sun M, Santos A, Jeong D, Jones L, Koustas K, Drekh M, Schmitz K, Haque N, Felisky JA, Guzman AE, Mellert K, Trese MT, Capone A, Drenser KA, Mitton KP. A survey of multigenic protein-altering variant frequency in Familial Exudative Vitreo-Retinopathy (FEVR) patients by targeted sequencing of seven FEVR-linked genes. Genes (Basel). 2022;13:495.
39. Costantini F, Shakya R. GDNF/Ret signaling and the development of the kidney. BioEssays. 2006;28:117–27.
40. Costantini F, Kopan R. Patterning a complex organ: branching morphogenesis and nephron segmentation in kidney development. Dev Cell. 2010;18:698–712.
41. Dai L, Li J, Xie L, Wang W, Lu Y, Xie M, Huang J, Shen K, Yang H, Pei C, Zhao Y, Zhang W. A Biallelic frameshift mutation in Nephronectin causes bilateral renal agenesis in humans. J Am Soc Nephrol. 2021;32:1871–9.
42. Darlow JM, Molloy NH, Green AJ, Puri P, Barton DE. The increased incidence of the RET p.Gly691Ser variant in French-Canadian vesicoureteric reflux patients is not replicated by a larger study in Ireland. Hum Mutat. 2009;30:E612–7.
43. de Bakker BS, de Jong KH, Hagoort J, de Bree K, Besselink CT, de Kanter FE, Veldhuis T, Bais B, Schildmeijer R, Ruijter JM, Oostra RJ, Christoffels VM, Moorman AF. An interactive three-dimensional digital atlas and quantitative database of human development. Science. 2016;354:aag0053.
44. de Bakker BS, van den Hoff MJB, Vize PD, Oostra RJ. The Pronephros; a fresh perspective. Integr Comp Biol. 2019;59:29–47.
45. Doan RN, Lim ET, De Rubeis S, Betancur C, Cutler DJ, Chiocchetti AG, Overman LM, Soucy A, Goetze S, Freitag CM, Daly MJ, Walsh CA, Buxbaum JD, Yu TW. Recessive gene disruptions in autism spectrum disorder. Nat Genet. 2019;51:1092–8.
46. Dobson MG, Darlow JM, Hunziker M, Green AJ, Barton DE, Puri P. Heterozygous nonsynonymous ROBO2 variants are unlikely to be sufficient to cause familial vesicoureteric reflux. Kidney Int. 2013;84:327–37.

47. Dudley AT, Robertson EJ. Overlapping expression domains of bone morphogenetic protein family members potentially account for limited tissue defects in BMP7 deficient embryos. Dev Dyn. 1997;208:349–62.
48. Elahi S, Homstad A, Vaidya H, Stout J, Hall G, Wu G, Conlon P Jr, Routh JC, Wiener JS, Ross SS, Nagaraj S, Wigfall D, Foreman J, Adeyemo A, Gupta IR, Brophy PD, Rabinovich CE, Gbadegesin RA. Rare variants in tenascin genes in a cohort of children with primary vesicoureteric reflux. Pediatr Nephrol. 2016;31:247–53.
49. Esquela AF, Lee SJ. Regulation of metanephric kidney development by growth/differentiation factor 11. Dev Biol. 2003;257:356–70.
50. Falardeau J, Chung WC, Beenken A, Raivio T, Plummer L, Sidis Y, Jacobson-Dickman EE, Eliseenkova AV, Ma J, Dwyer A, Quinton R, Na S, Hall JE, Huot C, Alois N, Pearce SH, Cole LW, Hughes V, Mohammadi M, Tsai P, Pitteloud N. Decreased FGF8 signaling causes deficiency of gonadotropin-releasing hormone in humans and mice. J Clin Invest. 2008;118:2822–31.
51. Fila M, Moriniere V, Eckart P, Terzic J, Gubler MC, Antignac C, Heidet L. Bi-allelic mutations in renin-angiotensin system genes, associated with renal tubular dysgenesis, can also present as a progressive chronic kidney disease. Pediatr Nephrol. 2020;35:1125–8.
52. Foster KJ, Zhang SQ, Braddock SR, Torti E, Chikarmane R, Sotelo-Avila C, Greenspon J. Retinoic acid receptor beta variant-related colonic hypoganglionosis. Am J Med Genet A. 2019;179:817–21.
53. Furlong RF, Holland PW. Were vertebrates octoploid? Philos Trans R Soc Lond Ser B Biol Sci. 2002;357:531–44.
54. Gbadegesin RA, Brophy PD, Adeyemo A, Hall G, Gupta IR, Hains D, Bartkowiak B, Rabinovich CE, Chandrasekharappa S, Homstad A, Westreich K, Wu G, Liu Y, Holanda D, Clarke J, Lavin P, Selim A, Miller S, Wiener JS, Ross SS, Foreman J, Rotimi C, Winn MP. TNXB mutations can cause vesicoureteral reflux. J Am Soc Nephrol. 2013;24:1313–22.
55. Ghosh AK, O'Bryan T. Ehlers-Danlos syndrome with reflux nephropathy. Nephron. 1995;70:266.
56. Gimelli S, Caridi G, Beri S, McCracken K, Bocciardi R, Zordan P, Dagnino M, Fiorio P, Murer L, Benetti E, Zuffardi O, Giorda R, Wells JM, Gimelli G, Ghiggeri GM. Mutations in SOX17 are associated with congenital anomalies of the kidney and the urinary tract. Hum Mutat. 2010;31:1352–9.
57. Gong KQ, Yallowitz AR, Sun H, Dressler GR, Wellik DM. A Hox-Eya-Pax complex regulates early kidney developmental gene expression. Mol Cell Biol. 2007;27:7661–8.
58. Grieshammer U, Le M, Plump AS, Wang F, Tessier-Lavigne M, Martin GR. SLIT2-mediated ROBO2 signaling restricts kidney induction to a single site. Dev Cell. 2004;6:709–17.
59. Grote D, Souabni A, Busslinger M, Bouchard M. Pax 2/8-regulated Gata 3 expression is necessary for morphogenesis and guidance of the nephric duct in the developing kidney. Development. 2006;133:53–61.
60. Grote D, Boualia SK, Souabni A, Merkel C, Chi X, Costantini F, Carroll T, Bouchard M. Gata3 acts downstream of beta-catenin signaling to prevent ectopic metanephric kidney induction. PLoS Genet. 2008;4:e1000316.
61. Gupta A, Bischoff A, Pena A, Runck LA, Guasch G. The great divide: septation and malformation of the cloaca, and its implications for surgeons. Pediatr Surg Int. 2014;30:1089–95.
62. Hanafusa H, Torii S, Yasunaga T, Nishida E. Sprouty1 and Sprouty2 provide a control mechanism for the Ras/MAPK signalling pathway. Nat Cell Biol. 2002;4:850–8.
63. Hartwig S, Bridgewater D, Di Giovanni V, Cain J, Mishina Y, Rosenblum ND. BMP receptor ALK3 controls collecting system development. J Am Soc Nephrol. 2008;19:117–24.
64. Heidet L, Decramer S, Pawtowski A, Moriniere V, Bandin F, Knebelmann B, Lebre AS, Faguer S, Guigonis V, Antignac C, Salomon R. Spectrum of HNF1B mutations in a large cohort of patients who harbor renal diseases. Clin J Am Soc Nephrol. 2010;5:1079–90.

65. Hoskins BE, Cramer CH, Silvius D, Zou D, Raymond RM, Orten DJ, Kimberling WJ, Smith RJ, Weil D, Petit C, Otto EA, Xu PX, Hildebrandt F. Transcription factor SIX5 is mutated in patients with branchio-oto-renal syndrome. Am J Hum Genet. 2007;80:800–4.
66. Hoyes AD, Ramus NI, Martin BG. Fine structure of the epithelium of the human fetal bladder. J Anat. 1972;111:415–25.
67. Hu MC, Wasserman D, Hartwig S, Rosenblum ND. p38MAPK acts in the BMP7-dependent stimulatory pathway during epithelial cell morphogenesis and is regulated by Smad1. J Biol Chem. 2004;279:12051–9.
68. Hu P, Deng FM, Liang FX, Hu CM, Auerbach AB, Shapiro E, Wu XR, Kachar B, Sun TT. Ablation of uroplakin III gene results in small urothelial plaques, urothelial leakage, and vesicoureteral reflux. J Cell Biol. 2000;151:961–72.
69. Huang Z, Xu L, Cai C, Zhou Y, Liu J, Xu Z, Zhu Z, Kang W, Cen W, Pei S, Chen D, Shi C, Wu X, Huang Y, Xu C, Yan Y, Yang Y, Xue T, He W, Hu X, Zhang Y, Chen Y, Bi C, He C, Xue L, Xiao S, Yue Z, Jiang Y, Yu JK, Jarvis ED, Li G, Lin G, Zhang Q, Zhou Q. Three amphioxus reference genomes reveal gene and chromosome evolution of chordates. Proc Natl Acad Sci USA. 2023;120:e2201504120.
70. Humbert C, Silbermann F, Morar B, Parisot M, Zarhrate M, Masson C, Tores F, Blanchet P, Perez MJ, Petrov Y, Khau Van Kien P, Roume J, Leroy B, Gribouval O, Kalaydjieva L, Heidet L, Salomon R, Antignac C, Benmerah A, Saunier S, Jeanpierre C. Integrin alpha 8 recessive mutations are responsible for bilateral renal agenesis in humans. Am J Hum Genet. 2014;94:288–94.
71. Hwang DY, Dworschak GC, Kohl S, Saisawat P, Vivante A, Hilger AC, Reutter HM, Soliman NA, Bogdanovic R, Kehinde EO, Tasic V, Hildebrandt F. Mutations in 12 known dominant disease-causing genes clarify many congenital anomalies of the kidney and urinary tract. Kidney Int. 2014;85:1429–33.
72. Hwang DY, Kohl S, Fan X, Vivante A, Chan S, Dworschak GC, Schulz J, van Eerde AM, Hilger AC, Gee HY, Pennimpede T, Herrmann BG, van de Hoek G, Renkema KY, Schell C, Huber TB, Reutter HM, Soliman NA, Stajic N, Bogdanovic R, Kehinde EO, Lifton RP, Tasic V, Lu W, Hildebrandt F. Mutations of the SLIT2-ROBO2 pathway genes SLIT2 and SRGAP1 confer risk for congenital anomalies of the kidney and urinary tract. Hum Genet. 2015;134:905–16.
73. Ichikawa I, Kuwayama F, Pope JCT, Stephens FD, Miyazaki Y. Paradigm shift from classic anatomic theories to contemporary cell biological views of CAKUT. Kidney Int. 2002;61:889–98.
74. Ikeda K, Watanabe Y, Ohto H, Kawakami K. Molecular interaction and synergistic activation of a promoter by Six, Eya, and Dach proteins mediated through CREB binding protein. Mol Cell Biol. 2002;22:6759–66.
75. Inman KE, Caiaffa CD, Melton KR, Sandell LL, Achilleos A, Kume T, Trainor PA. Foxc2 is required for proper cardiac neural crest cell migration, outflow tract septation, and ventricle expansion. Dev Dyn. 2018;247:1286–96.
76. Innoceta AM, Olivucci G, Parmeggiani G, Scarano E, Pragliola A, Graziano C. Chromosomal microarray analysis identifies a novel SALL1 deletion, supporting the Association of Haploinsufficiency with a mild phenotype of Townes-Brocks syndrome. Genes (Basel). 2023;14:258.
77. Jadeja S, Smyth I, Pitera JE, Taylor MS, van Haelst M, Bentley E, McGregor L, Hopkins J, Chalepakis G, Philip N, Perez Aytes A, Watt FM, Darling SM, Jackson I, Woolf AS, Scambler PJ. Identification of a new gene mutated in Fraser syndrome and mouse myelencephalic blebs. Nat Genet. 2005;37:520–5.
78. Jafari NV, Rohn JL. The urothelium: a multi-faceted barrier against a harsh environment. Mucosal Immunol. 2022;15:1127–42.
79. Jakubiuk-Tomaszuk A, Murcia Pienkowski V, Zietkiewicz S, Rydzanicz M, Kosinska J, Stawinski P, Szuminski M, Ploski R. Syndromic chorioretinal coloboma associated with het-

erozygous de novo RARA mutation affecting an amino acid critical for retinoic acid interaction. Clin Genet. 2019;96:371–5.
80. Jeanpierre C, Mace G, Parisot M, Moriniere V, Pawtowsky A, Benabou M, Martinovic J, Amiel J, Attie-Bitach T, Delezoide AL, Loget P, Blanchet P, Gaillard D, Gonzales M, Carpentier W, Nitschke P, Tores F, Heidet L, Antignac C, Salomon R. RET and GDNF mutations are rare in fetuses with renal agenesis or other severe kidney development defects. J Med Genet. 2011;48:497–504.
81. Jena N, Martin-Seisdedos C, McCue P, Croce CM. BMP7 null mutation in mice: developmental defects in skeleton, kidney, and eye. Exp Cell Res. 1997;230:28–37.
82. Jenkins D, Bitner-Glindzicz M, Malcolm S, Hu CC, Allison J, Winyard PJ, Gullett AM, Thomas DF, Belk RA, Feather SA, Sun TT, Woolf AS. De novo Uroplakin IIIa heterozygous mutations cause human renal adysplasia leading to severe kidney failure. J Am Soc Nephrol. 2005;16:2141–9.
83. Jenkins D, Bitner-Glindzicz M, Malcolm S, Allison J, de Bruyn R, Flanagan S, Thomas DF, Belk RA, Feather SA, Bingham C, Southgate J, Woolf AS. Mutation analyses of Uroplakin II in children with renal tract malformations. Nephrol Dial Transplant. 2006;21:3415–21.
84. Jones GE, Richmond AK, Navti O, Mousa HA, Abbs S, Thompson E, Mansour S, Vasudevan PC. Renal anomalies and lymphedema distichiasis syndrome. A rare association? Am J Med Genet A. 2017;173:2251–6.
85. Jordan P, Dorval G, Arrondel C, Moriniere V, Tournant C, Audrezet MP, Michel-Calemard L, Putoux A, Lesca G, Labalme A, Whalen S, Loeuillet L, Martinovic J, Attie-Bitach T, Bessieres B, Schaefer E, Scheidecker S, Lambert L, Beneteau C, Patat O, Boute-Benejean O, Molin A, Guimiot F, Fontanarosa N, Nizon M, Lefebvre M, Jeanpierre C, Saunier S, Heidet L. Targeted next-generation sequencing in a large series of fetuses with severe renal diseases. Hum Mutat. 2022;43:347–61.
86. Karam I, Droupy S, Abd-Alsamad I, Korbage A, Uhl JF, Benoit G, Delmas V. The precise location and nature of the nerves to the male human urethra: histological and immunohistochemical studies with three-dimensional reconstruction. Eur Urol. 2005;48:858–64.
87. Karam I, Droupy S, Abd-Alsamad I, Uhl JF, Benoit G, Delmas V. Innervation of the female human urethral sphincter: 3D reconstruction of immunohistochemical studies in the fetus. Eur Urol. 2005;47:627–633; discussion 634.
88. Kawakami K, Sato S, Ozaki H, Ikeda K. Six family genes--structure and function as transcription factors and their roles in development. BioEssays. 2000;22:616–26.
89. Kayumi S, Perez-Jurado LA, Palomares M, Rangu S, Sheppard SE, Chung WK, Kruer MC, Kharbanda M, Amor DJ, McGillivray G, Cohen JS, Garcia-Minaur S, van Eyk CL, Harper K, Jolly LA, Webber DL, Barnett CP, Santos-Simarro F, Pacio-Miguez M, Pozo AD, Bakhtiari S, Deardorff M, Dubbs HA, Izumi K, Grand K, Gray C, Mark PR, Bhoj EJ, Li D, Ortiz-Gonzalez XR, Keena B, Zackai EH, Goldberg EM, Perez de Nanclares G, Pereda A, Llano-Rivas I, Arroyo I, Fernandez-Cuesta MA, Thauvin-Robinet C, Faivre L, Garde A, Mazel B, Bruel AL, Tress ML, Brilstra E, Fine AS, Crompton KE, Stegmann APA, Sinnema M, Stevens SCJ, Nicolai J, Lesca G, Lion-Francois L, Haye D, Chatron N, Piton A, Nizon M, Cogne B, Srivastava S, Bassetti J, Muss C, Gripp KW, Procopio RA, Millan F, Morrow MM, Assaf M, Moreno-De-Luca A, Joss S, Hamilton MJ, Bertoli M, Foulds N, McKee S, MacLennan AH, Gecz J, Corbett MA. Genomic and phenotypic characterization of 404 individuals with neurodevelopmental disorders caused by CTNNB1 variants. Genet Med. 2022;24:2351–66.
90. Kim KM, Kogan BA, Massad CA, Huang YC. Collagen and elastin in the normal fetal bladder. J Urol. 1991;146:524–7.
91. Kitzler TM, Schneider R, Kohl S, Kolvenbach CM, Connaughton DM, Dai R, Mann N, Nakayama M, Majmundar AJ, Wu CW, Kari JA, El Desoky SM, Senguttuvan P, Bogdanovic R, Stajic N, Valivullah Z, Lek M, Mane S, Lifton RP, Tasic V, Shril S, Hildebrandt F. COL4A1 mutations as a potential novel cause of autosomal dominant CAKUT in humans. Hum Genet. 2019;138:1105–15.

92. Kiyozumi D, Sugimoto N, Sekiguchi K. Breakdown of the reciprocal stabilization of QBRICK/Frem1, Fras1, and Frem2 at the basement membrane provokes Fraser syndrome-like defects. Proc Natl Acad Sci USA. 2006;103:11981–6.
93. Kohl S, Hwang DY, Dworschak GC, Hilger AC, Saisawat P, Vivante A, Stajic N, Bogdanovic R, Reutter HM, Kehinde EO, Tasic V, Hildebrandt F. Mild recessive mutations in six Fraser syndrome-related genes cause isolated congenital anomalies of the kidney and urinary tract. J Am Soc Nephrol. 2014;25:1917–22.
94. Kohlhase J, Wischermann A, Reichenbach H, Froster U, Engel W. Mutations in the SALL1 putative transcription factor gene cause Townes-Brocks syndrome. Nat Genet. 1998;18:81–3.
95. Kohlhase J. Townes-Brocks syndrome. In: Adam MP, Mirzaa GM, Pagon RA, et al., editors. GeneReviews® (Internet). Seattle: Oxford University Press; last updated 2016.
96. Komaki F, Miyazaki Y, Niimura F, Matsusaka T, Ichikawa I, Motojima M. Foxc1 gene null mutation causes ectopic budding and kidney hypoplasia but not dysplasia. Cells Tissues Organs. 2013;198:22–7.
97. Kong XT, Deng FM, Hu P, Liang FX, Zhou G, Auerbach AB, Genieser N, Nelson PK, Robbins ES, Shapiro E, Kachar B, Sun TT. Roles of uroplakins in plaque formation, umbrella cell enlargement, and urinary tract diseases. J Cell Biol. 2004;167:1195–204.
98. Kosfeld A, Kreuzer M, Daniel C, Brand F, Schafer AK, Chadt A, Weiss AC, Riehmer V, Jeanpierre C, Klintschar M, Brasen JH, Amann K, Pape L, Kispert A, Al-Hasani H, Haffner D, Weber RG. Whole-exome sequencing identifies mutations of TBC1D1 encoding a Rab-GTPase-activating protein in patients with congenital anomalies of the kidneys and urinary tract (CAKUT). Hum Genet. 2016;135:69–87.
99. Kuechler A, Willemsen MH, Albrecht B, Bacino CA, Bartholomew DW, van Bokhoven H, van den Boogaard MJ, Bramswig N, Buttner C, Cremer K, Czeschik JC, Engels H, van Gassen K, Graf E, van Haelst M, He W, Hogue JS, Kempers M, Koolen D, Monroe G, de Munnik S, Pastore M, Reis A, Reuter MS, Tegay DH, Veltman J, Visser G, van Hasselt P, Smeets EE, Vissers L, Wieland T, Wissink W, Yntema H, Zink AM, Strom TM, Ludecke HJ, Kleefstra T, Wieczorek D. De novo mutations in beta-catenin (CTNNB1) appear to be a frequent cause of intellectual disability: expanding the mutational and clinical spectrum. Hum Genet. 2015;134:97–109.
100. Kumar JP. The sine oculis homeobox (SIX) family of transcription factors as regulators of development and disease. Cell Mol Life Sci. 2009;66:565–83.
101. Kumar S, Kimberling WJ, Weston MD, Schaefer BG, Berg MA, Marres HA, Cremers CW. Identification of three novel mutations in human EYA1 protein associated with branchio-oto-renal syndrome. Hum Mutat. 1998;11:443–9.
102. Kume T, Deng K, Hogan BL. Murine forkhead/winged helix genes Foxc1 (Mf1) and Foxc2 (Mfh1) are required for the early organogenesis of the kidney and urinary tract. Development. 2000;127:1387–95.
103. Lang RJ, Tonta MA, Zoltkowski BZ, Meeker WF, Wendt I, Parkington HC. Pyeloureteric peristalsis: role of atypical smooth muscle cells and interstitial cells of Cajal-like cells as pacemakers. J Physiol. 2006;576:695–705.
104. Lantieri F, Gimelli S, Viaggi C, Stathaki E, Malacarne M, Santamaria G, Grossi A, Mosconi M, Sloan-Bena F, Prato AP, Coviello D, Ceccherini I. Copy number variations in candidate genomic regions confirm genetic heterogeneity and parental bias in Hirschsprung disease. Orphanet J Rare Dis. 2019;14:270.
105. Lappin TR, Grier DG, Thompson A, Halliday HL. HOX genes: seductive science, mysterious mechanisms. Ulster Med J. 2006;75:23–31.
106. Lawson BAJ, Flegg MB. A mathematical model for the induction of the mammalian ureteric bud. J Theor Biol. 2016;394:43–56.
107. Lefevre JG, Short KM, Lamberton TO, Michos O, Graf D, Smyth IM, Hamilton NA. Branching morphogenesis in the developing kidney is governed by rules that pattern the ureteric tree. Development. 2017;144:4377–85.

108. Li X, Oghi KA, Zhang J, Krones A, Bush KT, Glass CK, Nigam SK, Aggarwal AK, Maas R, Rose DW, Rosenfeld MG. Eya protein phosphatase activity regulates Six1-Dach-Eya transcriptional effects in mammalian organogenesis. Nature. 2003;426:247–54.
109. Li Y, Yu M, Tan L, Xue S, Du X, Wu X, Xu H, Shen Q. Robo2 and Gen1 Coregulate ureteric budding by activating the MAPK/ERK signaling pathway in mice. Front Med (Lausanne). 2021;8:807898.
110. Liu J, Sun L, Shen Q, Wu X, Xu H. New congenital anomalies of the kidney and urinary tract and outcomes in Robo2 mutant mice with the inserted piggyBac transposon. BMC Nephrol. 2016;17:98.
111. Liu JL, Shen Q, Wu MY, Zhu GH, Li YF, Wang XW, Tang XS, Bi YL, Gong YN, Chen J, Fang XY, Zhai YH, Wu BB, Li GM, Sun YB, Gao XJ, Liu CH, Jiang XY, Hao S, Kang YL, Gong YL, Rong LP, Li D, Wang S, Ma D, Rao J, Xu H. Responsible genes in children with primary vesicoureteral reflux: findings from the Chinese Children Genetic Kidney Disease Database. World J Pediatr. 2021;17:409–18.
112. Lu W, van Eerde AM, Fan X, Quintero-Rivera F, Kulkarni S, Ferguson H, Kim HG, Fan Y, Xi Q, Li QG, Sanlaville D, Andrews W, Sundaresan V, Bi W, Yan J, Giltay JC, Wijmenga C, de Jong TP, Feather SA, Woolf AS, Rao Y, Lupski JR, Eccles MR, Quade BJ, Gusella JF, Morton CC, Maas RL. Disruption of ROBO2 is associated with urinary tract anomalies and confers risk of vesicoureteral reflux. Am J Hum Genet. 2007;80:616–32.
113. Mackie GG, Stephens FD. Duplex kidneys: a correlation of renal dysplasia with position of the ureteral orifice. J Urol. 1975;114:274–80.
114. Marcotte M, Sharma R, Bouchard M. Gene regulatory network of renal primordium development. Pediatr Nephrol. 2014;29:637–44.
115. Marose TD, Merkel CE, McMahon AP, Carroll TJ. Beta-catenin is necessary to keep cells of ureteric bud/Wolffian duct epithelium in a precursor state. Dev Biol. 2008;314:112–26.
116. McGregor L, Makela V, Darling SM, Vrontou S, Chalepakis G, Roberts C, Smart N, Rutland P, Prescott N, Hopkins J, Bentley E, Shaw A, Roberts E, Mueller R, Jadeja S, Philip N, Nelson J, Francannet C, Perez-Aytes A, Megarbane A, Kerr B, Wainwright B, Woolf AS, Winter RM, Scambler PJ. Fraser syndrome and mouse blebbed phenotype caused by mutations in FRAS1/Fras1 encoding a putative extracellular matrix protein. Nat Genet. 2003;34:203–8.
117. Mendelsohn C. Using mouse models to understand normal and abnormal urogenital tract development. Organogenesis. 2009;5:306–14.
118. Michelson M, Lidzbarsky G, Nishri D, Israel-Elgali I, Berger R, Gafner M, Shomron N, Lev D, Goldberg Y. Microdeletion of 16q24.1-q24.2-A unique etiology of Lymphedema-Distichiasis syndrome and neurodevelopmental disorder. Am J Med Genet A. 2022;188:1990–6.
119. Michos O, Panman L, Vintersten K, Beier K, Zeller R, Zuniga A. Gremlin-mediated BMP antagonism induces the epithelial-mesenchymal feedback signaling controlling metanephric kidney and limb organogenesis. Development. 2004;131:3401–10.
120. Michos O, Cebrian C, Hyink D, Grieshammer U, Williams L, D'Agati V, Licht JD, Martin GR, Costantini F. Kidney development in the absence of Gdnf and Spry1 requires Fgf10. PLoS Genet. 2010;6:e1000809.
121. Miller EM, Hopkin R, Bao L, Ware SM. Implications for genotype-phenotype predictions in Townes-Brocks syndrome: case report of a novel SALL1 deletion and review of the literature. Am J Med Genet A. 2012;158A:533–40.
122. Mitsioni AG, Siomou E, Bouba I, Petridi S, Siamopoulou A, Georgiou I. ROBO2 gene variants in children with primary nonsyndromic vesicoureteral reflux with or without renal hypoplasia/dysplasia. Pediatr Res. 2016;80:72–6.
123. Miyamoto N, Yoshida M, Kuratani S, Matsuo I, Aizawa S. Defects of urogenital development in mice lacking Emx2. Development. 1997;124:1653–64.
124. Miyazaki Y, Oshima K, Fogo A, Hogan BL, Ichikawa I. Bone morphogenetic protein 4 regulates the budding site and elongation of the mouse ureter. J Clin Invest. 2000;105:863–73.

125. Miyazaki Y, Oshima K, Fogo A, Ichikawa I. Evidence that bone morphogenetic protein 4 has multiple biological functions during kidney and urinary tract development. Kidney Int. 2003;63:835–44.
126. Motojima M, Tanaka M, Kume T. Foxc1 and Foxc2 are indispensable for the maintenance of nephron and stromal progenitors in the developing kidney. J Cell Sci. 2022;135:jcs260356.
127. Müller U, Wang D, Denda S, Meneses JJ, Pedersen RA, Reichardt LF. Integrin alpha8beta1 is critically important for epithelial-mesenchymal interactions during kidney morphogenesis. Cell. 1997;88:603–13.
128. Münch J, Engesser M, Schönauer R, Hamm JA, Hartig C, Hantmann E, Akay G, Pehlivan D, Mitani T, Coban Akdemir Z, Tüysuz B, Shirakawa T, Dateki S, Claus LR, van Eerde AM, Smol T, Devisme L, Franquet H, Attie-Bitach T, Wagner T, Bergmann C, Hohn AK, Shril S, Pollack A, Wenger T, Scott AA, Paolucci S, Buchan J, Gabriel GC, Posey JE, Lupski JR, Petit F, McCarthy AA, Pazour GJ, Lo CW, Popp B, Halbritter J. Biallelic pathogenic variants in roundabout guidance receptor 1 associate with syndromic congenital anomalies of the kidney and urinary tract. Kidney Int. 2022;101:1039–53.
129. Negrisolo S, Benetti E. PAX2 and CAKUT phenotypes: report on two new variants and a review of mutations from the Leiden open variation database. Int J Mol Sci. 2023;24:4165.
130. Neugebauer JM, Kwon S, Kim HS, Donley N, Tilak A, Sopory S, Christian JL. The prodomain of BMP4 is necessary and sufficient to generate stable BMP4/7 heterodimers with enhanced bioactivity in vivo. Proc Natl Acad Sci USA. 2015;112:E2307–16.
131. Newman J, Antonakopoulos GN. The fine structure of the human fetal urinary bladder. Development and maturation. A light, transmission and scanning electron microscopic study. J Anat. 1989;166:135–50.
132. Nicolaou N, Pulit SL, Nijman IJ, Monroe GR, Feitz WF, Schreuder MF, van Eerde AM, de Jong TP, Giltay JC, van der Zwaag B, Havenith MR, Zwakenberg S, van der Zanden LF, Poelmans G, Cornelissen EA, Lilien MR, Franke B, Roeleveld N, van Rooij IA, Cuppen E, Bongers EM, Giles RH, Knoers NV, Renkema KY. Prioritization and burden analysis of rare variants in 208 candidate genes suggest they do not play a major role in CAKUT. Kidney Int. 2016;89:476–86.
133. Nishimoto K, Iijima K, Shirakawa T, Kitagawa K, Satomura K, Nakamura H, Yoshikawa N. PAX2 gene mutation in a family with isolated renal hypoplasia. J Am Soc Nephrol. 2001;12:1769–72.
134. Nishimura H, Yerkes E, Hohenfellner K, Miyazaki Y, Ma J, Hunley TE, Yoshida H, Ichiki T, Threadgill D, Phillips JA 3rd, Hogan BM, Fogo A, Brock JW 3rd, Inagami T, Ichikawa I. Role of the angiotensin type 2 receptor gene in congenital anomalies of the kidney and urinary tract, CAKUT, of mice and men. Mol Cell. 1999;3:1–10.
135. Nishinakamura R, Matsumoto Y, Nakao K, Nakamura K, Sato A, Copeland NG, Gilbert DJ, Jenkins NA, Scully S, Lacey DL, Katsuki M, Asashima M, Yokota T. Murine homolog of SALL1 is essential for ureteric bud invasion in kidney development. Development. 2001;128:3105–15.
136. Norden PR, Sabine A, Wang Y, Demir CS, Liu T, Petrova TV, Kume T. Shear stimulation of FOXC1 and FOXC2 differentially regulates cytoskeletal activity during lymphatic valve maturation. elife. 2020;9:e53814.
137. Oshima K, Miyazaki Y, Brock JW 3rd, Adams MC, Ichikawa I, Pope JCt. Angiotensin type II receptor expression and ureteral budding. J Urol. 2001;166:1848–52.
138. Oswald J, Brenner E, Schwentner C, Deibl M, Bartsch G, Fritsch H, Radmayr C. The intravesical ureter in children with vesicoureteral reflux: a morphological and immunohistochemical characterization. J Urol. 2003;170:2423–7.
139. Oxburgh L, Chu GC, Michael SK, Robertson EJ. TGFbeta superfamily signals are required for morphogenesis of the kidney mesenchyme progenitor population. Development. 2004;131:4593–605.

140. Pavan M, Ruiz VF, Silva FA, Sobreira TJ, Cravo RM, Vasconcelos M, Marques LP, Mesquita SM, Krieger JE, Lopes AA, Oliveira PS, Pereira AC, Xavier-Neto J. ALDH1A2 (RALDH2) genetic variation in human congenital heart disease. BMC Med Genet. 2009;10:113.
141. Petrou P, Makrygiannis AK, Chalepakis G. The Fras1/Frem family of extracellular matrix proteins: structure, function, and association with Fraser syndrome and the mouse bleb phenotype. Connect Tissue Res. 2008;49:277–82.
142. Pitera JE, Woolf AS, Basson MA, Scambler PJ. Sprouty1 haploinsufficiency prevents renal agenesis in a model of Fraser syndrome. J Am Soc Nephrol. 2012;23:1790–6.
143. Pope JCT, Nishimura H, Ichikawa I. Role of angiotensin in the development of the kidney and urinary tract. Nephrologie. 1998;19:433–6.
144. Radmayr C, Schwentner C, Lunacek A, Karatzas A, Oswald J. Embryology and anatomy of the vesicoureteric junction with special reference to the etiology of vesicoureteral reflux. Ther Adv Urol. 2009;1:243–50.
145. Rasmussen M, Sunde L, Nielsen ML, Ramsing M, Petersen A, Hjortshoj TD, Olsen TE, Tabor A, Hertz JM, Johnsen I, Sperling L, Petersen OB, Jensen UB, Møller FG, Petersen MB, Lildballe DL. Targeted gene sequencing and whole-exome sequencing in autopsied fetuses with prenatally diagnosed kidney anomalies. Clin Genet. 2018;93:860–9.
146. Rastinejad F. Retinoic acid receptor structures: the journey from single domains to full-length complex. J Mol Endocrinol. 2022;69:T25–36.
147. Ravenscroft TA, Phillips JB, Fieg E, Bajikar SS, Peirce J, Wegner J, Luna AA, Fox EJ, Yan YL, Rosenfeld JA, Zirin J, Kanca O, Benke PJ, Cameron ES, Strehlow V, Platzer K, Jamra RA, Klockner C, Osmond M, Licata T, Rojas S, Dyment D, Chong JSC, Lincoln S, Stoler JM, Postlethwait JH, Wangler MF, Yamamoto S, Krier J, Westerfield M, Bellen HJ. Heterozygous loss-of-function variants significantly expand the phenotypes associated with loss of GDF11. Genet Med. 2021;23:1889–900.
148. Rosselot C, Spraggon L, Chia I, Batourina E, Riccio P, Lu B, Niederreither K, Dolle P, Duester G, Chambon P, Costantini F, Gilbert T, Molotkov A, Mendelsohn C. Non-cell-autonomous retinoid signaling is crucial for renal development. Development. 2010;137:283–92.
149. Rozen EJ, Schmidt H, Dolcet X, Basson MA, Jain S, Encinas M. Loss of Sprouty1 rescues renal agenesis caused by Ret mutation. J Am Soc Nephrol. 2009;20:255–9.
150. Ruf RG, Xu PX, Silvius D, Otto EA, Beekmann F, Muerb UT, Kumar S, Neuhaus TJ, Kemper MJ, Raymond RM Jr, Brophy PD, Berkman J, Gattas M, Hyland V, Ruf EM, Schwartz C, Chang EH, Smith RJ, Stratakis CA, Weil D, Petit C, Hildebrandt F. SIX1 mutations cause branchio-oto-renal syndrome by disruption of EYA1-SIX1-DNA complexes. Proc Natl Acad Sci USA. 2004;101:8090–5.
151. Rusu MC, Pop F, Petre N, Dobra MA. The sheath of Waldeyer is not a specific anatomical trait of the ureterovesical junction. Morphologie. 2018;102:6–11.
152. Sajithlal G, Zou D, Silvius D, Xu PX. Eya 1 acts as a critical regulator for specifying the metanephric mesenchyme. Dev Biol. 2005;284:323–36.
153. Sanna-Cherchi S, Khan K, Westland R, Krithivasan P, Fievet L, Rasouly HM, Ionita-Laza I, Capone VP, Fasel DA, Kiryluk K, Kamalakaran S, Bodria M, Otto EA, Sampson MG, Gillies CE, Vega-Warner V, Vukojevic K, Pediaditakis I, Makar GS, Mitrotti A, Verbitsky M, Martino J, Liu Q, Na YJ, Goj V, Ardissino G, Gigante M, Gesualdo L, Janezcko M, Zaniew M, Mendelsohn CL, Shril S, Hildebrandt F, van Wijk JAE, Arapovic A, Saraga M, Allegri L, Izzi C, Scolari F, Tasic V, Ghiggeri GM, Latos-Bielenska A, Materna-Kiryluk A, Mane S, Goldstein DB, Lifton RP, Katsanis N, Davis EE, Gharavi AG. Exome-wide Association Study identifies GREB1L mutations in congenital kidney malformations. Am J Hum Genet. 2017;101:789–802.
154. Sanyanusin P, Schimmenti LA, McNoe LA, Ward TA, Pierpont ME, Sullivan MJ, Dobyns WB, Eccles MR. Mutation of the PAX2 gene in a family with optic nerve colobomas, renal anomalies and vesicoureteral reflux. Nat Genet. 1995;9:358–64.

155. Schalkwijk J, Zweers MC, Steijlen PM, Dean WB, Taylor G, van Vlijmen IM, van Haren B, Miller WL, Bristow J. A recessive form of the Ehlers-Danlos syndrome caused by tenascin-X deficiency. N Engl J Med. 2001;345:1167–75.
156. Schild R, Knuppel T, Konrad M, Bergmann C, Trautmann A, Kemper MJ, Wu K, Yaklichkin S, Wang J, Pestell R, Muller-Wiefel DE, Schaefer F, Weber S. Double homozygous missense mutations in DACH1 and BMP4 in a patient with bilateral cystic renal dysplasia. Nephrol Dial Transplant. 2013;28:227–32.
157. Schonfelder EM, Knuppel T, Tasic V, Miljkovic P, Konrad M, Wuhl E, Antignac C, Bakkaloglu A, Schaefer F, Weber S. Mutations in Uroplakin IIIA are a rare cause of renal hypodysplasia in humans. Am J Kidney Dis. 2006;47:1004–12.
158. Schuchardt A, D'Agati V, Pachnis V, Costantini F. Renal agenesis and hypodysplasia in ret-k- mutant mice result from defects in ureteric bud development. Development. 1996;122:1919–29.
159. Sebe P, Fritsch H, Oswald J, Schwentner C, Lunacek A, Bartsch G, Radmayr C. Fetal development of the female external urinary sphincter complex: an anatomical and histological study. J Urol. 2005;173:1738–42. discussion 1742
160. Self M, Lagutin OV, Bowling B, Hendrix J, Cai Y, Dressler GR, Oliver G. Six2 is required for suppression of nephrogenesis and progenitor renewal in the developing kidney. EMBO J. 2006;25:5214–28.
161. Shafik A. Study of the effect of external urethral sphincter contraction on the mechanical activity of the ureterovesical junction and urinary bladder: recognition of the sphinctero-ureterovesical reflex. Urology. 1997;50:949–52.
162. Sharma R, Sanchez-Ferras O, Bouchard M. Pax genes in renal development, disease and regeneration. Semin Cell Dev Biol. 2015;44:97–106.
163. Sinibaldi L, Garone G, Mandarino A, Iarossi G, Chioma L, Dentici M, Merla G, Agolini E, Micalizzi A, Mancini C, Niceta M, Macchiaiolo M, Diodato D, Onesimo R, Blandino R, Delogu AB, De Rosa G, Trevisan V, Iademarco M, Zampino G, Tartaglia M, Novelli A, Bartuli A, Digilio MC, Calcagni G. Congenital heart defects in CTNNB1 syndrome: raising clinical awareness. Clin Genet. 2023;104:528–41.
164. Skinner MA, Safford SD, Reeves JG, Jackson ME, Freemerman AJ. Renal aplasia in humans is associated with RET mutations. Am J Hum Genet. 2008;82:344–51.
165. Smith RJH. Branchiootorenal spectrum disorder. In: Adam MP, Mirzaa GM, Pagon RA, et al., editors. GeneReviews((R)). University of Washington, Seattle; 1993.
166. Smyth I, Du X, Taylor MS, Justice MJ, Beutler B, Jackson IJ. The extracellular matrix gene Frem1 is essential for the normal adhesion of the embryonic epidermis. Proc Natl Acad Sci USA. 2004;101:13560–5.
167. Song R, Spera M, Garrett C, El-Dahr SS, Yosypiv IV. Angiotensin II AT2 receptor regulates ureteric bud morphogenesis. Am J Physiol Renal Physiol. 2010;298:F807–17.
168. Srour M, Caron V, Pearson T, Nielsen SB, Levesque S, Delrue MA, Becker TA, Hamdan FF, Kibar Z, Sattler SG, Schneider MC, Bitoun P, Chassaing N, Rosenfeld JA, Xia F, Desai S, Roeder E, Kimonis V, Schneider A, Littlejohn RO, Douzgou S, Tremblay A, Michaud JL. Gain-of-function mutations in RARB cause intellectual disability with progressive motor impairment. Hum Mutat. 2016;37:786–93.
169. Takamiya K, Kostourou V, Adams S, Jadeja S, Chalepakis G, Scambler PJ, Huganir RL, Adams RH. A direct functional link between the multi-PDZ domain protein GRIP1 and the Fraser syndrome protein Fras1. Nat Genet. 2004;36:172–7.
170. Tanagho EA, Hutch JA, Meyers FH, Rambo ON Jr. Primary Vesicoureteral Reflux: experimental studies of its etiology. J Urol. 1965;93:165–76.
171. Taylor RL, Soriano CS, Williams S, Dzulova D, Ashworth J, Hall G, Gale T, Lloyd IC, Inglehearn CF, Toomes C, Douzgou S, Black GC. Bi-allelic mutation of CTNNB1 causes a severe form of syndromic microphthalmia, persistent foetal vasculature and vitreoretinal dysplasia. Orphanet J Rare Dis. 2022;17:110.

172. Tinti M, Johnson C, Toth R, Ferrier DE, Mackintosh C. Evolution of signal multiplexing by 14-3-3-binding 2R-ohnologue protein families in the vertebrates. Open Biol. 2012;2:120103.
173. Tokhmafshan F, El Andalousi J, Murugapoopathy V, Fillion ML, Campillo S, Capolicchio JP, Jednak R, El Sherbiny M, Turpin S, Schalkwijk J, Matsumoto KI, Brophy PD, Gbadegesin RA, Gupta IR. Children with vesicoureteric reflux have joint hypermobility and occasional tenascin XB sequence variants. Can Urol Assoc J. 2020;14:E128–36.
174. Trieschmann G, Wilhelm C, Berweck S, Zech M. De novo retinoic acid receptor beta (RARB) variant associated with microphthalmia and dystonia. Eur J Med Genet. 2023;66:104802.
175. Ujiie N, Norden PR, Fang R, Beckmann L, Cai Z, Kweon J, Liu T, Tan C, Kuhn MS, Stamer WD, Aoto K, Quaggin SE, Zhang HF, Kume T. Differential roles of FOXC2 in the trabecular meshwork and Schlemm's canal in glaucomatous pathology. Life Sci Alliance. 2023;6:e202201721.
176. Unzaki A, Morisada N, Nozu K, Ye MJ, Ito S, Matsunaga T, Ishikura K, Ina S, Nagatani K, Okamoto T, Inaba Y, Ito N, Igarashi T, Kanda S, Ito K, Omune K, Iwaki T, Ueno K, Yahata M, Ohtsuka Y, Nishi E, Takahashi N, Ishikawa T, Goto S, Okamoto N, Iijima K. Clinically diverse phenotypes and genotypes of patients with branchio-oto-renal syndrome. J Hum Genet. 2018;63:647–56.
177. van der Ven AT, Connaughton DM, Ityel H, Mann N, Nakayama M, Chen J, Vivante A, Hwang DY, Schulz J, Braun DA, Schmidt JM, Schapiro D, Schneider R, Warejko JK, Daga A, Majmundar AJ, Tan W, Jobst-Schwan T, Hermle T, Widmeier E, Ashraf S, Amar A, Hoogstraaten CA, Hugo H, Kitzler TM, Kause F, Kolvenbach CM, Dai R, Spaneas L, Amann K, Stein DR, Baum MA, Somers MJG, Rodig NM, Ferguson MA, Traum AZ, Daouk GH, Bogdanovic R, Stajic N, Soliman NA, Kari JA, El Desoky S, Fathy HM, Milosevic D, Al-Saffar M, Awad HS, Eid LA, Selvin A, Senguttuvan P, Sanna-Cherchi S, Rehm HL, MacArthur DG, Lek M, Laricchia KM, Wilson MW, Mane SM, Lifton RP, Lee RS, Bauer SB, Lu W, Reutter HM, Tasic V, Shril S, Hildebrandt F. Whole-Exome sequencing identifies causative mutations in families with congenital anomalies of the kidney and urinary tract. J Am Soc Nephrol. 2018;29:2348–61.
178. van Eerde AM, Verhoeven VJ, de Jong TP, van de Putte EM, Giltay JC, Engelbert RH. Is joint hypermobility associated with vesico-ureteral reflux? An assessment of 50 patients. BJU Int. 2012;109:1243–8.
179. Verbitsky M, Krithivasan P, Batourina E, Khan A, Graham SE, Marasa M, Kim H, Lim TY, Weng PL, Sanchez-Rodriguez E, Mitrotti A, Ahram DF, Zanoni F, Fasel DA, Westland R, Sampson MG, Zhang JY, Bodria M, Kil BH, Shril S, Gesualdo L, Torri F, Scolari F, Izzi C, van Wijk JAE, Saraga M, Santoro D, Conti G, Barton DE, Dobson MG, Puri P, Furth SL, Warady BA, Pisani I, Fiaccadori E, Allegri L, Degl'Innocenti ML, Piaggio G, Alam S, Gigante M, Zaza G, Esposito P, Lin F, Simoes ESAC, Brodkiewicz A, Drozdz D, Zachwieja K, Miklaszewska M, Szczepanska M, Adamczyk P, Tkaczyk M, Tomczyk D, Sikora P, Mizerska-Wasiak M, Krzemien G, Szmigielska A, Zaniew M, Lozanovski VJ, Gucev Z, Ionita-Laza I, Stanaway IB, Crosslin DR, Wong CS, Hildebrandt F, Barasch J, Kenny EE, Loos RJF, Levy B, Ghiggeri GM, Hakonarson H, Latos-Bielenska A, Materna-Kiryluk A, Darlow JM, Tasic V, Willer C, Kiryluk K, Sanna-Cherchi S, Mendelsohn CL, Gharavi AG. Copy number variant analysis and genome-wide association study identify loci with large effect for vesicoureteral reflux. J Am Soc Nephrol. 2021;32:805–20.
180. Vincent C, Kalatzis V, Abdelhak S, Chaib H, Compain S, Helias J, Vaneecloo FM, Petit C. BOR and BO syndromes are allelic defects of EYA1. Eur J Hum Genet. 1997;5:242–6.
181. Vivante A, Kleppa MJ, Schulz J, Kohl S, Sharma A, Chen J, Shril S, Hwang DY, Weiss AC, Kaminski MM, Shukrun R, Kemper MJ, Lehnhardt A, Beetz R, Sanna-Cherchi S, Verbitsky M, Gharavi AG, Stuart HM, Feather SA, Goodship JA, Goodship TH, Woolf AS, Westra SJ, Doody DP, Bauer SB, Lee RS, Adam RM, Lu W, Reutter HM, Kehinde EO, Mancini EJ, Lifton RP, Tasic V, Lienkamp SS, Juppner H, Kispert A, Hildebrandt F. Mutations in TBX18 cause dominant urinary tract malformations via transcriptional dysregulation of ureter development. Am J Hum Genet. 2015;97:291–301.

182. Vivante A, Mann N, Yonath H, Weiss AC, Getwan M, Kaminski MM, Bohnenpoll T, Teyssier C, Chen J, Shril S, van der Ven AT, Ityel H, Schmidt JM, Widmeier E, Bauer SB, Sanna-Cherchi S, Gharavi AG, Lu W, Magen D, Shukrun R, Lifton RP, Tasic V, Stanescu HC, Cavailles V, Kleta R, Anikster Y, Dekel B, Kispert A, Lienkamp SS, Hildebrandt F. A dominant mutation in nuclear receptor interacting protein 1 causes urinary tract malformations via dysregulation of retinoic acid signaling. J Am Soc Nephrol. 2017;28:2364–76.
183. Wainwright EN, Wilhelm D, Combes AN, Little MH, Koopman P. ROBO2 restricts the nephrogenic field and regulates Wolffian duct-nephrogenic cord separation. Dev Biol. 2015;404:88–102.
184. Wang H, Li Q, Liu J, Mendelsohn C, Salant DJ, Lu W. Noninvasive assessment of antenatal hydronephrosis in mice reveals a critical role for Robo2 in maintaining anti-reflux mechanism. PLoS One. 2011;6:e24763.
185. Weber S, Moriniere V, Knuppel T, Charbit M, Dusek J, Ghiggeri GM, Jankauskiene A, Mir S, Montini G, Peco-Antic A, Wuhl E, Zurowska AM, Mehls O, Antignac C, Schaefer F, Salomon R. Prevalence of mutations in renal developmental genes in children with renal hypodysplasia: results of the ESCAPE study. J Am Soc Nephrol. 2006;17:2864–70.
186. Weber S, Taylor JC, Winyard P, Baker KF, Sullivan-Brown J, Schild R, Knuppel T, Zurowska AM, Caldas-Alfonso A, Litwin M, Emre S, Ghiggeri GM, Bakkaloglu A, Mehls O, Antignac C, Network E, Schaefer F, Burdine RD. SIX2 and BMP4 mutations associate with anomalous kidney development. J Am Soc Nephrol. 2008;19:891–903.
187. Wellik DM, Hawkes PJ, Capecchi MR. Hox11 paralogous genes are essential for metanephric kidney induction. Genes Dev. 2002;16:1423–32.
188. Wu XR, Kong XP, Pellicer A, Kreibich G, Sun TT. Uroplakins in urothelial biology, function, and disease. Kidney Int. 2009;75:1153–65.
189. Xiao J, Hao LW, Wang J, Yu XS, You JY, Li ZJ, Mao HD, Meng XY, Feng JX. Comprehensive characterization of the genetic landscape of familial Hirschsprung's disease. World J Pediatr. 2023;19:644–51.
190. Xu PX, Adams J, Peters H, Brown MC, Heaney S, Maas R. Eya1-deficient mice lack ears and kidneys and show abnormal apoptosis of organ primordia. Nat Genet. 1999;23:113–7.
191. Yang Y, Houle AM, Letendre J, Richter A. RET Gly691Ser mutation is associated with primary vesicoureteral reflux in the French-Canadian population from Quebec. Hum Mutat. 2008;29:695–702.
192. Yildirim-Toruner C, Subramanian K, El Manjra L, Chen E, Goldstein S, Vitale E. A novel frameshift mutation of FOXC2 gene in a family with hereditary lymphedema-distichiasis syndrome associated with renal disease and diabetes mellitus. Am J Med Genet A. 2004;131:281–6.
193. Yoshimura-Furuhata M, Nishimura-Tadaki A, Amano Y, Ehara T, Hamasaki Y, Muramatsu M, Shishido S, Aikawa A, Hamada R, Ishikura K, Hataya H, Hidaka Y, Noda S, Koike K, Wakui K, Fukushima Y, Matsumoto N, Awazu M, Miyake N, Kosho T. Renal complications in 6p duplication syndrome: microarray-based investigation of the candidate gene(s) for the development of congenital anomalies of the kidney and urinary tract (CAKUT) and focal segmental glomerular sclerosis (FSGS). Am J Med Genet A. 2015;167A:592–601.
194. Yosypiv IV, Boh MK, Spera MA, El-Dahr SS. Downregulation of Spry-1, an inhibitor of GDNF/Ret, causes angiotensin II-induced ureteric bud branching. Kidney Int. 2008;74:1287–93.
195. Zu S, Bartik Z, Zhao S, Sillen U, Nordenskjold A. Mutations in the ROBO2 and SLIT2 genes are rare causes of familial vesico-ureteral reflux. Pediatr Nephrol. 2009;24:1501–8.
196. Zweers MC, Bristow J, Steijlen PM, Dean WB, Hamel BC, Otero M, Kucharekova M, Boezeman JB, Schalkwijk J. Haploinsufficiency of TNXB is associated with hypermobility type of Ehlers-Danlos syndrome. Am J Hum Genet. 2003;73:214–7.

Prenatally Detected Vesicoureteral Reflux

Marie-Klaire Farrugia

Abstract Vesicoureteric reflux (VUR) diagnosed following investigation of prenatally-detected urinary tract dilatation (UTD), often remains asymptomatic and yet raises much parental anxiety and medical uncertainty. Previous studies suggest that "prenatal" VUR appears to have a different natural history to that of VUR diagnosed following investigation of recurrent febrile urinary tract infections (UTIs). Reports from Great Ormond Street (1997) and the Society for Fetal Urology registry (1999) highlighted the characteristics of VUR patients diagnosed following investigation of prenatal hydronephrosis, who were noted to be predominantly male with high-grade VUR and established renal uptake defects on DMSA. However, the management strategy tailored to this group of patients is not well-established, mainly due to the fact that studies on VUR management and outcome have included both prenatally-diagnosed and symptomatic patients, confounding the results. There is also a variation in diagnostic protocols following the findings of prenatal UTD, and indications for a micturating cystogram (MCUG) vary between institutions, making the incidence of asymptomatic VUR very variable. Studies focussing specifically on the asymptomatic cohort are few, small, and usually involve patients already on continuous antibiotic prophylaxis (CAP). Hence the true natural history of the condition is not known. A systematic review of 18 articles including 829 asymptomatic infants, mostly males with GIV–V VUR, revealed that 15.4% of infants developed at least one breakthrough UTI despite initiation of CAP from birth. The limited data available showed no conclu-

M.-K. Farrugia (✉)
Department of Paediatric Urology, Chelsea and Westminster Hospital and Imperial College (West London Children's Healthcare), London, UK
e-mail: m.farrugia@nhs.net

P. Puri, A. Yamataka (eds.), *Vesicoureteral Reflux*,
https://doi.org/10.1007/978-3-031-95091-9_6

sive benefit of CAP, primarily due to lack of a strong comparator cohort. The PREDICT trial is the only randomised controlled trial to date, and only included asymptomatic VUR patients, assigned to prophylaxis or no treatment. Febrile UTI's occurred in 21% of the prophylaxis group vs 35% of the no treatment group, and were more common in females, mostly in the first 6 months. Although the trial showed a small significant benefit of prophylaxis, this came at the expense of non-E Coli and resistant UTI's in the prophylaxis group. Importantly, there was no difference between the groups in the incidence of new scars at 2-year follow up. The authors concluded that prophylaxis might only be of benefit in girls, for the first year only. This chapter will expand on the evidence behind prenatal ultrasound findings which are indications for a postnatal VCUG; and further investigation and management once VUR is diagnosed in this (initially) asymptomatic patient group.

Keywords Vesicoureteric reflux · Prenatal diagnosis · Antenatal ultrasound · Urinary tract infection · Antibiotic prophylaxis · Renal scarring · Dysplasia · Micturating cystourethrogram · Antenatal hydronephrosis · Urinary tract dilation

Introduction

"Prenatally detected" vesicoureteric reflux (VUR) is defined as VUR diagnosed on investigation of urinary tract dilatation (UTD) detected on antenatal ultrasound scan. Improved antenatal ultrasound has led to a rise in the diagnosis of a prenatal VUR cohort, that appears to have a different natural history to that of VUR diagnosed as a result of investigation of recurrent febrile urinary tract infections (UTI's). Reports from Great Ormond Street (1997) and the Society for Fetal Urology registry (1999) highlighted the characteristics of VUR patients diagnosed following investigation of prenatal hydronephrosis, who were noted to be predominantly male with high-grade VUR and established renal uptake defects on DMSA. However, the management strategy tailored to this group of patients is not well-established, mainly due to the fact that studies on VUR management and outcome have included both prenatally-diagnosed and symptomatic patients,

Table 1 Characteristics of prenatally-detected and postnatally-diagnosed VUR

VUR	"Disease"	"Symptom"
Predominant gender	Male	Female
Age at presentation	Postnatal	Childhood
Ultrasound features	Upper tract dilatation	Normal
DMSA findings	Congenital uptake defects	Normal
Typical grade of VUR	IV–V	I–III
Spontaneous resolution	50% in the first 2 years	80–90%
Possible pathogenesis	Congenital urinary tract malformation	Bladder dysfunction

confounding the results. There is also a variation in diagnostic protocols following the findings of prenatal UTD, and indications for a micturating cystogram (MCUG) vary between institutions, making the incidence of asymptomatic VUR very variable. Demede et al. described two differing VUR patient groups in their review of "evidence-based medicine and vesicoureteral reflux" (Table 1) [1]. The congenital "reflux disease" patients are detected predominantly males with prenatal UTD, diagnosed with dilating IV–V VUR on postnatal MCUG, and renal uptake defects on DMSA. The second and more common form of VUR at the time, was defined as the "reflux symptom", usually detected following investigation of febrile UTI, more commonly in girls, who are found to have lesser VUR grades and normal kidneys. This distinction may explain the low incidence of VUR with concomitant chronic kidney disease (CKD) seen in 3–4 children/year/10^6 of age-related population, predominantly in males, and the high incidence of VUR without CKD seen in 10,000 children/year/10^6 of age related population, predominantly in female [2].

Prenatal Diagnosis: Why and When to Investigate

The gold standard technique for diagnosing VUR is the micturating (or voiding) cystourethrogram (MCUG/VCUG). Indications for a postnatal MCUG following antenatal ultrasound findings vary between institutions. The incidence of VUR appears to increase with the degree of dilatation; up to 40% of children with mild to moderate prenatal UTD will be found to have VUR, regardless of postnatal ultrasound findings (Table 2) [3]. However, the degree of dilatation does not correlate with the grade of VUR. In addition, a normal postnatal US does not exclude high-grade VUR. Visuri et al. reviewed the renal tract ultrasound scan findings in 180 infants with GIV-V VUR and concluded that a visible ureter and reduced renal length on postnatal ultrasound are significant risk factors for high-grade VUR, and would therefore be an indication for requesting an MCUG [4]. The Society for Fetal Urology (SFU) and American Urological Association (AUA) recommend an MCUG for SFU grade III–IV hydronephrosis, the presence of a hydroureter, or an

Table 2 Causes of prenatally-detected UTD

Aetiology	Incidence (%)
Transient/physiologic	50–70
Pelviureteric junction obstruction (PUJO)	10–30
Vesicureteric reflux (VUR)	10–40
Obstructive megaureter	5–15
Multicystic dysplastic kidney (MCDK)	2–5
Duplex systems/ureterocoele	4–7
Posterior urethral valves (PUV)	1–5
Other pathologies (urethral atresia/prune belly syndrome/polycystic kidneys)	Rare

abnormal bladder on fetal ultrasound [5]. The European Association of Urology (EAU) guidelines state that the use of MCUG is recommended in patients with ultrasound findings of bilateral high-grade hydronephrosis, dilated duplex kidneys/ureterocele, ureteric dilatation, abnormal bladders [6]. The common denominator between guidelines is that an MCUG should only be performed to exclude bladder outlet obstruction, and to diagnose conditions that may put the infant at risk of UTI and renal impairment, rather than to make a diagnosis of VUR per se. There is no evidence to support a VCUG for prenatally-diagnosed isolated hydronephrosis.

Indications for nuclear medicine studies (DMSA/MAG-3 renogram) following the diagnosis of VUR, also vary between institutions. The correlation between high-grade VUR and renal dysplasia is well known—and the finding of uptake defects on DMSA prior to the onset of febrile UTI's is prevalent in the prenatally-diagnosed group [7]. In a study to evaluate the characteristics of VUR in infants with prenatal hydronephrosis, Ransley's group in Great Ormond Street reported that of 155 consecutive patients, 75% were male, of whom half had bilateral VUR. 65% of patients with high-grade VUR had an abnormal DMSA, of whom 28% had focal damage and 72% generalized damage. Overall, there was a significantly greater prevalence of abnormal kidneys in males (40% vs 12% of females); 91% of abnormal kidneys were associated with severe reflux, that was significantly associated with males [8].

A DMSA may therefore be helpful to determine renal status in order to plan long-term follow-up, especially in patients with bilateral renal defects (Figs. 1, 2, and 3).

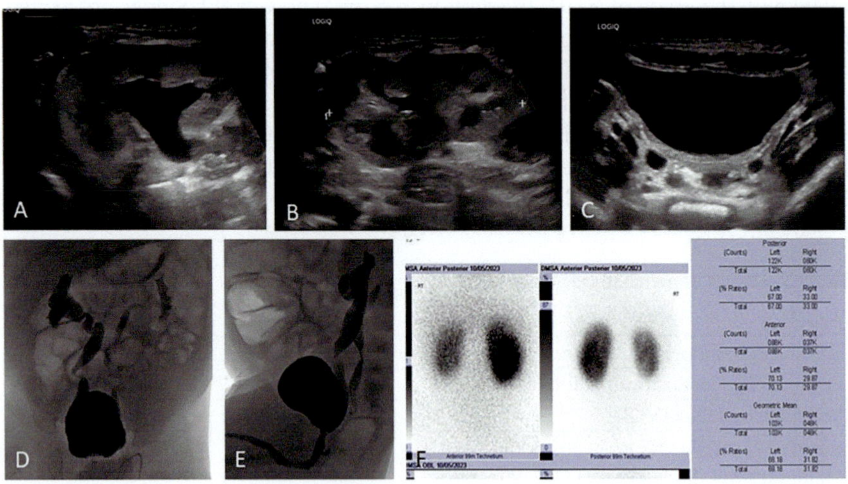

Fig. 1 Male infant with prenatally-detected bilateral hydronephrosis. Postnatal ultrasound (**a–c**) showing bilateral ureteric dilatation; MCUG (**d**, **e**) showed right GIV and left GIII VUR and normal posterior urethra, with evidence of right reduced function and scarring on DMSA (**f**)

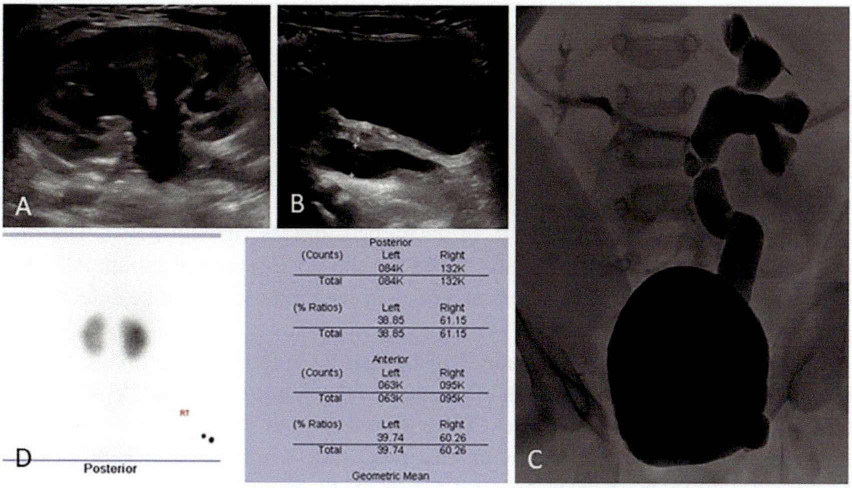

Fig. 2 Female infant with prenatally-detected left hydroureteronephrosis, confirmed postnatally (**a**, **b**). MCUG revealed left GIV and right G2 VUR (**c**) but no scarring on DMSA (**d**)

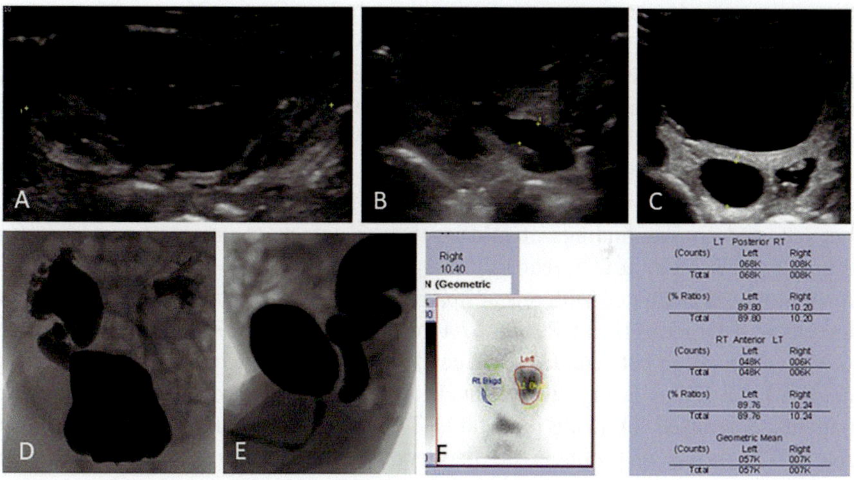

Fig. 3 Male infant with prenatally-detected right hydroureteronephrosis; noted to have right cystic dysplastic dilated kidney with ureteric dilatation, and a normal left kidney, on postnatal ultrasound (**a**–**c**). MCUG confirmed right GV and left GII VUR and a normal posterior urethra (**d**, **e**). DMSA showed poor uptake in the cystic dysplastic right kidney (**f**)

Demographics and Natural History

A number of studies in the literature sought to establish the clinical importance of asymptomatic VUR, in particular UTI risk and incidence of new scars. Whereas some studies report a "benign" course with likely spontaneous resolution and no new scars, others raise caution with reports of significant UTI risk despite prophylaxis, and development of new scars.

A study based on the Society for Fetal Urology hydronephrosis registry explored the natural history of 71 patients diagnosed with VUR following investigation of prenatal UTD [9]. The majority of patients were boys with bilateral high-grade VUR, and all patients were started on CAP. Outcomes revealed that Grades III to V reflux resolved at an average age of 0.9 and 2.1 years in 18% of renal units in boys and 37.5% in girls, respectively. UTI developed in 37% (mostly boys). The incidence of infection was significantly higher in the uncircumcised group. Although only a minority of patients underwent a nuclear medicine scan, uptake defects were identified in 63% [9].

Farhat et al. evaluated the natural history of 31 infants (54 refluxing ureters) diagnosed following investigation of prenatal UTD. VUR was grade IV–V in 48%, and again most patients were males. The authors reported a 50% chance of improvement (decrease in reflux grade by at least two grades) in high-grade reflux by age 16 months, using the Kaplan-Meier estimate. UTI developed in 26% of patients, while on CAP. There was no statistical difference between those who suffered a UTI who were circumcised, compared to those who were not [10]. A follow-up study by the same group reviewed outcomes of the same patient cohort at 4-year follow-up. Six patients underwent surgery and were excluded. Of the 25 remaining cases, reflux resolved in 13 patients (52%) and improved in 6 (24%): in particular, high-grade VUR resolved or improved in 59% of cases. Follow-up DMSA did not reveal new scars. The authors concluded that expectant management was effective in the majority of cases, and associated with a low UTI rate and no somatic growth retardation or hypertension [11].

Further retrospective case series confirmed a variable UTI rate on CAP (11–25%), but reported similar findings of DMSA uptake defects at presentation (14–34%) without progression at 2–7 year follow-up [12]. In the study by Silva et al., VUR resolution was evaluated with repeat imaging: at 48 months after diagnosis, 75% of the cases of Grade I–III VUR, and 37% of Grade IV–V VUR had resolved. There was no association between UTI and gender, grade of VUR or presence of cortical defects [13]. Evans et al. retrospectively evaluated UTI risk in 54 asymptomatic patients, diagnosed following prenatal UTD [14]. This study reported a higher UTI rate of 52%, whilst on prophylaxis. Bladder dysfunction was a significant risk factor for UTI. The authors reported that UTI occurred in 22% of boys after circumcision compared to 68% prior/without circumcision ($p < 0.05$) [14].

Four studies directly compared outcomes in the prenatal vs postnatally-diagnosed patient groups. The first of two retrospective studies by Ylinen et al. showed no difference in incidence of dysplasia at diagnosis (14%). During follow up, 38% of the antenatal cases developed a break-through UTI vs 47% in the postnatal group, whilst on prophylaxis. Focal renal scars developed during follow-up in 19% of renal units. New scars were observed in dilating VUR only, especially in grades IV and V, and these were exclusively in the postnatal patient group ($P < 0.005$) [15]. Chen et al. reviewed the outcome of 202 infants and similarly, did not find a difference in incidence of congenital dysplasia (28% vs 23%) between the prenatally-detected and postnatal group. Patients with high-grade VUR were more likely to suffer a break-through UTI when diagnosed following a UTI. New scars were also more prevalent in the UTI group; interestingly, half the boys who developed new scars had not had a breakthrough UTI [16].

Two prospective studies compared the outcome of a prenatally-detected VUR cohort versus those presenting with UTI. The first included 115 infants followed-up for a mean 62 months [17]. Renal status (parenchymal abnormality and function) remained unchanged 78%, improved in 5%, and deteriorated in 18%. Predictive factors for deterioration were recurrent febrile UTI, bilateral abnormality and reduced total glomerular filtration rate. In this study, deteriorated renal status was more common in cases diagnosed prenatally than in those detected after UTI—the authors speculated that this may be due the higher incidence of grade IV–V VUR in the antenatal group [17]. The second study did not show a difference in incidence of recurrent UTI (10.6%) or cortical defects (19%) between groups. Contrary to other studies, there was a higher VUR resolution in the postnatal group (73% vs 49%) [18].

It is challenging to reconcile the findings in these studies. There certainly appears to be a spontaneous resolution rate, even in the higher VUR grades, of up to 60% by 2 years. Incidence of UTI on prophylaxis varies between studies, from 10% (in a prospective study) to 52% (in a small retrospective study). Whereas three studies reported no progression of renal scarring at follow-up, others found a very consistent figure of 18–19% incidence of new scars, which appears to be unrelated to whether or not the patient suffered a break-through UTI. All patients were on prophylaxis.

Lower urinary tract dysfunction (LUTD) has been reported in children with VUR, including infants. Yeung et al. found abnormal urodynamics at 6 months of age in 57% of 42 infants diagnosed with moderate or severe VUR, compared with the dynamics in others with 'normal' lower urinary tracts and no history of VUR [19]. Godley et al. hypothesised that VUR may represent one component of a composite primary mal-development of the urinary tract, i.e. a sign of ipsilateral renal tract malformation, as opposed to the cause of it. They postulated that the mal-development, which includes LUTD, may extend to the kidney [20]. This hypothesis led to a study exploring the effect of early renal status and bladder function on VUR resolution at 16 months, which showed that VUR associated with normal kidneys would resolve by 16 months, whereas high-grade VUR with bilateral scarred kidneys, was a poor prognostic sign for the early outcome of VUR and for bladder function [20].

Pathophysiology

The pathophysiology of the two VUR entities is not well established. The study by Godley et al. was significant in showing associations that link the lower urinary tract, the competence of the vesico-ureteric junction (VUJ) and the kidneys. The embryologic explanation is that the trigone is formed from mesoderm as the mesonephric duct migrates caudally away from the ureteric bud. A primary embryological error affecting the mesonephric duct, or the ureteric bud, at a critical time may allow displacement of the VUJ and at the same time cause disorganization of the trigone with a potential for abnormal bladder outflow function. In turn, an abnormal location of the ureteric bud might be associated with anomalous renal differentiation, as shown by Mackie and Stephens [21]. Further, the nephrogenic mesenchyme is the tissue responsible for inducing the ureteric bud. Therefore, a primary mal-development involving uretero-trigonal structures and anomalous renal differentiation may account for patients with abnormal kidneys at the outset, LUTD and severe VUR through 'golf-hole' orifices with pronounced lateral displacement of the VUJ [22]. By contrast, delayed maturation or transient distortion of the intravesical ureter and trigonal muscular function may account for moderate, or even severe, VUR in infancy with normal kidneys and a good outcome.

Initial Management

Initial approach is conservative in all prenatally-diagnosed asymptomatic primary VUR patients. The conservative options include watchful waiting or continuous antibiotic prophylaxis (CAP). Use of CAP is not evidence-based in the prenatally-diagnosed cohort [23], but most current guidelines err on the side of caution and recommend starting CAP in infants diagnosed with grade III-V VUR [24]. The practice of recommending CAP is based on the assumption that prenatally-detected VUR is a risk factor for UTI, and hence raises the potential of acquired scarring. While this practice has been shown to be beneficial for infants with symptomatic VUR (i.e., VUR found after presentation with UTI), to date there has been only one recent trial evaluating this intervention in the asymptomatic VUR group [25].

A systematic review of 18 articles including 829 asymptomatic infants, of whom 473 (69.4%) were males and 48.7% had high grade (IV–V) VUR, revealed that 15.4% of infants developed at least one breakthrough UTI despite initiation of CAP from birth [26]. Forty-four percent of females developed a UTI while on CAP, versus 26% of males. The limited data available showed no conclusive benefit of CAP, primarily due to lack of a strong comparator cohort [26].

The PREDICT trial is the only prospective, randomized, controlled study to date, and compared the use of CAP vs no treatment for 24 months, in 292 infants (146 per group, 75% males) [25]. Most patients were diagnosed following investigation of prenatal UTD, and none had ever suffered a UTI. Further data analyses are planned at 5-year follow-up. Patients were 1–5 months of age, with grade III–V VUR (80.5% had grade IV or V VUR). In this study cohort, the use of CAP provided a significant but small benefit in preventing a first symptomatic UTI, which occurred in 21% of the CAP group and in 35.6% of the no-treatment group (hazard ratio, 0.55; 95% confidence interval [CI], 0.35–0.86; $p = 0.0008$). The time to the first UTI was 6.4 months in the prophylaxis group and 5.2 months in the untreated group, and most UTI's occurred within the first year. Interestingly, 64% of the infants in the no-treatment arm had no UTIs: it was necessary to treat seven infants for 2 years to prevent one UTI. Of note, Pseudomonas species, other non-Escherichia coli organisms, and antibiotic resistance, were more common in patients who suffered UTIs in the CAP arm vs the untreated group. In the subgroup analysis of the treatment effect in all combinations of participant, sex and VUR grade, CAP was mainly beneficial in female participants with grade IV or V VUR. The occurrence of new kidney scars at 2-year follow-up was similar (19%) between the two groups, and was unrelated to whether or not the patient had suffered a febrile UTI during the trial period. There was no difference in estimated GFR or serum creatinine between the two groups. The authors concluded that "although the trial showed a numerical benefit of primary CAP in young infants with VUR without preceding UTI, the results are of doubtful clinical benefit and we believe do not support the routine use of CAP in this population" [25].

The recent EAU/ESPU guideline update concluded that CAP may not be needed in every VUR patient, and suggested that a practical approach may be to use CAP until BBD resolution. The guidelines do not give any recommendations on the prenatal group, and only advise that initial medical management can be considered for a child with a febrile UTI and high-grade VUR [27].

Although circumcision is frequently offered in boys with VUR, the influence of circumcision on UTI risk is variable between studies [28]. The caveat is that a retractable foreskin has also been shown to reduce UTI risk [29, 30]. It is difficult to reconcile why some studies show a benefit of circumcision whereas others do not—this may be because the retractability in the non-circumcised group is often not documented.

Surgical Intervention

The previous section has highlighted that infants in both the CAP and observation groups are at risk of febrile UTI's. It is well-reported that recurrent febrile UTI's are a risk factor for new kidney scarring [31]—hence the consideration of surgical intervention in *symptomatic* patients. The question then arises as to whether surgery in infancy makes any difference to outcome—in terms of further UTI's and/or kidney function deterioration. Once again, there is a lack of articles specific to the prenatal group.

The Swedish infant high-grade reflux trial sought to answer this question, although the study was not limited to a prenatally-diagnosed cohort. Although the mean patient age was 2.3 (0.2–6.6) months, only 29% presented prenatally [32]. This was a prospective, randomized, controlled, multicentre trial, of 77 infants randomized to CAP ($n = 39$) or endoscopic injection treatment (with prophylaxis until resolution) ($n = 38$). 87% had abnormal scintigraphy, with more generalized damage in boys ($p = 0.0097$). 21% of infants developed a UTI, with no difference between the two treatment groups. Similarly to other studies, UTIs were more likely to occur in girls than in boys ($p = 0.039$) independent of treatment group [32].

Female sex and high post-void residual volume (PVR) was predictive of febrile UTI ($p = 0.039$ and 0.034). Kidney parenchyma deterioration was detected in eight children (10%) at follow-up, and correlated with recurrent UTI and VUR grade of the scarred renal unit. This study could not show any difference between endoscopic intervention and CAP in reducing the risk of UTI recurrence and kidney parenchyma deterioration [32].

Although the evidence for first-line endoscopic intervention is poor, surgery may be considered in symptomatic patients. Endoscopic anti-reflux procedures have been shown to be safe and effective in this age-group. Al Hindi et al. reported the prospective outcome of 30 children (50 renal units) with high-grade VUR who underwent endoscopic injection at a mean age of 6.3 ± 2.5 months. VUR resolution was seen in 76% of GIV VUR and 83% of GV VUR, at a mean follow-up of 6.5 years. Reported post-operative complications were haematuria, UTI and one case of ureteral obstruction. All the post-operative complications were managed conservatively; the ureteric obstruction resolved with conservative management within 8 weeks [33]. Vandersteen et al. and Cerwinka et al. reported a 0.3% and 0.6% rate of post-operative ureteric obstruction, respectively (all age groups) and therefore a post-operative ultrasound within the first 4 weeks is warranted to check for this [34, 35].

Ureteric reimplantation in infants below 1 year of age may be challenging due to the discrepancy between the grossly dilated ureter and the small infantile bladder, and concern regarding possible iatrogenic bladder dysfunction. De Jong investigated the bladder functional outcome of 49 neonates and infants with primary obstructive or refluxing megaureters who had undergone a Politano-Leadbetter procedure, at a mean follow-up of 7.3 years. No onset of voiding dysfunction was noted at follow-up, and bladder capacity for age was significantly increased. No postoperative ureteral obstruction was observed. The study concluded that early major reconstructions of the lower urinary tract do not damage the urodynamic properties of the bladder and pelvic floor, provided that the surgery is performed by specialized paediatric urological surgeons [36]. A further study from the same group compared urodynamic outcome in patients who had undergone ureteral reimplantation before or after 1 year of age. No significant difference in bladder capacity, compliance, or incidence of instability was found [37]. Upadhyay et al. reported similar outcomes in a 9.5-year follow-up study of 21 infants who had undergone ureteral reimplantation (half the patients had bilateral procedures) before 12 months of age [38].

Conclusion

VUR diagnosed following investigation of prenatally-detect UTD is known as "congenital VUR" and has a different natural history to VUR diagnosed following investigation of febrile UTI. It affects boys three times as much as girls, is high-grade and bilateral in up to 80%, and over 50% of patients have established kidney uptake defects on DMSA at presentation and prior to any UTI's [1]. An MCUG is indicated in patients with ultrasound features suspicious for bladder outlet obstruction, significant hydroureteronephrosis or renal hypodysplasia. In patients with high-grade VUR, a DMSA at baseline is helpful in identifying uptake defects, which are an indication for long-term follow-up, and may be of predictive value [27]. The driver for invasive imaging should be the underlying risk of obstruction, UTI or renal impairment, rather than to make a VUR diagnosis per se.

Although studies focussing on the natural history of congenital VUR are limited, and mainly include patients on prophylaxis, the evidence suggests that approximately one-third of patients will suffer at least one break-through UTI, and up to 19% may develop new scars, despite being on CAP. The PREDICT trial has shown that the figures in patients not initiated on CAP are very similar. The trial showed a significant but small difference in incidence of febrile UTI's at 2-year follow-up, and reported that most febrile UTI's occurred in the first 6–12 months of life, most commonly in females. Interestingly, 64% of the infants in the no-treatment arm did not suffer a UTI, and the occurrence of new kidney scarring was similar between the two groups. Infants in the CAP group were more likely to suffer UTI's with resistant or non E-coli organisms. Based on these findings, the PREDICT trial authors suggest that CAP could be omitted in male infants with asymptomatic reflux, after a comprehensive discussion with the family, while it could be recommended in females with dilating reflux and stopped at 12 months of age [25]. Indications for surgical intervention in prenatally-diagnosed VUR are not evidence based, and endoscopic or surgical treatment should only be considered in symptomatic patients [39].

References

1. Demède D, Cheikhelard A, Hoch M, Mouriquand P. Médecine factuelle et reflux vésico-urétéral. Ann Urol. 2006;40:161–74. https://doi.org/10.1016/j.anuro.2006.02.005.
2. Hewitt I, Montini G. Vesicoureteral reflux is it important to find? Pediatr Nephrol. 2021;36:1011–7. https://doi.org/10.1007/s00467-020-04573-9.
3. Nguyen HT, Herndon CDA, Cooper C, Gatti J, Kirsch A, Kokorowski P, et al. The Society for Fetal Urology consensus statement on the evaluation and management of antenatal hydronephrosis. J Pediatr Urol. 2010;6:212–31. https://doi.org/10.1016/j.jpurol.2010.02.205.
4. Visuri S, Kivisaari R, Jahnukainen T, Taskinen S. Postnatal imaging of prenatally detected hydronephrosis—when is voiding cystourethrogram necessary? Pediatr Nephrol. 2018;33:1751–7. https://doi.org/10.1007/s00467-018-3938-y.
5. Nguyen HT, Benson CB, Bromley B, Campbell JB, Chow J, Coleman B, et al. Multidisciplinary consensus on the classification of prenatal and postnatal urinary tract dilation (UTD classification system). J Pediatr Urol. 2014;10:982–98. https://doi.org/10.1016/j.jpurol.2014.10.002.
6. EAU. EAU guidelines on pediatric urology. n.d. https://D56bochluxqnzCloudfrontNet/Documents/Full-Guideline/EAU-Guidelines-on-Paediatric-Urology-2023Pdf. https://uroweb.org/guidelines/paediatric-urology
7. Peters C, Rushton HG. Vesicoureteral reflux associated renal damage: congenital reflux nephropathy and acquired renal scarring. J Urol. 2010;184:265–73. https://doi.org/10.1016/j.juro.2010.03.076.

8. Yeung CK, Godley ML, Dhillon HK, Gordon I, Duffy PG, Ransley PG. The characteristics of primary vesico-ureteric reflux in male and female infants with pre-natal hydronephrosis. Br J Urol. 1997;80:319–27.
9. Herndon CDA, McKenna PH, Kolon TF, Gonzales ET, Barker LA, Docimo SG. A multicenter outcomes analysis of patients with neonatal reflux presenting with prenatal hydronephrosis. J Urol. 1999;162:1203–8. https://doi.org/10.1097/00005392-199909000-00096.
10. Farhat W, McLorie G, Geary D, Capolicchio G, Bägli D, Merguerian P, et al. The natural history of neonatal vesicoureteral reflux associated with antenatal hydronephrosis. J Urol. 2000;164:1057–60. https://doi.org/10.1016/s0022-5347(05)67249-7.
11. Upadhyay J, McLorie GA, Bolduc S, Bägli DJ, Khoury AE, Farhat W. Natural history of neonatal reflux associated with prenatal hydronephrosis: long-term results of a prospective study. J Urol. 2003;169:1837–41. https://doi.org/10.1097/01.ju.0000062440.92454.cf.
12. McIlroy PJ, Abbott GD, Anderson NG, Turner JG, Mogridge N, Wells JE. Outcome of primary vesicoureteric reflux detected following fetal renal pelvic dilatation. J Paediatr Child Health. 2000;36:569–73. https://doi.org/10.1046/j.1440-1754.2000.00571.x.
13. Penido Silva JM, Oliveira EA, Diniz JSS, Bouzada MCF, Vergara RM, Souza BC. Clinical course of prenatally detected primary vesicoureteral reflux. Pediatr Nephrol. 2006;21:86–91. https://doi.org/10.1007/s00467-005-2058-7.
14. Evans K, Asimakadou M, Nwankwo O, Desai D, Cherian A, Mushtaq I, et al. What is the risk of urinary tract infection in children with antenatally presenting dilating vesico-ureteric reflux? J Pediatr Urol. 2015;11:93.e1–6. https://doi.org/10.1016/j.jpurol.2015.01.009.
15. Ylinen E, Ala-Houhala M, Wikström S. Risk of renal scarring in vesicoureteral reflux detected either antenatally or during the neonatal period. Urology. 2003;61:1238–42. https://doi.org/10.1016/S0090-4295(03)00229-2.
16. Chen JJ, Pugach J, West D, Naseer S, Steinhardt GF. Infant vesicoureteral reflux: a comparison between patients presenting with a prenatal diagnosis and those presenting with a urinary tract infection. Urology. 2003;61:442–6. https://doi.org/10.1016/S0090-4295(02)02275-6.
17. Sjöström S, Jodal U, Sixt R, Bachelard M, Sillén U. Longitudinal development of renal damage and renal function in infants with high grade vesicoureteral reflux. J Urol. 2009;181:2277–83. https://doi.org/10.1016/j.juro.2009.01.051.
18. Mohammadjafari H, Alam A, Mohammadi S, Mousavi SA, Kosaryan A, Khademloo M, et al. Outcome of vesicoureteral reflux in infants: impact of prenatal diagnosis. Iran J Pediatr. 2013;23:439–44.
19. Yeung CK, Godley ML, Dhillon HK, Duffy PG, Ransley PG. Urodynamic patterns in infants with normal lower urinary tracts or primary vesico-ureteric reflux. Br J Urol. 1998;81:461–7. https://doi.org/10.1046/j.1464-410X.1998.00567.x.
20. Godley ML, Desai D, Yeung CK, Dhillon HK, Duffy PG, Ransley PG. The relationship between early renal status, and the resolution of vesico-ureteric reflux and bladder function at 16 months. BJU Int. 2001;87:457–62.
21. Mackie GG, Stephens FD. Duplex kidneys: a correlation of renal dysplasia with position of the ureteral orifice. J Urol. 1975;114:274–80.
22. Lyon RP, Marshall S, Tanagho EA. The ureteral orifice: its configuration and competency. J Urol. 1969;102:504–9. https://doi.org/10.1016/S0022-5347(17)62184-0.
23. Montini G, Hewitt I. Urinary tract infections: to prophylaxis or not to prophylaxis? Pediatr Nephrol. 2009;24:1605–9. https://doi.org/10.1007/s00467-009-1213-y.
24. Peters CA, Skoog SJ, Arant BS, Copp HL, Elder JS, Hudson RG, et al. Summary of the AUA guideline on management of primary vesicoureteral reflux in children. J Urol. 2010;184:1134–44. https://doi.org/10.1016/j.juro.2010.05.065.
25. Morello W, Baskin E, Jankauskiene A, Yalcinkaya F, Zurowska A, Puccio G, et al. Antibiotic prophylaxis in infants with grade III, IV, or V vesicoureteral reflux. N Engl J Med. 2023;389:987–97. https://doi.org/10.1056/nejmoa2300161.
26. Leigh J, Rickard M, Sanger S, Petropoulos J, Braga LH, Chanchlani R. Antibiotic prophylaxis for prevention of urinary tract infections in the first year of life in children with vesicoure-

teral reflux diagnosed in the workup of antenatal hydronephrosis: a systematic review. Pediatr Nephrol. 2020;35:1639–46. https://doi.org/10.1007/s00467-020-04568-6.
27. Gnech M, 't Hoen L, Zachou A, Bogaert G, Castagnetti M, O'Kelly F, et al. Update and summary of the European Association of Urology/European Society of Paediatric Urology paediatric guidelines on vesicoureteral reflux in children. Eur Urol. 2024;85:433–42.
28. Morris BJ, Wiswell TE. Circumcision and lifetime risk of urinary tract infection: a systematic review and meta-analysis. J Urol. 2013;189:2118–24. https://doi.org/10.1016/j.juro.2012.11.114.
29. Holzman SA, Chamberlin JD, Davis-Dao CA, Le DT, Delgado VA, Macaraeg AM, et al. Retractable foreskin reduces urinary tract infections in infant boys with vesicoureteral reflux. J Pediatr Urol. 2021;17:209.e1–6. https://doi.org/10.1016/j.jpurol.2021.01.007.
30. Chen CJ, Satyanarayan A, Schlomer BJ. The use of steroid cream for physiologic phimosis in male infants with a history of UTI and normal renal ultrasound is associated with decreased risk of recurrent UTI. J Pediatr Urol. 2019;15:472.e1–6. https://doi.org/10.1016/j.jpurol.2019.06.018.
31. Chen MJ, Cheng HL, Chiou YY. Risk factors for renal scarring and deterioration of renal function in primary vesico-ureteral reflux children: a long-term follow-up retrospective cohort study. PLoS One. 2013;8:e57954. https://doi.org/10.1371/journal.pone.0057954.
32. Nordenström J, Sjöström S, Sillén U, Sixt R, Brandström P. The Swedish infant high-grade reflux trial: UTI and renal damage. J Pediatr Urol. 2017;13:146–54. https://doi.org/10.1016/j.jpurol.2016.12.023.
33. Al Hindi S, Mubarak M, Al Aradi H. High-grade vesicoureteral reflux in infants: our experience with endoscopic subureteric injections. Urologia. 2022;89:120–5. https://doi.org/10.1177/0391560320966187.
34. Vandersteen DR, Routh JC, Kirsch AJ, Scherz HC, Ritchey ML, Shapiro E, et al. Postoperative ureteral obstruction after subureteral injection of dextranomer/hyaluronic acid copolymer. J Urol. 2006;176:1593–5. https://doi.org/10.1016/j.juro.2006.06.101.
35. Kirsch AJ, Kaye JD, Cerwinka WH, Watson JM, Elmore JM, Lyles RH, et al. Dynamic hydrodistention of the ureteral orifice: a novel grading system with high interobserver concordance and correlation with vesicoureteral reflux grade. J Urol. 2009;182:1688–92. https://doi.org/10.1016/j.juro.2009.02.061.
36. de Jong TP. Treatment of the neonatal and infant megaureter in reflux, obstruction and complex congenital anomalies. Acta Urol Belg. 1997;65:45–7.
37. De Kort LMO, Klijn AJ, Uiterwaal CSPM, De Jong TPVM. Ureteral reimplantation in infants and children: effect on bladder function. J Urol. 2002;167:285–7. https://doi.org/10.1016/S0022-5347(05)65451-1.
38. Upadhyay J, Shekarriz B, Fleming P, González R, Barthold JS. Ureteral reimplantation in infancy: evaluation of long-term voiding function. J Urol. 1999;162:1209–12. https://doi.org/10.1016/S0022-5347(01)68135-7.
39. Puri P, Friedmacher F, Farrugia MK, Sharma S, Esposito C, Mattoo TK. Primary vesicoureteral reflux. Nat Rev Dis Primers 2024;10:75.

Vesicoureteral Reflux and Urinary Tract Infection

Per Brandström, Sverker Hansson, and Magnus Lindén

Abstract Urinary tract infection (UTI) is one of the most common bacterial infection in children affecting 1.7% of boys and 8.4% of girls before the age of 7 years. The diagnostic work up can be demanding, especially in infants where the symptoms are often vague and urine sampling for urinalysis and the mandatory urine culture is more challenging. Antibiotic treatment for 7–10 days is recommended in febrile UTI and 3–5 days in cystitis. It can safely be given orally to most children.

Vesicoureteral reflux (VUR) is often diagnosed after a UTI, but nowadays prenatal hydronephrosis is an increasing reason for detecting VUR, with growing awareness of the congenital nature of many of the kidney damages associated to VUR. New kidney scarring and deterioration of old preexisting damage is strongly associated to high grade VUR and recurrent febrile UTI. However, long-term consequences of kidney damage related to UTI and VUR, are rare and in most cases limited.

The objective of different guidelines for UTI in children is to identify children with high grade VUR and severe kidney damage. They also have a common aim to eliminate the discomfort of recurrent symptomatic UTI and reduce the risk for long-term complications.

Keywords Urinary tract infections · Vesicoureteral reflux · Kidney damage

P. Brandström (✉) · S. Hansson
Queen Silvia Children's Hospital, Sahlgrenska University Hospital, Gothenburg, Sweden

Inst of Clinical Science, Dept of Pediatrics, Sahlgrenska Academy, University of Gothenburg, Gothenburg, Sweden
e-mail: per.brandstrom@gu.se

M. Lindén
Department of Pediatrics, Halland Hospital, Halmstad, Sweden

Inst of Clinical Science, Dept of Pediatrics, Sahlgrenska Academy, University of Gothenburg, Gothenburg, Sweden

P. Puri, A. Yamataka (eds.), *Vesicoureteral Reflux*,
https://doi.org/10.1007/978-3-031-95091-9_7

Urinary Tract Infections in Studies and in Real Life

Urinary tract infection (UTI) is one of the most common bacterial infections in children and affects 1.7% of boys and 8.4% of girls before the age of 7 years with the highest incidence the first year of life [27, 30, 52]. In infants presenting symptoms are usually vague with fever, inadequate feeding or failure to thrive. The work-up in a child with suspected UTI starts with a urine sample. Adhesive bags to the perineum, nappy pads, mid-stream voided urine/clean catch and invasive methods with catheter or suprapubic aspiration are used. Most studies have strict criteria for urine sampling, at least for urine culture, that are not always complied with in everyday medical practice. Urinalysis with dipstick or microscopy can be performed independent of sampling technique. The leukocyte esterase test is often used in the initial evaluation of a suspected UTI in children. In many studies a positive urinalysis is required for a UTI diagnosis. These tests are more likely to be negative in infections with non-*E. coli* bacteria and in UTI with low bacterial counts. The use of a negative leukocyte esterase test to rule out a UTI has been questioned, as it will leave some children with a febrile UTI without proper treatment [55]. The advice is to view a positive leukocyte-esterase test as indicative for a UTI, although not a definite proof, while a negative test makes UTI unlikely, but does not rule it out completely. Nitrite test has a low sensitivity in children, while the specificity is high (99%). A positive nitrite test strongly supports the presence of bacteriuria, while a negative nitrite test is of little or no diagnostic help in children. There are additional urine biomarkers that have been studied for their ability to differentiate between UTI and other febrile infections. Neutrophil gelatinase-associated lipocalin and interleukine-8 are two of the more promising biomarkers, but they still have to find their way into clinical practice [1, 56, 65].

It is standard procedure and uniformly recommended in guidelines to always confirm a UTI in a child with a urine culture. Urine culture should not be performed on urine from nappy pads or urine bags, owing to the high risk of contamination. A positive urine culture requires growth of a single uropathogen, with some rare exceptions. The cut off for bacterial count, or colony forming units (CFU), is usually set to a fix number. Since this level is not standardized globally, studies are using different cut off limits, as shown in Table 1. Since urine normally is presumed to be sterile, any growth after bladder aspiration is considered positive in many guidelines. In clean catch urine, also referred to as midstream free voided urine, the lower limit of significant growth is set to 10^4–10^5 cfu/mL in most guidelines, while the limit from catheterized urine is often lower. With these limits there is a risk that a true UTI goes undetected when the number of bacteria is low, which is more likely in infections with non-*E. coli* strains [55, 63]. Moreover, in real life there are practical aspects to UTI in children that can make it challenging to implement results from scientific studies into clinical practice. For example, urine culture is not always done or even possible in some circumstances, leaving the physician to decide about treatment and follow-up based on less robust information.

Table 1 Summary of a selection of globally published guidelines on Urinary tract infections in children

		Diagnostic procedure/test			Treatment			Imaging		
Guidelines	Age	Urine collection in non-toilet trained	Significant bacteriuria	Blood test recommended	Route of administration in febrile UTI	Length of treatment (days) in febrile UTI	Prophylactic antibiotics recommended	RBUS	VCUG	DMSA
UK/NICE	0–16 years	1. MSU	Not defined	CRP *should not* be used for differentiating upper/lower UTI	<3 months: refer to hospital	10	No	<6 months: all children	<6 months if atypical or recurrence	<3 years if atypical or recurrence
		2. Pad			<1 month: iv			>6 months if atypical or recurrence	6–36 months: consider if [atypical or recurrence] + risk factor[b]	>3 years if recurrence
		3. Cath/SPA			<3 months and toxic: iv					
					>3 months oral					
USA/AAP[a]	2–24 months	Cath/SPA	Cath/SPA $\geq 5x10^4$	No recommendations given	Iv if toxic/unable to retain oral fluid	7-14	No	All children	If abnormal RBUS or complicated UTI	Not recommended
		MSU for screening			Otherwise oral				Consider if recurrence	
Italy[a]	2–36 months	Hospital-toxic: Cath/SPA	Cath/SPA $\geq 10^4$	<3 months and hospitalized: CRP, PCT, FBC, creat	Iv toxic/unable to retain oral fluid	10	Not routine	All children	If abnormal RBUS, recurrence or non-*E Coli* infection	If VUR grade 4-5
		Not toxic: MSU	MSU $\geq 5x10^4$		<3 months: iv		Consider if: VUR grade 4–5			
		Bag for screening			Otherwise oral		>3 febrile UTIs/1 year			
Canada	>2 months	Cath/SPA	SPA all growth	Creat if "complicated" UTI	Iv if toxic/unable to retain oral fluid	7–10	Not routine	<2 years all children	If abnormal RBUS	Only if UTI diagnosis is in doubt (acute scan)
		MSU for screening	Cath $\geq 5 \times 10^4$		Otherwise oral		VUR grade 4–5 and anomalies: discuss with urologist		<2 years if recurrence	
			MSU $\geq 10^5$							

(continued)

Table 1 (continued)

Guidelines	Age	Diagnostic procedure/test: Urine collection in non-toilet trained	Diagnostic procedure/test: Significant bacteriuria	Diagnostic procedure/test: Blood test recommended	Treatment: Route of administration in febrile UTI	Treatment: Length of treatment (days) in febrile UTI	Treatment: Prophylactic antibiotics recommended	Imaging: RBUS	Imaging: VCUG	Imaging: DMSA
ESPU/EAU	0–18 years	Cath/SPA/MSU	SPA all growth	<1 year: CRP/PCT, FBC, creat, electrolytes	<2 months: iv	7–14 (toilet trained, uncomplicated 7)	Consider if <1 year and in non-toilet trained girls	All children with febrile UTI	<1 year: all children	Alternative to VCUG (top-down) within 1–2 months from infection
		Bag for screening	Cath ≥10^3		Iv if toxic/ unable to retain oral fluid				>1 year: non-*E. coli* UTI, recurrent febrile UTI	
			MSU ≥10^5 (10^4 if sympt)		Otherwise oral				Alternative: DMSA (top-down model)	
Spain	0–18 years	Cath/SPA/MSU	SPA all growth	Optional: If <3 months blood culture	Iv if toxic/ unable to retain oral fluid	7–10	No Consider if obstructive uropathy	<6 months: all children		If atypical or recurrence
		Bag for screening	Cath ≥10^3		<3 months: iv			>6 months if atypical or recurrence		If UTI diagnosis is in doubt
			MSU ≥10^5 (10^4 if sympt)		Otherwise oral					
Sweden	0–18 years	1. SPA if <1 year	Not defined	CRP, creat, blood culture if iv	Iv if toxic/ unable to retain oral fluid	10	VUR≥ grade 3	<2 years: all children	<2 years if dilatation on RBUS or DMSA pathology	<2 years if abnormal RBUS, risk factor[c] or recurrence
		2. MSU (x2)			Otherwise oral		Recurrent UTI	>2 years: febrile UTI or recurrent cystitis (boys one, girls three)	>2 years if [recurrent febrile UTI or abnormal RBUS] + DMSA pathology	>2 years if abnormal RBUS or febrile recurrence
		3. Cath								

Asia	Not defined	Cath/SPA	SPA all growth	Consider PCT or CRP	<3 months: refer to hospital	7–14	VUR≥ grade 3	All children with febrile UTI	If abnormal RBUS and or abnormal DMSA	Severe acute pyelonephritis
		Bag for screening	Cath $\geq 5 \times 10^4$		<3 months and toxic: iv		Recurrent UTI		If febrile recurrence	Hypodysplasia on RBUS
			MSU $\geq 10^5$		>3 months oral		Urinary tract obstruction			If UTI diagnosis is in doubt (acute scan)
Switzerland	0–16 years	1. Cath/SPA	SPA all growth	Consider: CRP/PCT	<2 months: iv	7–10	Consider in: VUR grade 4–5	All children with febrile UTI	Risk factors[d]	Consider after interdisciplinary discussion
		2. MSU	Cath $\geq 10^3$	<3 months: FBC, electrolytes, creatinine	Iv if toxic/unable to retain oral fluid		Complex CAKUT or underlying bladder dysfunction		Abnormal RBUS	
		Bag for screening	MSU $\geq 10^5$		Otherwise oral				Recurrent pyelonephritis (2 or more episodes)	

Reprinted by permission from pp 1102–1103 in [8]

UK/NICE [38]; USA/AAP [46, 61]; Italy [5]; Canada [47]; ESPU/EAU [58, 64]; Spain [41]; Sweden [9]; Asia [70]; Switzerland [12]

[a]Guideline only considers febrile UTIs

[b]UK risk factors: dilatation on ultrasound (US), poor urine flow, non-*E. coli*, family history of VUR

[c]Swedish risk factors: dilatation on US, serum CRP ≥70 mg/mL, non-*E. coli*, increased serum creatinine

[d]Swiss risk factors: abnormal US, poor urine flow, oliguria, urinary retention, non-*E.coli*, treatment failure >48 h, abnormal creatinine or electrolytes

UTI urinary tract infection, *RBUS* renal ad bladder ultrasonography, *VCUG* voiding cystourethrography, *DMSA* 99Tc-dimercaptosuccuunic acid, *MSU* mid stream urine, *SPA* suprapubic aspiration, C-reactive protein, *PCT* procalcitonin, *FBC* full blood count, *CAKUT* congenital anomalies of the kidneys and urinary tract

Antibiotic treatment of UTI in children can safely be initiated orally if the child is not severely sick or vomiting and tolerates oral feeding. Most guidelines still recommend initial intravenous treatment in the youngest children, the limit usually set at or below 2–3 months of age. Most guidelines recommend a treatment duration of 7–10 days for febrile infections, 14 days in the most severe cases. In afebrile infections 3–5 days of treatment is sufficient [60]. The choice of antibiotic agent depends on local resistance pattern and access to child friendly preparations and will not be specified in this chapter. As most children are treated empirically before the results from urine culture is available, it is important to inform the parents that the child is expected to improve significantly within 48 h of treatment. If that is not the case the child should be reevaluated promptly. High alertness of the healthcare provider to change the antibiotic agent depending on the culture results and the resistance pattern is of utmost importance.

UTI and Identification of VUR

In some children VUR is suspected before birth from urinary tract dilatation detected on antenatal ultrasonography. These children are usually evaluated after birth with ultrasonography, and in those with persisting urinary tract dilatation, imaging is recommended to confirm the VUR diagnosis or to detect any obstruction of the urinary tract. To manage children with VUR with antibiotic prophylaxis before any UTI has occurred has been questioned. In a European randomized study on prophylaxis to infants with VUR prior to any UTI, the lower UTI recurrence rate seen in children treated with prophylaxis came at a cost of recurrences more often caused by non-*E. coli* or resistant strains [71]. The issue will not be further addressed in this chapter.

Most children with VUR have been identified after a urinary tract infection. Historically most guidelines recommended imaging to detect any grade of VUR after the first UTI, preferably with voiding cystourethrography (VCUG). Today most advocate a more selective approach in the management of children with UTI. The aim is to reduce the burden of invasive imaging without having children with significant VUR go undiagnosed. By identifying risk factors for clinically important VUR, further imaging to detect the presence and grade of VUR can be more selective. Earlier studies, where VCUG was performed in most children with a first time UTI, revealed VUR in about 30–40% of all children with UTI, but only half of them were dilating grade III to V, see Fig. 1 [25, 29].

Through the years clinical factors associated with UTI and correlated to a greater risk of significant VUR have been proposed. These include UTI with other bacteria than *E. coli*, urinary tract dilatation on ultrasonography and renal parenchymal defects, either from kidney engagement of the acute UTI or congenital parenchymal

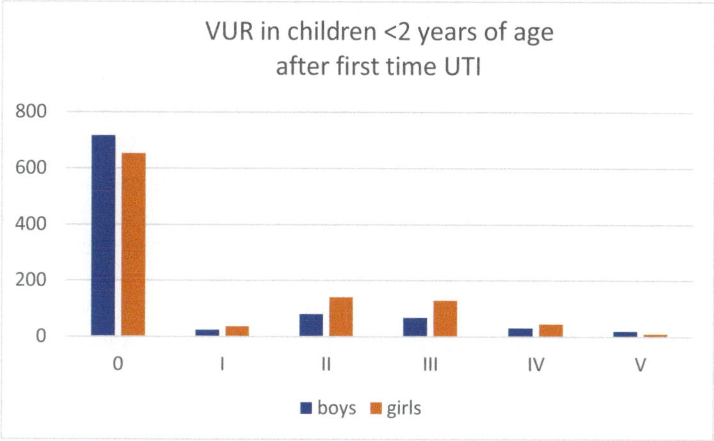

Fig. 1 VUR grade in 1953 of a total of 2309 children <2 years of age with first time UTI. From the results of a Swedish Quality Assurance study. [25]

defects. Inflammatory markers have been studied as indicators for acute pyelonephritis, implying kidney involvement in febrile UTI. Procalcitonin values ≥0.5 μg/L or CRP ≥70 mg/L have been shown to correlate with renal parenchymal involvement motivating more thorough follow-up [35, 43].

The gold standard for detecting renal parenchymal involvement at or after UTI is 99Tc-dimercaptosuccinic acid scan (DMSA). However, in the acute phase it is sometimes difficult to differentiate between preexisting congenital defects and acute parenchymal defects from the inflammatory response to the infection. Acute defects on DMSA are highly correlated to high grade VUR and have been proposed to be used to identify children who would benefit from more specific VUR assessment [42]. Permanent kidney scarring or defects were historically detected by intravenous urography, but today DMSA is preferred, preferably with at least 6 months interval since the last febrile UTI, to allow for acute uptake defects to resolve. Children with larger or bilateral permanent defects or scarring have been recommended for follow-up to reduce the risk of long-term sequelae, while the long-term effect of smaller restricted defects has been questioned. Most guidelines, however, do not recommend DMSA to be performed after childhood UTI, neither in the acute phase nor for follow-up, and reserve this investigation for children with more severe abnormalities on ultrasound or signs of decreased kidney function.

This shift towards lesser radiographic investigations after UTI in children, may delay the diagnosis of VUR. However, VUR poses little risk of progressive kidney damage in the absence of UTI. With attentive follow-up and prompt action at recurrent UTI, the risk for kidney deterioration in children with undetected VUR is diminished [6].

VUR, Renal Damage and Recurrent UTI

The association between UTI and congenital abnormalities of the kidney and urinary tract, especially its association to VUR and kidney scarring has been thoroughly evaluated. There is a strong correlation between dilating VUR and permanent renal damage in boys, where it is often congenital. In girls, the role of UTI and renal inflammation seem to be equally or more important, with VUR as a reinforcing factor [62]. Many studies have pointed out that the risk for kidney damage increases with increasing number of UTI recurrences [11, 31, 54].

The study by Alsaywid on boys with high grade VUR (IV or V), identified at evaluation after prenatal hydronephrosis or UTI, highlights the fact that UTI recurrences do occur also in boys with high grade VUR, and new renal damage is strongly related to the recurrence of infections [3].

There have been attempts to stratify the risk of UTI recurrence by identifying risk factors. One risk stratification and probability model for breakthrough infections in children with VUR on antibiotic prophylaxis was presented by Hidas et al. [28]. The risk factors they identified and included were high grade (IV or V) VUR, presentation of VUR after urinary tract infection and female gender. Bladder and bowel dysfunction also increases the risk of UTI recurrence, most pronounced in children with low grade VUR (I to III). The objective with their probability model was to aid physicians to better inform families about the 2-year risk of breakthrough infections and treatment strategies.

The risk for UTI recurrence is correlated not only to VUR grade but also to the timing of reflux during filling of the bladder. When reflux into the ureter starts early in the filling phase there is a higher risk of breakthrough infections, independent of the VUR grade [2]. The authors argue that cystogram reports should include the bladder volume at which the reflux is first noted, providing the clinician with prognostic information about recurrence risk and chances of VUR resolution.

Park reported higher risk for recurrences the earlier the child had its first UTI during their first year of life. Those with higher grade of VUR, bilateral VUR or a non-*E. coli* strain causing their first UTI, also had a significantly increased risk of recurrent UTIs [39].

UTI After VUR Correction

In a study by Chi et al. the number of UTI before surgical VUR correction with dextranomer/hyaluronic acid injection was the best predictor of postoperative recurrences. Furthermore, recurrent VUR was present in nearly half those with postoperative febrile urinary tract infections [14]. In a study by Sedberry-Ross up to 27% of patients with a successful endoscopic treatment suffered from recurrent febrile UTI and more than 90% of these children had delayed VUR recurrence [50]. Thus, recurrent UTI in children treated for VUR might indicate recurrence of VUR. These results are somewhat different from previous observations from an era where neo-implantation was the method of choice for VUR surgery in most centers. Children with VUR detected after a febrile UTI were still susceptible to UTI after surgical VUR correction, but most of their recurrent infections were afebrile. [7, 32].

How to Reduce UTI Recurrence and Renal Damage

The objective for most guidelines on children with VUR is to reduce the risk for kidney damage and future complications linked to this. It has been shown that antibiotic prophylaxis as well as surgical correction or reduction of VUR will reduce the UTI recurrence rate, and by doing so the risk of future renal damage is expected to be reduced as well. In the Swedish Reflux Trial, where antibiotic prophylaxis and endoscopic treatment of VUR both were superior to surveillance only in reducing the number of UTI recurrences, this was correlated to a significant (prophylaxis group) or trend for (endoscopic treatment) lower risk of new renal damage [11]. However, since new permanent kidney damage after UTI is a rare event, except in those with high grade VUR, most studies have not been able to demonstrate any significant results on lowering the rate of kidney damage with different management strategies. Nevertheless, management recommendations are focusing on lowering UTI recurrence rates with the aim of eliminating the discomfort of symptomatic UTI and reducing the risk for kidney damage.

For many years antibiotic prophylaxis was used to prevent recurrent UTI in all children with VUR, with very little scientific support. When more recent randomized studies on prophylaxis were performed, limited or no benefit was found of prophylactic antibiotics over surveillance only [18, 36, 40], or even negative effect with more recurrences in the treated group [26]. But in a few studies antibiotic prophylaxis lowered the risk of UTI recurrence in high grade VUR in girls [10] and boys [48]. The Randomized Intervention for Children with Vesicoureteral Reflux (RIVUR) trial found a protective effect in all VUR grades, [45] confirmed in a meta-analysis of available studies [16]. According to the latest studies, the RIVUR trial in USA and a large placebo-controlled study in Australia, prophylaxis will reduce the recurrence rate by up to 50% [15, 45]. Recurrences tend to be more frequent if the child is treated with a prophylactic agent to which the bacteria of a previous UTI was resistant [34].

On the downside of prophylaxis there is also an increased risk of multidrug resistance [51]. The risk of extended-spectrum beta-lactamase producing bacteria or other non-*E. coli* multidrug pathogens is greater if the child receives cephalosporin prophylaxis, the use of which should be discouraged [13]. The preferred prophylactic agents in many guidelines are trimethoprim-sulfamethoxazole or nitrofurantoin.

Circumcision in boys has been shown to reduce the UTI recurrence rate significantly and it can be redommended for uncircumcised boys with high grade VUR and recurrent UTI [57]. Additional non-surgical treatments have been proposed for childhood UTI including urotherapy based behavioral modification with timed voiding and biofeedback training for dysfunctional voiding, treatment of phimosis with topical steroids, cranberry juice, vitamin A, vitamin D, and clean intermittent catheterization for children with large post void residual urine. Published reports on these methods are usually small in patient numbers and are often lacking randomization and control group [69].

VUR, UTI and Bowel and Bladder Dysfunction

Bladder and bowel dysfunction (BBD), or dysfunctional elimination syndrome, increases the risk of UTI recurrences and breakthrough infections. It also plays an important role in delayed VUR resolution and reduces the success rate after VUR interventions with surgery and injection therapies. This correlation between bladder/sphincter dysfunction and UTI recurrence and delayed resolution of VUR was noted already in the International Reflux Study, implying the necessity of detection and treatment of these children [66]. Evaluating and treating children with BBD will be cost effective, by decreasing the number of UTI recurrences and the need for surgical interventions [33].

Contributing Factors to UTI Severity and Long-Term Consequences

Differences in severity of pediatric urinary tract infections can be attributed to different levels of bacterial virulence [59]. But there is also increasing interest and growing knowledge on how human genetic variation contributes to the risk for UTI and its consequences in children. The innate immune system is important in preventing UTI by different antimicrobial peptides and proteins in the urine. When a UTI occurs, the innate immune system regulates the reaction of host defense systems to the infection by modifying the intensity of symptoms from the inflammatory response and the degree of parenchymal scarring [23, 44, 49].

VUR is not the main risk factor for sequelae after UTI, but rather congenital anomalies of the kidney and urinary tract (CAKUT) and bladder-bowel dysfunction. Hence, many guidelines recommend ultrasonography of the urinary tract after pyelonephritis in children, although they differ in their recommendations to what extent all children should be assessed with ultrasonography, or if it should be reserved for a more restricted group of children at greater risk of kidney and urinary tract abnormalities [12, 38]. The sensitivity of ultrasonography, however, to detect even high grade VUR (IV and V) is poor [37].

Imaging of VUR, in addition to ultrasonography, is nowadays often not recommended unless the child has a complicated UTI or UTI recurrence [17]. The definition of a complicated or atypical UTI is not always stated but usually refers to a febrile infection with one or several risk factors, including severely sick child, non-*E. coli* infections, abnormal findings on ultrasound, abnormalities in the lower back or abdomen and defects on acute DMSA scan [4].

Girls prone to UTI continue to be susceptible to symptomatic UTI as adults, but the infections shift from febrile to afebrile [22]. This is also true for girls successfully treated for VUR, who continue to be susceptible to mainly afebrile UTI as adults, while recurrent UTI is a rare event in boys and adult men [7].

Permanent kidney damage after febrile UTI in children is found in approximately 15% [53]. Long-term complications from renal scarring after childhood UTI have been documented, with reduced kidney function, hypertension and pregnancy complications. Long-term follow-up data from Finland and Sweden have put these risks into a more realistic perspective. In a study of 1221 children after a first febrile UTI followed to a mean age of 24.5 years, a normal glomerular filtration rate (GFR) without any deterioration between 14.5 and 24.5 years was seen in those with unilateral scarring. For seven children with bilateral scars there was no deterioration over time although their GFR was significantly lower compared to those with unilateral scars. There was no increase in hypertension measured with 24 h ambulatory blood pressure monitoring (ABPM) [67, 68]. In another long-term study 86 women with recurrent UTI or kidney scarring in childhood were followed-up at a median age of 27 and later at 41 years. In those without scarring or unilateral scarring GFR was unchanged, while in those with bilateral scarring GFR dropped from a median of 96 mL/min/1.73 m^2 to 81 mL/min/1.73 m^2. Hypertension diagnosed with ABPM was found in 38% of women with kidney scarring and in 14% of those without scars. The degree of hypertension correlated to the extent of kidney damage seen on DMSA, and pregnancy related hypertension was only seen in women with kidney scarring [19–21]. In a Finnish study 1185 children were followed 6 to 17 years after UTI. New kidney damage was rare, but was found in 20% of those with high grade VUR. At follow-up at an age of 6 to 25 years all had normal estimated GFR from cystatin-C and were normotensive, none presented with proteinuria [24].

Conclusion

In all children, febrile UTI is a nasty, discomforting and potentially severe disease. It is often the event that leads to the identification of children with kidney or urinary tract anomalies. Recurrent UTI is associated with high grade VUR, and especially in combination with bladder and bowel dysfunction, it is correlated to an increased risk of kidney damage and long-term complications. With good access to proper evaluation and prompt treatment of UTI in children, such complications are rare. For most children the risk of progression of kidney damage and hypertension after childhood UTI appears to be very low. However, since it may take up to 30 to 40 years for long-term sequelae to manifest in patients with more pronounced or bilateral kidney scarring, we recommend they are monitored regarding renal function, blood pressure and proteinuria to counteract further kidney deterioration.

References

1. Abbasi A, Nabizadeh F, Gardeh M, Mohamed Ali K, Yousefifard M, Hosseini M. Discriminatory precision of neutrophil gelatinase-associated lipocalin in detection of urinary tract infection in children: a systematic review and meta-analysis. Arch Acad Emerg Med. 2020;8(1):e56.
2. Alexander SE, Arlen AM, Storm DW, Kieran K, Cooper CS. Bladder volume at onset of vesicoureteral reflux is an independent risk factor for breakthrough febrile urinary tract infection. J Urol. 2015;193(4):1342–6.
3. Alsaywid BS, Saleh H, Deshpande A, Howman-Giles R, Smith GH. High grade primary vesicoureteral reflux in boys: longterm results of a prospective cohort study. J Urol. 2010;184(4 Suppl):1598–603.
4. Alsaywid BS, Alyami FA, Alqarni N, Neel KF, Almaddah TO, Abdulhaq NM, Alajmani LB, Hindi MO, Alshayie MA, Alsufyani H, Alajlan SA, Albulushi BI, Labani SK. Urinary tract infection in children: a narrative review of clinical practice guidelines. Urol Ann. 2023;15(2):113–32.
5. Ammenti A, Alberici I, Brugnara M, Chimenz R, Guarino S, La Manna A, La Scola C, Maringhini S, Marra G, Materassi M, Morello W, Nicolini G, Pennesi M, Pisanello L, Pugliese F, Scozzola F, Sica F, Toffolo A, Montini G, Italian Society of Pediatric, N. Updated Italian recommendations for the diagnosis, treatment and follow-up of the first febrile urinary tract infection in young children. Acta Paediatr. 2020;109(2):236–47.
6. Bandari J, Docimo SG. Vesicoureteral reflux is a phenotype, not a disease: a population-centered approach to pediatric urinary tract infection. J Pediatr Urol. 2017;13(4):378–82.
7. Beetz R, Mannhardt W, Fisch M, Stein R, Thuroff JW. Long-term followup of 158 young adults surgically treated for vesicoureteral reflux in childhood: the ongoing risk of urinary tract infections. J Urol. 2002;168(2):704–7. discussion 707
8. Brandstrom P, Hansson S. Urinary tract infection in children. Pediatr Clin N Am. 2022;69(6):1099–114.
9. Brandstrom P, Linden M. How Swedish guidelines on urinary tract infections in children compare to Canadian, American and European guidelines. Acta Paediatr. 2021;110(6):1759–71.
10. Brandstrom P, Esbjorner E, Herthelius M, Swerkersson S, Jodal U, Hansson S. The Swedish Reflux Trial in Children: III. Urinary tract infection pattern. J Urol. 2010a;184(1):286–91.
11. Brandstrom P, Neveus T, Sixt R, Stokland E, Jodal U, Hansson S. The Swedish Reflux Trial in Children: IV. Renal damage. J Urol. 2010b;184(1):292–7.
12. Buettcher M, Trueck J, Niederer-Loher A, Heininger U, Agyeman P, Asner S, Berger C, Bielicki J, Kahlert C, Kottanattu L, Meyer Sauteur PM, Paioni P, Posfay-Barbe K, Relly C, Ritz N, Zimmermann P, Zucol F, Gobet R, Shavit S, Rudin C, Laube G, von Vigier R, Neuhaus TJ. Swiss consensus recommendations on urinary tract infections in children. Eur J Pediatr. 2021;180(3):663–74.
13. Cheng CH, Tsai MH, Huang YC, Su LH, Tsau YK, Lin CJ, Chiu CH, Lin TY. Antibiotic resistance patterns of community-acquired urinary tract infections in children with vesicoureteral reflux receiving prophylactic antibiotic therapy. Pediatrics. 2008;122(6):1212–7.
14. Chi A, Gupta A, Snodgrass W. Urinary tract infection following successful dextranomer/hyaluronic acid injection for vesicoureteral reflux. J Urol. 2008;179(5):1966–9.
15. Craig JC, Simpson JM, Williams GJ, Lowe A, Reynolds GJ, McTaggart SJ, Hodson EM, Carapetis JR, Cranswick NE, Smith G, Irwig LM, Caldwell PH, Hamilton S, Roy LP. Antibiotic prophylaxis and recurrent urinary tract infection in children. N Engl J Med. 2009;361(18):1748–59.
16. de Bessa J Jr, de Carvalho Mrad FC, Mendes EF, Bessa MC, Paschoalin VP, Tiraboschi RB, Sammour ZM, Gomes CM, Braga LH, Bastos Netto JM. Antibiotic prophylaxis for prevention of febrile urinary tract infections in children with vesicoureteral reflux: a meta-analysis of randomized, controlled trials comparing dilated to nondilated vesicoureteral reflux. J Urol. 2015;193(5 Suppl):1772–7.

17. Expert Panel on Pediatric, I, Karmazyn BK, Alazraki AL, Anupindi SA, Dempsey ME, Dillman JR, Dorfman SR, Garber MD, Moore SG, Peters CA, Rice HE, Rigsby CK, Safdar NM, Simoneaux SF, Trout AT, Westra SJ, Wootton-Gorges SL, Coley BD. ACR Appropriateness Criteria((R)) urinary tract infection-child. J Am Coll Radiol. 2017;14(5S):S362–71.
18. Garin EH, Olavarria F, Garcia Nieto V, Valenciano B, Campos A, Young L. Clinical significance of primary vesicoureteral reflux and urinary antibiotic prophylaxis after acute pyelonephritis: a multicenter, randomized, controlled study. Pediatrics. 2006;117(3):626–32.
19. Geback C, Hansson S, Himmelmann A, Sandberg T, Sixt R, Jodal U. Twenty-four-hour ambulatory blood pressure in adult women with urinary tract infection in childhood. J Hypertens. 2014;32(8):1658–64. discussion 1664
20. Geback C, Hansson S, Martinell J, Sandberg T, Sixt R, Jodal U. Renal function in adult women with urinary tract infection in childhood. Pediatr Nephrol. 2015;30(9):1493–9.
21. Geback C, Hansson S, Martinell J, Milsom I, Sandberg T, Jodal U. Obstetrical outcome in women with urinary tract infections in childhood. Acta Obstet Gynecol Scand. 2016a;95(4):452–7.
22. Geback C, Hansson S, Martinell J, Sandberg T, Jodal U. Urinary tract infection pattern in adult women followed from childhood. Pediatr Nephrol. 2016b;31(7):1107–11.
23. Godaly G, Ambite I, Puthia M, Nadeem A, Ho J, Nagy K, Huang Y, Rydstrom G, Svanborg C. Urinary tract infection molecular mechanisms and clinical translation. Pathogens. 2016;5(1):24
24. Hannula A, Perhomaa M, Venhola M, Pokka T, Renko M, Uhari M. Long-term follow-up of patients after childhood urinary tract infection. Arch Pediatr Adolesc Med. 2012;166(12):1117–22.
25. Hansson S, Bollgren I, Esbjorner E, Jakobsson B, Marild S. Urinary tract infections in children below two years of age: a quality assurance project in Sweden. The Swedish Pediatric Nephrology Association. Acta Paediatr. 1999;88(3):270–4.
26. Hari P, Hari S, Sinha A, Kumar R, Kapil A, Pandey RM, Bagga A. Antibiotic prophylaxis in the management of vesicoureteric reflux: a randomized double-blind placebo-controlled trial. Pediatr Nephrol. 2015;30(3):479–86.
27. Hellstrom A, Hanson E, Hansson S, Hjalmas K, Jodal U. Association between urinary symptoms at 7 years old and previous urinary tract infection. Arch Dis Child. 1991;66(2):232–4.
28. Hidas G, Billimek J, Nam A, Soltani T, Kelly MS, Selby B, Dorgalli C, Wehbi E, McAleer I, McLorie G, Greenfield S, Kaplan SH, Khoury AE. Predicting the risk of breakthrough urinary tract infections: primary vesicoureteral reflux. J Urol. 2015;194(5):1396–401.
29. Hoberman A, Charron M, Hickey RW, Baskin M, Kearney DH, Wald ER. Imaging studies after a first febrile urinary tract infection in young children. N Engl J Med. 2003;348(3):195–202.
30. Jakobsson B, Esbjorner E, Hansson S. Minimum incidence and diagnostic rate of first urinary tract infection. Pediatrics. 1999;104(2 Pt 1):222–6.
31. Jodal U. The natural history of bacteriuria in childhood. Infect Dis Clin N Am. 1987;1(4):713–29.
32. Jodal U, Smellie JM, Lax H, Hoyer PF. Ten-year results of randomized treatment of children with severe vesicoureteral reflux. Final report of the International Reflux Study in Children. Pediatr Nephrol. 2006;21(6):785–92.
33. Koff SA, Wagner TT, Jayanthi VR. The relationship among dysfunctional elimination syndromes, primary vesicoureteral reflux and urinary tract infections in children. J Urol. 1998;160(3 Pt 2):1019–22.
34. Lee JN, Byeon KH, Woo MJ, Baek HS, Cho MH, Jeong SY, Lee SM, Ham JY, Ha YS, Kim HT, Yoo ES, Kwon TG, Chung SK. Susceptibility of the index urinary tract infection to prophylactic antibiotics is a predictive factor of breakthrough urinary tract infection in children with primary vesicoureteral reflux receiving continuous antibiotic prophylaxis. J Korean Med Sci. 2019;34(21):e156.
35. Leroy S, Fernandez-Lopez A, Nikfar R, Romanello C, Bouissou F, Gervaix A, Gurgoze MK, Bressan S, Smolkin V, Tuerlinckx D, Stefanidis CJ, Vaos G, Leblond P, Gungor F, Gendrel D, Chalumeau M. Association of procalcitonin with acute pyelonephritis and renal scars in pediatric UTI. Pediatrics. 2013;131(5):870–9.

36. Montini G, Rigon L, Zucchetta P, Fregonese F, Toffolo A, Gobber D, Cecchin D, Pavanello L, Molinari PP, Maschio F, Zanchetta S, Cassar W, Casadio L, Crivellaro C, Fortunati P, Corsini A, Calderan A, Comacchio S, Tommasi L, Hewitt IK, Da Dalt L, Zacchello G, Dall'Amico R. Prophylaxis after first febrile urinary tract infection in children? A multicenter, randomized, controlled, noninferiority trial. Pediatrics. 2008;122(5):1064–71.
37. Nelson CP, Johnson EK, Logvinenko T, Chow JS. Ultrasound as a screening test for genitourinary anomalies in children with UTI. Pediatrics. 2014;133(3):e394–403.
38. NICE. Urinary tract infection in under 16s: diagnosis and management: NICE clinical guideline. National Institute for Health and Care Excellence: Guidelines: London; 2018.
39. Park S, Song SH, Lee C, Kim JW, Kim KS. Bacterial pathogens in first febrile urinary tract infection affect breakthrough infections in infants with vesicoureteral reflux treated with prophylactic antibiotics. Urology. 2013;81(6):1342–5.
40. Pennesi M, Travan L, Peratoner L, Bordugo A, Cattaneo A, Ronfani L, Minisini S, Ventura A. Is antibiotic prophylaxis in children with vesicoureteral reflux effective in preventing pyelonephritis and renal scars? A randomized, controlled trial. Pediatrics. 2008;121(6):e1489–94.
41. Pineiro Perez R, Cilleruelo Ortega MJ, Ares Alvarez J, Baquero-Artigao F, Silva Rico JC, Velasco Zuniga R, Martinez Campos L, Carazo Gallego B, Conejo Fernandez AJ, Calvo C, Grupo Colaborador de Infeccion Urinaria en, P. & Grupo colaborador de infeccion urinaria en. Recommendations on the diagnosis and treatment of urinary tract infection. An Pediatr (Barc). 2019;90(6):400 e1–400 e9.
42. Preda I, Jodal U, Sixt R, Stokland E, Hansson S. Normal dimercaptosuccinic acid scintigraphy makes voiding cystourethrography unnecessary after urinary tract infection. J Pediatr. 2007;151(6):581-4, 584 e1.
43. Preda I, Jodal U, Sixt R, Stokland E, Hansson S. Imaging strategy for infants with urinary tract infection: a new algorithm. J Urol. 2011;185(3):1046–52.
44. Ragnarsdottir B, Lutay N, Gronberg-Hernandez J, Koves B, Svanborg C. Genetics of innate immunity and UTI susceptibility. Nat Rev Urol. 2011;8(8):449–68.
45. Rivur Trial Investigators, Hoberman A, Greenfield SP, Mattoo TK, Keren R, Mathews R, Pohl HG, Kropp BP, Skoog SJ, Nelson CP, Moxey-Mims M, Chesney RW, Carpenter MA. Antimicrobial prophylaxis for children with vesicoureteral reflux. N Engl J Med. 2014;370(25):2367–76.
46. Roberts KB. Urinary tract infection: clinical practice guideline for the diagnosis and management of the initial UTI in febrile infants and children 2 to 24 months. Pediatrics. 2011;128(3):595–610.
47. Robinson JL, Finlay JC, Lang ME, Bortolussi R, Canadian Paediatric Society, I. D. & Immunization Committee, C. P. C. Urinary tract infections in infants and children: Diagnosis and management. Paediatr Child Health. 2014;19(6):315–25.
48. Roussey-Kesler G, Gadjos V, Idres N, Horen B, Ichay L, Leclair MD, Raymond F, Grellier A, Hazart I, de Parscau L, Salomon R, Champion G, Leroy V, Guigonis V, Siret D, Palcoux JB, Taque S, Lemoigne A, Nguyen JM, Guyot C. Antibiotic prophylaxis for the prevention of recurrent urinary tract infection in children with low grade vesicoureteral reflux: results from a prospective randomized study. J Urol. 2008;179(2):674–9. discussion 679
49. Schwaderer AL, Wang H, Kim S, Kline JM, Liang D, Brophy PD, McHugh KM, Tseng GC, Saxena V, Barr-Beare E, Pierce KR, Shaikh N, Manak JR, Cohen DM, Becknell B, Spencer JD, Baker PB, Yu CY, Hains DS. Polymorphisms in alpha-defensin-encoding DEFA1A3 associate with urinary tract infection risk in children with vesicoureteral reflux. J Am Soc Nephrol. 2016;27(10):3175–86.
50. Sedberry-Ross S, Rice DC, Pohl HG, Belman AB, Majd M, Rushton HG. Febrile urinary tract infections in children with an early negative voiding cystourethrogram after treatment of vesicoureteral reflux with dextranomer/hyaluronic acid. J Urol. 2008;180(4 Suppl):1605–9; discussion 1610
51. Selekman RE, Shapiro DJ, Boscardin J, Williams G, Craig JC, Brandstrom P, Pennesi M, Roussey-Kesler G, Hari P, Copp HL. Uropathogen resistance and antibiotic prophylaxis: a meta-analysis. Pediatrics. 2018;142(1)

52. Shaikh N, Morone NE, Bost JE, Farrell MH. Prevalence of urinary tract infection in childhood: a meta-analysis. Pediatr Infect Dis J. 2008;27(4):302–8.
53. Shaikh N, Ewing AL, Bhatnagar S, Hoberman A. Risk of renal scarring in children with a first urinary tract infection: a systematic review. Pediatrics. 2010;126(6):1084–91.
54. Shaikh N, Haralam MA, Kurs-Lasky M, Hoberman A. Association of renal scarring with number of febrile urinary tract infections in children. JAMA Pediatr. 2019;173(10):949–52.
55. Shaikh N, Osio VA, Wessel CB, Jeong JH. Prevalence of asymptomatic bacteriuria in children: a meta-analysis. J Pediatr. 2020;217(110-117):e4.
56. Shaikh N, Liu H, Kurs-Lasky M, Forster CS. Biomarkers for febrile urinary tract infection in children. Pediatr Nephrol. 2022;37(1):171–7.
57. Singh-Grewal D, Macdessi J, Craig J. Circumcision for the prevention of urinary tract infection in boys: a systematic review of randomised trials and observational studies. Arch Dis Child. 2005;90(8):853–8.
58. Stein R, Dogan HS, Hoebeke P, Kocvara R, Nijman RJ, Radmayr C, Tekgul S, European Association of, U. & European Society for Pediatric, U. Urinary tract infections in children: EAU/ESPU guidelines. Eur Urol. 2015;67(3):546–58.
59. Storm DW, Patel AS, Horvath DJ Jr, Li B, Koff SA, Justice SS. Relationship among bacterial virulence, bladder dysfunction, vesicoureteral reflux and patterns of urinary tract infection in children. J Urol. 2012;188(1):236–41.
60. Strohmeier Y, Hodson EM, Willis NS, Webster AC, Craig JC. Antibiotics for acute pyelonephritis in children. Cochrane Database Syst Rev. 2014;7:CD003772.
61. Subcommittee On Urinary Tract, I. Reaffirmation of AAP clinical practice guideline: the diagnosis and management of the initial urinary tract infection in febrile infants and young children 2–24 months of age. Pediatrics. 2016;138(6):e20163026
62. Swerkersson S, Jodal U, Sixt R, Stokland E, Hansson S. Relationship among vesicoureteral reflux, urinary tract infection and renal damage in children. J Urol. 2007;178(2):647–51. discussion 650–1
63. Swerkersson S, Jodal U, Ahren C, Sixt R, Stokland E, Hansson S. Urinary tract infection in infants: the significance of low bacterial count. Pediatr Nephrol. 2016;31(2):239–45.
64. t Hoen LA, Bogaert G, Radmayr C, Dogan HS, Nijman RJM, Quaedackers J, Rawashdeh YF, Silay MS, Tekgul S, Bhatt NR, Stein R. Update of the EAU/ESPU guidelines on urinary tract infections in children. J Pediatr Urol. 2021;17(2):200–7.
65. Valdimarsson S, Jodal U, Barregard L, Hansson S. Urine neutrophil gelatinase-associated lipocalin and other biomarkers in infants with urinary tract infection and in febrile controls. Pediatr Nephrol. 2017;32(11):2079–87.
66. van Gool JD, Hjalmas K, Tamminen-Mobius T, Olbing H. Historical clues to the complex of dysfunctional voiding, urinary tract infection and vesicoureteral reflux. The International Reflux Study in Children. J Urol. 1992;148(5 Pt 2):1699–702.
67. Wennerstrom M, Hansson S, Hedner T, Himmelmann A, Jodal U. Ambulatory blood pressure 16-26 years after the first urinary tract infection in childhood. J Hypertens. 2000a;18(4):485–91.
68. Wennerstrom M, Hansson S, Jodal U, Sixt R, Stokland E. Renal function 16 to 26 years after the first urinary tract infection in childhood. Arch Pediatr Adolesc Med. 2000b;154(4):339–45.
69. Yang SS, Chiang IN, Lin CD, Chang SJ. Advances in non-surgical treatments for urinary tract infections in children. World J Urol. 2012;30(1):69–75.
70. Yang SS, Tsai JD, Kanematsu A, Han CH. Asian guidelines for urinary tract infection in children. J Infect Chemother. 2021;27(11):1543–54.
71. Morello W, Baskin E, Jankauskiene A, Yalcinkaya F, Zurowska A, Puccio G, Serafinelli J, La Manna A, Krzemień G, Pennesi M, La Scola C, Becherucci F, Brugnara M, Yuksel S, Mekahli D, Chimenz R, De Palma D, Zucchetta P, Vajauskas D, Drozdz D, Szczepanska M, Caliskan S, Lombet J, Minoli DG, Guarino S, Gulleroglu K, Ruzgiene D, Szmigielska A, Barbi E, Ozcakar ZB, Kranz A, Pasini A, Materassi M, De Rechter S, Ariceta G, Weber LT, Marzuillo P, Alberici I, Taranta-Janusz K, Caldas Afonso A, Tkaczyk M, Català M, Cabrera Sevilla JE, Mehls O, Schaefer F, Montini G; PREDICT Study Group. Antibiotic Prophylaxis in Infants with Grade III, IV, or V Vesicoureteral Reflux. N Engl J Med. 2023;389(11):987–997.

Incidence and Classification of Vesicoureteral Reflux

David Coyle

Abstract In children with febrile urinary tract infections (UTI) it is estimated that between 28% and 36% have vesicoureteral (VUR) to some extent. The prevalence is higher in younger children range due to the propensity of VUR to improve or resolve with age. Such is the heritability of the condition that approximately 15% of siblings of an index case of VUR in a family will have VUR. From a pathophysiology standpoint, VUR can be thought of as being primary, due to anatomical factors related to ureteral implantation into the trigone, or secondary, which occurs in response to raised intra-vesical pressure. The radiological classification of VUR depends on the mode of imaging. The fluoroscopic classification derived from the International Study of Reflux in Children grades VUR from grade I to grade V, with grades I–II representing non-dilating VUR and grade III–V representing dilating VUR. The clinical behaviour and natural history of non-dilating VUR vs dilating VUR differ significantly. A separate, less granular, classification system exists for VUR diagnosed by radionuclide cystography.

Keywords Vesicoureteral · Incidence · Prevalence · Primary VUR · Secondary VUR

Introduction

In describing the incidence of vesicoureteral reflux (VUR), context is essential. This context can be provided by looking at the many ways VUR can be classified, i.e. primary versus secondary, dilating versus non-dilating, symptomatic versus screen-detected, etc. This chapter will look at the incidence and prevalence of VUR in the many contexts in which it is diagnosed. It will also examine variety of ways VUR can be classified, while recognizing detailed descriptions of its role in individual conditions, such as neurogenic bladder is addressed in separate chapters.

D. Coyle (✉)
Department of Pediatric Urology, Children's Health Ireland at Crumlin, Dublin, Ireland

P. Puri, A. Yamataka (eds.), *Vesicoureteral Reflux*,
https://doi.org/10.1007/978-3-031-95091-9_8

Incidence of Vesicoureteral Reflux

Demographics of VUR

There is little population-level data regarding the incidence or prevalence of VUR in the population at large, largely because best diagnostic investigations are invasive and come with ionizing radiation exposure. In a Japanese cohort of 2000 children screened for transcient urinary tract dilation (UTD) by dynamic ultrasonography during voiding, VUR was diagnosed in 0.8% [1]. This prevalence is probably an underestimate given that UTD on ultrasound lacks accuracy for the detection of VUR, particularly in its lower grades [2]. Venhola et al. found VUR in between 28% and 36% of patients in their cohort of children referred for evaluation after UTI regardless of the reliability of the UTI diagnosis, indicating that VUR was far more common in young children (their cohort were <5 years of age) than previously thought [3]. In a multi-centre prospective study the prevalence of VUR in 309 children under 2 years of age presenting with a first febrile UTI was 39% [4].

Ethnicity also contributes to the population-level prevalence of VUR. When Chand et al. looked at the records of all children undergoing voiding cystourethrography (VCUG) for all indications at their institution, they found Black children were approximately one third as likely to have VUR as White children. The male-to-female ratio of this series of 15,504 children was 1:2. Their data also show a significant fall-off in prevalence VUR with advancing age, especially over the age of 2 years [5]. This reflects what is known regarding the natural history of primary VUR from numerous studies, including the International Reflux Study in Children, whereby spontaneous resolution, particularly of lower grade, non-dilating VUR, may occur as children get older [6, 7].

VUR and Antenatal Urinary Tract Dilatation

Antenatal UTD is found in 1–2% of all pregnancies. There is significant variation between clinicians regarding the practice of screening babies with antenatally diagnosed UTD using VCUG. In one review of 34 studies the percentage of infants screened ranged from 11% to 100%, although the mean was 78% [8]. Following post-natal evaluation, between 12% and 38% of infants with an antenatal history of UTD are found to have VUR. Only 5% of with normal post-natal screening ultrasounds following a history of antenatal UTD have VUR, while closer to 40% of those in whom dilatation persists have VUR [9]. The radiological grade of reflux in this population follows a "rule of thirds", with one third having low grade (I–II) VUR, one third having intermediate grade (III) VUR and one third having high grade VUR (IV–V) [8].

Screen-Detected Familial VUR

VUR is a condition with a strong genetic component, with evidence supporting an autosomal dominant inheritance pattern. In a multiple gestation study, Kaefer et al. demonstrated concurrent VUR in 80% and 35% of monozygotic and dizygotic twins respectively, which rose to 100% and 50% when the younger patients were considered, mitigating the effects of age-related spontaneous resolution [10]. In a study from the United Kingdom comprising 265 cases where a newborn sibling of a child with VUR had a screening VCUG, VUR was detected in approximately 14% of cases, with 4.9% having dilating VUR. Of note, in this cohort, the negative predictive value of a normal postnatal urinary tract ultrasound in the sibling of an index case of VUR was 95.4% [11].

One series of 159 families with affected siblings found that sisters of female index cases had a higher incidence of VUR but brothers of male index cases had a higher grades of VUR [12]. UTIs are a relatively common occurrence in the siblings of index cases of VUR (approximately 10%) but no difference in the incidence of UTI has been demonstrated in screened versus unscreened individuals [13]. The question of whether siblings of children with VUR should be routinely screened for VUR is dealt with in another chapter.

VUR Co-occurring with Other Congenital Anomalies of the Kidney and Urinary Tract

The co-existence of VUR with other congenital anomalies of the kidney and urinary tract (CAKUT), which overall constitute approximately 50% of congenital anomalies, is well recognized. Duplex collecting systems are present in 0.8% of the population at autopsy and follow a similar autosomal dominant inheritance pattern seen in VUR [14]. Indeed, studies of families with VUR show a relatively high incidence of both VUR and duplication anomalies, especially in males between 4 and 15% [12, 15]. The VUR seen in duplex systems is primary in nature, and, as a result, typically affects the lower pole moiety of complete duplication anomalies, with a ureteral orifice lying high and lateral compared to that of the upper pole moiety.

In those with a multicystic dysplastic kidney, the contralateral upper urinary tract is affected by VUR in approximately 17% of cases, with obvious ramifications for the threshold to treat VUR surgically. The use of VCUG to screen the solitary functioning kidney for VUR in such cases in the absence of dilatation or a history of UTI should involved shared decision making with the patient's family [16].

Ureteropelvic junction obstruction (UPJO) is the most common cause of upper tract obstructive uropathy in children. In 2 large series, VUR is present in those with UPJO in between 11% and 18% of cases [17, 18]. Critically, the incidence of UTIs does not seem to differ between those with UPJO who have VUR and those who are not screened for it [18]. While VCUG is an important component in the evaluation of high risk UTD its routine use in patients with suspected or confirmed UPJ obstruction has been called into question.

In male infants born with posterior urethral valves (PUV) approximately 60–65% have VUR at diagnosis [19, 20]. The affected kidney is often poorly functioning. This is, at least in part, due to the "pop-off" nature of a refluxing system in PUV, the so-called Vesicoureteral Reflux Dysplasia (VURD) syndrome, seen in approximately 20% of cases of PUV [21]. This mechanism has traditionally been thought of as being protective in terms of bladder function however long-term follow-up has demonstrated worse bladder dynamics and less favourable continence in children with a "pop-off" mechanism than in those who do not [22].

Bladder-Bowel Dysfunction in VUR

Bowel and bladder dysfunction (BBD) refers to abnormalities in how the bladder fills and empties in association with lower urinary tract symptoms including urinary incontinence, as well as abnormal bowel habit with constipation and soiling. It is common in the paediatric population and is a risk factor for recurrent UTI, particularly when combined with VUR. In a prospective cohort study of children with and without VUR from the RIVUR (Randomized Intervention for VUR) and CUTIE (Careful UTI Evaluation) studies, BBD was found to be present in 46% of those without VUR (i.e. children with 1–2 febrile UTIs who did not meet the eligibility criteria for the RIVUR study) and 59% of those with VUR. In this study, children with BBD and any degree of VUR were at the highest risk of recurrent UTI [23]. A systematic review of the literature also found a pooled prevalence of BBD in 49% of children with primary VUR, where it increased the risk of recurrent UTIs by twofold [24]. Such is the prevalence and clinical importance of BBD in VUR that it is recommended that all children diagnosed with primary VUR are screened for BBD.

Reflux Nephropathy and Chronic Kidney Disease

CAKUT are the most common cause of chronic kidney disease (CKD) in younger children, accounting, together with congenital nephropathies, for over 50% of cases. In older children, acquired disease becomes proportionately more significant as a cause of childhood CKD. End-stage renal disease (ESRD), the point at which renal replacement therapy with either dialysis or transplantation becomes necessary, is the end-point of progression for CKD. In Europe CAKUT accounts for 34–43% of ESRD [25]. Over time reflux nephropathy has become a less prominent contributor to this morbidity, as obstructive nephropathies and renal dysplasia/hyposplasia become more prominent. In the United States, approximately 8.8% of paediatric patients who have had a transplant or are on dialysis have an underlying diagnosis of reflux nephropathy [26].

Classification of Vesicoureteral Reflux

Clinical Parameters

There are several ways of classifying vesicoureteral reflux, each with its own clinical relevance. At a pathological level, the distinction between primary and secondary VUR determines the focus of management. The radiological grade of depends on the modality used (nuclear medicine vs. fluoroscopy). In broader terms, most clinicians make a distinction between primary dilating and non-dilating VUR, as, with all other things equal, they represent clinically distinct entities. No one classification system for VUR serves the essential function of all classification systems: to predict clinical behaviour and guide management. That there is so much heterogeneity in practice regarding the management of VUR is in large part due to this.

Primary Versus Secondary VUR

Primary VUR may, particularly at low grades, be physiological. Ordinarily, backflow of urine from the bladder into the upper tract is prevented by a combination of an oblique course of the intramural ureter through the detrusor muscle of the bladder and the tone of the ureter at this junction. In VUR abnormal, faulty interaction between the ureteral and the metanephric mesenchyme during embryogenesis leads to abnormal lateral implantation of the ureter into the bladder with a shorter, less oblique transmural course of the ureter. Because the mechanism of ureteral budding is also critical to the normal formation of the kidney, renal dysplasia can co-occur alongside VUR [27, 28].

Secondary VUR is reflux that occurs in the context of raised bladder pressure, which overwhelms the anti-reflux mechanism of an otherwise anatomically normal ureterovesical junction. This may occur in the context of a lower urinary tract obstruction such as posterior urethral valves, or in lower urinary tract dysfunction, most classically in the neurogenic bladder of a child with spina bifida (Fig. 1). In certain conditions, the anatomical findings of primary VUR may co-exist with the conditions that give rise to secondary VUR. An excellent example of this is in children with anorectal malformations, where primary VUR may be present as a co-occurring congenital anomaly in the VACTERL association. Secondary VUR may also be present in this population of patients, where pelvic surgery, abnormal sacral anatomy and spinal cord anomalies all contribute to an increased risk of neurogenic lower urinary tract dysfunction [29].

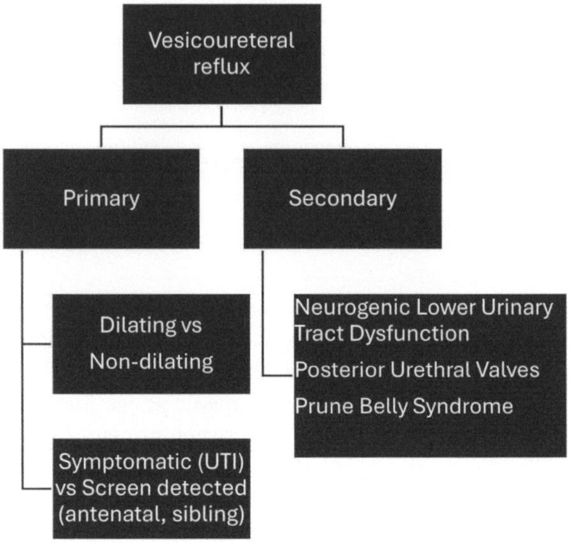

Fig. 1 Schematic classification of vesicoureteral reflux

Radiological Classification of VUR

The most commonly used techniques for radiologically assessing for the presence of VUR is VCUG and indirect radionuclide cystography (RNC). Lately the emergence of a radiation-sparing approach of direct cystography using ultrasonographic contrast has also been described, but this still requires the placement of a urethral catheter for filling (contrast-enhanced voiding urosonography [Ce-VUS]).

In 1985 the investigators in the International Study of Reflux in Children (ISRC) combined previous classification systems and described a standardized technique for VCUG, publishing the classification system which graded VUR severity from I to V, depending on the extent of contrast reflux into the upper tracts. This is the classification system still widely in use today (Fig. 2) [30]. In evaluating the VCUGs of those enrolled in the Randomized Intervention for Children with VesicoUreteral Reflux (RIVUR) trial, there was notable inter-observer variability in the grade of VUR between both local radiologists and reference radiologists for the study [31].

When VUR is evaluated by RNC, less granular detail results in three grades of VUR: mild, moderate and severe, corresponding to VCUG grade I, grades II/III, and grades IV/V respectively [32]. This technique does not require urethral catheterization but does require intravenous cannulation (Table 1).

Darge and Troeger (2002) adapted the ISRC classification system for Ce-VUS, depending on where microbubbles were seen on ultrasound (Table 1) [33]. Accepting its dependence on operator experience, Ce-VUS was comparable to VCUG in detection of VUR [34]. There is relatively little data demonstrating equivalence of the grading systems in terms of their ability to predict clinical outcome.

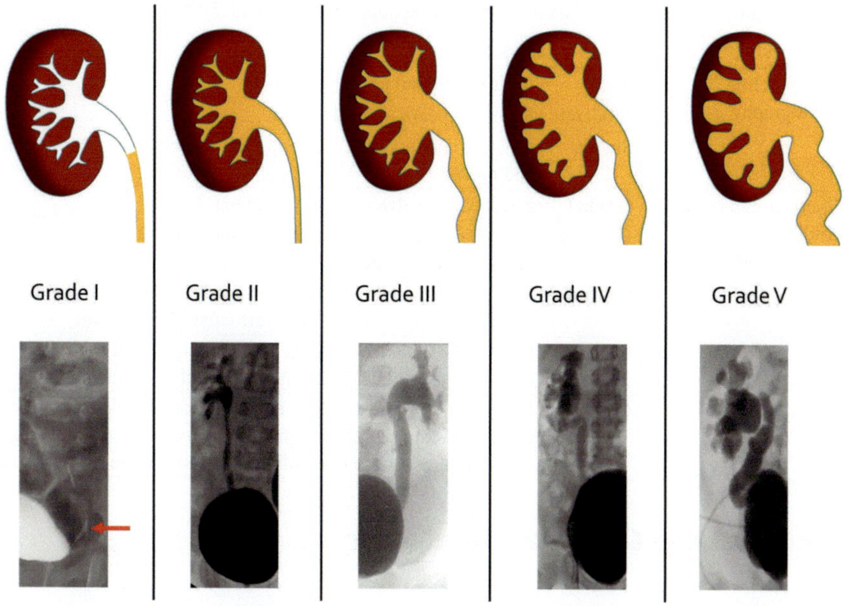

Fig. 2 ISRC classification of VUR: Grade I—Reflux involving the ureter only with varying degrees of dilatation; Grade II—Non-dilating reflux involving the renal pelvis with normal fornices; Grade III—moderate dilation of the collection system, normal or mildly deformed fornices, mild-to-moderate dilation of the ureter with or without kinking; Grade IV—Moderately dilated collecting system, blunted fornices, papillae still intact, moderate ureteral dilation with or without kinking; Grade V—Marked dilation of collecting system, loss of papillary impressions, intraparenchymal reflux, marked dilation of ureter with tortuosity

Dilating Versus Non-dilating VUR

A more simplified and clinically relevant classification of VUR is as dilating or non-dilating, based on the effect of VUR on the renal pelvis at VCUG. Thus, grades III through V all represent dilating VUR while grades I and II are non-dilating. Those with dilating VUR are at a significantly higher risk of reflux nephropathy (scarring/dysplasia) [35]. This is therefore the group at highest risk for long-term sequelae such as hypertension and chronic kidney disease. Female patients with renal scarring and VUR are also at higher risk of adverse obstetric events in pregnancy [36]. The clinical distinction between dilating and non-dilating VUR was recognized in the conception of the Swedish Reflux Trial, arising from expert panel review of the literature which concluded that more emphasis be placed on management of BBD and renal function preservation rather than on treatment of VUR itself. Thus, follow-up in those with non-dilating reflux was truncated where renal damage was absent [37, 38].

Table 1 Summary of components of VUR classification by RNC and Ce-VUS

Modality	Severity	Description
Radionuclide Cystography	Mild	Reflux confined to ureter
	Moderate	Reflux to pelvicalyceal system
	Severe	Reflux to pelvicalyceal system with dilated collecting system and ureter
Contrast-enhanced voiding urosonography	Grade I	Microbubbles detected only in ureter
	Grade II	Microbubbles detected in renal pelvis without significant renal pelvic dilatation
	Grade III	Microbubbles detected in the renal pelvis with significant renal pelvic dilatation + moderate calyceal dilatation
	Grade IV	Microbubbles detected in the renal pelvis with significant renal pelvic dilatation and significant calyceal dilatation
	Grade V	Microbubbles detected in the renal pelvis with significant renal pelvic dilatation, significant calyceal dilatation and loss of renal pelvis contour and dilated tortuous ureter

The "Refluxing Obstructed Megaureter"

Primary obstructed megaureter (POM) with concurrent VUR is a specific and seemingly paradoxical entity. It is uncommon—in one series it was found in 0.3% of the combined populations of children with VUR and those with POM. It should be suspected where radiological contrast during VCUG is diluted on refluxing into the ureter and drainage of the ureter into the bladder is slow or absent. Confirmation is by isotope renography with a urinary catheter *in situ*, to eliminate the confounding effects of VUR (Fig. 3). Unlike primary VUR without obstruction, non-operative management of this phenomenon is not recommended [39].

Future Directions

A better understanding of the natural history of VUR has changed how clinicians think about the classification of VUR, as a dynamic feature of the condition rather than a fixed one. The tendency of VUR, particularly non-dilating VUR, to spontaneously resolve has altered the threshold for many surgeons to offer operative management of VUR, and has led to a redirection of attention to other risk factors for recurrent UTIs in older children with a history of VUR, such as BBD.

Future and ongoing efforts are directed to predicting those whose VUR is less likely to resolve spontaneously, and those with VUR more likely to develop UTI and acquired reflux nephropathy.

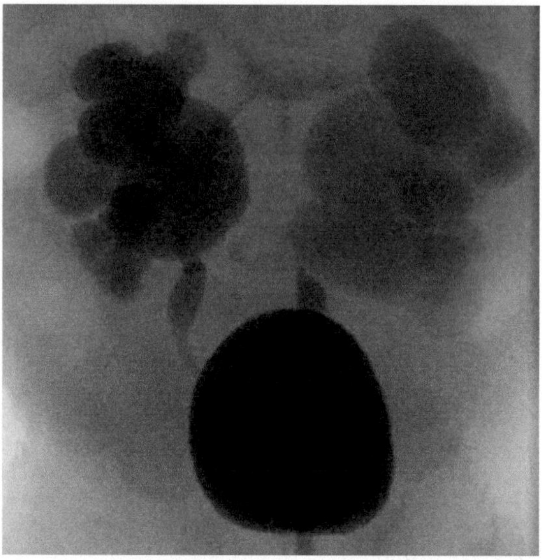

Fig. 3 Voiding cystourethrogram demonstrating high grade hydronephrosis with loss of the papillary impressions in keeping with grade V VUR, however the degree of ureteric dilatation is minor. A MAG3 renogram with a urethral catheter in situ demonstrated bilateral UPJ obstruction, confirming the presence of a refluxing obstructed system

References

1. Hiraoka M, Hori C, Tsukahara H, Kasuga K, Ishihara Y, Kotsuji F, Mayumi M. Vesicoureteral reflux in male and female neonates as detected by voiding ultrasonography. Kidney Int. 1999;55(4):1486–90.
2. Shaikh N, Spingarn RB, Hum SW. Dimercaptosuccinic acid scan or ultrasound in screening for vesicoureteral reflux among children with urinary tract infections. Cochrane Database Syst Rev. 2016;7(7):CD010657.
3. Venhola M, Hannula A, Huttunen NP, Renko M, Pokka T, Uhari M. Occurrence of vesicoureteral reflux in children. Acta Paediatr. 2010;99(12):1875–8.
4. Hoberman A, Charron M, Hickey RW, Baskin M, Kearney DH, Wald ER. Imaging studies after a first febrile urinary tract infection in young children. N Engl J Med. 2003;348(3):195–202.
5. Chand DH, Rhoades T, Poe SA, Kraus S, Strife CF. Incidence and severity of vesicoureteral reflux in children related to age, gender, race and diagnosis. J Urol. 2003;170(4 Pt 2):1548–50.
6. Zerati Filho M, Calado AA, Barroso U Jr, Amaro JL. Spontaneous resolution rates of vesicoureteral reflux in Brazilian children: a 30-year experience. Int Braz J Urol. 2007;33(2):204–12. discussion 13–5
7. Tamminen-Mobius T, Brunier E, Ebel KD, Lebowitz R, Olbing H, Seppanen U, Sixt R. Cessation of vesicoureteral reflux for 5 years in infants and children allocated to medical treatment. The International Reflux Study in Children. J Urol. 1992;148(5 Pt 2):1662–6.
8. Skoog SJ, Peters CA, Arant BS Jr, Copp HL, Elder JS, Hudson RG, et al. Pediatric vesicoureteral reflux guidelines panel summary report: clinical practice guidelines for screening siblings of children with vesicoureteral reflux and neonates/infants with prenatal hydronephrosis. J Urol. 2010;184(3):1145–51.
9. Nguyen HT, Benson CB, Bromley B, Campbell JB, Chow J, Coleman B, et al. Multidisciplinary consensus on the classification of prenatal and postnatal urinary tract dilation (UTD classification system). J Pediatr Urol. 2014;10(6):982–98.
10. Kaefer M, Curran M, Treves ST, Bauer S, Hendren WH, Peters CA, et al. Sibling vesicoureteral reflux in multiple gestation births. Pediatrics. 2000;105(4 Pt 1):800–4.

11. Singhal N, Gopal M, Ali A, McGlade F, Ahmed I, Harkensee C, et al. The prevalence of familial vesicoureteric reflux in infants with normal antenatal scans. Acta Paediatr. 2022;111(9):1808–13.
12. Pirker ME, Mohanan N, Colhoun E, Barton D, Green A, Puri P. Familial vesicoureteral reflux: influence of sex on prevalence and expression. J Urol. 2006;176(4 Pt 2):1776–80.
13. Nelson CP, Finkelstein JA, Logvinenko T, Schuster MA. Incidence of urinary tract infection among siblings of children with vesicoureteral reflux. Acad Pediatr. 2016;16(5):489–95.
14. Houat AP, Guimaraes CTS, Takahashi MS, Rodi GP, Gasparetto TPD, Blasbalg R, Velloni FG. Congenital anomalies of the upper urinary tract: a comprehensive review. Radiographics. 2021;41(5):E165.
15. Hunziker M, Mohanan N, Menezes M, Puri P. Prevalence of duplex collecting systems in familial vesicoureteral reflux. Pediatr Surg Int. 2010;26(1):115–7.
16. Erlich T, Lipsky AM, Braga LH. A meta-analysis of the incidence and fate of contralateral vesicoureteral reflux in unilateral multicystic dysplastic kidney. J Pediatr Urol. 2019;15(1):77 e1–e7.
17. Bomalaski MD, Hirschl RB, Bloom DA. Vesicoureteral reflux and ureteropelvic junction obstruction: association, treatment options and outcome. J Urol. 1997;157(3):969–74.
18. Suarez Arbelaez MC, Khanna K, Raymo A, Weber A, Lerendegui L, Nackeeran S, et al. Does preoperative screening VCUG affect the outcomes and complications of pyeloplasty in patients with ureteropelvic junction obstruction? J Pediatr Urol. 2024;20(1):76 e1–e7.
19. Cozzi DA, Morgante D, Frediani S, Iaconelli R, Ceccanti S, Mele E, Cozzi F. Posterior urethral valves: relationship between vesicoureteral reflux and renal function. Urology. 2011;77(5):1209–12.
20. Heikkila J, Rintala R, Taskinen S. Vesicoureteral reflux in conjunction with posterior urethral valves. J Urol. 2009;182(4):1555–60.
21. Narasimhan KL, Mahajan JK, Kaur B, Mittal BR, Bhattacharya A. The vesicoureteral reflux dysplasia syndrome in patients with posterior urethral valves. J Urol. 2005;174(4 Pt 1):1433–5. discussion 5
22. D'Oro A, Meyer T, Gong EM, Rosoklija I, Liu DB. Are pressure pop-offs beneficial to the bladder in boys with posterior urethral valves? J Pediatr Urol. 2020;16(4):488 e1–e8.
23. Keren R, Shaikh N, Pohl H, Gravens-Mueller L, Ivanova A, Zaoutis L, et al. Risk factors for recurrent urinary tract infection and renal scarring. Pediatrics. 2015;136(1):e13–21.
24. Meena J, Mathew G, Hari P, Sinha A, Bagga A. Prevalence of bladder and bowel dysfunction in toilet-trained children with urinary tract infection and/or primary vesicoureteral reflux: a systematic review and meta-analysis. Front Pediatr. 2020;8:84.
25. Harambat J, van Stralen KJ, Kim JJ, Tizard EJ. Epidemiology of chronic kidney disease in children. Pediatr Nephrol. 2012;27(3):363–73.
26. Brakeman P. Vesicoureteral reflux, reflux nephropathy, and end-stage renal disease. Adv Urol. 2008;2008:508949.
27. Tullus K. Vesicoureteric reflux in children. Lancet. 2015;385(9965):371–9.
28. Emma F, Goldstein. In: Emma F, Goldstein SL, Bagga A, Bates CM, Shroff R, editors. Pediatric nephrology. 8th ed. Cham: Springer; 2022.
29. Duci M, Midrio P, Castagnetti M, Gamba P, Faggin R, Fascetti-Leon F. Urinary tract anomalies in patients with anorectal malformations: the role of screening and clinical follow-up. Urology. 2020;143:216–20.
30. Lebowitz RL, Olbing H, Parkkulainen KV, Smellie JM, Tamminen-Mobius TE. International system of radiographic grading of vesicoureteric reflux. International Reflux Study in Children. Pediatr Radiol. 1985;15(2):105–9.
31. Schaeffer AJ, Greenfield SP, Ivanova A, Cui G, Zerin JM, Chow JS, et al. Reliability of grading of vesicoureteral reflux and other findings on voiding cystourethrography. J Pediatr Urol. 2017;13(2):192–8.
32. Reeves RA, Sandhu PK. Radionuclide cystography. Treasure Island: StatPearls; 2024.

33. Darge K, Troeger J. Vesicoureteral reflux grading in contrast-enhanced voiding urosonography. Eur J Radiol. 2002;43(2):122–8.
34. Paltiel HJ, Barnewolt CE, Chow JS, Bauer SB, Diamond DA, Stamoulis C. Accuracy of contrast-enhanced voiding urosonography using Optison for diagnosis of vesicoureteral reflux in children. J Pediatr Urol. 2023;19(1):135 e1–e8.
35. Shaikh N, Ewing AL, Bhatnagar S, Hoberman A. Risk of renal scarring in children with a first urinary tract infection: a systematic review. Pediatrics. 2010;126(6):1084–91.
36. Fitzpatrick A, Venugopal K, Scheil W, McDonald SP, Jesudason S. The spectrum of adverse pregnancy outcomes based on kidney disease diagnoses: a 20-year population study. Am J Nephrol. 2019;49(5):400–9.
37. Brandstrom P, Jodal U, Sillen U, Hansson S. The Swedish reflux trial: review of a randomized, controlled trial in children with dilating vesicoureteral reflux. J Pediatr Urol. 2011;7(6):594–600.
38. Jodal U, Lindberg U. Guidelines for management of children with urinary tract infection and vesico-ureteric reflux. Recommendations from a Swedish state-of-the-art conference. Swedish Medical Research Council. Acta Paediatr Suppl. 1999;88(431):87–9.
39. Somogyi R, Oberritter Z, Juhasz Z, Vajda P, Pinter AB. Combination of vesicoureteric reflux and vesicoureteric junction obstruction. Scand J Urol Nephrol. 2009;43(6):501–5.

Vesico-ureteral Reflux and Lower Urinary Tract Dysfunction

Tryggve Nevéus

Abstract Even though the relationship between VUR and conditions such as the neurogenic bladder and posterior urethral valves is clear we know less regarding the importance of LUT function in primary VUR. Still, studies indicate that LUT dysfunction, mainly detrusor overactivity or voiding dysfunction, is indeed overrepresented in infants and children with VUR and that treatment of the bladder may increase the chance for spontaneous VUR resolution. This may influence the management especially of infants with febrile UTIs and dilating VUR.

Keywords Vesico-ureteral reflux · Detrusor overactivity · Dysfunctional voiding · Urinary tract infections · Constipation

Background

Overview

This chapter is about the relationship between primary VUR and lower urinary tract (LUT) dysfunction. Neurogenic bladder, congenital obstruction and urinary tract infections (UTIs) will be only peripherally mentioned, since they, and their links to VUR, are dealt with in depth in other chapters.

Throughout the chapter the LUT terminology recommended by the International Children's Continence Society will be consistently adhered to [4]. This means, for instance, that the term "voiding dysfunction" refers *not* to any kind of LUT problem but specifically to dysfunction of the voiding phase.

T. Nevéus (✉)
Department of Women's and Children's Health, Uppsala University, Uppsala, Sweden
e-mail: Tryggve.neveus@kbh.uu.se

P. Puri, A. Yamataka (eds.), *Vesicoureteral Reflux*,
https://doi.org/10.1007/978-3-031-95091-9_9

The relationship between VUR and LUT dysfunction is complex and incompletely understood but probably highly relevant. The extreme and obvious examples are of course the neurogenic bladder and congenital obstructive malformation, which are often accompanied by VUR, but even without such grave conditions VUR and LUT dysfunction are often coexisting and treatment of the one may possibly influence the other.

But our knowledge regarding this relationship is hampered by our lack of knowledge of the prevalences of (1) LUT dysfunction in children without VUR and (2) VUR in children without UTIs or symptoms of LUT dysfunction. Obviously, invasive urodynamic investigations or VCUGs are rarely performed in the normal population. It may very well be the case that both LUT function anomalies and VUR are quite common among healthy children and that their coexistence may in many cases be coincidental.

Tools of Investigation

LUT dysfunction can be suspected in children with symptoms such as urgency, holding maneuvers or daytime incontinence. The suspicion can be further substantiated via noninvasive urodynamic investigations, which in toilet-trained children usually means a combination of a voiding chart (documenting incontinence episodes, voiding frequency and voided volumes during a few days), uroflow measurements and residual urine assessment. A good and validated noninvasive urodynamic screening tool for infants and toddlers before the age of bladder control is the four-hour voiding observation [18]. This child-friendly examination should be used more frequently than is today the case.

But to give a definite diagnosis of conditions such as detrusor overactivity, detrusor-sphincter dyssynergia, detrusor underactivity or outflow obstruction invasive examinations, i.e. cystometry, is needed. As will be clear from this chapter, invasive urodynamics are only rarely indicated in children with primary VUR.

One can not mention LUT dysfunction without also mentioning the bowel, since constipation and LUT dysfunction very often coexist, and eradication of concomitant constipation is a crucial part of managing LUT dysfunction. However, there is scant evidence for a connection between constipation *per se* and VUR. The possible link between constipation and VUR goes via the bladder. This said, it should be stressed that whenever the LUT is evaluated in a child after the first 2–3 years of life, the bowel should also be evaluated, looking for signs of constipation. So far the best way to do this is to classify the child according to the Rome IV criteria [8], and the best (although by no means perfect) way to detect constipation radiologically is to measure the transverse rectal diameter behind the bladder via ultrasound; is this diameter more than 3 cm then constipation is very probable [9]

The Relation Between LUT Dysfunction and VUR

Epidemiology

A substantial proportion of children with VUR have signs or symptoms of LUT dysfunction. Many of these children have increased risk of UTIs, which probably depends more on the LUT dysfunction than the VUR.

Cystometric abnormalities such as detrusor overactivity or detrusor-sphincter dyscoordination are found in 44–77% of infants with primary VUR [6, 20, 24, 35]. Looking at siblings of children with VUR detected after UTI researchers found that VUR was linked to detrusor overactivity [5]. And the normalization of VUR and LUT dysfunction tend to go hand in hand in children with both conditions [12]. On the other hand, Taskinen, examining children after a first pyelonephritis, found that detrusor overactivity was equally common in children with and without VUR [43]. So the matter is not yet conclusively settled.

Taking the opposite strategy, looking for VUR in children with proven LUT dysfunction, Ural et al found a reflux prevalence of 46% (and 60% of these had VUR grade III or more), the reflux risk being equal regardless of whether the urodynamic disturbance was detrusor overactivity or voiding dysfunction [46]. On the other hand, Hoebeke et al looked at 1000 children with various non-neurogenic LUT disturbances and found VUR in only 15%, regardless of the urodynamic findings [16].

In neurogenic bladder, or children with severe bladder bowel dysfunction (previously "Hinman bladder"), VUR is present in approximately 50% of cases [3, 29, 36]. The same is true for boys with posterior urethral valves [17]. But interestingly, when looking at children with cerebral paresis, VUR seems not to be overrepresented. In studies looking at CP patients with LUT symptoms or UTIs only very few were found to have VUR, even though their cystometries were pathological [39].

It is also unclear whether there is some sort of dose response-relationship or not. Some researchers have found a correlation between detrusor pressure and the reflux grade [11], whereas others have not [1, 6]. And the presence of overt LUT symptoms does not necessarily mean that the grade of VUR is higher [19].

Types of LUT Dysfunction

Overall, 45-75% of children with VUR have detrusor overactivity and 19–68% show dysfunctional voiding [6, 34]. As illustrated in Table 1, two general patterns of LUT dysfunction in infants with VUR have emerged [33]. Either (A) the bladder is small and uncompliant and shows detrusor overactivity or (B) it is large and voiding is incomplete and dyscoordinated. Pattern A is common among boys whereas B is

Table 1 LUT dysfunction patterns in infants with dilating reflux

	Bladder volume	Bladder compliance	Detrusor overactivity	Voiding	Residual urine
Boys	small	low	+++	Coordinated	no
Girls	large	high	+	Dyscoordinated	+++

more prevalent among girls. This might reflect congenital obstruction among the boys and may, incidentally, explain why girls with VUR have a higher risk for recurrent UTIs and acquired renal scarring than boys. It is frustrating that we do not know how common these two patterns are in normal infants.

The dyscoordination associated with VUR may be less likely to remit spontaneously than the detrusor overactivity [6]. There are data suggesting that boys with pattern 1 above often change to pattern 2 within a couple of years. This is reflected by the observation that perhaps a third of potty-trained children with dilating VUR have LUT problems, usually voiding difficulties [38]. Furthermore, in adults who as children had VUR, symptoms and signs of LUT dysfunction are common, both urgency, incontinence and voiding dysfunction [26].

In conclusion, although it is clear that neurogenic bladder dysfunction or congenital obstruction are linked to VUR, the situation is less clear for children without these conditions. Still, it is fair to assume that the coexistence of LUT and primary VUR in infants and children with febrile UTIs is not just coincidental. And, given the tendency for dysfunctional voiding with residual urine for these children, this may not be a benign combination. It may also certainly be argued that the LUT dysfunction is more crucial than the VUR as a risk factor for UTIs and renal damage in this group.

Correlation or Causation?

Given the possible link between VUR and LUT dysfunction the question regarding the cause behind this link invites itself.

In primary VUR, as explained elsewhere in this publication, the cause of VUR is not necessarily LUT dysfunction but a misplaced uretereal ostium without a substantial intramural part. This gives no immediate explanation why LUT dysfunction should be part of the condition.

Still, high intravesical pressures are considered likely causes behind severe primary reflux in infants [34], although the pressure need not be high at the actual moment of reflux. Indeed, it has long been known that VUR can happen during low intravesical pressure, possibly even as a result of backward ureteral peristalsis [47]. The reflux may occur both during filling and emptying as well as with or without overactive detrusor contractions [47].

In cases of congenital obstruction it is logical to assume that the increased intravesical pressure itself may be guilty of destroying the valve mechanism. The same may be said regarding the neurogenic bladder. Extra evidence for the role of LUT dysfunction causing VUR in these situations comes from the observation that ureteral reimplantation into a noncompliant high-pressure bladder without bladder augmentation carries a high risk for VUR recurrence [15]. Still, interestingly, VUR may not be apparent at birth in children with myelomeningocele [27], indicating that it takes time for the bladder to damage the valve. Linsenmeyer found that VUR occurred in children with neurogenic bladder either if the bladder was severely trabeculated or the ureteral orifice was misplaced as in primary VUR [29]. In the former case high intravesical pressure is probably causing the VUR while in latter case the association may be just coincidental and the children would have VUR regardless of the neurogenic bladder.

Again, we can conclude that the picture is most clear regarding congenital urethral obstruction or the neurogenic bladder, whereas we know less regarding the arrow of causation in the (possible) link between primary VUR and LUT dysfunction. Probably, LUT dysfunction should not be regarded as a central cause behind primary VUR but as an added risk factor in predisposed individuals.

The Consequences of LUT Dysfunction in Children with VUR

Effects on VUR Resolution

It is reasonably clear that the presence of LUT dysfunction adversely affects the chances of VUR resolution [10, 24, 38, 40]. This has been observed both in infants [40] and older children [38]. The greatest chance of VUR resolution may be in children whose reflux appear only at high bladder pressure or high bladder filling [23].

Possibly, LUT dysfunction also adversely affects the chances of successful anti-reflux treatment. Koff et al found that unsuccessful ureteral reimplantation only happened in children with bladder-bowel dysfunction [24], but the picture is less clear for injection treatment: in some studies LUT dysfunction was a predictor of poor treatment results [7] but in others no such connection was found [25]. But children with neurogenic bladder do have a greater risk of unsuccessful injection treatment than if the reflux was primary [30].

UTI Risk

The most clinically relevant consequence of LUT dysfunction in children with (or without) VUR is an increased risk for UTIs [2, 24, 41]. In fact, LUT dysfunction is a greater risk factor for recurrent UTIs than the VUR *per se*, [41] although the risks of the two conditions are probably additive [21, 32, 41]. This is true both in infants and older children. Within LUT dysfunction residual urine constitutes the greatest risk. The ultimate consequence of this is that LUT dysfunction increases the risk for renal scarring [38, 41], even though it is unclear whether this increased risk is due only to the febrile UTIs as such or partly to the LUT dysfunction subjecting the kidneys to increased pressure. The bottom line here is that it is often more important to look for signs of LUT dysfunction, such as residual urine, in children with UTIs than it is to look for VUR.

Effects on VUR of LUT Treatment

Given the assumption that LUT dysfunction is linked to primary VUR and the observation that the former may delay the resolution of the latter, efforts have been spent looking at whether treatment of the bladder may promote reflux resolution. Results in infants have been largely negative. Sillén et al found that early potty-training of children with dilating reflux and large bladder volumes (group B above) decreased UTIs but did not make the reflux go away [37]. The situation may be different in older children, as several authors have found encouraging results in uncontrolled studies when treating detrusor overactivity with anticholinergics [1, 14] or voiding dysfunction with biofeedback [22]. But, sadly, no randomized, controlled study has so far been performed in any pediatric age group.

The situation is possibly different in children with neurogenic bladder, but even here the situation is not clear-cut. Sillén et al found that VUR in newborn children with myelomeningocele almost universally disappeared during CIC treatment [36], and delayed CIC start has been associated with increased VUR persistence [28]. In boys with posterior urethral valves and VUR, the latter will have a 66% chance of disappearing without specific treatment, just by incision of the valve [45].

It has been claimed that treatment of VUR may help against LUT dysfunction, but this is not based on controlled studies. Kraft et al found that 40% of children with detrusor overactivity and VUR could stop treatment of the former when corrected for the latter [25]. On the other hand, De Kort et al found that cystometry results did not differ between children with dilating VUR surgically corrected during infancy or in later childhood [13].

Recommendations and Clinical Relevance

So where does this lead us? Which clinical recommendations can be given?

Should We Evaluate the Bladder in Children with VUR?

The VUR guidelines of both the European Association of Urology (EAU) and American Urologic Association (AUA) underline the importance of evaluating LUT function in children with VUR [31, 44], but this evaluation does not include invasive urodynamics, except that the EAU guidelines recommend video cystography if LUT dysfunction is therapy-resistant.

Obviously, urodynamic evaluations are crucial in children with suspected spinal dysraphism or obstructive malformations, regardless of VUR. The main reasons for evaluating LUT function in other children are not VUR *per se* but (1) recurrent UTIs or (2) symptoms such as urgency or incontinence. This evaluation can usually be made noninvasively, only proceeding to cystometry (or cystoscopy) in case of consistent grave pathology on uroflow and residual urine measurements.

In potty-trained children with UTIs LUT function has usually been, or should have been, noninvasively evaluated before looking for VUR. This includes the bowel. Only rarely is a VCUG needed in this situation, but should a VCUG have been performed and VUR found, then this does not diminish the need for LUT evaluation.

In infants, VUR is usually either found because of febrile UTIs or antenatal hydronephrosis. In the former case one could argue for performing noninvasive urodynamics, i.e. four-hour voiding observation, since it gives information regarding the chance for spontaneous VUR resolution, whereas the value of this examination is lower without a history of febrile UTI.

What Should We Do When We Find LUT Dysfunction in a Child with VUR?

In the AUA guidelines it is emphasized that LUT or bowel disturbances should be treated before considering VUR correction [31]. The ESPU guidelines on UTIs in children underlines the importance of evaluating LUT function but gives no specific recommendations as to children with concomittant VUR and LUT dysfunction [42]

It should be kept in mind that LUT dysfunction in a child with VUR probably means that the chance of spontaneous VUR resolution is low but that this possibly increases if the LUT dysfunction is treated. Thus, one sensible strategy for infants with dilating VUR and a history of febrile UTIs, who are found to have LUT dysfunction with consistent residual urine, is to encourage early potty-training and give antibiotic prophylaxis until the child has achieved bladder control. But if there are breakthrough infections correction of the VUR is encouraged regardless of LUT function. In older children with VUR, UTIs and LUT dysfunction treatment of the latter is even more important, but this is true irrespective of the VUR.

References

1. Acar B, Arikan FI, Germiyanoglu C, Dallar Y. Influence of high bladder pressure on vesicoureteral reflux and its resolution. Urol Int. 2009;82(1):77–80.
2. Alexander SE, Arlen AM, Storm DW, Kieran K, Cooper CS. Bladder volume at onset of vesicoureteral reflux is an independent risk factor for breakthrough febrile urinary tract infection. J Urol. 2015;193:1342–6.
3. Allen TD. The non-neurogenic neurogenic bladder. J Urol. 1977;117:232–8.

4. Austin P, Bauer S, Bower W, Chase J, Franco I, Hoebeke P, et al. The standardization of terminology of lower urinary tract function in children and adolescents: update report from the standardization committee of the International Children's Continence Society. J Urol. 2014;191(6):1863–5.
5. Bachelard M, Sillén U, Hansson S, Hermansson G, Jodal U, Jacobsson B. Urodynamic pattern in asymptomatic infants: siblings of children with vesicoureteral reflux. J Urol. 1999;162(5):1733–8.
6. Batinic D, Milosevic D, Topalovic-Grkovic M, Nizic L, Vrljicak K, Batinic D, et al. Vesicoureteral reflux and urodynamic dysfunction. Urol Int. 2013;90(4):480–3.
7. Baydilli N, Selvi I, Pinarbasi AS, Akinsal EC, Demirturk HC, Tosun H, et al. Additional VCUG-related parameters for predicting the success of endoscopic injection in children with primary vesicoureteral reflux. J Pediatr Urol. 2021;17(1):68.e1–8.
8. Benninga MA, Faure C, Hyman PE, St James Roberts I, Schechter NL, Nurko S. Childhood functional gastrointestinal disorders: neonate/toddler. Gastroenterology. 2016;150(6):1443–55.e2.
9. Burgers R, de Jong TPVM, Benninga MA. Rectal examination in children: digital versus transabdominal ultrasound. J Urol. 2013;190:667–72.
10. Cakmak O, Tarhan H, Akarken I, Dogan HS, Yavascan O, Sahin H, et al. Can we predict vesicoureteral reflux resolution in patients with non-neurogenic lower urinary tract dysfunction? Int J Urol. 2019;26(6):638–42.
11. Capitanucci ML, Silveri M, Mosiello G, Zaccara A, Capozza N, De Gennaro M. Prevalence of hypercontractility in male and female infants with vesico-ureteral reflux. Eur J Pediatr Surg. 2000;10(3):172–6.
12. Chandra M, Maddix H, McVicar M. Transient urodynamic dysfunction of infancy: relationship to urinary tract infections and vesicoureteral reflux. J Urol. 1996;155:673–7.
13. de Kort LMO, Klijn AJ, Uiterwaal CSPM, de Jong TPVM. Ureteral reimplantation in infants and children: effect on bladder function. J Urol. 2002;167(1):285–7.
14. Fast AM, Nees SN, Van Batavia JP, Combs AJ, Glassberg KI. Outcomes of targeted treatment for vesicoureteral reflux in children with nonneurogenic lower urinary tract dysfunction. J Urol. 2013;190(3):1028–32.
15. Granata C, Buffa P, Di Rovasenda E, Mattioli G, Scarsi PL, Podesta E, et al. Treatment of vesico-ureteric reflux in children with neuropathic bladder: a comparison of surgical and endoscopic correction. J Pediatr Surg. 1999;34:1836–8.
16. Hoebeke P, van Laecke E, Van Camp C, Raes A, Vande WJ. One thousand video-urodynamic studies in children with non-neurogenic bladder sphincter dysfunction. BJU Int. 2001;87(6):575–80.
17. Holmdahl G. Bladder dysfunction in boys with posterior urethral valves. Scand j Urol Nephrol. 1997;188(Suppl):1–36.
18. Holmdahl G, Hanson E, Hanson M, Hellström A-L, Hjälmås K, Sillén U. Four-hour voiding observation in healthy infants. J Urol. 1996;156:1809–12.
19. Hong YK, Altobelli E, Borer JG, Bauer SB, Nguyen HT. Urodynamic abnormalities in toilet trained children with primary vesicoureteral reflux. J Urol. 2011;185(5):1863–8.
20. Karami H, Razi A, Mazloomfard MM, Javanmard B. Is there any role for urodynamic study in children with high-grade vesicoureteral reflux? Urology. 2012;79(4):888–91.
21. Keren R, Shaikh N, Pohl H, Gravens-Mueller L, Ivanova A, Zaoutis L, et al. Risk factors for recurrent urinary tract infection and renal scarring. Pediatrics. 2015;136(1):e13–21.
22. Kibar Y, Ors O, Demir E, Kalman S, Sakallioglu O, Dayanc M. Results of biofeedback treatment on reflux resolution rates in children with dysfunctional voiding and vesicoureteral reflux. Urology. 2007;70(3):563–7.
23. Knudson MJ, Austin JC, McMillan ZM, Hawtrey CE, Cooper CS. Predictive factors of early spontaneous resolution in children with primary vesicoureteral reflux. J Urol. 2007;178:1684–8.
24. Koff SA, Wagner TT, Jayanthi VR. The relationship among dysfunctional elimination syndromes, primary vesicoureteral reflux and urinary tract infections in children. J Urol. 1998;160(3 Pt 2):1019–22.

25. Kraft KH, Molitierno JAJ, Dewhurst L, Geers C, Gunderson K, Scherz HC, et al. Is endoscopic injection therapy a reasonable treatment option for low- grade vesicoureteral reflux in association with overactive bladder. Urology. 2011;78:675–8.
26. Lahdes-Vasama TT, Roihuvuo-Leskinen HM, Koskimäki JE, Tammela TL. Urodynamical findings on women with voiding problems and earlier vesico-ureteral reflux. Neurourol Urodyn. 2009;28(8):1015–21.
27. Levitt SB, Sandler HJ. The absence of vesicoureteral reflux in the neonate with myelodysplasia. J Urol. 1975;114(1)
28. Li Y, Wen YB, He X, Li Y, Wu J, Feng J, et al. Application of clean intermittent catheterization for neurogenic bladder in infants less than 1 year old. Neuro Rehabil. 2018;42(4):377–82.
29. Linsenmeyer TA, House JG, Millis SR. The role of abnormal congenitally displaced ureteral orifices in causing reflux following spinal cord injury. J Spinal Cord Med. 2004;27(2):116–9.
30. Perez-Brayfield M, Kirsch AJ, Hensle TW, Koyle MA, Furness P, Scherz HC. Endoscopic treatment with dextranomer/hyaluronic acid for complex cases of vesicoureteral reflux. J Urol. 2004;172(4 Pt 2):1614–6.
31. Peters CA, Skoog SJ, Arant BS Jr, et al. Summary of the AUA guideline on management of primary vesicoureteral reflux in children. J Urol. 2010;184(3):1134–44.
32. Shaikh K, Hoberman A, Keren R, Gotman N, Docimo SG, Mathews R, et al. Recurrent urinary tract infections in children with bladder and bowel dysfunction. Pediatrics. 2016;137(1):e20152982.
33. Sillén U. Vesicoureteral reflux in infants. Pediatr Nephrol. 1999;13(4):355–61.
34. Sillén U, Hjälmås K, Aili M, Bjure J, Hanson E, Hansson S. Pronounced detrusor hypercontractility in infants with gross bilateral reflux. J Urol. 1992;148:598–9.
35. Sillén U, Bachelard M, Hansson S, Hermansson G, Jacobson B, Hjälmås K. Video cystometric recording of dilating reflux in infancy. J Urol. 1996a;155:1711–5.
36. Sillén U, Hansson E, Hermansson G, Hjälmås K, Jacobsson B, Jodal U. Development of the urodynamic pattern in infants with myelomeningocele. Br J Urol. 1996b;78:596–601.
37. Sillén U, Holmdahl G, Hellström A-L, Sjöström S, Sölsnes E. Treatment of bladder dysfunction and high grade vesicoureteral reflux does not influence the spontaneous resolution rate. J Urol. 2007;177(1):325.
38. Sillén U, Brandström P, Jodal U, Holmdahl G, Sandin A, Sjöberg I, et al. The Swedish reflux trial in children: V. Bladder dysfunction. J Urol. 2010;194:298–304.
39. Silva JA, Alvares RA, Barboza AL, Monteiro RT. Lower urinary tract dysfunction in children with cerebral palsy. Neurourol Urodyn. 2009;28(8):959–63.
40. Sjöström S, Sillén U, Jodal U, Sameby L, Sixt R, Stokland E. Predictive factors for resolution of congenital high grade vesicoureteral reflux in infants: results of univariate and multivariate analyses. J Urol. 2010;183(3):1177–84.
41. Sjöström S, Sillén U, Bachelard M, Johansson E, Brandström P, Hellström A-L, et al. Bladder/bowel dysfunction in pre-school children following febrile urinary tract infection in infancy. Pediatr Nephrol. 2021;36:1489–97.
42. Stein R, Dogan HS, Hoebeke P, Kocvara R, Nijman RJ, Tekgül S. Urinary tract infections in children: EAU/ESPU guidelines. Eur Urol. 2015;67:546–58.
43. Taskinen S, Rintala R. Post-pyelonephritic renal scars are not associated with high voiding pressures. J Pediatr Urol. 2007;3(1):40–4.
44. Tekgül S, Riedmiller H, Hoebeke P, Kocvara R, Nijman RJ, Radmayr C, et al. EAU guidelines on vesicoureteral reflux in children. Eur Urol. 2012;62(3):534–42.
45. Tourchi A, Kajbafzadeh AM, Aryan Z, Ebadi M. The management of vesicoureteral reflux in the setting of posterior urethral valve with emphasis on bladder function and renal outcome: a single center cohort study. Urology. 2014;83(1):199–205.
46. Ural Z, Ulman I, Avanoglu A. Bladder dynamics and vesicoureteral reflux: factors associated with idiopathic lower urinary tract dysfunction in children. J Urol. 2008;179:1564–7.
47. Wahll L, Bachelard M, Sjöström S, Sillén U. Is the mode of occurrence of vesicoureteral reflux correlated to bladder function and spontaneous resolution? J Pediatr Urol. 2009;5(3):170–7.

Pathogenesis of Vesicoureteral Reflux Associated Renal Parenchymal Damage

B. Chertin, G. Raisin, and P. Puri

Abstract Vesicoureteral reflux (VUR) can cause congenital or acquired renal nephropathy. Both forms predispose their carriers to renal damage ranging from mild hypertension to end stage renal disease in the most severe cases. Congenital VUR nephropathy is characterized by kidney dysplasia thought to be a result of high pressure on the developing kidney while acquired VUR nephropathy is characterized by irreversible renal scarring facilitated by recurring insults to the renal parenchyma by bacterial infection. The mechanisms for the development of parenchymal damage in both VUR forms are complex. The following chapter will try to summarize what is known so far about the elaborate physiological processes behind both entities.

Keywords Vesicoureteral reflux · Renal parenchymal damage · Congenital renal dysplasia · Urinary tract infections · Renal scarring · Pathogenesis · Risk factors

Introduction

Vesicoureteral reflux (VUR) is the most common congenital urinary tract abnormality in childhood. The prevalence of VUR is 1% to 2% in the pediatric population and 30% to 40% in children who present with a urinary tract infection (UTI) [1]. VUR renal damage can be congenital or acquired. Congenital VUR is associated with parenchymal damage caused by high pressure on the developing kidney and is characterized by kidney dysplasia [2]. Acquired VUR is caused by recurring insults to the renal parenchyma, facilitated by bacterial infection, which may result in

B. Chertin (✉) · G. Raisin
Departments of Urology & Pediatric Urology, Shaare Zedek Medical Center, Faculty of Medicine, Hebrew University, Jerusalem, Israel
e-mail: chertinb@szmc.org.il

P. Puri
Beacon Consultants Clinic, University College Dublin, Dublin, Ireland

P. Puri, A. Yamataka (eds.), *Vesicoureteral Reflux*,
https://doi.org/10.1007/978-3-031-95091-9_10

irreversible renal scarring [1, 2]. Both etiologies put the patients at risk for hypertension, proteinuria and chronic kidney disease with progressive renal failure, including end stage renal disease [1].

Risk Factors and Parenchymal Insult

The parenchymal damage in congenital reflux nephropathy (CRN) is caused by a high-pressure sterile reflux affecting normal prenatal renal development and resulting in focal renal dysplasia. Abnormal bladder dynamics during gestation and early postnatal period is thought to play a role in these changes; clinical and experimental evidence shows that immature animals, typically males, have abnormal bladder function due to incomplete sphincter relaxation; Animal VUR models have demonstrated a pattern of mild bladder outlet obstruction in male but not female sheep fetuses, suggesting that the immature male sphincter is partially obstructive [2]. In addition, previous studies have noted high pressure voiding in male infants and even more so in those with VUR. This pattern seems to disappear with VUR resolution in the fetal reflux model, although the causality is unknown [1–3]. In acquired reflux nephropathy (ARN), the parenchymal damage is the result of a complex interaction of host and bacterial factors that leads to acute alterations in renal function and may lead to permanent renal scarring. Risk factors for renal impairment in acquired renal scaring (ARS) include high reflux grade, bladder-bowel disorder (BBD), recurrent pyelonephritic episodes and delayed initiation of antibiotic therapy [1].

Damage Detection

Renal Imaging

Technetium-99m dimercaptosuccinic acid (DMSA) is a nuclear agent that shows most effectively the renal cortical tissue. It is currently considered the clinical gold standard to detect acquired renal scarring. Sites of new onset renal scarring correspond to sites of acute pyelonephritis on initial DMSA renal scan, confirming the role of the infection/inflammation process in the etiology of ARN [2]. Although a good tool for assessing renal damage in RN, many aspects of renal function are not assessed by DMSA scan, including concentrating ability, acid-base handling, and sodium and water homeostasis [2]. A study examining Diffusion-weighted magnetic resonance imaging (DW-MRI) for the detection of acute renal parenchymal lesions, have found DW-MRI had greater sensitivity for acute lesions detection compared to DMSA renal scan, but both modalities have found the same number of parenchymal scarring on follow up scans [4]. Currently, the role of DW-MRI as a low radiation alternative to renal scan is not fully understood.

Markers

Both serum and urinary markers are a well-established tool of early detection as well as monitoring for disease progression. Erythropoietin was previously suggested as a useful marker in predicting chronic renal failure in diabetic patients with overt nephropathy and normal renal function but did not prove efficient for renal damage assessment in RN [5]. Connective tissue growth factor (CTGF), a humoral factor secreted by infiltrating renal cells, who stimulates renal fibroblast proliferation and extracellular matrix (ECM) synthesis, was found to play a key role in the development and progression of diabetic renal fibrosis, with urinary levels being associated with the stage of diabetic nephropathy [6]. In a study by Gultekin et al. urinary CTGF levels were found to be significantly increased in children with VUR, independent on the presence of renal scarring, suggesting its potential as a marker for renal fibrosis in VUR patients [6]. Though additional studies examining various markers have been performed, currently, there are not highly specific urinary or serum biochemical markers of RN.

Pathogenesis of Renal Parenchymal Damage in ARN

The classic histological findings in ARN kidneys are interstitial infiltration with chronic inflammatory cells, tubular basement membrane thickening, epithelial-cell atrophy, collapse of the tubular lumen, dilatation of other tubules with atrophic epithelium, eosinophilic casts, medial and intimal thickening of the arteries and arterioles, periglomerular fibrosis, and compensatory hypertrophy in adjacent unscarred renal tissue [7]. The pathogenesis of renal scarring has not been clearly understood. The initiating event in pyelonephritis is bacterial invasion of the renal parenchyma, which elicits inflammatory and immune responses. Inflammation releases toxic enzymes, such as lysozymes, into the lumen of renal tubules. At the same time, the infiltrating lymphocytes, monocytes/macrophages and mast cells activate and produce reactive oxygen species (ROS), which generates oxygen radicals that are toxic not only to the bacteria but also to the surrounding tubular cells. Tubular cell death occurs, further spreading the inflammatory process into the interstitium thus expanding the magnitude of renal damage. In addition, focal ischemia results from intravascular aggregation of granulocytes and edema [8]. The resulting damage causes interstitial inflammation, collagen deposition and disruption of the normal tubular arrangement. As a result, permanent parenchymal damage and scar formation occur, which are accompanied by tubular atrophy and interstitial fibrosis [7, 9]. Though not entirely understood, some key players in this intricate process have been previously studied and their roles are described below.

Macrophage Colony Stimulating Factor (M-CSF)

M-CSF is a hematopoietic cytokine that is macrophage chemoattractant as well as it serves as a growth and differentiation factor for macrophages. It has been documented to play a pivotal role in the development of nephritis via macrophage activation [8]. A study by Rolle et al. demonstrated increased immunoreactivity and mRNA expression of M-CSF in the refluxing kidney compared to control kidney [8]. They speculated that cytokines released during inflammation stimulate renal tissue to produce M-CSF, which may act as chemotactic signal for monocyte-macrophages. The activated macrophages and renal tubular epithelium release numerous substances, such as nitric oxide, free oxygen radicals, and lysozymes, which induce tissue injury and ultimately leading to renal scarring.

Nitric Oxide (NO)

NO is synthesised from the guanidino nitrogen of L-arginine by NO synthase (NOS). Three distinct isoforms of NOS have been identified: inducible (iNOS), endothelial (eNOS), and neuronal NOS (nNOS) [7]. iNOS is involved in non-specific immunity and participates in the complex mechanism of tissue injury as a mediator of inflammatory processes and apoptosis. In the kidney, iNOS is present in glomerular mesangial and tubular epithelial cells and has been reported to induces immunologic injury to glomerular cells and enhances accumulation of extracellular matrix in the glomerulus and tubulointerstitial space [7]. In their study, Chertin et al. have demonstrated identical immunolocalization of iNOS and TGF-ß1 in severe RN kidneys. They hypothesized that macrophage-stimulating overproduction of pro-inflammator cytokines and iNOS may trigger apoptosis, ultimately leading to tubular atrophy and renal tissue loss and dysfunction in RN [7] (Fig. 1).

Mast Cells (MCs)

Mast cells secrete many fibrogenic factors and have been implicated in chronic inflammatory processes with fibrous tissue deposition [10]. The granules in MCs contain various inflammatory mediators and chemotactic factors. Based on their neutral serine protease contents, MCs have been subtyped as tryptase positive MCs- a profibrogenic factor, stimulating type I collagen production by fibroblasts and inducing chemotaxis in fibroblasts, or chymase-positive MCs- which releases the matrix-bound transforming growth factor (TGF)-b1 and is an efficient converter of angiotensin I into angiotensin II [10]. A study by Solari et al. showed increased

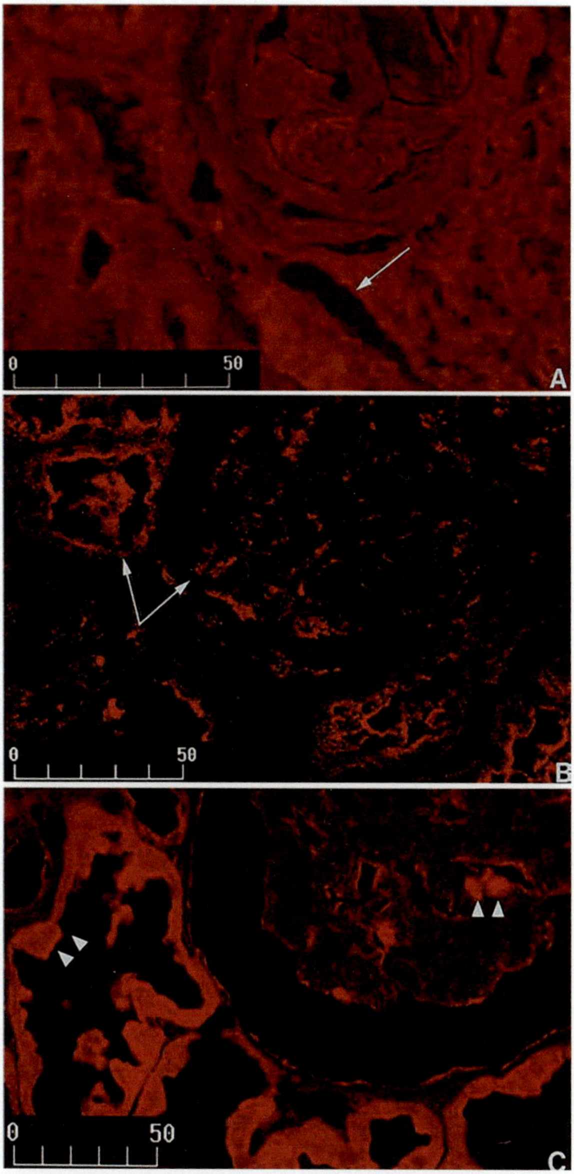

Fig. 1 (**a**) Control kidney shows weak immunoreactivity for inducible nitric-oxide synthase (iNOS) in proximal tubules (arrow); (**b**) Reflux nephropathy (RN) kidney shows strong immunoreactivity for iNOS in glomerulus and proximal tubules (arrows); (**c**) Strong immunoreactivity for transforming growth factor-ß1 in glomerulus and proximal tubule of RN kidney similar to iNOS (arrowheads)

immunoreactivity of MCs and fibrosis in the renal interstitium of kidneys with RN with the number of infiltrating tryptase-positive MCs correlating with the degree of interstitial renal scarring [10]. Though further studies are required, it seems that MCs may play a role in the pathogenesis of RN.

Angiotensin-Converting Enzyme (ACE) and Angiotensin II

ACE converts the inactive decapeptide angiotensin I (Ang I) to the active octapeptide angiotensin II (Ang II), a potent vasoconstrictor. In the kidney, ACE is found in the epithelial cells of the proximal renal tubule. ACE increases production of the components of extracellular matrix (ECM) mediated through Ang II. Two studies by Chertin et al. found upregulation of both ACE and Ang II receptors in the RN kidneys [11, 12] (Fig. 2). They suggested that Overexpression of Ang II receptors causes not only increased fluid and sodium reabsorption with alteration of the glomerular-tubular balance, but also an influx of

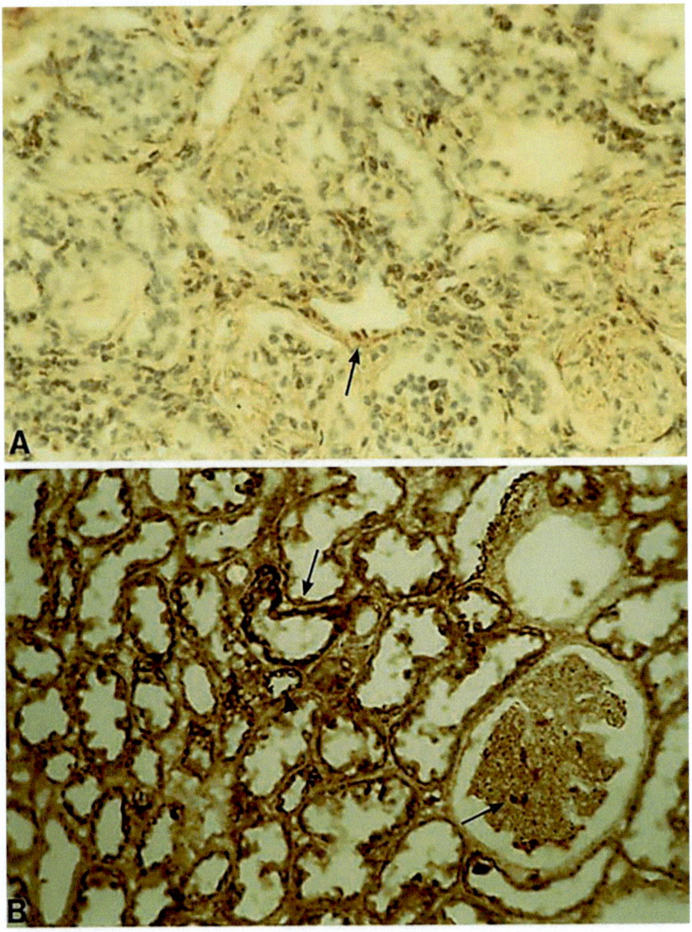

Fig. 2 (**a**) Control kidney: weak angiotensin-converting enzyme (ACE) staining in proximal tubules (arrow). (**b**) Reflux nephropathy strong ACE immunoreactivity in glomerulus and proximal tubules (arrows) and moderate-to-strong in distal tubules (arrowhead)

pro-inflammatory cytokines such as transforming growth factor- b into the tubulointerstitial space. These processes may lead to a reduction in tubular fraction volume with tubular atrophy, dilatation, and hypertrophic changes ultimately leading to interstitial fibrosis [11, 12].

Cyclooxygenase-2 (COX-2)

Another key player studied for its part in the pathogenesis of RN is COX2. COX-2, an enzyme responsible for prostaglandin synthesis, is a key enzyme in the regulation of renin synthesis and its overproduction has been reported to be among the mediators of altered renal function and glomerular damage following subtotal renal ablation. In a study by Solari et al, COX2 was found to be over expressed in RN kidneys, they suggest the this over expression may trigger over production of renin, resulting in increased secretion of angiotensin II [13].

Epidermal Growth Factor (EGF)

EGF is produced by tubular kidney cells. It plays an important role in the modulation of renal tubular cell growth and has been reported to be decreased following acute and chronic tubular injury [14, 15]. Moreover, it has been demonstrated that the administration of EGF during acute tubular injury attenuates tubular damage and accelerates tubular regeneration [16]. EGF expression was previously examined in RN kidneys and found to be downregulated. This may indicate EGF has an important role in the pathogenesis of tubular damage, by triggering the overproduction of proinflammatory and profibrotic cytokines in RN patients [14].

Insulin-Like Growth Factor-1 (IGF-1)

IGF-1, a peptide growth factor produced by collecting ducts, has been shown to enhance proliferation and reduce apoptosis of tubular cells following renal injury. A study by Chertin et al. found its expression to be downregulated in RN kidneys suggesting its role in RN pathogenesis by increasing interstitial collagen deposition and tubular apoptosis [17] (Fig. 3).

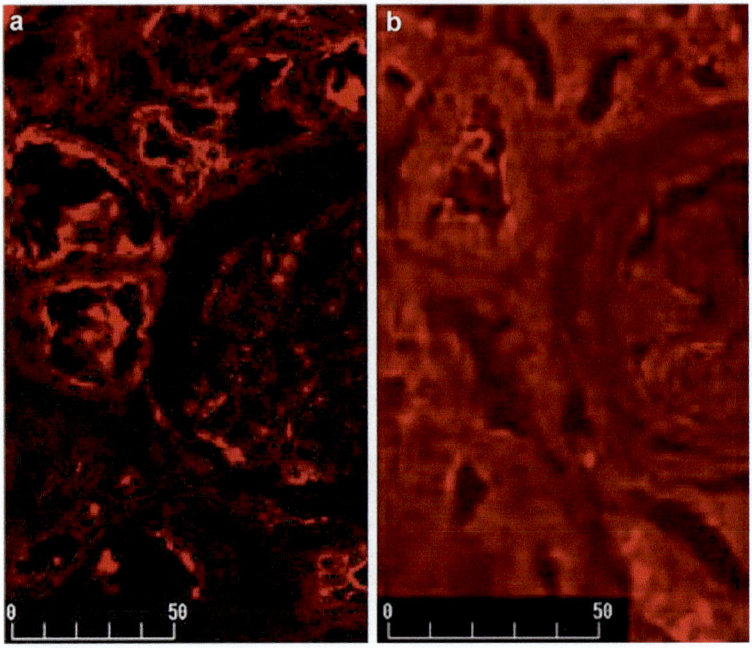

Fig. 3 (**a**) Strong IGF-1 immunoreactivity demonstrated in the proximal tubules and moderate immunoreactivity in the glomeruli of normal kidney. (**b**) IGF-1 immunoreactivity markedly reduced in the proximal tubules and glomeruli of RN kidney

Genetics

Familial clustering of VUR and observations of sex dependent differences in VUR prevalence support the hypothesis that VUR is a genetic disorder [18, 19]. Until this day, no candidate gene study managed to discover a high prevalence gene mutation in the VUR population, supporting the assumption that VUR is a genetically heterogeneous disorder.

Few studies have examined genetics as a predisposing factor to renal scaring in RN; Genetic polymorphism of TGF-β1, a potent fibrogenic cytokine who promotes fibrosis, was studied in RN children by Solari et al. [20, 21]. They have found a significant association between coding region 10 and the polymorphic variant 509 of the TGF- β1 gene in renal scarring following vesicoureteral reflux. In another study by Solari et al., TNF-α, a proinflammatory cytokine promoting interstitial infiltration of inflammatory cells, was also studied for gene polymorphism in RN children [22]. They have discovered a significant association of TNF-α gene polymorphism in patients with reflux nephropathy, suggesting its involvement in the pathogenesis of renal scarring. Larger studies are needed to further understand the genetic basis of ARN scar formation and renal damage predisposition.

Pathogenesis or Renal Parenchymal Damage in CRN

The classic histological finding in CRN kidneys is focal dysplasia [2]. It is identified by the presence of primitive ducts associated with increased mesenchyme and reflects intrauterine maldevelopment [11]. Unlike CRN kidneys, ARN kidneys contain no dysplastic features.

It is presumed that two factors are responsible for the damage seen in CRN kidneys. high grade reflux and abnormal bladder dynamics especially high-pressure voiding [11, 19, 23]. Both factors are assumed to create mechanical forces that alter the cell-cell signaling involved in cell differentiation, growth and apoptosis, similar to changes observed in an obstructive system [2]. The high pressure of non-infected urine on the renal parenchyma leads to local ischemia with the release of proinflammatory cytokines, toxic metabolites, and ROS. Local inflammation occurs, and a process of architectural remodeling is initiated, leading to renal scar development [23]. These factors are potentially responsible for early focal disruption of normal nephron formation, thus granting CRN kidneys their unique histological appearance.

A further investigation into RN pathogenesis and its genetic basis might further shed light on the management, treatment and prevention of such prevalent disease.

Conclusions

The pathogenesis of renal parenchymal damage in vesicoureteral reflux is a complex and not well understood process that involves many key players. A better understanding of these processes has the potential to assist in the development of better markers for diagnosis and follow up of reflux nephropathy as well as a potential cure.

References

1. Hunziker M, Colhoun E, Puri P. Prevalence and predictors of renal functional abnormalities of high grade vesicoureteral reflux. J Urol. 2013;190(4 SUPPL):1490–4. https://doi.org/10.1016/j.juro.2013.01.068.
2. Peters C, Rushton HG. Vesicoureteral reflux associated renal damage: congenital reflux nephropathy and acquired renal scarring. J Urol. 2010;184(1):265–73. https://doi.org/10.1016/j.juro.2010.03.076.
3. Mattoo TK. Vesicoureteral reflux and reflux nephropathy; 2011. https://doi.org/10.1053/j.ackd.2011.07.006.
4. Bosakova A, et al. Diffusion-weighted magnetic resonance imaging is more sensitive than dimercaptosuccinic acid scintigraphy in detecting parenchymal lesions in children with acute pyelonephritis: a prospective study. J Pediatr Urol. 2018;14(3):269.e1–7. https://doi.org/10.1016/j.jpurol.2018.02.014.

5. Cascio S, Solari V, Reen DJ, Puri P. The significance of serum erythropoietin levels in assessing the severity of renal damage in children with reflux nephropathy. In: Journal of Urology. Lippincott Williams and Wilkins; 2004. p. 1607–9. https://doi.org/10.1097/01.ju.0000138521.04892.ab.
6. Dilay Gültekin N, Benzer M, Tekin-Neijmann Ş. Is there any relation between connective tissue growth factor and scar tissue in vesicoureteral reflux? Turk J Pediatr. 2019;61(1):71–8. https://doi.org/10.24953/turkjped.2019.01.011.
7. Chertin B, Rolle U, Farkas A, Puri P. The role of nitric oxide in reflux nephropathy. Pediatr Surg Int. 2002:630–4. https://doi.org/10.1007/s00383-002-0858-4.
8. Rolle U, Shima H, Puri P. Nitric oxide, enhanced by macrophage-colony stimulating factor, mediates renal damage in reflux nephropathy. Kidney Int. 2002;62(2):507–13. https://doi.org/10.1046/j.1523-1755.2002.00485.x.
9. Demir M, Yagmur I, Pelit ES, Kati B, Ördek E, Çiftçi H. Is there a relationship between renal scarring and neutrophil-to-lymphocyte ratio in patients with vesicoureteral reflux? Archivio Italiano di Urologia e Andrologia. 2021;93(4):436–40. https://doi.org/10.4081/aiua.2021.4.436.
10. Solari V, Unemoto K, Piaseczna Piotrowska A, Puri P. Increased expression of mast cells in reflux nephropathy. Pediatr Nephrol. 2004;19(2):157–63. https://doi.org/10.1007/s00467-003-1323-x.
11. Chertin B, Solari V, Reen DJ, Farkas A, Puri P. Up-regulation of angiotensin-converting enzyme (ACE) gene expression induces tubulointerstitial injury in reflux nephropathy. Pediatr Surg Int. 2002:635–9. https://doi.org/10.1007/s00383-002-0857-5.
12. Chertin B, et al. Upregulation of angiotensin II receptors in reflux nephropathy. In: Journal of Pediatric Surgery. W.B. Saunders; 2002. p. 251–5. https://doi.org/10.1053/jpsu.2002.30266.
13. Solari V, Piotrowska AP, Cascio S, Unemoto K, Chertin B, Puri P. Cyclooxygenase-2 up-regulation in reflux nephropathy. In: Journal of Urology. Lippincott Williams and Wilkins; 2003. p. 1624–7. https://doi.org/10.1097/01.ju.0000085810.37816.65.
14. Chertin B, Farkas A, Puri P. Epidermal growth factor and monocyte chemotactic peptide-1 expression in reflux nephropathy. Eur Urol. 2003;44(1):144–9. https://doi.org/10.1016/S0302-2838(03)00190-8.
15. El-Dydamony EM, Abdelaal MA, Kasim SA, Ameen DR, Abd El-Fattah DA. Urinary epidermal growth factor and monocyte chemotactic protein-1 as biomarkers of renal injury in patients with obstructed nephropathy. Archivio Italiano di Urologia e Andrologia. 2022;94(4):443–6. https://doi.org/10.4081/aiua.2022.4.443.
16. Grandaliano G, et al. MCP-1 and EGF renal expression and urine excretion in human congenital obstructive nephropathy. Kidney Int. 2000;58(1):182–92. https://doi.org/10.1046/j.1523-1755.2000.00153.x.
17. Chertin B, Farkas A, Puri P. Insulin-like growth factor-1 expression in reflux nephropathy. In: Pediatric Surgery International. Springer; 2004. p. 283–9. https://doi.org/10.1007/s00383-003-1127-x.
18. Puri P, Gosemann J-H, Darlow J, Barton DE. Genetics of vesicoureteral reflux. Nat Rev Urol. 2011;8(10):539–52. https://doi.org/10.1038/nrurol.2011.113.
19. Puri P, Friedmacher F, Farrugia M-K, Sharma S, Esposito C, Mattoo TK. Primary vesicoureteral reflux. Nat Rev Dis Primers. 2024;10(1):75. https://doi.org/10.1038/s41572-024-00560-8.
20. Solari V, Owen D, Puri P. Association of transforming growth factor-beta1 gene polymorphism with reflux nephropathy. J Urol. 2005;174(4 Pt 2):1609–11.; discussion 1611. https://doi.org/10.1097/01.ju.0000179385.64585.dc.
21. Yoneda A, Oue T, Puri P. Angiotensin-converting enzyme genotype distribution in familial vesicoureteral reflux. Pediatr Surg Int. 2001;17(4):308–11. https://doi.org/10.1007/s003830100600.

22. Solari V, Ennis S, Cascio S, Puri P, Austin P, Furness PD. Tumor necrosis factor-α gene polymorphism in reflux nephropathy. J Urol. 2004;172(4):1604–6. https://doi.org/10.1097/01.ju.0000140210.12175.69.
23. Colceriu MC, Aldea PL, Răchişan AL, Clichici S, Sevastre-Berghian A, Mocan T. Vesicoureteral reflux and innate immune system: physiology, physiopathology, and clinical aspects. MDPI; 2023. https://doi.org/10.3390/jcm12062380.

Diagnosis of Vesicoureteral Reflux

Mayu Nakagawa, Amane Endo, and Yutaka Tanami

Abstract Voiding cystourethrography (VCUG) is the gold standard for diagnosing vesicoureteral reflux (VUR). This chapter serves as a practical guide for clinicians performing VCUG for VUR diagnosis. It emphasizes the importance of a standardized approach to maximize diagnostic yield while minimizing patient discomfort and radiation exposure. Given that about one-third of children with urinary tract infections (UTIs) have VUR, not all children with UTIs need VUR imaging. This chapter also explores alternative imaging modalities for VUR detection, including Renal and bladder ultrasonography (US), dimercaptosuccinic acid scan, and contrast-enhanced US. Additionally, the chapter highlights the limitations and considerations for each imaging modality in diagnosing VUR and associated conditions.

Keywords Voiding cystourethrography · Renal and bladder ultrasound · Technetium-99m mercaptoacetyltriglycine renogram · Vesicoureteral reflux · Diagnosis · Urinary tract infections · Ultrasound · Contrast-enhanced Voiding Urosonography · Dimercaptosuccinic acid Scan · Grading of reflux

Introduction

Vesicoureteral reflux (VUR) investigation is recommended for asymptomatic newborns with significant urinary tract dilation (UTD) detected prenatally or for children who have recurrent febrile urinary tract infections (UTIs) [1].

M. Nakagawa (✉) · A. Endo
Department of Pediatrics, Faculty of Medicine, Juntendo University, Tokyo, Japan
e-mail: mnakaga@juntendo.ac.jp; aendo@juntendo.ac.jp

Y. Tanami
Division of Radiology, Saitama Children's Medical Center, Saitama, Japan
e-mail: tanami.yutaka@saitama-pho.jp

P. Puri, A. Yamataka (eds.), *Vesicoureteral Reflux*,
https://doi.org/10.1007/978-3-031-95091-9_11

Common imaging techniques for diagnosing suspected VUR include renal and bladder ultrasound (RBUS), voiding cystourethrogram (VCUG), and nuclear renal scans, such as the technetium-99m mercaptoacetyltriglycine (MAG3) renogram or the dimercaptosuccinic acid (DMSA) scan. Newer methods for investigating VUR include contrast-enhanced voiding urosonography and positional instillation of contrast cystography [1].

Prenatally Detected UTD

In the prenatal period, UTD observed in conditions such as VUR (15–21% of cases) can lead to UTIs in up to 30% of patients [2]. Overall, 10–40% of patients with high-grade VUR (grade III to V) frequently exhibit congenital dysplasia and/or acquired post-infectious damage in the affected kidney; therefore, investigations should be appropriately targeted [3].

The initial investigation is an RBUS, typically performed between 72 h and 4 weeks of age. This timing is due to the fact that an RBUS conducted within the first 72 h might not fully capture the extent of upper tract dilatation, a result of perinatal dehydration in the newborn infant [1]. Indications for a postnatal VCUG following prenatal ultrasonography findings vary across institutions [1]. The Society for Fetal Urology and the American Urological Association recommend a VCUG for cases of grade III and IV hydronephrosis according to Society for Fetal Urology standards, particularly under urgent conditions if bilateral, and in the presence of a hydroureter or an abnormal bladder observed on fetal ultrasonography [4]. The European Association of Urology and the European Society of Pediatric Urology (EAU/ESPU) guidelines advise VCUG use in patients with ultrasonography findings of bilateral high-grade hydronephrosis, duplex kidneys with hydronephrosis, ureterocele, ureteric dilatation, and abnormal bladders, as well as in cases presenting renal cortical abnormalities on RBUS, characterized by cortical thinning, irregularity, and increased echogenicity [5].

A DMSA renal scan, performed after the diagnosis of congenital VUR but before any febrile UTI, is useful to establish renal dysplasia at baseline and may assist in predicting the likelihood of breakthrough UTIs [5].

Febrile UTI

UTIs are common in children and may indicate an associated urinary tract abnormality, especially if febrile [6]. The risk of recurrence is remarkably high in the first 6–12 months after the initial UTI [7], and the prevalence of VUR is reported to be

30% in these children [8]. Between 10–40% of children with VUR develop renal scarring after a UTI, leading to damage [8]. The severity of VUR directly correlates with renal damage risk [7, 9]. The primary goal in preventing UTI is to avoid renal scarring.

International guidelines recommend an RBUS exam after the first culture-positive febrile UTI in children under 2 years of age [5]. Guidelines agree that a VCUG is indicated in the presence of an abnormal RBUS or recurrent infections [1]. EAU/ESPU and British guidelines specify that urosepsis, non-Escherichia coli UTI, failure to respond to sensitive antibiotics, and poor urine flow with or without a palpable bladder also indicate a need for VCUG [5].

An indirect technetium-99m MAG3 renogram is an alternative to VCUG for toilet-trained children [1]. A DMSA scan is best obtained from 3 months of age to ensure full glomerular filtration rate maturity in infants. Renal scarring is a significant risk factor for breakthrough febrile UTIs and is useful in predicting symptomatic VUR resolution [10].

Delaying a DMSA scan for 4–6 months after a kidney infection allows the acute episode to subside, so that any persistent cortical defects can be assumed to represent permanent renal scarring [7, 11]. The "top-down" approach involves an early DMSA scan at the time of infection, with the reasoning that a normal DMSA renal scan avoids an unnecessary VCUG in over 50% of patients [5, 7].

Ultrasonography

Ultrasound (US) is commonly used to evaluate postnatal hydronephrosis and UTIs in children, but it has limited sensitivity for detecting VUR [12]. The presence or level of UTD on US does not always correspond to the VUR grade, and a normal ultrasound cannot exclude VUR [1]. Nonetheless, abnormal findings like UTD, renal parenchymal changes, and bladder abnormalities may indicate potential VUR, necessitating further tests [1]. In the Randomized Intervention for Children with Vesicoureteral Reflux (RIVUR) study, 11% of VUR patients exhibited an abnormal US examination, characterized by hydronephrosis or ureteral duplication [13]. Figure 1 illustrates the upper renal portion of the duplicated kidney with reflux into the lower kidney. The renal resistive index from color Doppler US has also been employed to monitor children with VUR, although it has not gained broad acceptance due to its poor correlation with VUR [14]. Color-flow Doppler sonography has been utilized to detect retrograde ureteral jets at the ureterovesical junction as an indicator of VUR. A strong correlation was observed with VCUG [15], but detecting ureteral jets was not adequately sensitive for VUR diagnosis. Moreover, the procedure requires the child to urinate in a supine position, which can be difficult.

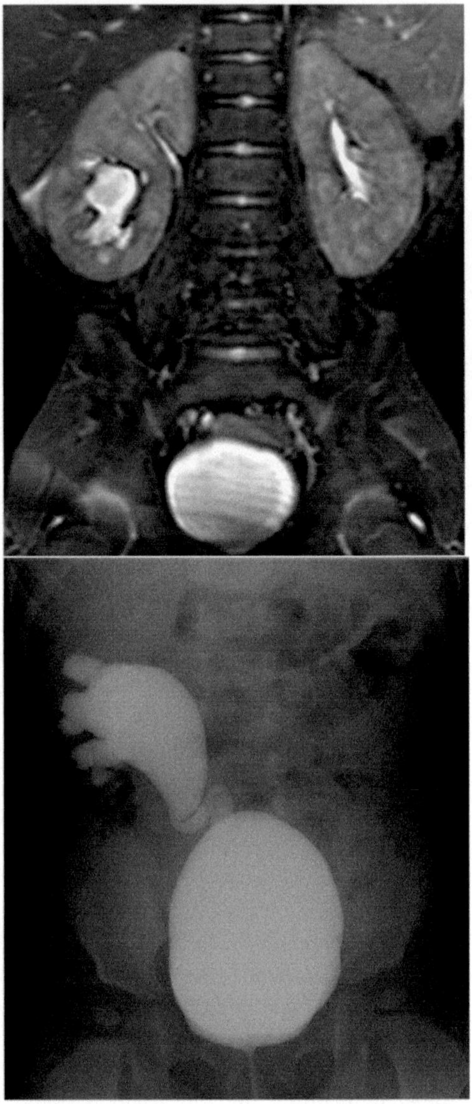

Fig. 1 The upper renal side of the duplicated kidney with reflux into the lower kidney. A 1-year-old girl in whom VCUG shows reflux into the right lower kidney, that is, dropping the lily sign. MRI depicts the upper renal side of the duplicated kidney

Voiding Cystourethrogram

Timing

VCUG is the benchmark for diagnosing VUR [16], providing anatomical details of the genitourinary tract and facilitating the grading of VUR. It should be reserved for children with a high suspicion of VUR (see the "Introduction" section). VCUG is not recommended following ureteroneocystostomy or endoscopic treatment, as the long-term clinical success rates for both procedures are considered very high [17–19]. Follow-up imaging after endoscopic sub-ureteral transurethral injection is subject to debate: some authors recommend a follow-up study planned 3–12 months after surgical intervention, while others suggest follow-up only after a febrile UTI [17–19].

VCUGs for evaluating congenital anomalies can be performed at any time. Previous recommendations [20, 21] to delay VCUG after a UTI to allow resolution of the inflammatory process may not be necessary. Spencer et al. reported that early VCUGs (within a week of diagnosis) did not exacerbate illness and had outcomes similar to those of late VCUGs [22]. However, according to a recent meta-analysis, the timing of VCUG has only minor, if not negligible, effects on the results [23].

Radiation

The ALARA principle, or as low as reasonably achievable, is applied to minimize radiation exposure with respect to time, distance, and shielding. Exposure time should be managed with protocols, experienced personnel, and tools such as stop-watches [24], and pulsed fluoroscopy should be used to reduce radiation exposure. The distance between the subject and the radiation source should be increased to decrease the radiation dose. Shielding also helps protect patients and workers from radiation [24, 25]. High-quality image-capture technology is used to reduce the radiation dose. Modern techniques in fluoroscopic VCUGs have lower radiation doses compared to radionucleotide cystography [26]. Ward et al. found radiation exposure eight times lower using grid-controlled variable-rate pulsed fluoroscopy [27].

Preparation and Sedation

VCUG can be a traumatizing test for patients and parents because of catheterization or fear of the unknown [28, 29]. Parental anxiety can affect their children's fear, distress, and pain during the procedure. Education and preparation for parents and children can help reduce anxiety and stress [30, 31]. Allowing a calm parent to accompany the child during the procedure decreases patient distress [32, 33]. Providing support and distractions such as toys, videos, and balloons can help children cope with this procedure. Notably, children are more cooperative and calmer during invasive procedures when supported by their parents. Therefore, child life specialists can be beneficial during VCUGs [30, 34]. Sedation can be used in certain situations; however, it should not alter the voiding phase or test outcomes. The use of sedation is acceptable in cases in which less-invasive methods fail to create a relaxed atmosphere for the child and/or family. Moreover, a randomized trial of sedation versus placebo showed no significant between-group difference in the volume infused during the filling or voiding phases [35]. Sedation should follow the guidelines for preparation, monitoring, and recovery recommended by the American Academy of Pediatrics.

Sterile Catheterization

Urethral catheterization should be performed using strict aseptic techniques. An 8-French feeding tube should be used instead of an indwelling catheter to avoid confusion with the ureterocele [12]. A larger catheter should be selected for older children and a smaller catheter for premature or very small infants. The catheter is advanced no further than 1–2 cm after obtaining urine to prevent bladder injury and tube knot formation [12]. Moreover, a urine dip test should be performed, and cultures should be sent for specimens positive for leukocytes and/or nitrites. Lidocaine jelly should be applied before catheterization in older children to decrease sensation [36]. Notably, the use of local anesthetics, such as lidocaine gel applied 1–4 min before catheterization, may reduce discomfort [37]. The external sphincter is the most common site of resistance in men. Applying gentle, steady posterior pressure can help advance the catheter when the patient takes a deep breath. Leaving the catheter in place during voiding can help determine whether the residual contrast in the upper tracts is due to a continuous reflex or secondary obstruction [38, 39].

Whether the catheter should be left during the voiding phase of VCUG is still debated. Leaving the catheter in place during voiding can have benefits, such as avoiding re-catheterization for cyclic examinations and allowing for repeated examinations or bladder distension.

Contrast Material

Low-osmolarity contrast materials are recommended for imaging. A dilute contrast is preferred when outlining the presence of a urethrocele to avoid obscuring the detection. Warm (body temperature) contrast materials are ideal for minimizing distress and bladder effects, especially in children [12]. Receptors in the bladder mucosa and trigone can trigger a sensitive cooling reflex that affects bladder function [40, 8]. This reflex is usually suppressed by age 4 [8]. Furthermore, the contrast media should be slowly infused under gravity to reduce bladder spasms and potential adverse reactions. The prewarmed iodinated contrast agent (concentration 100 to 150 mg iodine/ml) should be instilled into the bladder by gravity from a height of between 50 cm and 100 cm above the table [28]. In the case of recent bladder surgery, a lower height should be considered to reduce bladder filling pressure [41].

The estimated bladder capacity is as follows: for patients aged <2 years, weight (kg) × 7; patients aged >2–14 years, (age in years × 30) + 30; and patients aged

>14 years, 500 mL. The bladder is filled until voiding occurs. If bladder filling reaches >2 times the bladder capacity and no voiding occurs, subsequent evaluation of the patient with a videourodynamic study should be considered.

Images

No universal protocol exists for conducting VCUG; however, it is crucial to include specific views in imaging protocols. These should encompass an early filling image, bilateral steep oblique images of the ureterovesical junction (UVJ), including the trigone or the presumed location of the distal ureters when the bladder is full [12]. Additionally, voiding images of the urethra and post-void images of the kidneys and bladder are necessary [12, 28]. If pathology is detected, further images may be required to delineate the abnormality [28]. Additional views of the bladder and kidneys during repeated filling and voiding can detect subtle abnormalities such as intermittent VUR [12, 28]. If reflux is identified, delayed imaging of the kidneys can be used to determine the extent to which the system drains [12].

Additionally, the scout image should encompass the spine and pelvis to assess for spinal dysraphism, sacral agenesis, scoliosis, or other potential abnormalities [12]. Furthermore, evaluations for masses, stones, and foreign bodies are essential. Colonic gas patterns and stool volume should be evaluated, as constipation may play a significant role in the underlying urological problems.

Early Filling Image
An early filling anteroposterior view of the bladder may reveal a ureterocele or filling defect representing a bladder mass, clot, or other pathology [12, 28]. Correct catheter placement is confirmed during this phase of the study [12].

Full Bladder Image
The full bladder is evaluated using steep oblique images coned to the bladder and the expected location of the distal ureters [12]. These images evaluate low-grade VUR, everting ureteroceles, diverticula, or other bladder anomalies. Additional assessments include bladder capacity, contour, presence of trabeculations, and emptying capability [39]. Figure 2 demonstrates the classic appearance of a neurogenic bladder with high-grade VUR. If present, VURs should be reported according to the International Reflux Study Committee classification (Figs. 3, 4 and 5).

The grade of reflux is determined according to the most severe VUR, which typically, but not always, coincides with the peak of voiding [42]. Reflux is most likely to occur during voiding, and approximately 20% of reflux cases are undetected if voiding does not occur [39]. Intrarenal reflux may be observed on VCUGs (Fig. 5) and can be identified by contrast observed within the renal parenchyma and the collecting system. This should be reported as it has prognostic implications for renal scarring, hypertension, and long-term renal function [43, 44].

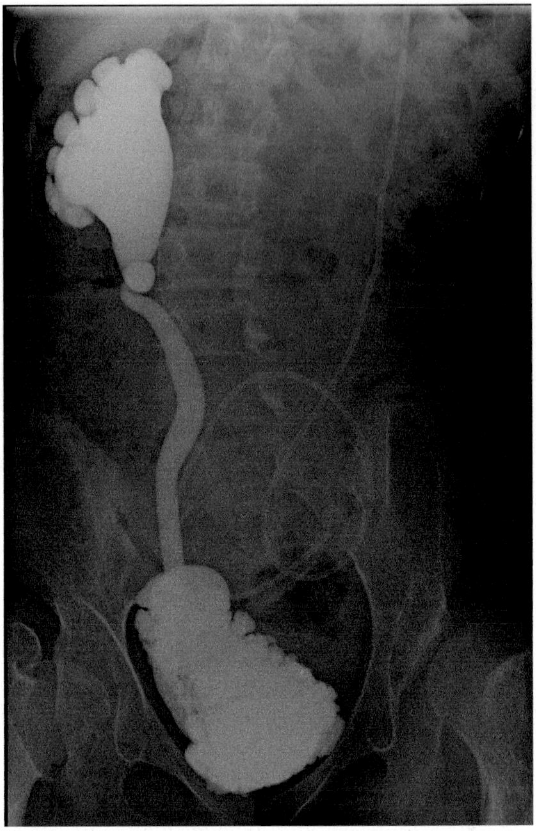

Fig. 2 VCUG image of a 13-year-old girl with neurogenic bladder. The bladder has a "Christmas tree-like" vertical morphology

Voiding Images

For males, voiding images should be obtained in the anterior oblique position, while for females, the AP position is recommended [39]. During voiding, the caliber of the urethra should be evaluated, in addition to the presence of VUR [11]. Figure 6 illustrates VUR associated with a posterior urethral valve.

Coordinated voiding between the bladder neck, the external sphincter, and the caliber of the bladder neck should be assessed, particularly in girls and patients with a neurogenic bladder [11] (Fig. 7).

Post-void Images

Post-void images of the kidneys in an AP view are obtained to assess for VUR [12]. A quickly draining VUR may be missed if there are delays in obtaining post-void images. If a high-grade VUR (grades IV or V) is present, imaging should be delayed for approximately 15 min after voiding to assess potential obstruction at the UVJ [12]. Additionally, post-void bladder images are evaluated for complete emptying. It is essential to acknowledge that most infants do not empty completely [45]. Moreover, it is critical to note the presence of contrast in the vagina as although this could be a normal pooling artifact from supine voiding [12]. It might also account

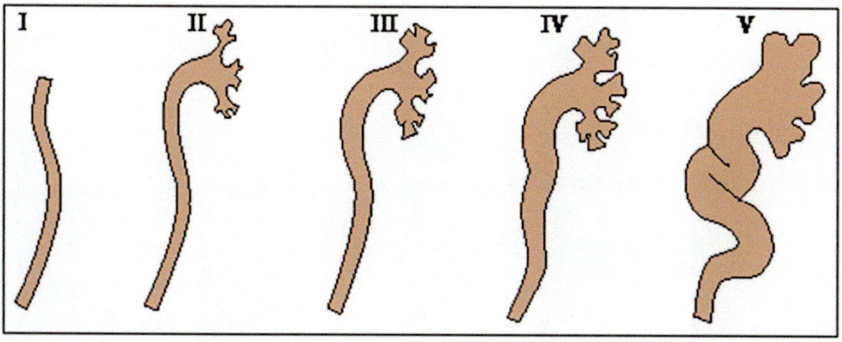

Fig. 3 International Reflux Study Committee classification. Grade I: Ureter only. Grade II: Ureter, pelvis, and calyces; no dilatation; normal calyceal fornices. Grade III: Mild or moderate dilatation and/or tortuosity of the ureter and mild or moderate dilatation of the renal pelvis and no or only slight blunting of the fornices. Grade IV: Moderate dilatation and/or tortuosity of the ureter and moderate dilatation of the renal pelvis and calyces; blunting of the sharp angle of the fornices but maintenance of papillary impressions in most calyces. Grade V: Gross dilatation and tortuosity of the ureter, severe dilatation of the renal pelvis and calyces, and papillary impressions no longer visible in most calyces

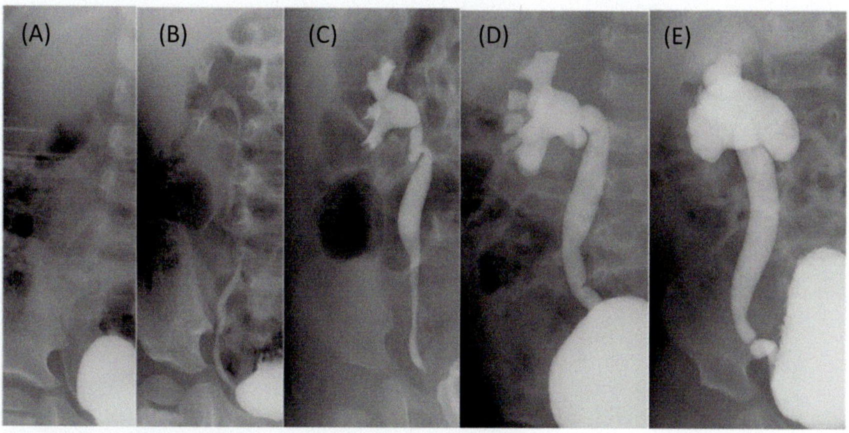

Fig. 4 Representative images of VUR by grade on VCUG imaging. (**a**) 3-year-old girl with VUR grade I. (**b**) A 3-year-old boy VUR grade II. (**c**) A 5-month-old girl with VUR grade III. (**d**) A 3-month-old girl with VUR grade IV. (**e**) A 5-month-old girl with VUR grade V

for symptoms of post-void wetness, vaginitis, or false-positive bacterial growth in non-catheterized urine samples [11].

Cyclic VCUG

Cyclic VCUGs entail filling the bladder and having the patient void multiple times. The catheter is commonly left in place throughout the procedure. Repeated imaging of the bladder and kidneys during voiding and post-void is conducted. As VUR can be intermittent, cyclic studies increase the yield of detecting VUR by up to 20% [40,

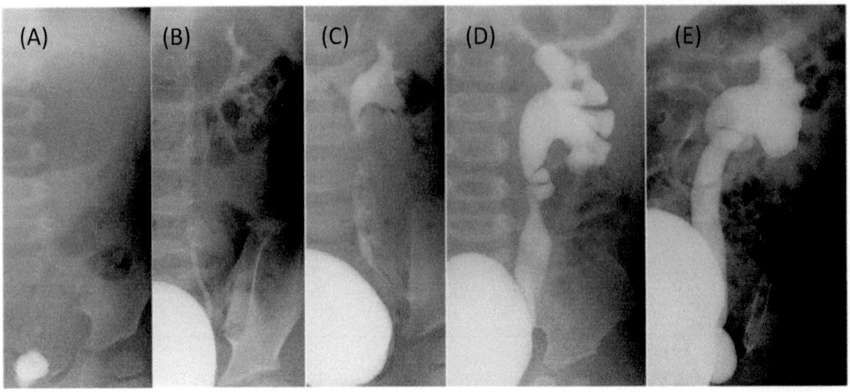

Fig. 5 Representative images of VUR by grade on VCUG imaging. (**a**) A 1-year-old boy with VUR grade I. (**b**) A 2-year-old boy with VUR grade II. (**c**) A 1-year-old boy with VUR grade III. (**d**) An 8-month-old boy with VUR grade IV. (**e**) A 10-month-old boy with VUR grade V

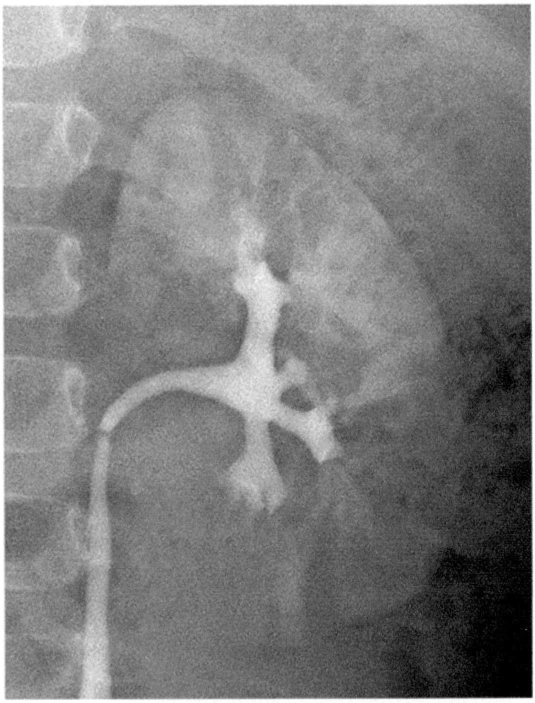

Fig. 6 Intrarenal reflux on VCUG. A 1-year-old boy demonstrates severe regurgitation into the left renal parenchyma as observed on VCUG

46], most of which are grade II or higher. Additionally, the VUR grade may be higher during the second cycle [40, 46]. Cyclic studies are recommended for children under 5 years, children with suspected VUR, and patients with a suspected ectopic ureter. Additionally, cyclic studies should be conducted in children who spontaneously void at low volumes, as this may result from bladder spasms, and reflux may occur at higher volumes in a normal physiological state for these

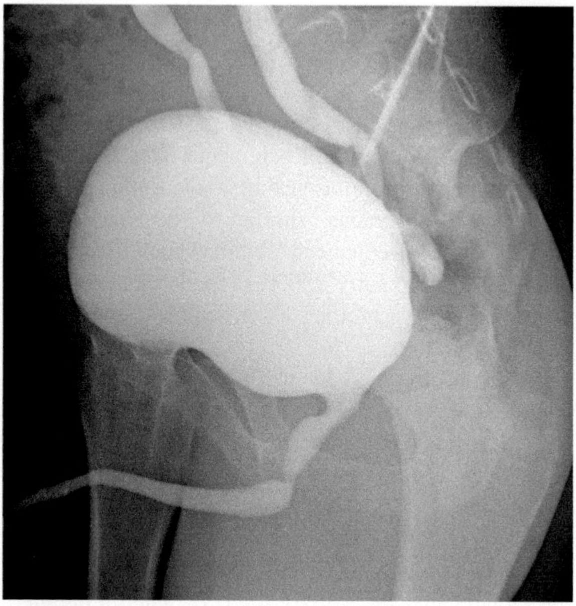

Fig. 7 A 7-year-old boy with a posterior urethral valve. The posterior urethra shows circumferential stenosis.

children. Failure to conduct a VCUG for the second voiding cycle may result in overlooking a refluxing ureter [11]. Several cycles with the patient in an oblique position may enhance the detection of the refluxing ectopic ureter [11].

VCUG Report

In VCUG reports, the bladder volume and timing of VUR onset should also be included, as these may impact clinical decisions. Volume at onset of VUR may be standardized as a percentage of the patient's predicted bladder capacity. Earlier onset of VUR has a lower rate of spontaneous resolution and an increased risk of breakthrough UTIs, regardless of grade, compared to late VUR onset at a higher filling volume [28, 47, 48]. Late filling VUR is a VUR onset at over 75% of estimated bladder capacity. Filling VUR refers to VUR occurring before voiding. While voiding, VUR (or "high-pressure VUR") characterizes VUR as onset during or after micturition [47, 49–51].

Complications

Catheter-related complications include dysuria, perineal discomfort, urinary retention, hematuria, creation of a false passage, perforation, and knotting of the catheter, all of which may require surgery [11]. In addition, catheters may be mistakenly placed in the vagina, ureteral orifice, prostatic utricle, or ureterocele, leading to misinformation [52]. Instrumentation may also cause UTIs. If absorbed, patients may also develop an allergic reaction to latex or contrast material.

Contrast-Enhanced Voiding Urosonography (VUS)

Contrast-enhanced VUS is a well-established intracavitary application of ultrasound contrast agents used in children to detect and grade VUR and urethral imaging [53–55]. The depiction of echogenic microbubbles in the ureters or pelvicalyceal system confirms the presence of VUR. Reflux with contrast-enhanced VUS is classified into five grades, similar to the international reflux grading system for VCUG. Contrast-enhanced VUS has been used in Europe in clinical practice since the 1990s. In the early 2000s, second-generation ultrasound contrast agents, composed of inert gas-filled microbubbles with better back-scattering properties, became available.

Since its approval by the Food and Drug Administration in 2016, contrast-enhanced VUS has been reported as an alternative test to VCUG in some national guidelines for VUR detection [56]. The European Society of Pediatric Radiology Task Force strongly encourages contrast-enhanced VUS as the first-line technique when possible and VCUG when contrast-enhanced VUS is not available or if the urinary tract cannot be adequately analyzed by US (for example, in the presence of an ectopic kidney, severe scoliosis, complicated CAKUT—congenital anomalies of the kidneys and the urinary tract) or when a detailed morphological study of the male urethra is required.

According to currently published literature, contrast-enhanced VUS exhibits good accuracy, with a sensitivity of 90% and specificity of 92.8% in detecting VUR [57]. Contrast-enhanced VUS does not involve ionizing radiation, allowing repeated filling and emptying cycles without concern for radiation exposure [58]. VCUG remains an option, especially in scenarios like preoperative assessment, and stands as the gold standard for evaluating urethral pathology.

DMSA Scan

A DMSA scan is the gold standard for diagnosing acute pyelonephritis (APN) and renal scarring. Single-photon emission computed tomography DMSA scintigraphy is superior to planar imaging for detecting renal cortical damage [59, 60]. DMSA scintigraphy also exhibits greater sensitivity compared to US, intravenous urography, and computed tomography in diagnosing renal scarring [61–63]. Notably, cortical defects identified on a DMSA scan performed during or shortly after APN may result from pre-existing lesions (acquired or congenital reflux nephropathy) or an acute inflammatory response associated with APN. Moreover, delaying the DMSA scan until at least 4–6 months after a UTI permits the resolution of the acute inflammatory response, at which point persistent cortical defects are believed to signify permanent renal scarring [7, 11]. Figure 8 illustrates bilateral VUR with a right-side predominance on VCUG. The DMSA scan reveals atrophy of the right kidney and scarring with a superior pole predominance in the left kidney.

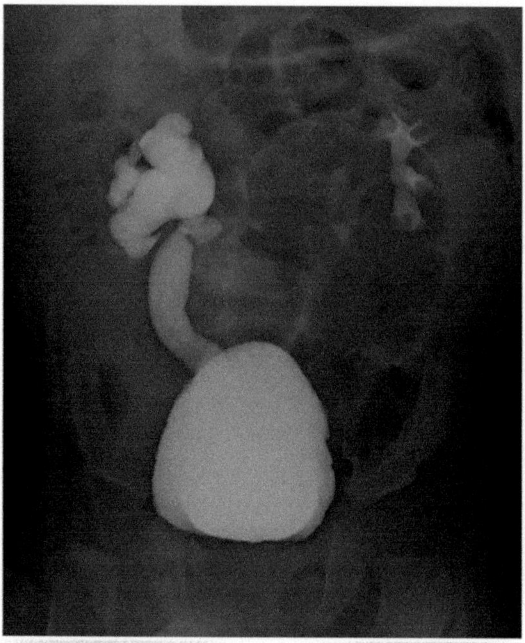

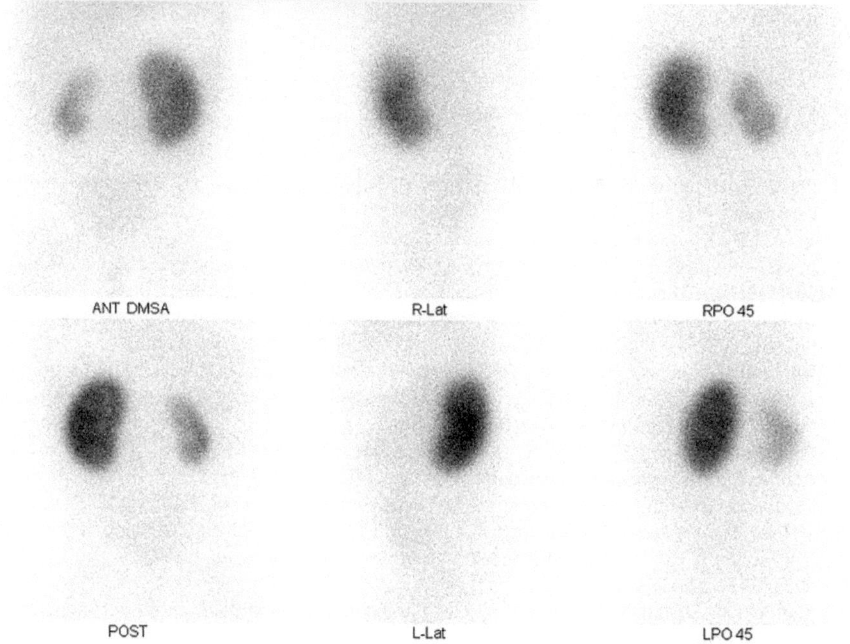

Fig. 8 A 3-month-old boy with VCUG showing bilateral VUR with right predominance. DMSA scan shows atrophy of the right kidney and scarring with superior pole predominance in the left kidney

Hansson et al. suggested using a DMSA renal scan as an initial evaluation after a child's UTI diagnosis [64]. This "top-down" approach is an alternative to VCUG after UTI, also called the "bottom-up" approach [5].

Although an acute-phase DMSA scan is highly specific for diagnosing APN, its findings are unreliable for predicting high-grade VUR [61]. Pooled data from 21 studies involving 4047 participants showed that with VCUG as the reference test, acute-phase DMSA scan exhibited good sensitivity (94%) but poor specificity (45%) in predicting high-grade VUR. Moreover, DMSA scans are associated with radiation exposure. Given its poor specificity in predicting high-grade VUR, inability to detect permanent renal scarring, cost, limited availability, and variability in interpretation, acute-phase DMSA scan has limited diagnostic utility for VUR.

Other Imaging Modalities

For patients with clinical suspicion that VUR may be associated with or be secondary to BBD, initial investigations will include bladder emptying studies and a plain abdominal x-ray. Video-urodynamics are more invasive investigations (involving the measurement of abdominal and bladder pressures using catheters under x-ray visualization) indicated when more complex forms of bladder dysfunction are suspected. They do not usually have a role in the management of primary VUR.

References

1. Puri P, Friedmacher F, Farrugia MK, Sharma S, Esposito C, Mattoo TK. Primary vesicoureteral reflux. Nat Rev Dis Primers. 2024;10(1):75.
2. Visuri S, Kivisaari R, Jahnukainen T, Taskinen S. Postnatal imaging of prenatally detected hydronephrosis-when is voiding cystourethrogram necessary? Pediatr Nephrol. 2018;33(10):1751–7.
3. Mohanan N, Colhoun E, Puri P. Renal parenchymal damage in intermediate and high grade infantile vesicoureteral reflux. J Urol. 2008;180(4 Suppl):1635–8. discussion 8.
4. Nguyen HT, Benson CB, Bromley B, Campbell JB, Chow J, Coleman B, et al. Multidisciplinary consensus on the classification of prenatal and postnatal urinary tract dilation (UTD classification system). J Pediatr Urol. 2014;10(6):982–98.
5. Gnech M, t Hoen L, Zachou A, Bogaert G, Castagnetti M, O'Kelly F, et al. Update and summary of the European Association of Urology/European Society of Paediatric Urology Paediatric Guidelines on Vesicoureteral Reflux in Children. Eur Urol. 2024;85(5):433–42.
6. t Hoen LA, Bogaert G, Radmayr C, Dogan HS, Nijman RJM, Quaedackers J, et al. Update of the EAU/ESPU guidelines on urinary tract infections in children. J Pediatr Urol. 2021;17(2):200–7.
7. Mattoo TK, Shaikh N, Nelson CP. Contemporary management of urinary tract infection in children. Pediatrics. 2021;147(2)
8. Goodman TR, Kilborn T, Pearce R. Warm or cold contrast medium in the micturating cystourethrogram (MCUG): which is best? Clin Radiol. 2003;58(7):551–4.
9. Hunziker M, Colhoun E, Puri P. Prevalence and predictors of renal functional abnormalities of high grade vesicoureteral reflux. J Urol. 2013;190(4 Suppl):1490–4.

10. Loukogeorgakis SP, Burnand K, MacDonald A, Wessely K, De Caluwe D, Rahman N, Farrugia MK. Renal scarring is the most significant predictor of breakthrough febrile urinary tract infection in patients with simplex and duplex primary vesico-ureteral reflux. J Pediatr Urol. 2020;16(2):189 e1–e7.
11. Ditchfield MR, Summerville D, Grimwood K, Cook DJ, Powell HR, Sloane R, et al. Time course of transient cortical scintigraphic defects associated with acute pyelonephritis. Pediatr Radiol. 2002;32(12):849–52.
12. Cubillos J. Principles of Voiding Cystourethrography (VCUG). In: Lane S, Palmer JSP, editors. Pediatric and adolescent urologic imaging. Springer; 2014.
13. Hoberman A, Chesney RW, Investigators RT. Antimicrobial prophylaxis for children with vesicoureteral reflux. N Engl J Med. 2014;371(11):1072–3.
14. Radmayr C, Klauser A, Maneschg C, Bartsch G, Frauscher F. Importance of the renal resistive index in children suffering from vesicoureteral reflux. Eur Urol. 1999;36(1):75–9.
15. Oak SN, Kulkarni B, Chaubal N. Color flow Doppler sonography: a reliable alternative to voiding cystourethrogram in the diagnosis of vesicoureteral reflux in children. Urology. 1999;53(6):1211–4.
16. Johnin K, Kobayashi K, Tsuru T, Yoshida T, Kageyama S, Kawauchi A. Pediatric voiding cystourethrography: an essential examination for urologists but a terrible experience for children. Int J Urol. 2019;26(2):160–71.
17. Diamond DA, Mattoo TK. Endoscopic treatment of primary vesicoureteral reflux. N Engl J Med. 2012;366(13):1218–26.
18. Arlen AM, Scherz HC, Filimon E, Leong T, Kirsch AJ. Is routine voiding cystourethrogram necessary following double hit for primary vesicoureteral reflux? J Pediatr Urol. 2015;11(1):40:e1–5.
19. Nelson CP, Finkelstein JA, Logvinenko T, Schuster MA. Incidence of urinary tract infection among siblings of children with vesicoureteral reflux. Acad Pediatr. 2016;16(5):489–95.
20. Andrich MP, Majd M. Diagnostic imaging in the evaluation of the first urinary tract infection in infants and young children. Pediatrics. 1992;90(3):436–41.
21. McDonald A, Scranton M, Gillespie R, Mahajan V, Edwards GA. Voiding cystourethrograms and urinary tract infections: how long to wait? Pediatrics. 2000;105(4):E50.
22. Spencer JD, Bates CM, Mahan JD, Niland ML, Staker SR, Hains DS, Schwaderer AL. The accuracy and health risks of a voiding cystourethrogram after a febrile urinary tract infection. J Pediatr Urol. 2012;8(1):72–6.
23. Mazzi S, Rohner K, Hayes W, Weitz M. Timing of voiding cystourethrography after febrile urinary tract infection in children: a systematic review. Arch Dis Child. 2020;105(3):264–9.
24. Connolly B, Racadio J, Towbin R. Practice of ALARA in the pediatric interventional suite. Pediatr Radiol. 2006;36(Suppl 2):163–7.
25. Bevelacqua JJ. Practical and effective ALARA. Health Phys. 2010;98(Suppl 2):S39–47.
26. Lee RS, Diamond DA, Chow JS. Applying the ALARA concept to the evaluation of vesicoureteric reflux. Pediatr Radiol. 2006;36(Suppl 2):185–91.
27. Ward VL, Strauss KJ, Barnewolt CE, Zurakowski D, Venkatakrishnan V, Fahey FH, et al. Pediatric radiation exposure and effective dose reduction during voiding cystourethrography. Radiology. 2008;249(3):1002–9.
28. Frimberger D, Mercado-Deane MG, Section On U, Section OR. Establishing a standard protocol for the voiding cystourethrography. Pediatrics. 2016;138(5)
29. Phillips DA, Watson AR, MacKinlay D. Distress and the micturating cystourethrogram: does preparation help? Acta Paediatr. 1998;87(2):175–9.
30. Salmon K, McGuigan F, Pereira JK. Brief report: optimizing children's memory and management of an invasive medical procedure: the influence of procedural narration and distraction. J Pediatr Psychol. 2006;31(5):522–7.
31. Srivastava T, Betts G, Rosenberg AR, Kainer G. Perception of fear, distress and pain by parents of children undergoing a micturating cystourethrogram: a prospective study. J Paediatr Child Health. 2001;37(3):271–3.

32. Zelikovsky N, Rodrigue JR, Gidycz CA, Davis MA. Cognitive behavioral and behavioral interventions help young children cope during a voiding cystourethrogram. J Pediatr Psychol. 2000;25(8):535–43.
33. Salmon K, Pereira JK. Predicting children's response to an invasive medical investigation: the Influence of effortful control and parent behavior. J Pediatr Psychol. 2002;27(3):227–33.
34. Stokland E, Andreasson S, Jacobsson B, Jodal U, Ljung B. Sedation with midazolam for voiding cystourethrography in children: a randomised double-blind study. Pediatr Radiol. 2003;33(4):247–9.
35. Herd DW, McAnulty KA, Keene NA, Sommerville DE. Conscious sedation reduces distress in children undergoing voiding cystourethrography and does not interfere with the diagnosis of vesicoureteric reflux: a randomized controlled study. AJR Am J Roentgenol. 2006;187(6):1621–6.
36. Gerard LL, Cooper CS, Duethman KS, Gordley BM, Kleiber CM. Effectiveness of lidocaine lubricant for discomfort during pediatric urethral catheterization. J Urol. 2003;170(2 Pt 1):564–7.
37. Poonai N, Li J, Langford C, Lepore N, Taddio A, Gerges S, et al. Intraurethral lidocaine for urethral catheterization in children: a randomized controlled trial. Pediatrics. 2015;136(4):e879–86.
38. Ditchfield MR, Grattan-Smith JD, de Campo JF, Hutson JM. Voiding cystourethrography in boys: does the presence of the catheter obscure the diagnosis of posterior urethral valves? AJR Am J Roentgenol. 1995;164(5):1233–5.
39. Fernbach SK, Feinstein KA, Schmidt MB. Pediatric voiding cystourethrography: a pictorial guide. Radiographics. 2000;20(1):155–68. discussion 68–71
40. Agrawalla S, Pearce R, Goodman TR. How to perform the perfect voiding cystourethrogram. Pediatr Radiol. 2004;34(2):114–9.
41. Damasio MB, Donati F, Bruno C, Darge K, Mentzel HJ, Kljucevsek D, et al. Update on imaging recommendations in paediatric uroradiology: the European Society of Paediatric Radiology workgroup session on voiding cystourethrography. Pediatr Radiol. 2024;54(4):606–19.
42. Berrocal T, Lopez-Pereira P, Arjonilla A, Gutierrez J. Anomalies of the distal ureter, bladder, and urethra in children: embryologic, radiologic, and pathologic features. Radiographics. 2002;22(5):1139–64.
43. Rolleston GL, Maling TM, Hodson CJ. Intrarenal reflux and the scarred kidney. Arch Dis Child. 1974;49(7):531–9.
44. Hannerz L, Wikstad I, Johansson L, Broberger O, Aperia A. Distribution of renal scars and intrarenal reflux in children with a past history of urinary tract infection. Acta Radiol. 1987;28(4):443–6.
45. Sillen U. Bladder function in healthy neonates and its development during infancy. J Urol. 2001;166(6):2376–81.
46. Papadopoulou F, Efremidis SC, Oiconomou A, Badouraki M, Panteleli M, Papachristou F, Soteriou I. Cyclic voiding cystourethrography: is vesicoureteral reflux missed with standard voiding cystourethrography? Eur Radiol. 2002;12(3):666–70.
47. Arlen AM, Cooper CS. New trends in voiding cystourethrography and vesicoureteral reflux: who, when and how? Int J Urol. 2019;26(4):440–5.
48. Alexander SE, Arlen AM, Storm DW, Kieran K, Cooper CS. Bladder volume at onset of vesicoureteral reflux is an independent risk factor for breakthrough febrile urinary tract infection. J Urol. 2015;193(4):1342–6.
49. Ji D, Ridley DE, Grattan-Smith JD, Williams JP, Arlen AM, Kirsch AJ, et al. Accuracy of subjective vesicoureteral reflux timing assessment: supporting new voiding cystourethrogram guidelines. Pediatr Radiol. 2020;50(7):953–7.
50. Arsanjani A, Alagiri M. Identification of filling versus voiding reflux as predictor of clinical outcome. Urology. 2007;70(2):351–4.
51. Han DS, Cambareri G, Alagiri M, Chiang G. Reflux timing is a predictor of successful endoscopic treatment of vesicoureteral reflux. Urology. 2019;124:237–40.

52. Rathaus V, Konen O, Shapiro M, Grunebaum M. Malposition of catheters during voiding cystourethrography. Eur Radiol. 2001;11(4):651–4.
53. Darge K. Voiding urosonography with US contrast agent for the diagnosis of vesicoureteric reflux in children: an update. Pediatr Radiol. 2010;40(6):956–62.
54. Duran C, Beltran VP, Gonzalez A, Gomez C, Riego JD. Contrast-enhanced voiding urosonography for vesicoureteral reflux diagnosis in children. Radiographics. 2017;37(6):1854–69.
55. Ntoulia A, Aguirre Pascual E, Back SJ, Bellah RD, Beltran Salazar VP, Chan PKJ, et al. Contrast-enhanced voiding urosonography. Part 1: Vesicoureteral reflux evaluation. Pediatr Radiol. 2021;51(12):2351–67.
56. Ammenti A, Alberici I, Brugnara M, Chimenz R, Guarino S, La Manna A, et al. Updated Italian recommendations for the diagnosis, treatment and follow-up of the first febrile urinary tract infection in young children. Acta Paediatr. 2020;109(2):236–47.
57. Chua ME, Mendoza JS, Ming JM, Dy JS, Gomez O. Diagnostic accuracy of contrast-enhanced voiding urosonogram using second-generation contrast with harmonic imaging (CEVUS-HI) study for assessment of vesicoureteral reflux in children: a meta-analysis. World J Urol. 2019;37(10):2245–55.
58. Novljan G, Kenig A, Rus R, Kenda RB. Cyclic voiding urosonography in detecting vesicoureteral reflux in children. Pediatr Nephrol. 2003;18(10):992–5.
59. Applegate KE, Connolly LP, Davis RT, Zurakowski D, Treves ST. A prospective comparison of high-resolution planar, pinhole, and triple-detector SPECT for the detection of renal cortical defects. Clin Nucl Med. 1997;22(10):673–8.
60. Yen TC, Tzen KY, Lin WY, Chen WP, Lin CY. Identification of new renal scarring in repeated episodes of acute pyelonephritis using Tc-99m DMSA renal SPECT. Clin Nucl Med. 1998;23(12):828–31.
61. Lavocat MP, Granjon D, Allard D, Gay C, Freycon MT, Dubois F. Imaging of pyelonephritis. Pediatr Radiol. 1997;27(2):159–65.
62. Ahmed M, Eggleston D, Kapur G, Jain A, Valentini RP, Mattoo TK. Dimercaptosuccinic acid (DMSA) renal scan in the evaluation of hypertension in children. Pediatr Nephrol. 2008;23(3):435–8.
63. Elison BS, Taylor D, Van der Wall H, Pereira JK, Cahill S, Rosenberg AR, et al. Comparison of DMSA scintigraphy with intravenous urography for the detection of renal scarring and its correlation with vesicoureteric reflux. Br J Urol. 1992;69(3):294–302.
64. Hansson S, Dhamey M, Sigstrom O, Sixt R, Stokland E, Wennerstrom M, Jodal U. Dimercaptosuccinic acid scintigraphy instead of voiding cystourethrography for infants with urinary tract infection. J Urol. 2004;172(3):1071–3. discussion 3–4

Radioisotope Imaging Techniques in the Detection of Vesicoureteric Reflux

Lorenzo Biassoni

Abstract Evaluation of vesico-ureteric reflux (VUR) with radionuclide imaging techniques has evolved, with the introduction of new ways to improve sensitivity in the detection of VUR. These examinations include techniques that make use of a bladder catheter (direct isotope cystogram) and techniques with no catheter (indirect radionuclide cystogram). The direct isotope cystogram (DIC) is slowly fading away, leaving more room to the radiological micturating cystogram. The indirect radionuclide cystogram (IRC) has been recently improved, with more comprehensive acquisition and processing protocols. The IRC explores bladder emptying in a physiological condition. It offers a complete evaluation of the excretory system, including renal parenchymal integrity and contribution to total renal parenchymal function, drainage and completeness/timing of bladder emptying, with the possible detection of VUR during physiological micturition. The study can also be used as a screening test for bladder function if a non-invasive urodynamic bladder contraction assessment with a flow meter is performed during bladder emptying.

Keywords Vesicoureteral reflux · Radioisotope renography · Cystogram · Kidney scarring

Introduction

Radionuclide imaging techniques to diagnose vesicoureteric reflux (VUR) have been used in clinical practice for more than 50 years as they represent an attractive lower radiation alternative to the radiological micturating cysto-urogram (MCUG), that at the time delivered a high radiation dose to the patient [1, 2]. With the much-improved technology of the recent fluoroscopy units, high quality radiological images can be produced with a low radiation dose and an exquisite anatomical detail

L. Biassoni (✉)
Department of Radiology, Great Ormond Street Hospital for Children, London, UK
e-mail: Lorenzo.Biassoni@gosh.nhs.uk

P. Puri, A. Yamataka (eds.), *Vesicoureteral Reflux*,
https://doi.org/10.1007/978-3-031-95091-9_12

of the urinary excretory system [3]. The only inconvenience is the use of a bladder catheter, which can be particularly unpleasant in older children.

At the same time, radionuclide imaging to detect VUR has evolved toward a much more physiological, less invasive form, with more advanced ways of processing the acquired raw data. Controversy still exists on the diagnostic yield of a more modern non-invasive way of performing the radionuclide cystogram [4, 5]; however, reports in the last decade suggest that a modified form of the radionuclide cystogram retains good diagnostic value with minimal inconvenience for the patient [6].

The currently available radionuclide imaging techniques to identify the possible presence of VUR in paediatrics include the direct isotope cystogram (DIC) and the indirect radionuclide cystogram (IRC).

Direct Isotope Cystogram

The European Association of Nuclear Medicine has published a set of guidelines on the acquisition and interpretation of the DIC [7]. This examination requires the use of a bladder catheter, which is sited in the bladder prior to the start. Antibiotic cover is required: if the child is already on prophylactic antibiotics, the usual dose that is taken once a day is doubled and also increased to twice a day, and this is for three days (the day before the test, the day of the test, and the day after the test) before reverting to the normal prophylactic dose. If the child is not on prophylactic antibiotics, then a treatment dose of antibiotics is initiated prior to the test.

The child is placed supine on the gamma camera couch; the catheter is connected via a three-way tap to a bag of saline; this is run to fill the bladder. The dynamic acquisition of the images covers both the bladder filling and emptying phases. The radiotracer used is [^{99m}Tc]Tc-pertechnetate. This is placed in a syringe and instilled in the bladder as soon as the administration of saline begins. The gamma camera acquires dynamic images continuously at a rate of 1 frame/s for 10 min with a 128 × 128 matrix, a zoom as necessary (maximum of 2), and a low energy general purpose collimator. The acquisition is stopped when the bladder is empty or 30 s after VUR is identified (Fig. 1a, b).

The main strength of the DIC is its high sensitivity, due to the continuous acquisition of the images, and the low radiation dose (approximately 0.02 mSv).

The disadvantages are the poor anatomy, especially the lack of visualization of the urethra, which is necessary to exclude posterior urethral valves in a young male patient, the inability to see the possibly dilated ureters behind the bladder, and the inconvenience of having to insert a bladder catheter, which can be traumatic in older patients.

Currently, the clinical use of the DIC is decreasing as the latest fluoroscopy units deliver a low radiation dose with excellent anatomical delineation of the urethra, of the bladder contour, and—if VUR is present—of the ureters and pelvicalyceal system. A DIC is still performed in a young female patient (younger than 1 year of

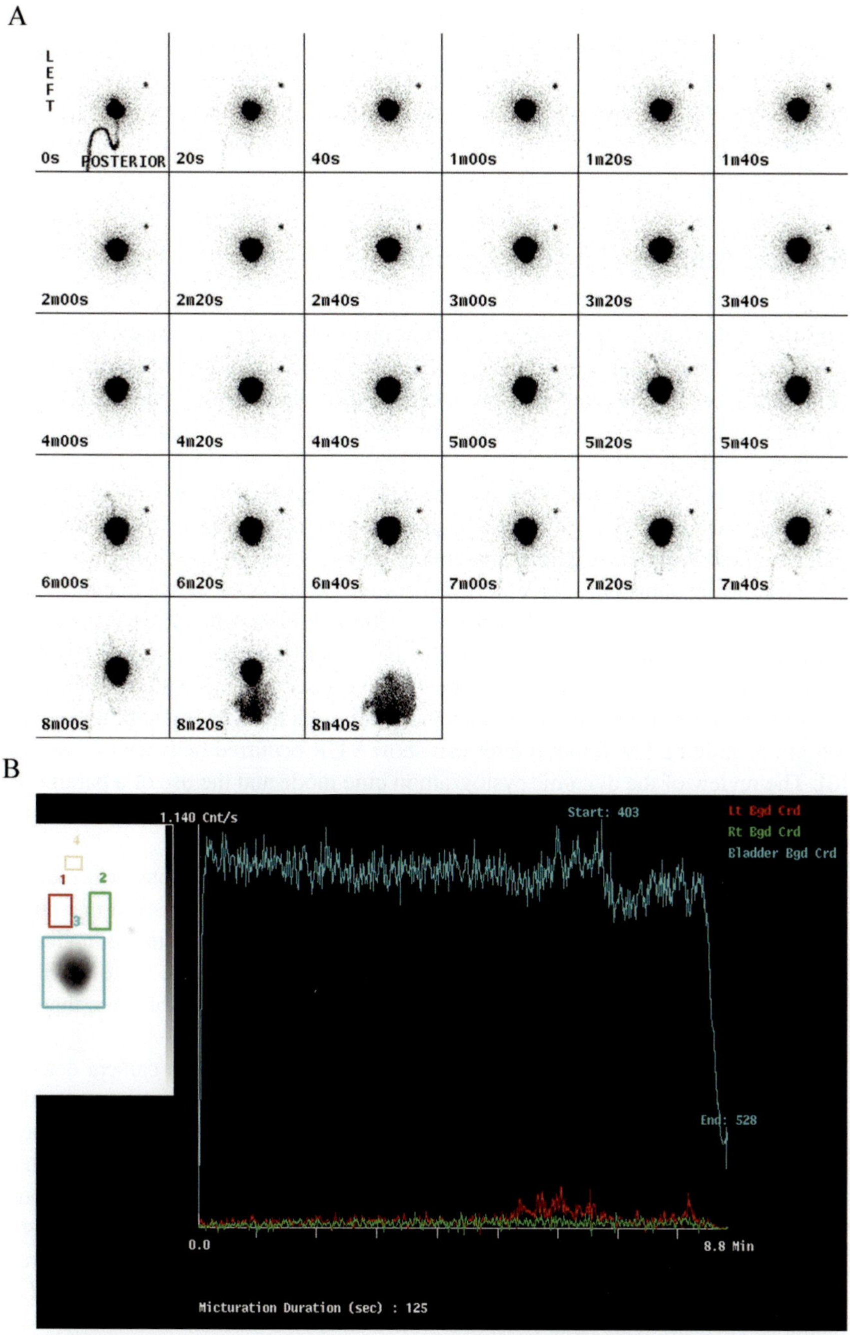

Fig. 1 (**a** and **b**) Nine months old female patient with a history of an atypical urinary tract infection. The direct bladder catheter shows a left VUR (**a**), confirmed on the time activity curves (**b**)

age), where a detailed anatomical visualization of the urethra is not usually required. Young male patients investigated for VUR in infancy may require a radiological MCUG to be certain the VUR is not related to outflow obstruction such as posterior urethral valves. The clinical decision will be made in conjunction with the ultrasound findings.

Indirect Radionuclide Cystogram

The IRC allows imaging of the micturition phase under physiological conditions. It's done in fully toilet trained patients (usually 3 years of age and above), as the child must be able to void on command to allow the radiographer to start the dynamic cystogram once the computer linked to the gamma camera has been programmed, and not before.

Despite its physiological nature and its good acceptance by the patient, the IRC has not replaced the MCUG in most paediatric radiology departments, even among toilet trained children in whom anatomical detail is not required, in view of the perceived lower sensitivity for VUR [5]. However, it has been shown that the sensitivity for VUR can be increased by the acquisition of more than one dynamic cystogram during the patient's visit. VUR can be intermittent, and if it has not been demonstrated on a cystogram, it can be shown on another cystogram. Also, comparison of the last frame of a dynamic cystogram with the first frame of a new cystogram acquired a few minutes later can show VUR occurred between cystograms [6]. The review of the dynamic cystogram in cine mode and the use of a parametric image with compressed counts over the bladder and kidneys can be of further help to confirm or exclude the presence of VUR.

The IRC is preceded by a radionuclide dynamic renography with either [^{99m}Tc]Tc-diethylene-triamine-penta-acetic acid (DTPA) or [^{99m}Tc]Tc-mercapto-acetyl-triglycine (MAG3); the latter is the preferred radiopharmaceutical in view of its higher extraction efficiency by the renal parenchyma. Once the radiotracer has been taken up, handled and mostly (or completely) excreted in the bladder, then the IRC can begin when the child wants to micturate.

The child sits on a commode with the back against the gamma camera detector (Fig. 2) and voids freely when instructed. A dynamic acquisition is commenced with a low energy general purpose collimator, a matrix of 128 × 128, a frame rate of 1 frame/s, and a zoom as necessary (maximum of 2.0). The acquisition is stopped when the child empties the bladder or doesn't feel the need to continue voiding. If a significant amount of radiotracer is still seen in the bladder or in the pelvicalyceal system, a second cystogram is acquired when the child wants to void again [8]. Sometimes, a third cystogram can be acquired if VUR has not been demonstrated yet and a significant amount of radiotracer persists in the renal collecting system and in the bladder.

The images are then processed and displayed: usually a screen capture image, with dynamic images reformatted as 5 or 10 s/frame summed images, is produced. A series of compressed images can be useful to increase the sensitivity for VUR (Fig. 3).

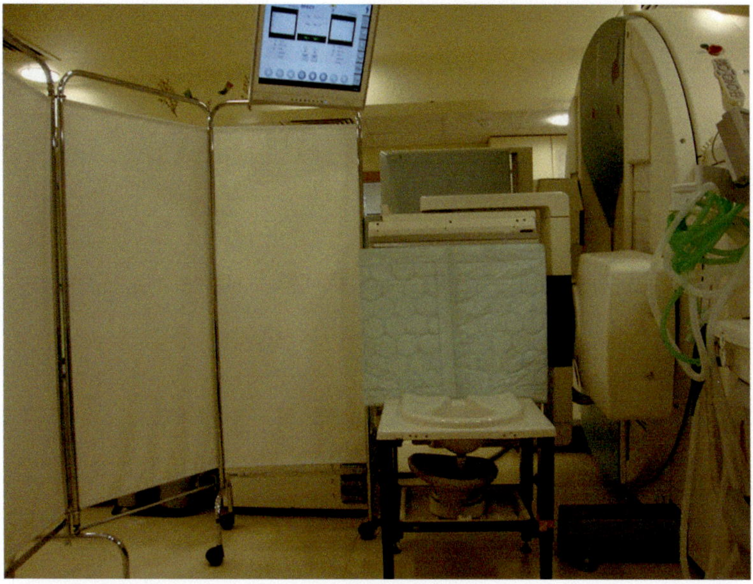

Fig. 2 Set up for the IRC in use at Great Ormond Street Hospital for Children. The child sits on the commode with the back against the gamma camera detector and voids in a bowl

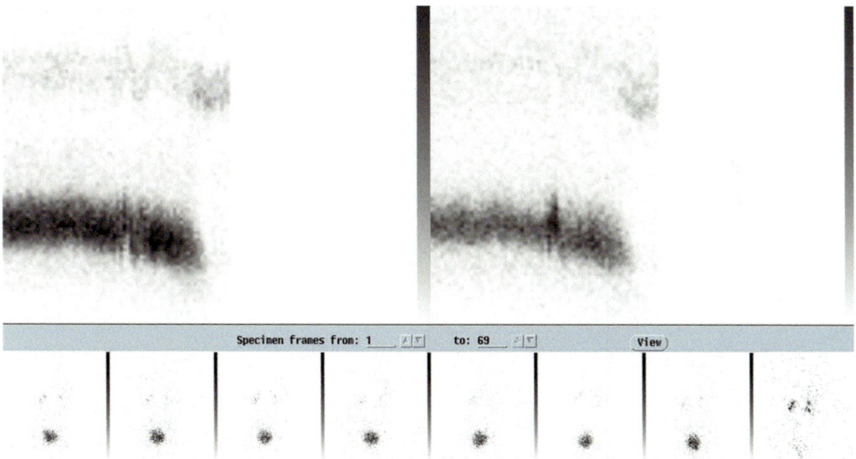

Fig. 3 The compressed image demonstrates in a graphic form the increased counts over the kidneys and the reduced counts in the bladder, consistent with bilateral VUR with bladder emptying

The most frequent use of the MAG3/IRC examination is in toilet trained children with a history of recurrent urinary tract infections. In this group of patients the test can assess the renal parenchymal function, the drainage, the timing and completeness of bladder emptying, and the possible presence of VUR (Figs. 4a, b and 5a–c)

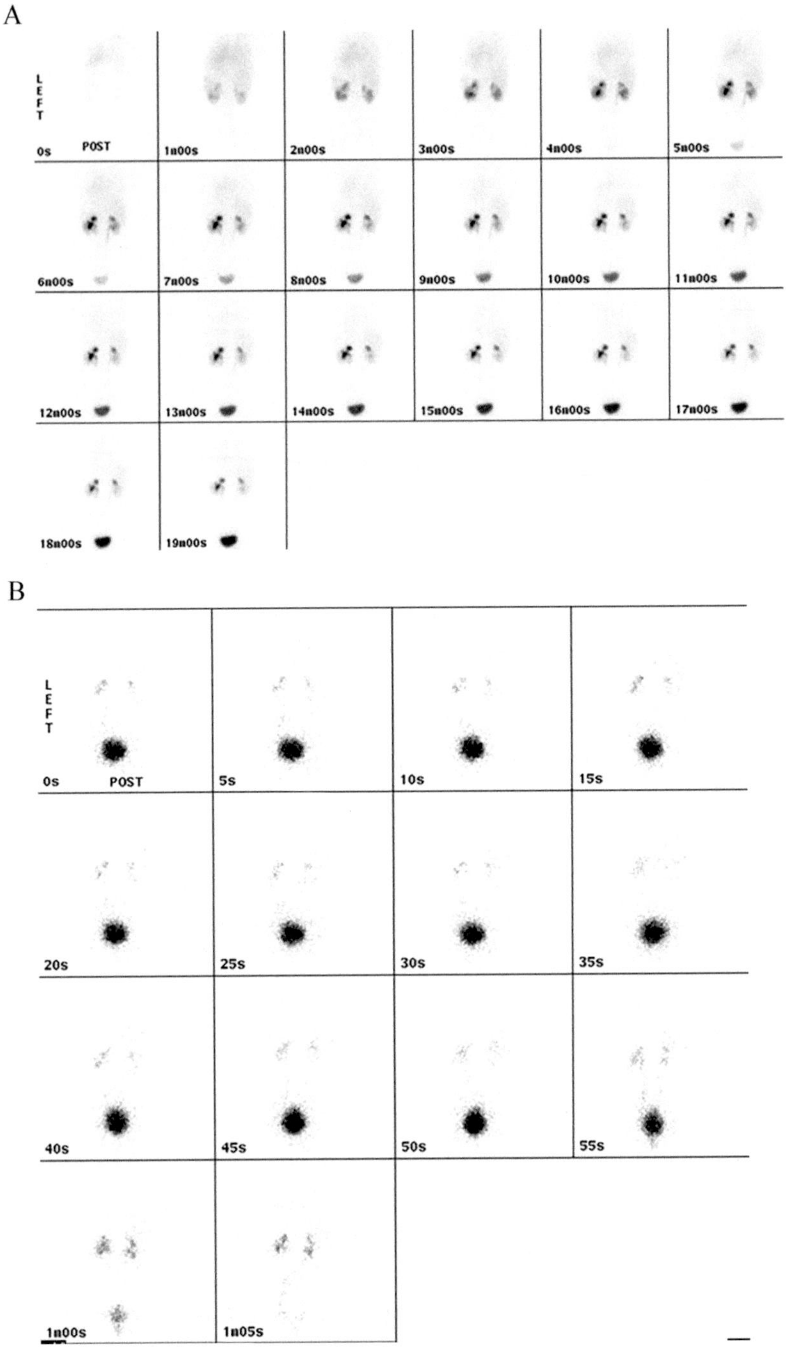

Fig. 4 (**a** and **b**) Seven years old female patient with a history of chronic kidney disease and recurrent urinary tract infections. The [^{99m}Tc]Tc-MAG3 dynamic renography (**a**) shows bilateral renal damage, worse on the right than the left. The IRC shows bilateral VUR (**b**)

A

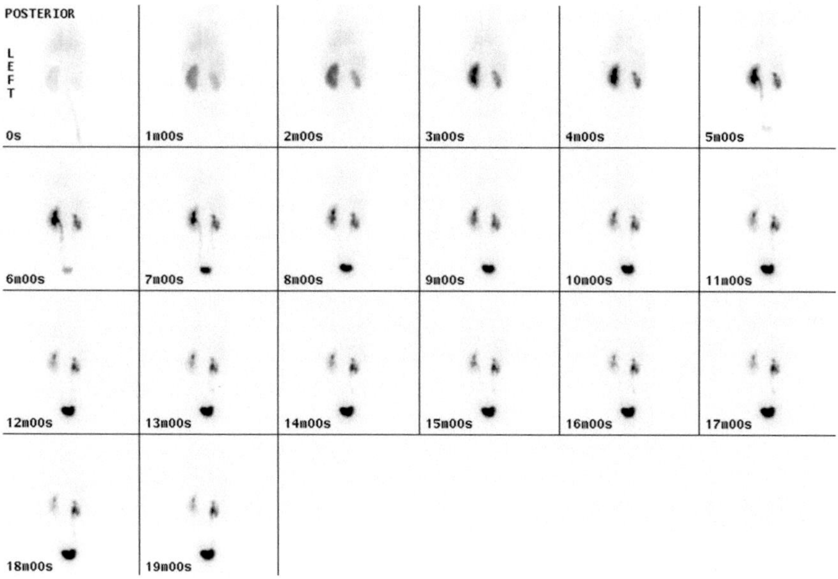

B

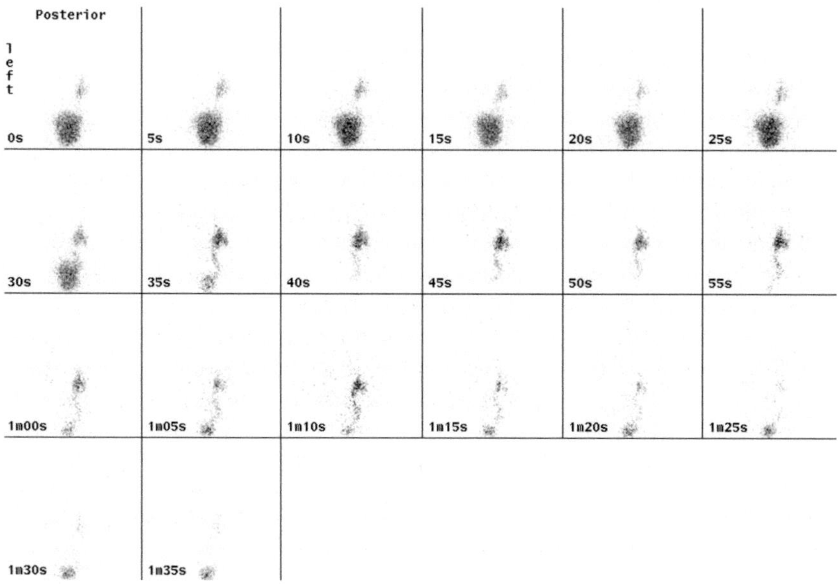

Fig. 5 (**a**–**c**) Four years old female with right hydronephrosis, right ureteric re-implantation two years prior, and recurrent urinary tract infections. The [^{99m}Tc]Tc-MAG3 dynamic renography (**a**) shows significantly reduced parenchymal function in the right kidney (24% contribution to total renal function; left kidney 76%). There is some urinary stasis in the right pelvicalyceal system at the end of the dynamic renography with further although incomplete drainage after change of posture and micturition. The IRC with the time activity curves (**b** and **c**) shows complete bladder emptying in physiological time with a voided volume of 132 mL and a significant right sided VUR

c

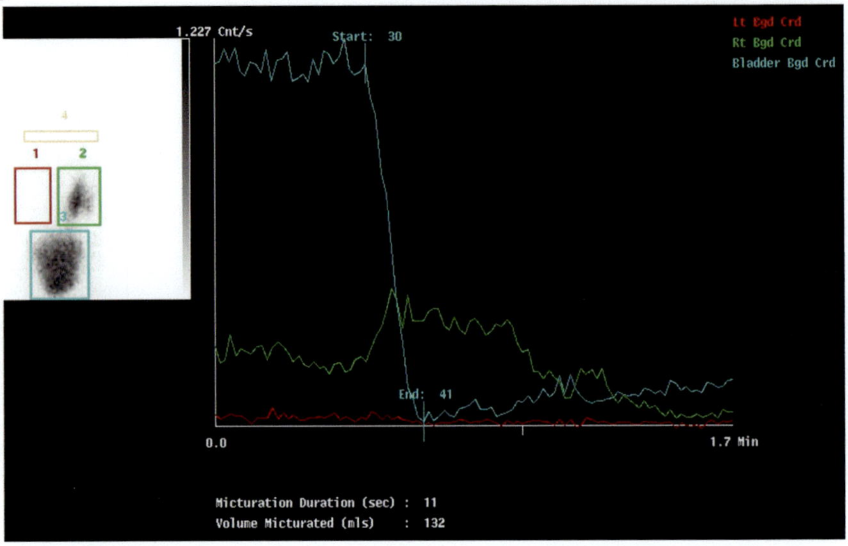

Fig. 5 (continued)

The main advantages of the MAG3/IRC are the following:

- It is a completely physiological test, very well tolerated by the child, with no need to insert a bladder catheter;
- It provides a comprehensive evaluation of the urinary tract, informing on relative parenchymal renal function and the possible presence of gross renal scarring (small scars can be missed), on drainage from the upper tracts, on the time and completeness of bladder emptying, and the possible presence of VUR;
- The acquisition of more than one cystogram acquisition allows the possible demonstration of VUR that has happened in between cystograms (Fig. 6a–c); again, this increases the sensitivity of the test for VUR;
- Sometimes VUR is shown during the dynamic renography or cystography when no bladder emptying has occurred yet (Fig. 7a–c): this is likely due to ineffective bladder contractions. Further evaluation of bladder function may reveal the presence of an unstable bladder;
- The radiation dose is low (usually around 0.5–0.7 mSv).

The main disadvantages are a lower sensitivity for VUR in comparison to the radiological MCUG, the inability to demonstrate the anatomy of the urethra and to grade

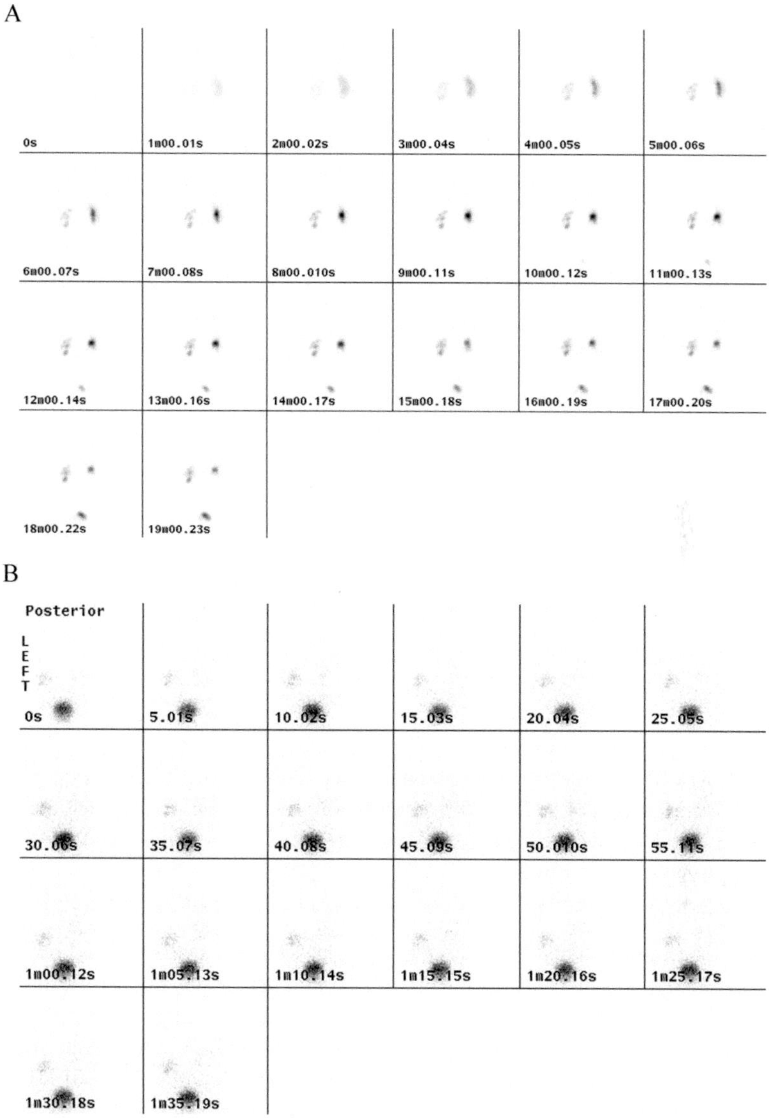

Fig. 6 (**a**–**c**) Five years old female with recurrent urinary tract infections, failure to thrive, left upper pole heminephrectomy 5 years ago, left deflux injection two years ago. The [^{99m}Tc]Tc-MAG3 dynamic renography (**a**) shows a reduced parenchymal function in the left kidney (24%) and a normal right kidney contributing 76% to total renal function. There is some residual urinary stasis in the pelvicalyceal system bilaterally at the end of the dynamic renography with the patient supine with good drainage after change of posture and micturition. The first IRC (**b**) shows some residual urinary stasis in the left pelvicalyceal system with no significant VUR. The second IRC, performed a few minutes later (**c**), shows a significant amount of tracer in the left pelvicalyceal system at the start, consistent with a left VUR occurred between the first and the second IRC. This case illustrates the increased sensitivity of the IRC for VUR when more than one dynamic cystogram is performed during the patient's visit

C

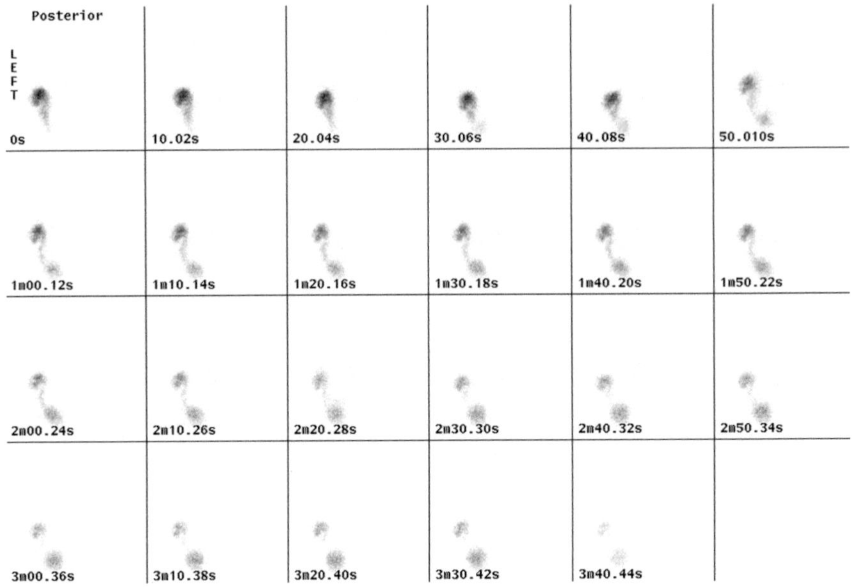

Fig. 6 (continued)

VUR. However, it is worth noticing that the two tests explore bladder emptying and the possible presence of VUR in different conditions: the MCUG is performed with a catheter filled bladder under external pressure; the IRC explores micturition under entirely physiological conditions.

The sensitivity of the IRC for VUR can decrease in the following conditions:

- Persisting radiotracer in the pelvicalyceal system and ureters at the end of the dynamic renography and during the dynamic cystogram, due to a dilated and possibly atonic collecting system, with loss of physiologic peristalsis;
- A small voided volume at the end of the micturition phase. One of the formulae to estimate the functional bladder capacity is [(age in years + 2) × 30] mL. If the voided volume is much smaller than expected and the pre-test likelihood of VUR is high, a negative IRC cannot exclude VUR;
- Significant motion during the acquisition of the images;
- A non-toilet trained child; in this case, usually the child voids before been asked to, with consequent loss of a significant portion of the micturition phase.

As the presence of VUR is related to the effectiveness of the valve mechanism at the vesicoureteric junction, in cases when this mechanism is only minimally compromised (shorter ureteric tunnel in the bladder wall, for example) VUR can be intermittently demonstrated on IRC; that is, in the same patient the IRC sometimes shows VUR and sometimes doesn't (Fig. 7).

A

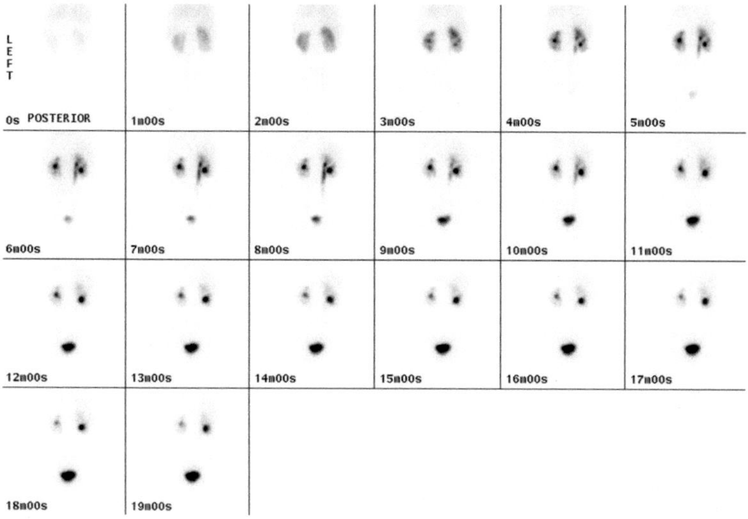

B

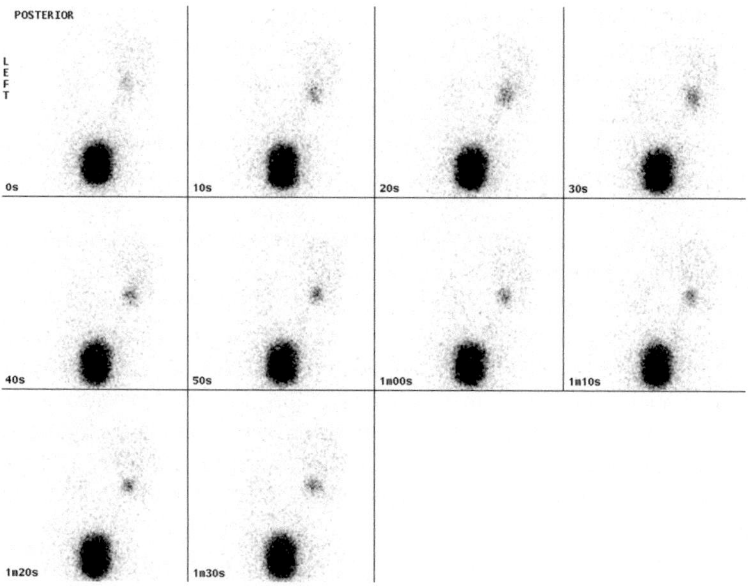

Fig. 7 (**a–d**) Six years old female patient with a history of recurrent febrile urinary tract infections and a right duplex kidney. The [^{99m}Tc]Tc-MAG3 dynamic renography (**a**) shows slightly reduced parenchymal function in the left kidney (43% contribution to total renal function, right kidney 57%) with a focal scar at the left upper pole. The right duplex kidney shows mild diffusely reduced parenchymal function in the lower moiety and good function in the upper moiety. There is some urinary stasis in the lower moiety collecting system at the end of the dynamic renography with the child supine. The first IRC (**b**) shows VUR in the right lower moiety with no bladder emptying; the second IRC shows bladder emptying with a voided volume of 205 mL and no VUR (**c**). This case shows that VUR can be intermittent: VUR with no bladder emptying could be due to ineffective bladder contractions, sometimes associated to bladder instability

c

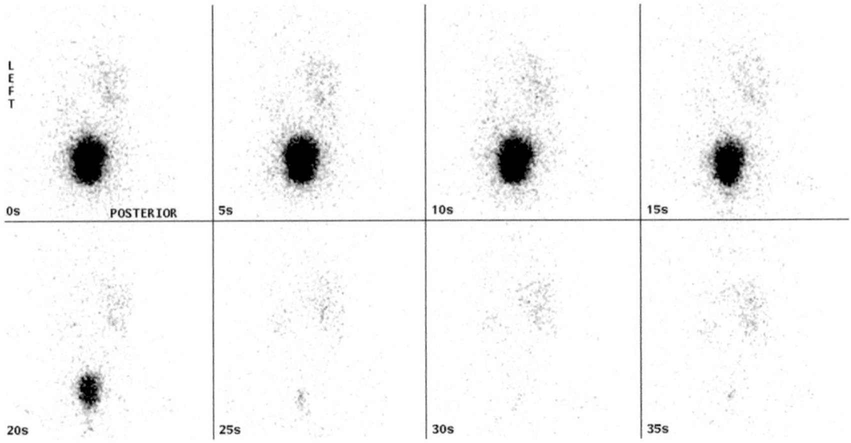

Fig. 7 (continued)

The IRC can also provide information on bladder function [9]. The duration in time of the micturition can be measured, as well as the voided volume of urine. A prolonged micturition or an incomplete micturition with a significant bladder residue—especially if confirmed on a repeat dynamic cystogram a few minutes later—raise the possibility of bladder dysfunction. A large voided volume, in excess of what is expected for the child's age, can be a sign of a pathologically distended bladder.

The contemporaneous use of a flow meter during the micturition phase can provide further information on bladder function (Fig. 8a–c). The use of this device permits the identification of voiding patterns with a bladder contraction curve. A low amplitude curve or a fractionated voiding can be signs of a dysfunctional voiding, which may be due to a detrusor—sphincter dyssynergia. The demonstration of a dysfunctional bladder, with incomplete emptying, is of clinical interest especially in patients with recurrent urinary tract infections and renal parenchymal scarring: the identification of the bladder as the likely culprit for recurrent infections and renal damage allows to instigate the appropriate treatment and helps avoiding possible further renal damage.

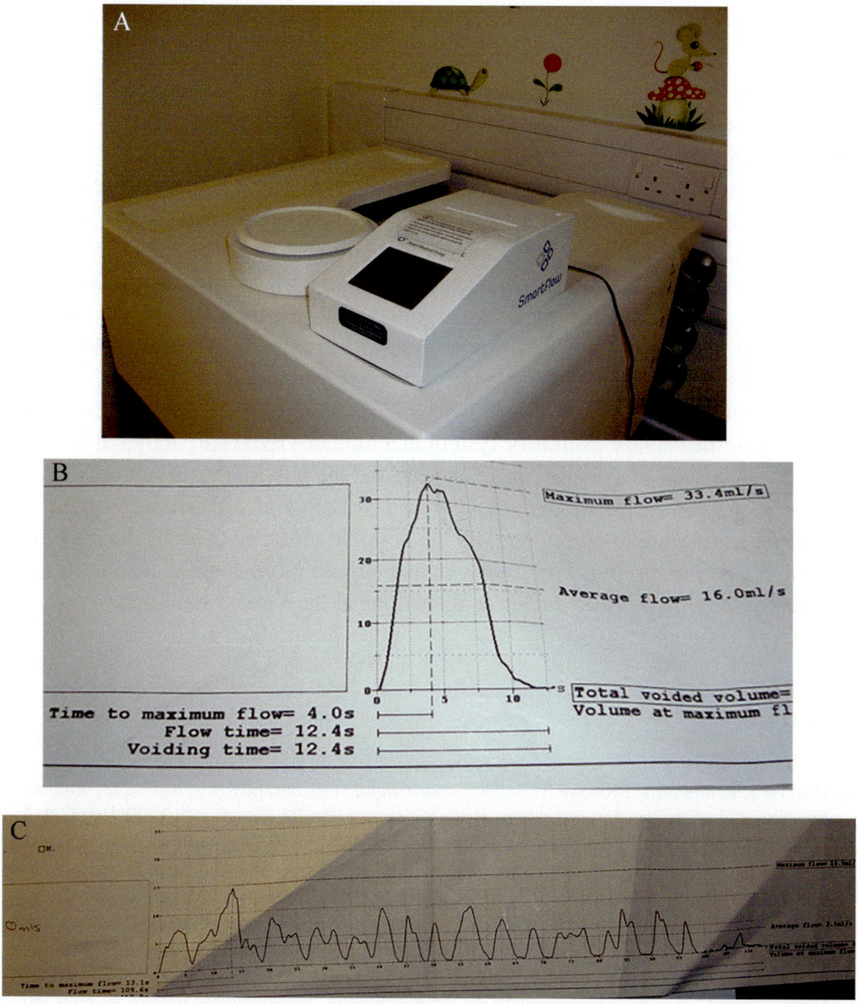

Fig. 8 (**a–c**) A flow meter (**a**) can be used during the micturition phase; this generates a bladder contraction curve. A normal curve is presented (**b**) as well as a grossly abnormal one (**c**), which shows multiple low amplitude bladder contractions, in keeping with bladder dysfunction (with permission)

Conclusion

The IRC is a low radiation well-tolerated examination to look for the possible presence of VUR during physiological bladder emptying. The child needs to be toilet trained (usually at least three years of age or older) to co-operate with the test. The use of IRC in clinical practice is still controversial in some countries or with some groups because of the reduced sensitivity for VUR in comparison with the radiological MCUG. However, with repeated acquisitions of the dynamic cystogram until the bladder and the upper tracts are empty, and with a better processing of the raw data, the sensitivity for VUR can significantly increase. The use of the IRC, especially if coupled with a flow meter study to assess bladder contraction, as a screening test for bladder function requires further evaluation.

In summary, the MAG3/IRC can offer the referring clinician a comprehensive evaluation of the urinary excretory system that includes renal parenchymal function (with the evaluation of the split renal function and the possible visualisation of gross renal scars), drainage from the pelvicalyceal system and ureters, the timing and completeness of bladder emptying, and the possible presence of VUR during physiological bladder emptying. The study can also offer a more detailed information on bladder contraction if a flow meter study is done at the same time.

References

1. Gordon I, Peters AM, Morony S. Indirect radionuclide cystography: a sensitive technique for the detection of vesico-ureteral reflux. Pediatr Nephrol (Berlin, Germany). 1990;4(6):604–6.
2. Dalirani R, Mahyar A, Sharifian M, Mohkam M, Esfandiar N, Ghehsareh AA. The value of direct radionuclide cystography in the detection of vesicoureteral reflux in children with normal voiding cystourethrography. Pediatr Nephrol (Berlin, Germany). 2014;29(12):2341–5.
3. Hiorns MP, Saini A, Marsden PJ. A review of current local dose-area product levels for paediatric fluoroscopy in a tertiary referral centre compared with national standards. Why are they so different? Br J Radiol. 2006;79(940):326–30.
4. De Sadeleer C, De Boe V, Keuppens F, Desprechins B, Verboven M, Piepsz A. How good is technetium-99m mercaptoacetyltriglycine indirect cystography? Eur J Nucl Med. 1994;21(3):223–7.
5. Capone V, Taroni F, Pavesi MA, Castellani M, Consonni D, Berrettini A, et al. Voiding cystourethrography and (99M)TC-MAG3 renal scintigraphy in pediatric vesicoureteral reflux: what is the role of indirect cystography? J Pediatr Urol. 2019;15(5):514.e1–e6.
6. Keir MJ, Lambert HJ, Coulthard MG. Maximizing the sensitivity of the indirect radionuclide cystogram: a retrospective audit. Pediatr Nephrol (Berlin, Germany). 2013;28(11):2137–41.
7. Fettich J, Colarinha P, Fischer S, Frökier J, Gordon I, Hahn K, et al. Guidelines for direct radionuclide cystography in children. Eur J Nucl Med Mol Imag. 2003;30(5):B39–44.
8. Gordon I, Colarinha P, Fettich J, Fischer S, Frökier J, Hahn K, et al. Guidelines for indirect radionuclide cystography. Eur J Nucl Med. 2001;28(3):16–20.
9. Vlajković M, Ilić S, Bogićević M, Rajić M, Ristić L, Petronijević V, et al. Radionuclide voiding patterns in children with vesicoureteral reflux. Eur J Nucl Med Mol Imag. 2003;30(4):532–7.

Medical Management of Primary Vesicoureteral Reflux

Tej K. Mattoo and Dunya Mohammad

Abstract Primary vesicoureteral reflux (VUR) is diagnosed mostly after a urinary tract infection (UTI). It is also diagnosed during postnatal evaluation of antenatally diagnosed hydronephrosis or other congenital anomalies of the kidney and urinary tract. VUR is associated with recurrent UTI and renal scarring, which is also called reflux nephropathy. Prevention of UTI and renal scars and the preservation of renal function in cases with renal scars are the most important treatment objectives in children with VUR Until recently, most children with VUR were treated with long-term antimicrobial prophylaxis or surgical correction. However, lately a third option of surveillance-only has become acceptable. As a result, it is necessary to evaluate the risk factors for UTI recurrence and renal scarring for individual patients before deciding on any or no intervention for VUR. The important risk factors that need to be considered include severity of VUR, coexisting renal scarring, patient age and sex, presence of bladder-bowel dysfunction, socioeconomic factors and parental choice. Patients with renal scarring should be monitored and treated for potential complications such as hypertension, proteinuria, and progressive CKD. Appropriate counseling of patients during discharge from pediatric care is recommended.

Keywords Vesicoureteral reflux (VUR) · Urinary tract infection (UTI) · Bladder-bowel dysfunction (BBD) · Renal scarring · Reflux nephropathy · Antimicrobial prophylaxis · Medical management · Chronic kidney disease

---

T. K. Mattoo (✉)
Division of Pediatric Nephrology, Wayne Pediatrics, Departments of Pediatrics and Urology, Wayne State University School of Medicine, Detroit, MI, USA
e-mail: Tmattoo@med.wayne.edu

D. Mohammad
Division of Pediatric Nephrology, Department of Pediatrics, University of South Alabama, Mobile, AL, USA

P. Puri, A. Yamataka (eds.), *Vesicoureteral Reflux*,
https://doi.org/10.1007/978-3-031-95091-9_13

Introduction

Vesicoureteral reflux (VUR) may be primary or secondary. Primary VUR is present at birth in about 1.3% of healthy children [1]. In most cases, the primary VUR is diagnosed after a urinary tract infection (UTI). The incidence of VUR diagnosed after UTI is 36–49% in newborns and infants and it gradually decreases with age to about 10% at 14 years and 5% in adults [1, 2]. Primary VUR is also diagnosed during follow-up for antenatally diagnosed hydronephrosis, screening of siblings, when indicated, as well as during the evaluation of patients with other congenital anomalies of kidney and urinary tract (CAKUT). Secondary VUR may be present at birth as is seen in some infants with posterior urethral values (PUV) or it may occur later co due to neurogenic bladder, obstructive uropathy, decompression of ureterocoele, correction of uretero-vesical junction obstruction, and bladder bowel dysfunction (BBD).

Children with VUR detected after UTI are predominantly females whereas VUR diagnosed during follow-up of antenatally diagnosed hydronephrosis is seen more often in males. [3] Primary VUR is less common and typically less severe in African American as compared to Caucasian children [4]. Eighty-one percent of 607 children in the Randomized Intervention in Children with VUR (RIVUR) trial who were enrolled at 19 clinical sites across the United States from inpatient, outpatient as well as Emergency Department settings, were Caucasians. [5]

Primary VUR generally improves with time, and the rate of resolution is better with low-grade VUR at the time of diagnosis. VUR is associated with recurrent UTI and renal scarring, which is also called as reflux nephropathy. A systematic review of 33 studies on 4891 patients less than 19 years old revealed that VUR was associated with an increased risk of developing acute pyelonephritis (APN) (relative risk [RR] 1.5, 95% CI 1.1–1.9) and kidney scarring (RR 2.6, 95% CI 1.7–3.9); Grade III or higher VUR was associated with increased risk of kidney scarring compared with lower grades (RR 2.1, 95% CI 1.4–3.2). [6] The complications of renal scarring include hypertension, proteinuria, progressive CKD and pregnancy-related complications [3].

In the past, the standard of care for VUR was long-term antimicrobial prophylaxis until its resolution or surgical correction in selected cases. However, recent studies have revealed that the significance of VUR and UTI for renal scarring as well as the role of long-term antimicrobial prophylaxis for the prevention of renal scarring in such cases may have been overestimated. As a result, surveillance-only has become another option in the management of VUR.

Management Objectives

The core objectives for VUR management are prevention of recurrent UTI and renal scarring, also called reflux nephropathy (RN). The renal scarring may be new, or it could be the worsening of the pre-existing renal scars. The management is driven by individual risk factors that include the severity of VUR, risk factors for UTI and presence or absence of renal scarring. The duration of medical management is based on multiple factors that include the prospects for VUR resolution and patient's clinical course and is tailored to cover the time period during which the VUR is most likely to cause UTI recurrence or renal scarring. Patient monitoring for UTI and renal scarring, prevention and prompt treatment of UTI, treatment of constipation and or BBD, and management of complications associated with renal scarring are important elements of VUR management.

Pre-treatment Considerations

With the recently available surveillance-only option, it has become essential to evaluate the risk factors for UTI recurrence and renal injury for an individual patient before committing to long-term antibiotic prophylaxis or surgical intervention. The risk factors that need to be considered for each patient are summarized in Table 1 and are elaborated below.

Table 1 Pretreatment Considerations for VUR in Children

Severity of VUR (high-grade VUR)		
	Longer time and lower probability for resolution	
	Higher risk of UTI and renal scarring	
Patient age		
	Risk and morbidity of UTI in younger children is higher	
	Renal scarring can occur at any age	
Risk of UTI recurrence (high)		
	Females at all ages except in young male infants	
	Patients with BBD	
	Presence of other CAKUT anomalies	
	Uncircumcised male infants	
	Recent UTI or antibiotic treatment	
Risk of renal scarring (high)		
	High-grade VUR	
	Recurrent UTI	
	Delayed diagnosis or antibiotic treatment for cute pyelonephritis	
Anticipated duration of treatment		
	Patient's clinical course	
	Prospects of VUR resolution (high with)	
		Low-grade VUR
		Unilateral VUR
		Younger age
		Noon-white race
Constipation/ bladder bowel dysfunction.		
	Risk factor for UTI	
	Delays VUR resolution	
Risk of antibiotic resistance		
Socio-economic and other factors		

VUR vesicoureteral reflux, *UTI* urinary tract infection, *BBD* bladder-bowel dysfunction, *CAKUT* congenital anomalies of kidney and urinary tract

Severity of VUR

VUR, particularly high-grade, is a risk factor for UTI and renal scarring. A recent two-year, multi-site prospective cohort study that included 500 children; 305 with VUR in the Randomized Intervention for Vesicoureteral Reflux (RIVUR) study and 195 with no VUR in the Careful Urinary Tract Infection Evaluation (CUTIE) study, reported that the rates of recurrent febrile UTI were higher in children with VUR (25.4%) as compared to no VUR (17.3%) [7].

Renal scarring occurs with APN with or without VUR, but the risk is higher in presence of VUR, particularly a high-grade VUR. The odds ratio of renal scarring with APN in presence of VUR versus no VUR is 2.8 for patients and 3.7 for renal units [8]. A meta-analysis of the published data revealed that renal damage (per 100 renal units) occurred in 6.2% in those with grades I–III VUR and 47.9% in those with grades IV and V VUR [9]. In the RIVUR study, the proportion of new scars in renal units with grade IV VUR was significantly higher than in units with no VUR (OR, 24.2; 95% CI, 6.4 to 91.2) [10]. RIVUR study did not include patients with grade V VUR.

Patient Age

Younger age is a particular concern for UTI recurrence because of a non-specific clinical presentation, higher morbidity with a febrile illness, including febrile convulsions and septicemia, a higher likelihood of hospitalization for IV antibiotic administration and hydration, difficulty in getting urine specimens with a potential need for a catheterized or suprapubic urine specimen, and parental anxiety and family disruption. However, the occurrence of renal scarring is not limited to younger children only. Many recent studies, including the Randomized Intervention for Vesicoureteral Reflux (RIVUR) trial have shown that older children may be at higher risk of kidney scarring. [10] This is also validated by the occurrence of renal scarring with APN in adult kidneys.

Risk of UTI Recurrence

UTI at any age is more common in females as compared to males except for early infancy when it is more common in boys. Besides presence of a VUR, the other risk factors for UTI include use of diapers, other CAKUT anomalies, BBD, circumcision status in young boys, and recent antibiotic treatment [11]. Also, the risk of UTI recurrence in the first 6–12 months after the initial UTI is about 12–30% [12, 13].

Risk of Renal Scarring

Besides a high-grade VUR, the other risk factors for renal scarring are recurrent UTI and delayed antibiotic treatment. The reported prevalence of renal scarring after febrile UTI is about 15% [14]. It ranges from 3% after the first UTI to 29% after > three febrile UTIs [15, 16]. In the RIVUR study, children with a second UTI had significantly more renal scars [OR], 2.85; 95% confidence interval [95% CI], 1.38 to 5.92) as compared to those with a single UTI [10]. A post hoc analysis of RIVUR and Careful Urinary Tract Infection Evaluation (CUTIE) studies revealed that the odds of renal scarring after a second febrile UTI was 11.8 (95% CI, 4.1–34.4) times greater than after a single febrile infection, and the odds of renal scarring after three or more febrile infections was 13.7 (95% CI, 3.4–54.4) times greater than after a single febrile infection [17].

A multivariate analysis of 158 children with febrile UTI showed that a delay of greater than 48 hours in the initiation of antibiotic treatment was associated with an increased risk of acute lesions on renal scan [18]. The RIVUR study revealed that delayed initiation of antibiotic treatment was associated with an increased risk of scarring, with the odds ratio of new renal scarring 74% lower among children whose treatment started within 24 hours of onset of fever, compared to those whose treatment started after 72 hours of fever [17]. Other risk factors associated with increased risk of renal scarring with UTI include Non-*E. coli* UTI, bladder and bowel dysfunction and genetic predisposition [7, 19, 20].

Anticipated Duration of Treatment

The rate of resolution of VUR is better for low-grade VUR, younger age, non-white race, and in the absence of bladder bowel dysfunction [21]. In a study in 735 children with primary VUR and a follow-up of 6 to 411 months; the median resolution times for VUR resolution were 38 months for grade I/II, 98 months for grade III and 156 months for grade IV/V VUR [22]. Schwab and colleagues reported that grades I-III VUR resolve at a rate of 13% per year for the first 5 years of follow-up and 3.5% per year during subsequent years; grades IV and V VUR resolve at a rate of 5% per year [23]. According to another study, patients whose reflux improved while being managed medically were younger than those who did not improve, and the younger the patient the sooner the reflux resolved. The spontaneous resolution rates were 92.3%, 76.2%, 61.7%, and 32.0% for grades I, II, III, and IV, respectively [24].

After a systematic review of published literature on the resolution of VUR, Elder and colleagues reported that increasing age at presentation and the presence of bilateral VUR decrease probability of resolution and that bilateral grade IV VUR has a particularly low chance of spontaneous resolution [25]. A study that evaluated the racial differences in VUR resolution reported that mean time to spontaneous resolution in black children was significantly shorter at 14.6 months as compared 21.4 months in white children [26].

Bladder-Bowel Dysfunction

BBD predisposes to recurrent UTI, induces and perpetuates VUR, and may contribute to permanent renal damage. The presence of BBD in patients with primary VUR increases the risk of recurrent UTIs [relative risk (RR): 2.1; 1.7–2.5] [27]. In one study, dilating reflux and female sex were identified as risk factors for the development of BBD [28].

In a study of 366 children with symptoms of BBD, VUR was present in 20% of the patients who underwent cystourethrography [29]. In the RIVUR study, BBD was identified in 56% of 126 toilet-trained children (<6 years of age) with grade I to IV VUR [5]. A recent study reported a pooled prevalence of BBD at 41% (95% CI: 26–55; nine studies, 920 patients, $I^2 = 96.0\%$) in children without primary VUR as compared to 49% (43–56; 30 studies, 5060 patients, $I^2 = 96.0\%$) in those with primary VUR.

BBD increases the risk of febrile UTI in children with VUR on antimicrobial prophylaxis (44% with BBD and 3% without BBD) and it delays VUR resolution at 24 months (31% with BBD and 61% without BBD) [8]. The frequency of postoperative UTI is greater in children with BBD (22%) compared to those without BBD (5%) [8]. BBD can also adversely affected the results of ureteric reimplantation [30]. The frequency of UTI after open or endoscopic surgical correction of VUR is greater in children with BBD (22%) compared to those without BBD (5%) [8]. BBD is a relative contraindication for surgical correction of VUR because of a higher likelihood of treatment failure and the potential for recurrent UTI [8].

In a recent retrospective study in children between 4 and 18 years of age with first time APN and no CAKUT, 47% of the cases were identified as being constipated, which is considerably higher than the estimated prevalence of constipation in childhood (16%) [31].

Risk of Antibiotic Resistance

In a study, children who received medication for more than four weeks in the preceding six months had significantly more resistant E. Coli as compared to those who did not receive any such treatment [odds ratio (OR) = 13.9; 95% CI 8.2–23.5] [32]. In the RIVUR study 76% of subjects with UTI recurrence during the study and receiving TMP-SMX were resistant to this medication versus 28% of subjects receiving placebo ($P < .001$). The proportion of TMP-SMX-resistant recurrent UTI decreased over time. [33] A recent meta-analysis revealed that children with VUR who were treated with prophylaxis were more likely to have a multidrug-resistant infection (33% vs 6%, P < .001) and were more likely to receive broad-spectrum antibiotics (68% vs 49%, P = .004). Those receiving prophylaxis had 6.4 times the odds (95% confidence interval: 2.7–15.6) of developing a multidrug-resistant infection. One multidrug-resistant infection would develop for every 21 reflux patients treated with prophylaxis [34]. In a compliant patient, de novo antibiotic resistance caused by its prolonged administration may lead to UTI recurrences by a resistant pathogen [35].

Socio-economic and Other Factors

Family acceptance is essential for any or no intervention for VUR. Compliance with daily administration of the medication over a prolonged period of time is questionable. In once study, 97% of the parents reported compliance with low-dose daily antimicrobial prophylaxis and yet the medicine was found in only 31% of patient urines [36] The medication expense may be important in certain situations though according to one study in the U.S., the prophylaxis was associated with marginally higher costs as compared to placebo [37], while another study reported that prophylaxis was more cost effective than observation in children with high grade (grade IV), but not low grade VUR [38].

Medical Versus Surgical Management

Surgical correction of VUR was common until the concept of antimicrobial prophylaxis for childhood UTI was introduced in 1970s. Subsequent studies, particularly the landmark Birmingham study and the International Reflux Study in Children revealed that there was no difference in outcome between children managed surgically or medically [39, 40]. As a result, the management of VUR evolved into a long-term antimicrobial prophylaxis until VUR resolution or surgical intervention in selected cases with breakthrough UTIs on prophylaxis, non-resolution of VUR, allergy to antimicrobial agents, and patient/parent non-compliance with the medical management [41]. However, with the recent knowledge, surveillance-only has become another viable option for the management of VUR.

Medical Management

The medical management of VUR consists of surveillance-only or antimicrobial prophylaxis and the selection is made on the basis of individual risk factors for UTI and renal scarring and parental choice.

Surveillance Only

Watchful waiting is a viable option in children with VUR, particularly in those with no history of UTI or a low risk of UTI recurrence or renal scarring. It consists of a regimen of surveillance and prompt treatment of intercurrent episodes of UTI. The caregiver needs to be vigilant and must seek medical attention whenever there are symptoms suggestive of UTI or unexplained fever. Caregiver's social situation should be assessed for compliance because surveillance puts the onus on caregivers to promptly recognize a potential UTI and seek medical attention. This is particularly true in preverbal children who constitute the majority of cases diagnosed with VUR and UTI. Depending on the clinical course, particularly the occurrence of UTI, and the prevailing risk factors for UTI recurrence and renal scarring, intervention with antimicrobial prophylaxis or surgical procedure might be necessary in some cases.

Antimicrobial Prophylaxis

In the recent past, the use of long-term antimicrobial prophylaxis has declined substantially and is being used selectively on the basis of patient characteristics. The RIVUR trial in 607 children, aged two months to six years with grade I to IV VUR showed that children with grade III or IV VUR were more likely to have febrile or symptomatic UTI than those with grade I or II VUR (23 versus 14 percent). Patients had a lower risk of recurrent febrile or symptomatic UTI for children assigned to prophylactic antibiotics (trimethoprim-sulfamethoxazole [TMP-SMX]) versus those assigned to placebo. Prophylactic antibiotics decrease the risk of febrile, recurrent UTI (hazard ratio 0.50, 95% CI 0.34–0.74) [5]. Nearly twice as many children receiving placebo than children receiving prophylaxis were categorized as treatment failures (defined by two febrile UTIs, one febrile UTI and three symptomatic UTIs, four symptomatic UTIs, or new or worsening kidney scarring) [5]. Similar results were reported by another placebo-controlled-double-blind (PRIVENT study) trial [42]. However, other randomized studies showed either no or a female-restricted beneficial effect with prophylaxis [43].

The American Academy of Pediatrics Subcommittee on Urinary Tract Infection created a data set from six published studies with data for 1091 infants 2 to 24 months of age according to grade of VUR. Data analysis did not detect a statistically significant benefit of prophylaxis in preventing recurrence of febrile UTI/pyelonephritis in infants with grades I to IV VUR or no VUR. Only 5 infants were found to have grade V VUR and hence were not included for analysis [44]. Systematic reviews and meta-analyses have also reported mixed results, some concluding that prophylaxis is effective, while others reporting it as ineffective for the prevention of UTI recurrence. These variations in results have been attributed to significant differences in study designs, including patient inclusion and exclusion criteria [45].

Very recently, in a study in 292 young infants (77.7% male) with grade III-V VUR with other CAKUT anomalies, the first UTI occurred in 31 of 146 participants (21.2%) in the prophylaxis group and 52 of 146 participants (35.6%) in the untreated group; the between-group difference was significant (hazard ratio, 0.55; 95% confidence interval, 0.35 to 0.86; P = 0.008) [46, 47].

None of the above-mentioned studies, including the RIVUR trial, demonstrated any beneficial effect of antimicrobial prophylaxis for the prevention of renal scarring. However, none of these studies were powered to evaluate renal scarring as the primary outcome and a significant degree of heterogeneity exists among these studies, including differences in methodology and study populations [45]. Interestingly, a post-hoc analysis of RIVUR data revealed that the recurrent UTI associated new renal scarring occurred in 5 of 244 (2%) patients on antibiotic prophylaxis and 13 of 245 (5%) on placebo. The study revealed that compared to antibiotic prophylaxis, placebo was associated with a higher risk of recurrent urinary tract infection associated new renal scarring (OR 3.1, 95% CI 1.0–8.8, p = 0.04) after adjusting for age, sex, race, index urinary tract infection, bowel bladder dysfunction, duplication, hydronephrosis, VUR grade and baseline renal scarring. The study also revealed that new renal scarring developed in a proportion of subjects without recurrent UTI [48].

In a meta-analysis that evaluated the effect of antibiotic prophylaxis on UTI-related renal scarring prospective Seven RCTs (1427 subjects) randomized controlled trials (RCTs) performed and published between 1946 and August 2016. Our results show no influence of antibiotic prophylaxis in preventing renal scarring in subjects with VUR (pooled risk ratio, 0.79; 95% confidence interval, 0.51–1.24 [49].

Published Guidelines for Prophylaxis

The American Urological Association (AUA) recommends continuous antibiotic prophylaxis in children under one year of age and a selective approach in older children based on patient age, severity of VUR, recurrence of UTI, presence of BBD and renal cortical anomalies [50]. The European Association of Urology/European Society of Pediatric Urology, the Swedish and the Italian Society of Pediatric Nephrology as well as the Asian and the Swiss guidelines also recommend a more selective approach based on a combination of patient age, severity of VUR, and the presence of renal scarring [43].

Limitations with Prophylaxis

The most important limitations with prolonger prophylaxis are patient compliance and antibiotic resistance. Secondary analysis of the RIVUR study data revealed that patients who took TMP/SMZ <70% of the time were 2.5 times more likely to have a recurrent UTI (95%CI 1.1–5.6) and were at highest risk for renal scarring (OR = 24.2, 95%CI 3.0–197) as compared to more adherent patients [51]. Side

Table 2 Antimicrobial Agents Recommended for Prophylaxis in Some Countries [43]

Antimicrobial agent	EAU/ESPU 2015	NICE 2018	Swiss 2021	ISPN 2011	Asian 2021	Italian 2019
Trimethoprim[a]	✓	✓	✓			
Trimethoprim- sulfamethoxazole[b]	✓		✓	✓	✓	
Nitrofurantoin[c]	✓	✓	✓	✓	✓	✓
Cephalexin		✓		✓	✓	
Amoxicillin		✓	✓			
Cefaclor	✓					
Cefixime	✓					
Ceftibuten[c]	✓					✓
Cefuroxime axetil	✓					
Cefadroxil				✓		
Amoxicillin-clavulanic acida						✓

[a]Not recommended <6 weeks
[b]Not recommended <2 months
[c]Not recommended <3 months
EAU/ESPU European Association of Urology/European Society of Pediatric Urology
NICE National Institute of Health and Care Excellence (NICE), U.K.
ISPN Indian Society of Pediatric Nephrology

effects other than antibiotic resistance don't seem as significant. The RIVUR study revealed that long-term prophylaxis with TMP/SMZ was not associated with an increased risk of skin and soft tissue infections, pharyngitis or sinopulmonary infections [35], or excessive weight gain [52]. Another RIVUR study reported no abnormalities in blood chemistries, renal function or complete blood count results in children receiving long-term TMP/SMZ prophylaxis for a duration of two years [53].

Selection of Antimicrobial Agent

The selection of antimicrobial agent for prophylaxis depends on local profile for drug sensitivity. As a result, different antibiotics are recommended by guidelines in different countries (Table 2). In the U.S., TMP-SMX, TMP alone, nitrofurantoin, or cephalexin are used. In view of increasing resistance of *E. Coli*, ampicillin or amoxicillin are less effective as prophylactic agents [54–56], and are not generally prescribed beyond the first two months of life. During the first 2 months of life, it is advisable to avoid TMP-SMZ because it may worsen hyperbilirubinemia and promote neurotoxicity.

The prophylactic dose of antimicrobials is one-fourth to one-half of the therapeutic dose for acute infection. The dosage for commonly used antimicrobials for UTI prophylaxis is shown in Table 3. In toilet trained children, antibiotic prophylactic medication is generally administered at bedtime, though this recommendation is not evidence-based.

Table 3 Dosage of antimicrobial agents used for prophylaxis [43]

Antimicrobial agent	Dose
Trimethoprim–sulfamethoxazole	2 mg TMP/kg/day
Nitrofurantoin	1–2 mg/kg/dose
Cephalexin	10 mg/kg/dose
Amoxicillin (infants <2 months)	10 mg/kg/dose

Duration of Treatment

The duration of prophylaxis is determined by periodic reassessment of risk factors for UTI and renal scarring and the probability of VUR resolution. Treatment duration may be short-term until a VCUG can be obtained in cases with a recently diagnosed UTI to long-term in those with a high-grade VUR and UTI. Other factors that impact the duration include the age of the patient, status of toilet-training, frequency of UTI, presence of BBD, and presence and severity of renal scarring.

Bladder Bowel Dysfunction

Management of BBD is necessary to prevent recurrence of UTI and renal injury and to promote resolution of VUR. Combined results from the RIVUR and CUTIE studies, revealed that toilet-trained children with VUR and BBD exhibit the greatest benefit from antimicrobial prophylaxis [57].

Conservative management of BBD consists of treatment of constipation and voiding behavior modification (urotherapy). Constipation is managed by dietary measures, stool softeners, and behavioral therapy and voiding behavior modification by timed voiding schedule, increased hydration and optimization of relaxation and contraction of pelvic floor muscles. About 50% of children with BBD improve with behavioral changes and constipation treatment only [58]. Timed, frequent and complete voiding every two to three hours is a crucial part of management.

Patients who fail conservative management may benefit from pharmacologic therapy. This includes anticholinergic medication for detrusor overactivity causing overactive bladder or alpha-blockers to help with bladder emptying and reduce post-void residual (PVR) urine volumes. A combination of the two may be used when overactive bladder (OAB) coexists with functional bladder outlet obstruction [58]. Anticholinergic medications may however worsen constipation. Other interventions include pelvic floor relaxation measures, including Kegel exercises for older children and biofeedback for younger children, electrical stimulation therapy (neuromodulation), or botulinum toxin injections. Continuous intermittent catheterization may be necessary in extreme cases, as seen in Hinman's syndrome where there is functional bladder outlet obstruction from a non-neurogenic neurogenic bladder.

Hypertension

Of all the complications of renal scarring caused by APN, the one that is most likely to manifest in pediatric age group is hypertension. In a study in 159 healthy children who underwent DMSA renal scan for the evaluation of newly diagnosed hypertension of unknown etiology, 33 (21%) with a median age of 11 years had renal scarring; 22 had unilateral scarring and 11 had bilateral scarring. Included in the study were 18 (55%) females and 15 (45%) males. Only five of the 33 patients (15%) with abnormal DMSA scans had a past history of UTI. Of the patients with abnormal DMSA scans, voiding cystourethrogram (VCUG) was done in 20 patients, six (30%) of whom showed presence of VUR [59].

Children with renal scarring should have blood pressure checked during routine office visits. For those with hypertension, angiotensin converting enzyme inhibitors (ACEI) or angiotensin II receptor blockers (ARB) are preferred due to their renoprotective effect. Patients should also receive the routine counseling for other risk factors that may include weight control, dietary sodium restriction, caffeinated and energy drinks, increased physical activity. In patients with a unilateral poorly functioning scarred kidney, surgical removal of the affected kidney should be considered though this may not normalize the blood pressure.

Proteinuria

Proteinuria due to renal scarring caused by APN is less likely to occur in the pediatric age group, particularly in children with unilateral renal scarring. Proteinuria is more likely to manifest in adult life, males particularly who are also at a high risk of hypertension and CKD as compared to females with renal scarring, who present mostly with recurrent UTI [3] Studies have revealed that in addition to lowering blood pressure, ACEIs, reduce proteinuria due to reflux nephropathy. In a study by Lama et al. [60], 15.5% of children with VUR and reflux nephropathy had microalbuminuria. Treatment with an ACEI (captopril) for two years was associated with decreased microalbuminuria. Of note, GFR, serum creatinine, and BP remained stable. Notably, it is not known whether this antiproteinuric effect slows down the progressive loss of renal function.

Patient Follow-Up

Follow-up care of patients with VUR includes monitoring for UTI, re-assessment of risk factors for UTI and renal scarring, status of VUR resolution and new renal scarring or worsening of pre-existing renal scars, BP changes, presence of proteinuria and assessment of renal function in patients with bilateral significant scarring are essential. The AUA, in its updated guidelines in 2017 recommends annual renal ultrasound examination to monitor renal growth and voiding cystography 12 to 24 months or longer in those with high grade VUR (grades III-V), BBD and older age. DMSA renal imaging is recommended selectively for the patients with abnormal renal ultrasound examination, detection of new renal scarring or monitoring of existing scarring [61]. Patients with progressive CKD need proper monitoring of renal function and interventions, depending on the severity of kidney disease.

Conclusion

Prevention of UTI and renal scars and the preservation of renal function in cases with renal scars are the most important treatment objectives in children with VUR. Watchful waiting is an acceptable management option, particularly in patients with low-grade VUR and a low risk of UTI or renal scarring. Antimicrobial prophylaxis reduces the recurrence of UTI but its role in the prevention of renal scarring remains to be determined. It should be used cautiously because of the risk of causing drug resistance. Patients with renal scarring should be monitored for potential complications such as hypertension, proteinuria, and progressive CKD. Appropriate counseling of patients during discharge from pediatric follow-up is recommended.

References

1. Williams G, Fletcher JT, Alexander SI, Craig JC. Vesicoureteral reflux. J Am Soc Nephrol. 2008;19(5):847–62.
2. Bailey RR. The relationship of vesico-ureteric reflux to urinary tract infection and chronic pyelonephritis-reflux nephropathy. Clin Nephrol. 1973;1(3):132–41.
3. Mattoo TK. Vesicoureteral reflux and reflux nephropathy. Adv Chronic Kidney Dis. 2011;18(5):348–54.
4. Chand DH, Rhoades T, Poe SA, Kraus S, Strife CF. Incidence and severity of vesicoureteral reflux in children related to age, gender, race and diagnosis. J Urol. 2003;170(4 Pt 2):1548–50.
5. Hoberman A, Chesney RW, Investigators RT. Antimicrobial prophylaxis for children with vesicoureteral reflux. N Engl J Med. 2014;371(11):1072–3.
6. Shaikh N, Ewing AL, Bhatnagar S, Hoberman A. Risk of renal scarring in children with a first urinary tract infection: a systematic review. Pediatrics. 2010;126(6):1084–91.
7. Keren R, Shaikh N, Pohl H, et al. Risk factors for recurrent Urinary Tract Infection and renal scarring. Pediatrics. 2015;136(1):e13–21.
8. Peters CA, Skoog SJ, Arant BS, et al. Summary of the AUA guideline on management of primary vesicoureteral reflux in children. J Urol. 2010;184(3):1134–44.
9. Skoog SJ, Peters CA, Arant BS, et al. Pediatric vesicoureteral reflux guidelines panel summary report: clinical practice guidelines for screening siblings of children with vesicoureteral reflux and neonates/infants with prenatal Hydronephrosis. J Urol. 2010;184(3):1145–51.
10. Mattoo TK, Chesney RW, Greenfield SP, et al. Renal scarring in the randomized intervention for children with vesicoureteral reflux (RIVUR) trial. Clin J Am Soc Nephrol. 2016;11(1):54–61.

11. Mattoo TK, Shaikh N, Nelson CP. Contemporary Management of Urinary Tract Infection in children. Pediatrics. 2021;147(2)
12. Conway PH, Cnaan A, Zaoutis T, Henry BV, Grundmeier RW, Keren R. Recurrent urinary tract infections in children: risk factors and association with prophylactic antimicrobials. JAMA. 2007;298(2):179–86.
13. Dai B, Liu Y, Jia J, Mei C. Long-term antibiotics for the prevention of recurrent urinary tract infection in children: a systematic review and meta-analysis. Arch Dis Child. 2010;95(7):499–508.
14. Snodgrass WT, Shah A, Yang M, et al. Prevalence and risk factors for renal scars in children with febrile UTI and/or VUR: a cross-sectional observational study of 565 consecutive patients. J Pediatr Urol. 2013;9(6 Pt A):856–63.
15. Shaikh N, Craig JC, Rovers MM, et al. Identification of children and adolescents at risk for renal scarring after a first Urinary Tract Infection: a meta-analysis with individual patient data. JAMA Pediatr. 2014;168(10):893–900.
16. Roberts KB. Urinary tract infections and renal damage: focusing on what matters. JAMA Pediatr. 2014;168(10):884–5.
17. Shaikh N, Mattoo TK, Keren R, et al. Early antibiotic treatment for pediatric febrile Urinary Tract Infection and renal scarring. JAMA Pediatr. 2016;170(9):848–54.
18. Fernandez-Menendez JM, Malaga S, Matesanz JL, Solis G, Alonso S, Perez-Mendez C. Risk factors in the development of early technetium-99m dimercaptosuccinic acid renal scintigraphy lesions during first urinary tract infection in children. Acta Paediatrica (Oslo, Norway: 1992). 2003;92(1):21–6.
19. Ragnarsdottir B, Svanborg C. Susceptibility to acute pyelonephritis or asymptomatic bacteriuria: host-pathogen interaction in urinary tract infections. Pediatr Nephrol. 2012;27(11):2017–29.
20. Ching C, Schwartz L, Spencer JD, Becknell B. Innate immunity and urinary tract infection. Pediatr Nephrol. 2020;35(7):1183–92.
21. Silva JM, Diniz JS, Lima EM, Vergara RM, Oliveira EA. Predictive factors of resolution of primary vesico-ureteric reflux: a multivariate analysis. BJU Int. 2006;97(5):1063–8.
22. Silva JM, Santos Diniz JS, Marino VS, et al. Clinical course of 735 children and adolescents with primary vesicoureteral reflux. Pediatr Nephrol. 2006;21(7):981–8.
23. Schwab CW Jr, Wu HY, Selman H, Smith GH, Snyder HM 3rd, Canning DA. Spontaneous resolution of vesicoureteral reflux: a 15-year perspective. J Urol. 2002;168(6):2594–9.
24. Huang FY, Tsai TC. Resolution of vesicoureteral reflux during medical management in children. Pediatr Nephrol. 1995;9(6):715–7.
25. Elder JS, Peters CA, Arant BS Jr, et al. Pediatric vesicoureteral reflux guidelines panel summary report on the management of primary vesicoureteral reflux in children. J Urol. 1997;157(5):1846–51.
26. Skoog SJ, Belman AB. Primary vesicoureteral reflux in the black child. Pediatrics. 1991;87(4):538–43.
27. Meena J, Mathew G, Hari P, Sinha A, Bagga A. Prevalence of bladder and bowel dysfunction in toilet-trained children with urinary tract infection and/or primary vesicoureteral reflux: a systematic review and meta-analysis. Front Pediatr. 2020;8:84.
28. Gaither TW, Cooper CS, Kornberg Z, Baskin LS, Copp HL. Risk factors for the development of bladder and bowel dysfunction. Pediatrics. 2018;141(1)
29. Schulman SL, Quinn CK, Plachter N, Kodman-Jones C. Comprehensive management of dysfunctional voiding. Pediatrics. 1999;103(3):E31.
30. Koff SA, Wagner TT, Jayanthi VR. The relationship among dysfunctional elimination syndromes, primary vesicoureteral reflux and urinary tract infections in children. J Urol. 1998;160(3 Pt 2):1019–22.
31. Axelgaard S, Kristensen R, Kamperis K, Hagstrom S, Jessen AS, Borch L. Functional constipation as a risk factor for pyelonephritis and recurrent urinary tract infection in children. Acta Paediatr. 2023;112(3):543–9.

32. Allen UD, MacDonald N, Fuite L, Chan F, Stephens D. Risk factors for resistance to "first-line" antimicrobials among urinary tract isolates of Escherichia coli in children. CMAJ. 1999;160(10):1436–40.
33. Nelson CP, Hoberman A, Shaikh N, et al. Antimicrobial resistance and urinary tract infection recurrence. Pediatrics. 2016;137(4):e20152490.
34. Selekman RE, Shapiro DJ, Boscardin J, et al. Uropathogen resistance and antibiotic prophylaxis: a meta-analysis. Pediatrics. 2018;142(1)
35. Desai S, Fisher B. Impact of trimethoprim-sulfamethoxazole Urinary Tract Infection prophylaxis on non-UTI infections. Pediatr Infect Dis J. 2019;38(4):396–7.
36. Bollgren I. Antibacterial prophylaxis in children with urinary tract infection. Acta Paediatr Suppl. 1999;88(431):48–52.
37. Palmer LS, Seideman CA, Lotan Y. Cost-effectiveness of antimicrobial prophylaxis for children in the RIVUR trial. World J Urol. 2018;36(9):1441–7.
38. Shaikh N, Rajakumar V, Peterson CG, et al. Cost-utility of antimicrobial prophylaxis for treatment of children with vesicoureteral reflux. Front Pediatr. 2019;7:530.
39. Listed NA. Prospective trial of operative versus non-operative treatment of severe vesicoureteric reflux in children: five years' observation. Birmingham Reflux Study Group. Br Med J. 1987;295:237–41.
40. Jodal U, Smellie JM, Lax H, Hoyer PF. Ten-year results of randomized treatment of children with severe vesicoureteral reflux. Final report of the International Reflux Study in Children. Pediatr Nephrol. 2006;21(6):785–92.
41. Diamond DA, Mattoo TK. Endoscopic treatment of primary vesicoureteral reflux. N Engl J Med. 2012;366(13):1218–26.
42. Craig JC, Simpson JM, Williams GJ, et al. Antibiotic prophylaxis and recurrent urinary tract infection in children. N Engl J Med. 2009;361(18):1748–59.
43. Mattoo TK, Mohammad D. Primary vesicoureteral reflux and renal scarring. Pediatr Clin N Am. 2022;69(6):1115–29.
44. Subcommittee on Urinary Tract Infection SCoQI, Management, Roberts KB. Urinary tract infection: clinical practice guideline for the diagnosis and management of the initial UTI in febrile infants and children 2 to 24 months. Pediatrics. 2011;128(3):595–610.
45. Mattoo TK, Carpenter MA, Moxey-Mims M, Chesney RW, For The RTI. The RIVUR trial: a factual interpretation of our data. Pediatr Nephrol. 2015;30:707–12.
46. Morello W, Baskin E, Jankauskiene A, et al. Antibiotic prophylaxis in infants with grade III, IV, or V vesicoureteral reflux. N Engl J Med. 2023;389(11):987–97.
47. Mattoo TK. Selective antimicrobial prophylaxis for vesicoureteral reflux. N Engl J Med. 2023;389(11):1043–4.
48. Wang HH, Kurtz M, Logvinenko T, Nelson C. Why does prevention of recurrent Urinary Tract Infection not result in less renal scarring? A deeper dive into the RIVUR trial. J Urol. 2019;202(2):400–5.
49. Hewitt IK, Pennesi M, Morello W, Ronfani L, Montini G. Antibiotic prophylaxis for Urinary Tract Infection-related renal scarring: a systematic review. Pediatrics. 2017;139(5)
50. Peters C, Skoog, SJ, Arant BS et al. Management and Screening of Primary Vesicoureteral Reflux in Children (2010, amended 2017); https://www.auanet.org/guidelines/vesicoureteral-reflux-guideline. 2017. Accessed 25 Aug 2020.
51. Gaither TW, Copp HL. Antimicrobial prophylaxis for urinary tract infections: implications for adherence assessment. J Pediatr Urol. 2019;15:387.e1–8.
52. Edmonson MB, Eickhoff JC. Weight gain and obesity in infants and young children exposed to prolonged antibiotic prophylaxis. JAMA Pediatr. 2017;171(2):150–6.
53. Nadkarni MD, Mattoo TK, Gravens-Mueller L, et al. Laboratory findings after Urinary Tract Infection and antimicrobial prophylaxis in children with vesicoureteral reflux. Clin Pediatr (Phila). 2020;59(3):259–65.

54. Sullivan TD, Ellerstein NS, Neter E. The effects of ampicillin and trimethoprim/sulfamethoxazole on the periurethral flora of children with urinary tract infection. Infection. 1980;8 Suppl 3:S 339-41.
55. Ellerstein NS, Sullivan TD, Baliah T, Neter E. Trimethoprim/sulfamethoxazole and ampicillin in the treatment of acute urinary tract infections in children: a double-blind study. Pediatrics. 1977;60(2):245–7.
56. Practice parameter: the diagnosis, treatment, and evaluation of the initial urinary tract infection in febrile infants and young children. American Academy of Pediatrics. Committee on Quality Improvement. Subcommittee on Urinary Tract Infection. Pediatrics. 1999; 103(4 Pt 1):843–52.
57. Shaikh N, Hoberman A, Keren R, et al. Recurrent Urinary Tract infections in children with bladder and bowel dysfunction. Pediatrics. 2016;137(1):1–7.
58. Santos JD, Lopes RI, Koyle MA. Bladder and bowel dysfunction in children: an update on the diagnosis and treatment of a common, but underdiagnosed pediatric problem. Can Urol Assoc J. 2017;11(1-2Suppl1):S64–s72.
59. Ahmed M, Eggleston D, Kapur G, Jain A, Valentini RP, Mattoo TK. Dimercaptosuccinic acid (DMSA) renal scan in the evaluation of hypertension in children. Pediatr Nephrol. 2008;23(3):435–8.
60. Lama G, Salsano ME, Pedulla M, Grassia C, Ruocco G. Angiotensin converting enzyme inhibitors and reflux nephropathy: 2-year follow-up. Pediatr Nephrol. 1997;11(6):714–8.
61. Peters CA, Skoog SJ, Arant Jr. BS, Copp HL, Elder JS, Hudson RG, Khoury AE, Lorenzo AJ, Pohl HG, Shapiro E, Snodgrass WT. The practice guidelines committee would like to acknowledge the contributions of Dr. Aaron Martin to the 2017 guideline amendment. Management and screening of primary vesicoureteral reflux in children (2017). 2017. https://www.auanet.org/guidelines-and-quality/guidelines/vesicoureteral-reflux-guideline. Accessed 10/30/2023.

New Renal Parenchymal Damage Following Breakthrough Urinary Tract Infection in Patients Treated with Antibiotic Prophylaxis

Josefin Nordenström, Per Brandström, and Yvonne Simrén

Abstract Children with VUR have an increased risk of contracting a febrile urinary tract infection (UTI). Febrile UTIs may cause a renal scar, with the degree of renal damage being affected by a complex interaction of host defence mechanisms and bacterial virulence factors. However, not all renal parenchymal damages in children with VUR are infectious in origin. Renal scars seen in boys are mainly congenital dysplasia, associated with high grade VUR, and recurrent urinary tract infections are rare in boys. Girls have more frequently recurrent UTIs and their renal parenchymal damages are more often post-infection scars. New scars are mostly seen in children under 5 years of age and more frequently in children with high grade VUR.

Continuous antibiotic prophylaxis (CAP) has routinely been used in children with VUR to prevent recurrent UTIs and possibly also post-infectious scars. Its'

J. Nordenström (✉)
Department of Pediatrics, Institute of Clinical Science at Sahlgrenska Academy, University of Gothenburg, Gothenburg, Sweden

The Department of Pediatric Surgery/Urology, Pediatric Uro-Nephrologic Center, Queen Silvia Children's Hospital, Sahlgrenska University Hospital, Gothenburg, Sweden
e-mail: josefin.nordenstrom@vgregion.se

P. Brandström
Department of Pediatrics, Institute of Clinical Science at Sahlgrenska Academy, University of Gothenburg, Gothenburg, Sweden

The Department of Pediatric Nephrology, Pediatric Uro-Nephrologic Center, Queen Silvia Children's Hospital, Sahlgrenska University Hospital, Gothenburg, Sweden
e-mail: per.brandstrom@gu.se

Y. Simrén
Department of Radiology, Institute of Clinical Sciences at Sahlgrenska Academy, University of Gothenburg, Gothenburg, Sweden

The Department of Pediatric Radiology, Queen Silvia Children's Hospital, Sahlgrenska University Hospital, Gothenburg, Sweden
e-mail: yvonne.simren@vgregion.se

P. Puri, A. Yamataka (eds.), *Vesicoureteral Reflux*,
https://doi.org/10.1007/978-3-031-95091-9_14

effectiveness has been questioned after several RCTs and meta-analyses that have failed to reveal the efficacy of CAP in reducing the risk of renal scarring.

This chapter aims to describe the current knowledge regarding the risk of renal scarring in children with VUR and ongoing treatment with antibiotic prophylaxis.

Keywords Vesicoureteral reflux · Antibiotic prophylaxis · Urinary tract infection · Renal damage · Renal scar

Introduction

Vesicoureteral reflux (VUR) is diagnosed in 30–40% of children after a first febrile urinary tract infection (UTI), the prevalence being even higher during the infant year [1, 2]. The fear of UTI related renal damage has been a driving force for a considerable amount of research during the last decades and still, the puzzle of VUR, febrile UTI and renal parenchymal damage is not solved.

Febrile UTIs may cause a renal scar, with the degree of renal damage being affected by a complex interaction of host defence mechanisms and bacterial virulence factors. However, not all renal parenchymal damages in children with VUR are infectious in origin. Renal scars seen in boys are mainly congenital dysplasia, associated with high grade VUR, and recurrent urinary tract infections are rare in boys. Girls have more frequently recurrent UTIs and their renal parenchymal damages are more often post-infection scars [3, 4]. New scars are mostly seen in children under 5 years of age and more frequently in children with high grade VUR [5].

Continuous antibiotic prophylaxis (CAP) has routinely been used in children with VUR to prevent recurrent UTIs and possibly also post-infectious scars. Its' effectiveness has been questioned after several RCTs and meta-analyses that have failed to reveal the efficacy of CAP in reducing the risk of renal scarring [6–10].

This chapter aims to describe the current knowledge regarding the risk of renal scarring in children with VUR and ongoing treatment with antibiotic prophylaxis.

Challenges with Prophylaxis

The hallmark of a breakthrough UTI is a symptomatic infection in a child on prophylactic treatment aimed to prevent the child from UTI recurrence. This chapter addresses the child on a daily low dose of prophylactic antibiotics.

Breakthrough infections occur as a result of non-adherence to prescribed prophylaxis or resistance towards the used agent [11]. When children are prescribed an antibiotic to which their initial UTI was resistant, there is a greater risk of new recurrences with bacteria resistant to the prophylactic agent used. Also, prophylaxis increases the risk of multidrug resistant bacteria in recurrent infections. However, the drugs available and suitable for long term prophylaxis are limited, giving the physician few options.

One important factor for the occurrence of UTI recurrences is non-adherence to prescribed treatment [12]. In a registry study of the real-life situation, not more than 17% of children with VUR were compliant to the prophylactic antibiotics. Among patients on prophylactic therapy, 58% were diagnosed with a UTI within 1 year of treatment [13]. This compliance rate from reality can be compared with the one in a study setting, where patients have a stringent follow-up protocol and high adherence rate. As an example, in the RIVUR trial, 77% of parents reported administration of medication in 75% of the time and 85% of the parents in at least 50% of the time [14].

There have been trials of alternative prophylactic measures such as cranberry juice and treatment with probiotic bacteria, with lactobacilli or low virulent E. coli, often with contradictory results in children. Although some interventions to prevent recurrent UTI have been tried with promising results, they do not provide a definitive effective answer so far [15].

Prophylaxis and Recurrent UTIs

Several trials have failed to detect a significant decrease in UTI recurrences with CAP compared to observation alone [7–9, 16]. Some of the investigators concluded that there was no benefit with prophylaxis, and in a couple of studies recurrences were even more frequent in the children on prophylaxis than in those without. Unfortunately, these results are hard to compare, due to the differences regarding study context, first line care or referral centres, population size, age and sex distribution, circumcision status, VUR-grade, UTI definition, and type and dose of prophylactic agent. Hence, also the results of meta-analyses of such divergent studies should be interpreted with caution [17].

However, the investigators of the latest and largest studies on antibiotic prophylaxis to prevent recurrent UTI in children with VUR, did find a substantial decrease in recurrent UTI in children on prophylaxis compared to placebo or no treatment [10, 18]. This has been reaffirmed in meta-analyses performed after these studies were published [19, 20]. The RIVUR study identified three groups of children that would especially benefit from prophylaxis: girls with VUR grade I-III with BBD/constipation; uncircumcised boys with VUR grade I-III; and boys and girls with VUR grade IV. The Swedish Reflux Trial including children 1–2 years of age, found a similar reduction in UTI recurrences in girls with dilating VUR grade III-IV on antibiotic prophylaxis, while no benefit was detected among the boys, as recurrences are very rare in boys at this age [21].

Prophylaxis and Renal Scarring

Most studies of antibiotic prophylaxis in children with VUR have been designed to detect a reduction in recurrent UTI. With the reduction of UTI recurrences in children on prophylaxis seen in some of the studies, one could expect less renal scarring in children on prophylaxis. Since renal scarring in itself is such a rare event, the studies have been insufficiently powered to be able to draw any convincing conclusions on the effect of prophylaxis on the rate of acquired scarring.

In the Swedish Reflux Trial, the lower UTI rate was associated with less renal scarring, although not strong enough to rule out the effect of chance [4]. In the first reports from the RIVUR trial, there was no difference in the development of permanent kidney damage between the groups. However, further complementary analyses revealed that prophylaxis in fact lowers the risk of new renal scarring associated with recurrent UTI [22].

A study on patients with VUR and on prophylactic antibiotics reported new renal inflammatory changes on acute DMSA scan in at the most 17% of patients after a single breakthrough infection, however they did not report the degree of permanent scarring [23]. Shaik et al. reported even higher rates of renal scarring on a late follow-up 99mTc dimercaptosuccinic acid (DMSA) scan of 18, 27 and 69% in children with VUR grade I-II, III and IV-V respectively [24].

Risk Factors for New Renal Damage

It has been well established that VUR is an independent risk factor for recurrent UTI, a risk that increases with the severity of the reflux. In the RIVUR trial, new renal scarring was strongly correlated to the number of recurrent UTIs [25]. The same correlation between renal scarring and recurrent UTI was seen in the Swedish Reflux Trial [4]. In the RIVUR trial, the incidence of renal scarring was 2.8% after 1 febrile UTI, but as high as 25.7% after 2 febrile UTIs and 28.6% after 3 or more febrile UTIs. As stated by the authors, only a minority of children will have 2 or more febrile UTIs, but those who do, have a considerably higher risk of renal scarring compared with children with only one febrile UTI.

The concept of new renal scarring always being attributed to recurrent UTI was refuted by the results from the RIVUR trial, where half of the new scars developed in children without documented recurrent UTI during the study follow-up [22]. The cause of these scars has eluded the investigators. There may have been UTI episodes during the follow-up that did not fulfil the study criteria of a symptomatic UTI, still initiating an inflammatory response/cascade in the kidney. The explanation for this might be found in the growing evidence that congenital differences in the factors and function of the innate immune system will determine the degree of symptoms and scarring from an infection [26].

In an attempt to determine the role of treatment delay in the development of renal scarring Hewitt et al. studied 287 children with febrile UTI, all with parenchymal uptake defects on acute DMSA [27]. There was a span of treatment delay after fever onset of less than one day to over 5 days. They found no difference in scarring formation comparing duration of the delay. Karavanaki, on the other hand, found that a treatment delay of more than 72 hours strongly correlated to formation of permanent scars [28]. Also, Shaikh et al. reported an association between delay in treatment of febrile UTIs and permanent renal scarring in their study population [29].

When comparing the placebo group of the RIVUR trial (VUR I-IV) with the CUTIE (Careful Urinary Tract Infection Evaluation) study cohort (no VUR) it was once again demonstrated that children with VUR have a higher rate of recurrent UTI than children with no VUR (25.4% vs. 17.3%), with dilating VUR having the highest rates (28.9%). The other factor that strongly affected the UTI recurrence rate was bladder and bowel dysfunction (BBD). The highest risk of recurrent UTI was seen in children with BBD and any grade of VUR (56%), followed by children with BBD without VUR (35%). Non-potty-trained children with no VUR had the lowest risk of recurrent UTI (10%). At the end of the 2-year follow-up, 4.3% had new renal scars in the no-VUR group vs. 8.4% in the VUR group. Even though twice the proportion in the VUR group, the difference did not reach statistical significance [30]. The presence of BBD has been increasingly recognized as a significant contributor to UTI. A recent meta-analysis showed that the prevalence of BBD was high in both children with and without VUR (49% and 41%, respectively) and that the risk of UTI was increased two-fold in the presence of BBD in children with VUR [31]. It has also been shown that the presence of BBD significantly delays the resolution of VUR [32–34] and that BBD increases the risk of both UTI and renal scarring [32, 35, 36].

Reflux "Disease" and Reflux "Symptomatology"

To view VUR as two distinct clinical conditions can possibly be a key to understand why results from different trials regarding prophylaxis, recurrent UTIs and renal damages are discrepant and varying. The study populations are often mixed and heterogenous in age, sex and grade of VUR. Therefore, clear conclusions are hard to draw. It has been suggested to describe one group of children with VUR as a "symptomatology" group, consisting of the more common form of VUR, usually grade I-III, detected predominantly in girls in the follow-up after a febrile UTI. The symptomatology group have normal kidneys and most often an excellent long-term outcome regardless surveillance or active (medical/surgical) treatment. The second, "disease" group are often detected antenatally, usually in boys, have VUR grade IV-V and often poorly functioning, dysplastic kidneys. It is this small subgroup of VUR patients who is at risk of impaired renal function and renal failure [37–39]. In most trials investigating the risk of UTI and renal damage, the first group, with a more favorable prognosis, is dominating the study sample, affecting the results and the conclusions you can make.

Imaging of Renal Damage

The management of children with renal involvement of UTI is dependent on an accurate diagnosis and characterization of renal damage. The diagnosis of new renal damage following a breakthrough infection is especially challenging since the method needs to differentiate between acute and chronic renal scars as well as congenital damage/dysplasia [23]. DMSA scintigraphy is today considered the golden standard to detect both acute and permanent renal damage and is used in most centres managing this patient group [40].

Children with VUR on prophylaxis have usually had a previous evaluation of both morphology and function of the kidneys. In centres where renal scintigraphy is unavailable there are alternative methods to be used. A renal ultrasound (US) has limited value in detecting acute and permanent renal damage due to its low sensitivity and specificity but plays an important role in the detection of congenital malformations. Computed tomography (CT) delivers ionizing radiation and requires intravenous (IV) contrast. A promising alternative for both morphological and functional evaluation without any radiation burden is the magnetic resonance imaging (MRI), which can detect even small renal parenchymal defects. It does require IV contrast for evaluation of renal function and sedation or anaesthesia in younger children, although infants below 6 months can often be examined after feeding [41].

DMSA is a highly sensitive but nonspecific method to evaluate renal damage after UTI. The drawbacks of the method are the low spatial resolution and limited ability to differentiate between acute and chronic or congenital changes. Studies performed as part of the RIVUR study showed that the reproducibility is contradictive when the question goes beyond normal or not normal, with a high dependency on standardization of the method and interpretation of findings [42].

Acute Damage and Renal Scarring

On DMSA scans, acute lesions often appear as large polar hypoactive areas, without deformity of the outlines and with indistinct margins. Renal scarring is defined in Guidelines of nuclear medicine as a decreased uptake of tracer associated with loss of contour or cortical thinning [43]. The differentiation between acute and chronic renal damage is not always possible based only on these characteristics. Therefore, a late scan is useful to confirm permanent renal damage (Fig. 1) [44]. However, in the absence of a previous scan the characteristics of the lesion can be helpful [40]. Since it takes 2–6 months for the resolution of acute findings, most guidelines recommend the follow-up scan to be performed no earlier than 6 months after the acute

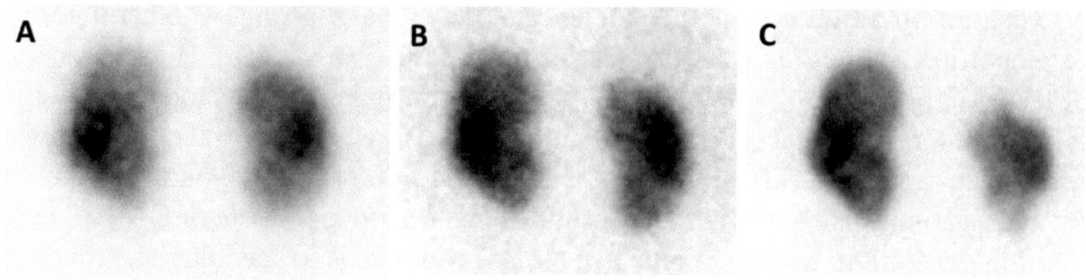

Fig. 1 DMSA images of a girl with right sided high grade VUR and recurrent pyelonephritis. (**a**) A first DMSA scan after the first pyelonephritis at the age of 8 months shows a small uptake defect at the lower pole of the right kidney. (**b**) A follow up DMSA scan was performed three years later after recurrent breakthrough-infections while on antibiotic prophylaxis. This scan shows new uptake defect in the apical pole and a more delineated defect in the caudal pole of the right kidney. The uptake in left kidney is noted as irregular. (**c**) At nine years of age, a follow-up scan shows progression of the uptake defects in the right kidney, thus progression of renal damage. There had been no new pyelonephritis for the past 3 year. No progression was seen in the left kidney

infection. The disadvantage of waiting further with the follow-up scan is that a recurrent UTI might complicate the interpretation of the late scan.

Congenital Renal Damage

The differentiation between congenital renal damage and postinfectious renal scarring is difficult. The use of prenatal imaging has revealed that part of the imaging findings that earlier were reported on as scars, actually were congenital damage [45]. On DMSA scans, general parenchymal changes can point to congenital hypo/dysplasia in contrast to the focal or multifocal areas that are seen in acute or permanent renal damage. This differentiation is important as children with congenital renal damage at presentation have an increased risk to progress to end-stage renal disease [45].

Summary

Studies have shown that recurrent, febrile urinary tract infections can cause non-congenital renal scarring, particularly in girls and in high grade VUR. CAP has been demonstrated to reduce the risk for recurrent infections and remains the first line treatment for high-grade reflux (grade III-V) with an aim to prevent UTI and its associated morbidity, while awaiting spontaneous resolution of VUR.

The Swedish reflux trial managed to show significantly more recurrent febrile UTIs and new renal damage in girls on surveillance [4]. Apart from that, several recent randomized studies have failed to reveal the efficacy of CAP in reducing risk of renal scarring [7–10]. Not even the RIVUR trial was able to reveal between-group differences in the incidence of new renal scarring, whether in terms of proportion of children (6% and 7%) or renal units (4% vs. 4%). However, none of these studies, including the RIVUR trial, were sufficiently powered to study the efficacy of CAP in renal scarring prevention, which was once again confirmed by a recent meta-analysis [46]. It has been estimated that 8000 patients would be required for such an analysis [47] why these results do not disprove the role of CAP in renal scarring prevention. Instead, a selective use of prophylaxis to specific risk groups at greatest risk of contracting ascending symptomatic UTI, namely children with dilating VUR grade 3–5, especially those with bowel and bladder dysfunction in addition to VUR, can be expected to reduce the risk of acquired renal damage. And from the reports on scarring related to treatment delay in febrile UTI, the relevant action for clinicians is to avoid any delay in testing for UTI in febrile children.

One can also argue that the close follow-up and aggressive treatment in a randomized study setup may prevent the onset of some pyelonephritis episodes, which could have otherwise led to scarring.

Even if the lack of difference in renal scarring between treatment and placebo groups may advocate the possibility of managing VUR children without CAP, with a very close and careful follow-up, such an approach is not always realistic in clinical practice [14, 47]. Moreover, the morbidity of a recurrent urinary tract infection, even in the absence of renal scarring, should not be underestimated, causing suffering to the child and considerable concern to the parents.

The management of VUR must continue to be tailored, based on the risk for further infections and renal scarring, with the likelihood of spontaneous resolution and parental preferences in mind. Early identification and appropriate treatment of associated bowel bladder dysfunction is central. Both antibiotic prophylaxis and surgical interventions should be used in a selective manner to optimize the risk-benefit ratio, by defining children with high risk of recurrent ascending UTI, with the aim to reduce recurrent pyelonephritis and repeated hospital admissions. The genetic profile of the innate immune system associated with renal scarring and other factors responsible for congenital and acquired renal parenchymal damage in children with VUR need to be further studied. Possibly, boys and girls should be managed differently, with respect to their differences in infection patterns and types of renal damage, and with the suggested two VUR groups in mind—"symptomatology" group and "disease" group. Regardless, we should aim for an equal and effective management of children with VUR to minimize the risk of UTI and permanent kidney damage. To reach this goal it is crucial that the families have access to an affordable and well operating health system for children.

References

1. Tullus K. Vesicoureteric reflux in children. Lancet. 2015;385(9965):371–9.
2. Hannula A, et al. Vesicoureteral reflux in children with suspected and proven urinary tract infection. Pediatr Nephrol. 2010;25(8):1463–9.

3. Wennerstrom M, et al. Primary and acquired renal scarring in boys and girls with urinary tract infection. J Pediatr. 2000;136(1):30–4.
4. Brandstrom P, et al. The Swedish reflux trial in children: IV. Renal damage. J Urol. 2010;184(1):292–7.
5. Olbing H, et al. New renal scars in children with severe VUR: a 10-year study of randomized treatment. Pediatr Nephrol. 2003;18(11):1128–31.
6. Mattoo TK, et al. Renal scarring in the randomized intervention for children with vesicoureteral reflux (RIVUR) trial. Clin J Am Soc Nephrol. 2016;11(1):54–61.
7. Garin EH, et al. Clinical significance of primary vesicoureteral reflux and urinary antibiotic prophylaxis after acute pyelonephritis: a multicenter, randomized, controlled study. Pediatrics. 2006;117(3):626–32.
8. Montini G, et al. Prophylaxis after first febrile urinary tract infection in children? A multicenter, randomized, controlled, noninferiority trial. Pediatrics. 2008;122(5):1064–71.
9. Pennesi M, et al. Is antibiotic prophylaxis in children with vesicoureteral reflux effective in preventing pyelonephritis and renal scars? A randomized, controlled trial. Pediatrics. 2008;121(6):e1489–94.
10. Craig JC, et al. Antibiotic prophylaxis and recurrent urinary tract infection in children. N Engl J Med. 2009;361(18):1748–59.
11. Bollgren I. Antibacterial prophylaxis in children with urinary tract infection. Acta Paediatr Suppl. 1999;88(431):48–52.
12. Gaither TW, Copp HL. Antimicrobial prophylaxis for urinary tract infections: implications for adherence assessment. J Pediatr Urol. 2019;15(4):387 e1–8.
13. Hensle TW, et al. Part 2: examining pediatric vesicoureteral reflux: a real-world evaluation of treatment patterns and outcomes. Curr Med Res Opin. 2007;23(Suppl 4):S7–13.
14. Lee T, Park JM. Vesicoureteral reflux and continuous prophylactic antibiotics. Investig Clin Urol. 2017;58(Suppl 1):S32–7.
15. Tewary K, Narchi H. Recurrent urinary tract infections in children: preventive interventions other than prophylactic antibiotics. World J Methodol. 2015;5(2):13–9.
16. Hari P, et al. Antibiotic prophylaxis in the management of vesicoureteric reflux: a randomized double-blind placebo-controlled trial. Pediatr Nephrol. 2015;30(3):479–86.
17. Greenfield SP, et al. Vesicoureteral reflux and antibiotic prophylaxis: why cohorts and methodologies matter. J Urol. 2016;196(4):1238–43.
18. Hoberman A, Chesney RW, Investigators RT. Antimicrobial prophylaxis for children with vesicoureteral reflux. N Engl J Med. 2014;371(11):1072–3.
19. de Bessa J Jr, et al. Antibiotic prophylaxis for prevention of febrile urinary tract infections in children with vesicoureteral reflux: a meta-analysis of randomized, controlled trials comparing dilated to nondilated vesicoureteral reflux. J Urol. 2015;193(5 Suppl):1772–7.
20. Wang HH, et al. Efficacy of antibiotic prophylaxis in children with vesicoureteral reflux: systematic review and meta-analysis. J Urol. 2015;193(3):963–9.
21. Brandstrom P, et al. The Swedish reflux trial in children: III. Urinary tract infection pattern. J Urol. 2010;184(1):286–91.
22. Wang HH, et al. Why does prevention of recurrent urinary tract infection not result in less renal scarring? A deeper dive into the RIVUR trial. J Urol. 2019;202(2):400–5.
23. Szlyk GR, et al. Incidence of new renal parenchymal inflammatory changes following breakthrough urinary tract infection in patients with vesicoureteral reflux treated with antibiotic prophylaxis: evaluation by 99MTechnetium dimercapto-succinic acid renal scan. J Urol. 2003;170(4 Pt 2):1566–8. discussion 1568–9
24. Shaikh N, et al. Identification of children and adolescents at risk for renal scarring after a first urinary tract infection: a meta-analysis with individual patient data. JAMA Pediatr. 2014;168(10):893–900.
25. Shaikh N, et al. Association of renal scarring with number of febrile urinary tract infections in children. JAMA Pediatr. 2019;173(10):949–52.

26. Kosmeri C, Kalaitzidis R, Siomou E. An update on renal scarring after urinary tract infection in children: what are the risk factors? J Pediatr Urol. 2019;15(6):598–603.
27. Hewitt IK, et al. Early treatment of acute pyelonephritis in children fails to reduce renal scarring: data from the Italian Renal Infection Study Trials. Pediatrics. 2008;122(3):486–90.
28. Karavanaki KA, et al. Delayed treatment of the first febrile urinary tract infection in early childhood increased the risk of renal scarring. Acta Paediatr. 2017;106(1):149–54.
29. Shaikh N, et al. Early antibiotic treatment for pediatric febrile urinary tract infection and renal scarring. JAMA Pediatr. 2016;170(9):848–54.
30. Keren R, et al. Risk factors for recurrent urinary tract infection and renal scarring. Pediatrics. 2015;136(1):e13–21.
31. Meena J, et al. Prevalence of bladder and bowel dysfunction in toilet-trained children with urinary tract infection and/or primary vesicoureteral reflux: a systematic review and meta-analysis. Front Pediatr. 2020;8:84.
32. Peters CA, et al. Summary of the AUA guideline on management of primary vesicoureteral reflux in children. J Urol. 2010;184(3):1134–44.
33. Sillén U, et al. The Swedish reflux trial in children: v. Bladder dysfunction. J Urol. 2010;184(1):298–304.
34. Nordenstrom J, et al. The Swedish infant high-grade reflux trial – bladder function. J Pediatr Urol. 2017;13(2):139–45.
35. Shaikh N, et al. Recurrent urinary tract infections in children with bladder and bowel dysfunction. Pediatrics. 2016;137(1)
36. Nordenstrom J, et al. The Swedish infant high-grade reflux trial: UTI and renal damage. J Pediatr Urol. 2017;13(2):146–54.
37. Demède D, Mouriquand P. The Vesicoureteric maze: the reasons of misunderstanding. In: Lima M, Manzoni G, editors. Pediatric urology. Milano: Springer; 2015.
38. Fanos V, Cataldi L. Antibiotics or surgery for vesicoureteric reflux in children. Lancet. 2004;364(9446):1720–2.
39. Hewitt I, Montini G. Vesicoureteral reflux is it important to find? Pediatr Nephrol. 2021;36(4):1011–7.
40. Rushton HG. The evaluation of acute pyelonephritis and renal scarring with technetium 99m-dimercaptosuccinic acid renal scintigraphy: evolving concepts and future directions. Pediatr Nephrol. 1997;11(1):108–20.
41. Majd M, et al. Acute pyelonephritis: comparison of diagnosis with 99mTc-DMSA, SPECT, spiral CT, MR imaging, and power Doppler US in an experimental pig model. Radiology. 2001;218(1):101–8.
42. Mattoo TK, et al. Interobserver variability for interpretation of DMSA scans in the RIVUR trial. J Pediatr Urol. 2017;13(6):616.e1–6.
43. Vali R, et al. SNMMI Procedure Standard/EANM Practice Guideline on Pediatric [99mTc]Tc-DMSA Renal Cortical Scintigraphy: An Update. 2021 [cited 2021 May 24]; Available from: https://s3.amazonaws.com/rdcms-snmmi/files/production/public/FileDownloads/ProcedureStandards/SNMMI%20EANM%20DMSA%20guideline_final.pdf
44. Risdon RA, et al. Renal pathology and the 99mTc-DMSA image during the evolution of the early pyelonephritic scar: an experimental study. J Urol. 1994;151(3):767–73.
45. Edefonti A, et al. Febrile urinary tract infections: clinical and laboratory diagnosis, imaging, and prognosis. Semin Nucl Med. 2014;44(2):123–8.
46. Hewitt IK, et al. Antibiotic prophylaxis for urinary tract infection-related renal scarring: a systematic review. Pediatrics. 2017;139(5)
47. Greenfield SP. Editorial comment. J Urol. 2015;193(5 Suppl):1777.

Antibiotic Prophylaxis for Reflux: The Effect on Patient Community and Global Environment

Christopher J. Corbett and Martin A. Koyle

Abstract Continuous antibiotic prophylaxis (CAP) is frequently utilized in the management of vesicoureteral reflux with the goal of preventing urinary tract infections (UTI), and more importantly permanent renal damage, which can have long term negative effects including kidney disease and hypertension. Although the utilization of CAP has been found to decrease the risk of UTIs, the decreased risk of developing renal scarring in the long run has been controversial. Moreover, the price to pay for implementing CAP has been the association with a marked increase in developing bacterial resistance. Thus, the potential benefits of prescribing CAP must be weighed against long term complications of antibiotic usage, both on an individual and global level. Hopefully, ongoing and future studies will continue to emerge with the goal of better identifying patients who are most likely to benefit from CAP in order to maximize their utility while minimizing the risk of side effects and complications.

Keywords Antibiotic prophylaxis · Antibiotic resistance · Vesicoureteral reflux

Introduction

The management of vesicoureteral reflux (VUR) has evolved over time as we have developed a better appreciation of its natural progression, the sequelae of VUR, and the ways in which it may be observed or treated. The focus of treatment in this patient population is to prevent long-term effects of urinary tract infections (UTIs) in the setting of VUR, which may have the potential to lead to long term kidney

C. J. Corbett
Division of Pediatric Urology, Children's National Medical Center, Washington, DC, USA

M. A. Koyle (✉)
Department of Urology, University of Minnesota Faculty of Medicine and Masonic Children's Hospital, Minneapolis, Minnesota, USA

P. Puri, A. Yamataka (eds.), *Vesicoureteral Reflux*,
https://doi.org/10.1007/978-3-031-95091-9_15

damage, reflux nephropathy, and renal scarring [1, 2]. Prevention of renal scarring and kidney damage may have important implications in avoiding the long-term development of chronic kidney disease (CKD) or hypertension [3, 4]. Based on our current understanding of VUR and high rates of spontaneous resolution over time, especially in lower grades of VUR, continuous antibiotic prophylaxis (CAP) has previously been one of the mainstays of treatment in this population in the vast majority of cases [5]. Other management strategies include observation, endoscopic management, and surgical reconstruction using open and/or minimally invasive options.

The randomized intervention for vesicoureteral reflux (RiVUR) study was conducted to more rigorously assess the utility of CAP in children with VUR. The study was a randomized, double-blinded, placebo controlled trial that sought to expand upon prior studies that were limited by their lack of control groups or were not blinded [6, 7]. Children were randomized to placebo or CAP with trimethoprim-sulfamethoxazole; primary outcome was prevention of recurrent UTIs, while secondary outcomes included renal scarring, treatment failure, and the development of antibiotic resistance. They found that UTI recurrence was decreased by 50% in the treatment arm, with even higher rates of reduction in children with concurrent bladder and bowel dysfunction, as well as children whose original UTI presentation included fevers [6]. While the original study found no significant difference in rates of renal scarring between the two cohorts, when further analyzed, renal scarring secondary to recurrent UTIs did decrease with CAP [7, 8]. However, the RiVUR study also identified higher rates of antibiotic resistance in the treatment group in children presenting with recurrent UTIs [6].

Since the RiVUR study was published, several systematic reviews, including a Cochrane Review, have called into question the utility and potential benefits of CAP. In the recent review by Autore et al., this conclusion was drawn in considering the limited data in prevention of renal scarring with CAP and the emergence of more antibiotic resistant UTIs [9]. Similar findings were reported in the Cochrane review [10]. In consideration of the risks and benefits of CAP, the most important intervention is the prompt treatment of febrile UTIs to prevent renal scarring [11]. This begs the question as to the importance of patient/caregiver education and compliance with treatment options.

As the pendulum begins to swing away from the use of CAP in children with VUR, the utilization of AI, machine learning, and predictive modeling may allow for the better selection of patients who serve to benefit most from CAP. As the optimal management of these children is considered, it is important to reflect on the broader implications of CAP. These considerations include broader implications of CAP on an individual's well-being, as well as on the patient population, those without VUR, and even on the environment, with the downstream effects CAP may have on drug development, and antibiotic resistance. Here, we hope to highlight the broader implications of CAP using a patient-centered, population-centered, and globally-centered viewpoint.

Current Prescribing Patterns and Antibiotic Selection

The prevalence of VUR is difficult to predict as typically there are few or no symptoms attributed directly to VUR, and more often it is found on workup for antenatal hydronephrosis or in infants presenting with a febrile UTI. Although prior estimates suggested rates of VUR approaching 2% in the population, some studies suggest rates may be significantly higher, especially in those presenting with a UTI [12]. Based on the natural course of VUR in many patients, CAP remains one of the most common management strategies in kids with VUR. Studies have found that approximately 75% of kids with VUR will ultimately be managed with CAP, though despite its high rate of utilization, many patients and families may not be compliant with management, with several studies reporting low rates of adherence with the recommended CAP regimen [13, 14]. Many factors may contribute to poor rates of adherence, including the prolonged duration CAP may be recommended, either until resolution of VUR or a child has completed toilet training, cost of antibiotics, side effects, or lack of communication and understanding by providers and families about the rationale for CAP.

Important considerations for the use of CAP in the management of VUR include duration of treatment and antibiotic selection, as this may alter patient adherence and risks of side effects from treatment and the development of antibiotic resistance. VUR resolves spontaneously in a majority of affected patients, and sterile reflux poses minimal risk to the kidneys and development of permanent renal scarring [15]. Therefore, patients most likely to benefit from CAP include those with a grade of VUR that is more likely to spontaneously resolve over time who have developed UTIs; those with incidentally found sterile reflux, or those with higher grades of VUR less likely to resolve over time are more likely to be affected by side effects of CAP, or to require more invasive treatments to assist in the resolution of VUR and prevent permanent renal damage, respectively. Other factors that contribute to the decision to use CAP include age, gender, and the presence of renal scarring on prior diagnostic imaging [1].

Antibiotic selection may be dependent on several factors, including patient age, prior urine culture results and resistance patterns, ease of administration, and provider preference. Antibiotics frequently selected for CAP include amoxicillin, amoxicillin-clavulanic acid, trimethoprim-sulfamethoxazole, cephalosporins, and nitrofurantoin. In the review by Autore et al. they noted two separate studies comparing UTI recurrence in patients on trimethoprim-sulfamethoxazole, one with cephalosporins, and the other with macrobid, with no significant difference noted in either study [9]. In contrast, one study recommended the use of amoxicillin-clavulanic acid as first line for CAP, with cephalosporins or nitrofurantoin remaining second line therapy, due to developing resistance patterns and antibiotic-specific side effects [16]. Other important considerations in antibiotic selection include dosing and changing antibiotics in the setting of a breakthrough UTI. In both a Cochrane Review and the guidelines by Autore et al. there were no conclusions regarding antibiotic dosage, with the expert opinion being utilization of a dose one-fourth to one-third of that for treatment [9, 10]. For breakthrough UTIs, one study showed no significant difference in recurrent UTIs with continuation of the original CAP regimen compared with changing to a new antibiotic regimen [17].

Penicillin derivatives, sometimes with the use of beta-lactamase inhibitors, and cephalosporins are frequently utilized, often readily available and generic antibiotics that may be used for CAP in children with VUR. Amoxicillin, amoxicillin-clavulanic acid, cefadroxil, and cephalexin are all antibiotics within this class that can be taken once daily as CAP for VUR [18]. Young children on CAP are unlikely to be able to take solid pills, and consideration of liquid formulations is necessary when considering the burden of treatment in these patients. Both amoxicillin and amoxicillin-clavulanic acid are not shelf stable, and benefit from refrigeration for storage, which poses challenges to individuals with limited access to electricity, refrigerated storage, or who reside in warmer climates. Poor shelf stability also necessitates more frequent refills of medications. Cephalexin and cefadroxil, both first generation cephalosporins, are also limited by these storage restrictions.

Trimethoprim, trimethoprim-sulfamethoxazole, and nitrofurantoin are also commonly used regimens for CAP in the VUR population. Trimethoprim is a diaminopyrimidine antibiotic that may be taken once daily, is more shelf stable and may be safely stored at room temperature. Similarly, trimethoprim-sulfamethoxazole—with an added sulfonamide component, is also shelf stable at room temperature and taken once daily. A major limitation is the presence of the sulfamethoxazole, which should be avoided in patients with sulfa allergies. It should also be avoided in children less than 2 months of age as it may increase the risk of jaundice in young infants. Lastly, nitrofurantoin may also be taken once daily, is shelf stable at room temperature, but should also be avoided in infants less than 1 month in age. Additional antibiotic considerations, including the risks of developing antibiotic resistance, will be explored later.

The Pros and Cons of Antibiotic Prophylaxis

In considering the overall utility of CAP in children with VUR, it is important to take into account the potential benefits and risks in both the near and long term to both the patient and family. Potential benefits include the prevention of recurrent UTIs, which may require repeated courses of antibiotics with side effects, and potentially necessitating hospitalization, as well as renal scarring, which can lead to chronic kidney damage and hypertension, with even more downstream effects. The utilization of CAP may also help avoid the progression to more invasive treatments, including both endoscopic surgical interventions as well as ureteral reimplant. Multiple psychosocial aspects of CAP should be taken into consideration as well, including the psychological distress families may encounter when considering the risks of permanent kidney damage. Potential risks and complications should be weighed as well, including the risk of antimicrobial resistance, the short and long term effects of long term antibiotic use, and even the financial considerations of CAP.

Several studies have found higher rates of renal scarring in children who have delayed treatment of febrile UTIs [11, 19]. Infants and young children are unable to verbalize their symptoms, and UTIs may be more challenging to diagnose promptly as a result, which is a critical reason behind the utilization of CAP in avoiding febrile UTIs. Several studies, including the rigorously conducted RIVUR trial found a decreased rate of UTIs in children on CAP, and these findings are supported in several systematic reviews, including two Cochrane reviews [10, 20]. In the more recent systematic review by Autore et al. they have found that although pooled data demonstrated a decreased risk of recurrent UTIs, the large size of the RIVUR trial skewed the pooled data towards significance [9]. When looking at individual trials, one study out of France found that CAP was associated with a decreased risk of recurrent UTIs in boys, and boys with grade III VUR [21]. The presence of bladder and bowel dysfunction is also an important risk factor in developing UTIs in patients with VUR, and CAP may be more beneficial in this population, though correction of bladder and bowel dysfunction should also remain a key focus of treatment [22].

Although studies have demonstrated a decreased risk of recurrent UTIs in children on CAP, the lack of evidence demonstrating decreased risk of permanent renal scarring while on CAP suggests its utilization may have fewer long term clinically significant benefits. Both the RIVUR trial and the Swedish reflux trial found no statistically significant difference in rates of renal scarring between control groups and those on CAP [9, 23]. However, on further analysis of the RIVUR trial cohort, they found that renal scarring associated with recurrent UTIs was decreased in the cohort receiving CAP, after accounting for individuals who developed renal scarring despite not developing recurrent UTIs [8]. Therefore, instead of focusing on treatment with CAP in patients with VUR, focus should instead be on preventing recurrent UTIs, which can increase the risk of permanent renal scarring, and prompt treatment of UTIs [11, 24] .

An important consideration in the utilization of CAP is whether it may be useful in preventing progression in management of VUR towards more invasive interventions, such as endoscopic or open surgical management. Compared with CAP, which may be quickly discontinued if side effects are encountered or desired by the family, these more invasive interventions may have more lasting side effects that are not readily reversible, and often include the added risks associated with surgery and anesthesia. In comparing surgical reimplantation with medical management, the European branch of the International reflux study noted fewer febrile UTIs in the cohort managed surgically, but long term renal growth outcomes were not significantly different between the two groups [25, 26]. However, a small portion of patients in the surgically managed cohort did develop postoperative obstruction [10]. Similarly, the Cochrane review found that endoscopic management, both with or without antibiotics, when compared with CAP, had little difference in rates of UTIs and kidney damage in the long term [10]. Overall, existing evidence suggests that long term renal outcomes may not differ between those with VUR managed surgically, either endoscopically or with reimplantation, when compared with CAP. These results may prove important then, when considering long term management in children with VUR, and increase the weight that should be placed when considering potential complications and side effects from different management options.

An additional consideration is the psychological toll that a diagnosis like VUR, and the uncertain long term effects it may have on a patient, can have on both patient and family. The non-specific symptoms associated with UTIs and concern about long term renal scarring and its sequelae for untreated UTIs may result in an anxious or hypervigilant state for caregivers that may have long term psychological consequences. Invasive procedures may have long term psychological consequences on both patients and caregivers, and the early age at which many children undergo surgical correction of VUR can make it challenging to assess measurable variables and study long term outcomes in this population. Studies have already looked at decisional regret in caregivers of children undergoing other types of urologic surgical procedures, such as hypospadias, and have found that for some procedures, decisional regret affects the majority of caregivers [27]. Future studies may address the paucity of data with regards to decision making and the psychological toll it exacts on patients and families for other urologic procedures, including the management of VUR.

As more evidence suggests minimal benefits with the utilization of CAP in patients with VUR, it is important to consider the side effects and potential complications associated with CAP, both prolonged usage and for short durations. The development of antibiotic resistant organisms remains one of the biggest challenges encountered with the use of CAP. Developing resistance patterns can make UTIs more challenging to treat, and in some situations necessitate hospitalization for IV antibiotics. With new antibiotic resistant organisms, we may soon run out of potential antibiotics to treat bacteria. Other possible long term complications from CAP use include immunologic changes that may predispose patients to certain diseases, alteration of gut microbiota, or changes in growth patterns. Some of these downstream effects even pose risks on a population level.

On a population level, antibiotic resistance is developing at an alarming rate. Studies have found an increased risk in children on antibiotic prophylaxis for the development of antibiotic resistant infections up to 24 times higher than for children who are not on prophylactic antibiotics [28]. Several population based studies out of Europe demonstrated alarmingly high resistance rates to commonly prescribed empiric antibiotics, including amoxicillin-clavulanic acid and trimethoprim-sulfamethoxazole; in one study, multidrug resistant organisms accounted for over 5% of resistant organisms [29, 30]. A Belgian study found that over a 20 year period, E. Coli resistance to amoxicillin-clavulanic acid more than doubled, with increasing annual resistance rates of approximately 2% in both kids who did and did not have previous exposure to antibiotics [31]. In the US, a retrospective study from 1999 to 2011 found that rates of antibiotic resistance to 3rd generation cephalosporins, or those that were extended-spectrum beta-lactamase producers, more than doubled in this time period [32].

Antimicrobial resistance is widely cited as a complication following the use of CAP in children with VUR. In the RIVUR trial, amongst children on CAP with trimethoprim-sulfamethoxazole who had a recurrent E.Coli UTI, almost two-thirds had strains of the bacteria that were resistant to the antibiotic, compared with only 19% in the control arm [6]. Similar risks were reported by Cochrane reviews, with children on CAP more than 2 times more likely to develop resistant organisms [10, 20]. In a more recent meta-analysis, the chance of preventing a UTI was similar to the chance of developing antimicrobial resistance, with a number needed to treat of 21 for either outcome to occur [33]. However, not all CAP regimens appear to pose the same risk of the development of resistant UTIs. The guidelines by Autore et al. noted an increased risk of developing antimicrobial resistance in children using cephalosporins for CAP, and therefore recommended against its use [9]. The Cochrane review by Williams and Craig noted two studies with lower rates of bacterial resistance in patients on nitrofurantoin compared with trimethoprim-sulfamethoxazole [20]. Thus, although there is an overall high relative risk of developing antimicrobial resistance on CAP, treatment regimens, specifically with nitrofurantoin, may pose an overall lower risk of the development of new resistant organisms, though other side effects of the medication limit its utility.

These evolving resistance patterns have immediate implications for patients, the benefits of CAP, and empiric management of subsequent infections. Treatment failure and progression of treatment is common due to antibiotic resistance. Children who present to the ER or primary care clinic may be treated empirically for a urinary tract infection. One study looking at outcomes of children treated empirically with discordant antibiotics found that most children improved, while 2% required an escalation of their care [34]. Although most of the patients in this study had positive outcomes, and the authors found that empiric treatment in the setting of rising antimicrobial resistance was appropriate, the potential long term implications and worsening resistance patterns are significant. Persistent antimicrobial resistance runs the risk of increasing patient morbidity and mortality, which may serve as drivers in future healthcare costs [35].

The utilization of CAP may also drive other unwanted side effects in patients. An increasingly studied area remains the role of the gut microbiome in human health and the effects antibiotics can have on this critical balance. Several studies have sought to understand the role of low dose CAP on the gut microbiome specifically in children with urinary tract malformations including VUR. One pilot study out of Austria evaluated the microbiome over a 70 day span, noting no significant difference between the treatment and control arm [36]. A second study out of Japan noted an initial alteration in the microbiome after treatment for a UTI; after treatment and placement into the control or CAP group, patients ultimately experienced a recovery in their gut microbiome, with no significant difference in overall diversity of the gut microbiome, though one bacteria was noted to comprise a smaller portion of the microbiome in the CAP cohort [37]. In contrast, an analysis of the gut microbiota of a cohort of patients from the PREDICT trial noted a rise in opportunistic pathogens in the composition of the gut microbiome following management with CAP [38]. Given the variability in findings from these studies, additional research is needed to better understand the potential effects of the microbiome from antibiotics in this unique patient cohort.

Additional downstream effects of both changes to the gut microbiome and from the utilization of antibiotics are an additional consideration when weighing the potential risks, both personally and on a population level, of management of VUR with CAP. Weight gain, for example, has been noted to be associated with the administration of antibiotics in animal models [28]. The immunologic effects from the exposure to antibiotics has long term implications for both our innate defenses to fight off these new, resistant pathogens and may lead to an increased risk of the development of certain autoimmune diseases [39, 40]. However, the effects from CAP on these immunologic diseases may not be as significant. One study noted that children with VUR who received therapeutic doses of antibiotics for UTI were at risk for developing asthma, in contrast to children on CAP who did not exhibit the same risk for the development of childhood asthma [41]. Similar to those studies assessing changes in the gut microbiome, low dose prophylaxis may not enact the same physiologic and immunologic changes as noted with therapeutic doses of antibiotics.

On a patient and provider level, the overall utility of CAP remains highly contested. Although the American Urologic Association guidelines currently recommend CAP in infants with VUR following a febrile UTI, and in those with grade III-IV VUR, regardless of a history of febrile UTI, the overall evidence is less certain, and weighing the risks and benefits with families is important before making a management decision. While there is good evidence that CAP can reduce the risk of recurrent UTIs, its effectiveness in preventing renal scarring is less clear, and may have more limited utility targeted to the highest risk patients. In contrast, the development of antimicrobial resistance may place individuals at higher risk from UTIs caused by resistant organisms, where delays in appropriate treatment may place patients at an even greater risk of renal scarring and permanent renal damage. Other downstream effects of antibiotic exposure, including changes to the gut microbiome and subsequent sequelae, may or may not occur following exposure to only low dose prophylactic antibiotics based on the existing data. Additional studies and longer follow-up of existing cohorts may help further elucidate the full risk-benefit balance of CAP in patients with VUR.

Global Implications of Continuous Antibiotic Prophylaxis

While a patient-centered approach to treatment is critical, one cannot ignore the more global effects of CAP in VUR patients, both its limitations in utilization as well as the consequences of its use. One of the most critical concerns on a global level is antibiotic resistance. This has wide-reaching implications, with access to safe care and antibiotics, as well as treatment failure necessitating costly, intensive inpatient treatment which is not readily available across the globe, and also the financial and environmental consequences of drug development necessary to combat resistant superbugs. On the other hand, the pressure placed on an already strained system may yield new innovations and discoveries that may improve the quality of care we provide patients in the long term.

On a global scale, the implications of antibiotic resistance are frightening in the near future. For example, there have been multiple reports of carbapenem-resistant UTIs in children without recent hospitalizations [42]. With emergence of resistant pathogens, healthcare costs will only further rise as these infections necessitate more intensive, inpatient hospitalizations, which are also associated with greater risks and side effects to patients [35]. These infections are also responsible for millions of deaths globally each year, and it is estimated that by 2050, antimicrobial resistance will be responsible for 10 million deaths annually [40]. These staggering numbers cannot be ignored, and pose a real risk to patients and entire populations.

The utilization of CAP, and the effects of antimicrobial resistance, require special consideration in low income countries. As noted, several antibiotics utilized for CAP are not shelf stable or require refrigeration, which can pose significant logistical hurdles where access to electricity and/or refrigeration is limited. Antibiotic resistance also poses a greater threat to individuals in lower income countries. Individuals are less likely to have access to good nutrition, sanitation, and medical care that we take for granted in higher income countries, and places individuals at higher risk when faced with these superbugs [40]. Additional factors that increase the risk of exposure to resistant organisms relate to the infrastructure in these countries. In low and middle income countries where access to formal healthcare is limited and may require traveling large distances, over the counter antibiotics are frequently obtained on request or as an alternative to seeing a doctor, and often without any oversight [43, 44]. Economically, these countries may rely more heavily on growing livestock or fish, necessitating antibiotic usage in these animals, which spurs on the development of resistant organisms. Wastewater and sewage infrastructure is also often less developed, and combined with less antibiotic oversight and limited access to antibiotics used to treat these resistant organisms, patients are much more likely to have higher morbidity and mortality from antimicrobial resistant organisms [45].

Our disposal of antibiotics into the environment is a major driving force in the development of antimicrobial resistant organisms. Treatment of infections with antibiotics will select for mutations in bacteria that can be transferred to other organisms and is one of the key environments that drives the development of antimicrobial resistance [45]. When bacteria in the environment are faced with antibiotic byproducts or antimicrobial waste, this can place similar pressure on these organisms and fuel the development of resistance. Key sources of antibiotics in the environment include human consumption and excretion, but also wastewater from hospitals, use of antibiotics in agriculture, and managing and treating livestock. These environmental drivers and exposures pose a significant risk in fueling the growth of antimicrobial resistance. For example, the majority of antibiotic sales in the US are for use in agriculture and livestock, with most antibiotics used for livestock also used for treating infections in humans. Contact with uncooked meat or animal waste can lead to the transmission of resistance bacteria, and there is growing evidence that this use of antibiotics is further driving the development of antimicrobial resistance [46]. A study out of Sweden noted high levels of multidrug resistant E. Coli in untreated hospital wastewater samples [47]. Curbing the development of new resistant organisms will not only require judicious use of antibiotics, but also ensuring proper disposal of wastewater and other sources contaminated with antibiotics.

The development of new antibiotics is simultaneously driven by increasing bacterial resistance, while also serving as a driving force of resistance. In a review by Larsson and Flach, they noted that antimicrobial waste was much higher in areas polluted by drug manufacturing compared with excreted antibiotics in wastewater; combined with the higher levels of resistant bacteria and low fecal contamination noted in these wastewater regions, this presents strong evidence that this is only hastening the development of resistant organisms [45]. Of course, contamination of groundwater and other sources of human exposure with these medical byproducts can present more risks, including those to the gut microbiome as discussed previously. In addition, pharmaceutical manufacturing costs are frequently cheaper in low and middle income countries, where poor waste management only increases the risk of contamination with byproducts and waste, such as in China and India, two of the largest producers of antibiotics [45]. These downstream consequences ultimately require greater investment into the safe development, manufacturing, and disposal of antibiotics and their byproducts to avoid more significant consequences.

In contrast, the development of antimicrobial resistance also serves as a force for scientific advancement. Worsening resistance patterns will necessitate the development of new drugs to treat these serious infections. However, as Huemer et al. note, pharmaceutical companies have focused less on the development of new antibiotics. Reasons for this include the high investment costs associated with drug development and concern that these new medications may not be profitable, instead focusing their efforts on creating new treatments for heart disease, cancer, high blood pressure, and other disease processes that have great financial potential [35]. Fortunately, this may instead result in the development of new technology and treatment strategies that have the potential to not only treat new and resistant infections, but implications for treatment in other disease processes as well.

This same forward thinking mindframe is also being used in the development of new tools to risk stratify patients with VUR and select those most likely to benefit from CAP to avoid some of the risks and complications with treatment. For example, prior studies have assessed distal ureteral diameter as an indicator of outcomes in patients with VUR, and have found that it can help identify patients who are likely to have spontaneous resolution of reflux, as well as those who are more likely to experience a breakthrough UTI [48, 49]. More recent studies and reviews have looked for genetic differences and biomarkers that can affect the innate immune system of the bladder, placing certain individuals at greater risk of developing a UTI [39]. Now, with the advent of AI and machine learning in scientific research, we are capable of developing predictive models that can more accurately risk stratify patients and improve care. For example, Bertsimas et al. developed a machine learning model utilizing the RIVUR data and were able to cut the prescription of CAP by more than 50% while still minimizing the risk of recurrent UTIs [50]. Learning from these studies and the rapid advancements in medical research will allow "personalization" in the care of patients with VUR to the optimal therapeutic option.

Conclusion

CAP remains a readily available, minimally invasive, and easily reversible management strategy for children who present with VUR. Several Cochrane and systematic reviews have closely analyzed the existing literature, and while CAP may help decrease the risk of recurrent UTIs in this population, its utility in preventing permanent renal scarring is less certain, though perhaps no less efficacious than more invasive treatments and with the inherent risks of the development of resistance and potential side effects related to the antibiotics. Further analyses of existing studies, as well as the development of new tools for risk stratifying patients with VUR, may ultimately allow for better selection of patients most likely to benefit from CAP, or those at greatest risk of developing recurrent UTIs. A more selective utilization may also help avoid the side effects of long term, low dose antibiotics, both on an individual and population level. We must carefully weigh the risks of antimicrobial side effects and the development of resistant organisms, as it can have significant implications for both the treatment and outcomes seen for these patients, as well as those all over the world.

References

1. Läckgren G, Cooper CS, Neveus T, Kirsch AJ. Management of Vesicoureteral Reflux: what have we learned over the last 20 years? Front Pediatr. 2021;9:650326.
2. Mattoo TK. Vesicoureteral reflux and reflux nephropathy. Adv Chronic Kidney Dis. 2011;18(5):348–54.
3. Xie M, Xu X, Cao Z, Xiao H. Do various treatment modalities of vesicoureteral reflux have any adverse effects in pediatric patients? A meta-analysis. Urol Int. 2021;105(11–12):1002–10.
4. Smellie JM, Prescod NP, Shaw PJ, Risdon RA, Bryant TN. Childhood reflux and urinary infection: a follow-up of 10-41 years in 226 adults. Pediatr Nephrol. 1998;12(9):727–36.
5. Hsu YL, Lin CL, Wei CC. Association between vesicoureteral reflux, urinary tract infection and antibiotics exposure in infancy and risk of childhood asthma. PLoS One. 2021;16(9):e0257531.
6. RIVUR Trial Investigators, Hoberman A, Greenfield SP, et al. Antimicrobial prophylaxis for children with vesicoureteral reflux. N Engl J Med. 2014;370(25):2367–76.
7. Damm T, Mathews R. The RiVUR study outcomes and implications on the management of Vesicoureteral Reflux. Arch Nephrol Ren Stud. 2022;2(1):1–5.
8. Wang HH, Kurtz M, Logvinenko T, Nelson C. Why does prevention of recurrent urinary tract infection not result in less renal scarring? A deeper dive into the RIVUR Trial. J Urol. 2019;202(2):400–5.

9. Autore G, Bernardi L, Ghidini F, et al. Antibiotic prophylaxis for the Prevention of urinary tract infections in children: guideline and recommendations from the Emilia-Romagna Pediatric Urinary Tract Infections (UTI-Ped-ER) Study Group. Antibiotics (Basel). 2023;12(6):1040. Published 2023 Jun 12
10. Williams G, Hodson EM, Craig JC. Interventions for primary vesicoureteric reflux. Cochrane Database Syst Rev. 2019;2(2):CD001532. Published 2019 Feb 20
11. Shaikh N, Mattoo TK, Keren R, et al. Early antibiotic treatment for pediatric febrile urinary tract infection and renal scarring. JAMA Pediatr. 2016;170(9):848–54.
12. Sargent MA. What is the normal prevalence of vesicoureteral reflux? Pediatr Radiol. 2000;30(9):587–93.
13. Hensle TW, Hyun G, Grogg AL, Eaddy M. Part 2: examining pediatric vesicoureteral reflux: a real-world evaluation of treatment patterns and outcomes. Curr Med Res Opin. 2007;23(Suppl 4):S7–S13.
14. Mattoo TK. Are prophylactic antibiotics indicated after a urinary tract infection? Curr Opin Pediatr. 2009;21(2):203–6.
15. Lee T, Park JM. Vesicoureteral reflux and continuous prophylactic antibiotics. Investig Clin Urol. 2017;58(Suppl 1):S32–7.
16. Ammenti A, Alberici I, Brugnara M, et al. Updated Italian recommendations for the diagnosis, treatment and follow-up of the first febrile urinary tract infection in young children. Acta Paediatr. 2020;109(2):236–47.
17. Shish L, Kieran K. Optimal management of continuous antibiotic prophylaxis after initial breakthrough uti in children with vesicoureteral reflux. J Urol. 2021;206:e460–1.
18. Robinson J. Antibiotic prophylaxis in vesicoureteral reflux: a practice revisited. Can Pharm J (Ott). 2013;146(2):84–7.
19. Coulthard MG, Lambert HJ, Vernon SJ, Hunter EW, Keir MJ, Matthews JN. Does prompt treatment of urinary tract infection in preschool children prevent renal scarring: mixed retrospective and prospective audits. Arch Dis Child. 2014;99(4):342–7.
20. Williams G, Craig JC. Long-term antibiotics for preventing recurrent urinary tract infection in children. Cochrane Database Syst Rev. 2019;4(4):CD001534. Published 2019 Apr 1
21. Roussey-Kesler G, Gadjos V, Idres N, et al. Antibiotic prophylaxis for the prevention of recurrent urinary tract infection in children with low grade vesicoureteral reflux: results from a prospective randomized study. J Urol. 2008;179(2):674–9.
22. Su D, Shen Q, Zhai Y, et al. Risk factors for breakthrough urinary tract infection in children with vesicoureteral reflux receiving continuous antibiotic prophylaxis. Transl Pediatr. 2022;11(1):1–9.
23. Brandström P, Nevéus T, Sixt R, Stokland E, Jodal U, Hansson S. The Swedish reflux trial in children: IV. Renal damage. J Urol. 2010;184(1):292–7.
24. Shaikh N, Haralam MA, Kurs-Lasky M, Hoberman A. Association of renal scarring with number of febrile urinary tract infections in children. JAMA Pediatr. 2019;173(10):949–52.
25. Olbing H, Hirche H, Koskimies O, et al. Renal growth in children with severe vesicoureteral reflux: 10-year prospective study of medical and surgical treatment: the International Reflux Study in Children (European branch). Radiology. 2000;216(3):731–7.
26. Jodal U, Smellie JM, Lax H, Hoyer PF. Ten-year results of randomized treatment of children with severe vesicoureteral reflux. Final report of the International Reflux Study in Children. Pediatr Nephrol. 2006;21(6):785–92.
27. Vavilov S, Smith G, Starkey M, Pockney P, Deshpande AV. Parental decision regret in childhood hypospadias surgery: a systematic review. J Paediatr Child Health. 2020;56(10):1514–20.
28. Cooper CS. Fat, demented and stupid: an unrecognized legacy of pediatric urology? J Pediatr Urol. 2017;13(4):341–4.
29. Alberici I, Bayazit AK, Drozdz D, et al. Pathogens causing urinary tract infections in infants: a European overview by the ESCAPE study group. Eur J Pediatr. 2015;174(6):783–90.
30. Esposito S, Maglietta G, Di Costanzo M, et al. Retrospective 8-year study on the antibiotic resistance of uropathogens in children hospitalised for urinary tract infection in the Emilia-Romagna Region, Italy. Antibiotics (Basel). 2021;10(10):1207. Published 2021 Oct 4

31. Dejonckheere Y, Desmet S, Knops N. A study of the 20-year evolution of antimicrobial resistance patterns of pediatric urinary tract infections in a single center. Eur J Pediatr. 2022;181(9):3271–81.
32. Logan LK, Braykov NP, Weinstein RA, Laxminarayan R, CDC Epicenters Prevention Program. Extended-Spectrum β-lactamase-producing and third-generation cephalosporin-resistant Enterobacteriaceae in children: trends in the United States, 1999–2011. J Pediatric Infect Dis Soc. 2014;3(4):320–8.
33. Selekman RE, Shapiro DJ, Boscardin J, et al. Uropathogen resistance and antibiotic prophylaxis: a meta-analysis. Pediatrics. 2018;142(1):e20180119.
34. Wang ME, Lee V, Greenhow TL, et al. Clinical response to discordant therapy in third-generation cephalosporin-resistant UTIs. Pediatrics. 2020;145(2):e20191608.
35. Huemer M, Mairpady Shambat S, Brugger SD, Zinkernagel AS. Antibiotic resistance and persistence-implications for human health and treatment perspectives. EMBO Rep. 2020;21(12):e51034.
36. Strasser C, Spindelboeck W, Kashofer K, Oswald J, Haid B. Low-dose antibiotic prophylaxis has no significant impact on the stability of the intestinal microbiome in children with urogenital tract malformations under 1 year of age. J Pediatr Urol. 2020;16(4):456.e1–7.
37. Akagawa Y, Kimata T, Akagawa S, et al. Impact of long-term low dose antibiotic prophylaxis on gut microbiota in children. J Urol. 2020;204(6):1320–5.
38. Morello W, D'Amico F, Serafinelli J, et al. Low-dose antibiotic prophylaxis induces rapid modifications of the gut microbiota in infants with vesicoureteral reflux. Front Pediatr. 2021;9:674716. Published 2021 Jun 17
39. Sorić Hosman I, Cvitković Roić A, Lamot L. A systematic review of the (un)known host immune response biomarkers for predicting recurrence of urinary tract infection. Front Med (Lausanne). 2022;9:931717. Published 2022 Jul 4
40. Baquero F. Threats of antibiotic resistance: an obliged reappraisal. Int Microbiol. 2021;24(4):499–506.
41. Hsu YL, Lin CL, Wei CC. Association between vesicoureteral reflux, urinary tract infection and antibiotics exposure in infancy and risk of childhood asthma. PLoS One. 2021;16(9):e0257531. Published 2021 Sep 21
42. Suh W, Kim BN, Kang HM, Yang EA, Rhim JW, Lee KY. Febrile urinary tract infection in children: changes in epidemiology, etiology, and antibiotic resistance patterns over a decade. Clin Exp Pediatr. 2021;64(6):293–300.
43. Belachew SA, Hall L, Selvey LA. Non-prescription dispensing of antibiotic agents among community drug retail outlets in Sub-Saharan African countries: a systematic review and meta-analysis. Antimicrob Resist Infect Control. 2021;10(1):13. Published 2021 Jan 14
44. Adhikari B, Pokharel S, Raut S, et al. Why do people purchase antibiotics over-the-counter? A qualitative study with patients, clinicians and dispensers in central, eastern and western Nepal. BMJ Glob Health. 2021;6(5):e005829.
45. Larsson DGJ, Flach CF. Antibiotic resistance in the environment. Nat Rev Microbiol. 2022;20(5):257–69.
46. Martin MJ, Thottathil SE, Newman TB. Antibiotics overuse in animal agriculture: a call to action for health care providers. Am J Public Health. 2015;105(12):2409–10.
47. Kraupner N, Hutinel M, Schumacher K, et al. Evidence for selection of multi-resistant E. Coli by hospital effluent. Environ Int. 2021;150:106436.
48. Cooper CS, Birusingh KK, Austin JC, Knudson MJ, Brophy PD. Distal ureteral diameter measurement objectively predicts vesicoureteral reflux outcome. J Pediatr Urol. 2013;9(1):99–103.
49. Arlen AM, Leong T, Guidos PJ, Alexander SE, Cooper CS. Distal ureteral diameter ratio is predictive of breakthrough febrile urinary tract infection. J Urol. 2017;198(6):1418–23.
50. Bertsimas D, Li M, Estrada C, Nelson C, Scott Wang HH. Selecting children with vesicoureteral reflux who are Most likely to benefit from antibiotic prophylaxis: application of machine learning to RIVUR. J Urol. 2021;205(4):1170–9.

Endoscopic Treatment of Vesicoureteral Reflux

Prem Puri

Abstract Vesicoureteral reflux (VUR) is the most common urological disorder in children, affecting 1–2% of the pediatric population and 30–50% of children presenting with urinary tract infection (UTI). The association of VUR, UTI, and renal parenchymal damage is widely recognized. The introduction of endoscopic treatment of vesicoureteral reflux in the early 1980s was a radical departure from the standard long-term antibiotic prophylaxis and open surgical intervention in the management of VUR in children. Since the approval of dextranomer/hyaluronic acid (Deflux®) by the US Food and Drug Administration (FDA) in 2001 as an acceptable tissue augmenting substance for submucosal injection into the refluxing ureteral orifice, the 15 min day care endoscopic procedure has gained worldwide popularity in the management of VUR in children. Over the years, multiple studies have demonstrated safety and long-term efficacy of this minimally invasive outpatient procedure.

Keywords Vesicoureteral reflux · Urinary tract infections · Reflux nephropathy · Ureter · Voiding cystography · Endoscopic treatment · Dextranomer-hyaluronic acid copolymer · Vantris

Introduction

Vesicoureteral reflux (VUR), the retrograde flow of urine from the bladder into the ureter and collecting system of the kidney, is one of the most common urinary tract abnormalities, affecting approximately 1–2% of the pediatric population, 30–50% of children presenting with urinary tract infection (UTI), and 7–35% of neonates with prenatally detected hydronephrosis [1–3]. The hereditary and familial nature of

P. Puri (✉)
Beacon Consultants Clinic, University College Dublin, Dublin, Ireland

P. Puri, A. Yamataka (eds.), *Vesicoureteral Reflux*,
https://doi.org/10.1007/978-3-031-95091-9_16

VUR is well recognized with an estimated prevalence of 26–50% in screened siblings and up to 66% in offspring of index patients [4–12]. The association of VUR, UTI, and renal parenchymal damage is well established and reflux nephropathy remains a major cause of childhood hypertension, growth impairment, and end-stage renal disease [13, 14]. Therefore, timely intervention is essential in infants and children with VUR in order to reduce the risk of permanent renal injury and to minimize sequelae of reflux nephropathy.

The management of VUR has been controversial. The main goals of treatment of children with VUR are to prevent renal parenchymal damage and prevent urinary tract infections. There are two main treatment approaches: non-surgical and surgical management. The choice of management depends on the presence of renal scars, the clinical course, the grade of VUR, ipsilateral renal function, bilaterality, bladder function, associated anomalies of the urinary tract, age, gender, compliance, side effects of antibiotics, antimicrobial resistance and parental preference [3, 15].

A number of prospective studies have shown that spontaneous resolution of reflux is much less likely in patients with high-grade reflux, presence of renal scarring, or bladder dysfunction, irrespective of observation length [16, 17]. Furthermore, the success of antibacterial treatment for VUR is largely dependent on patient compliance and involves the risk of antibiotic-resistant uropathogens, accompanied by potential breakthrough UTIs [18]. A meta-analysis including 17,972 children with primary reflux has demonstrated a lack of efficacy for continuous antibiotic prophylaxis (CAP) in terms of decreasing the incidence of UTIs and renal parenchymal damage [19].

Various anti-reflux procedures have been described for the surgical correction of VUR. Ureteral reimplantation (open, laparoscopic, or robotic-assisted operations) has a high success rate [3, 15, 19], but these remain invasive procedures that usually require 2–3 days inpatient hospitalization and temporary urinary catheter drainage.

The introduction of endoscopic treatment of vesicoureteral reflux by Puri and O'Donnell was a radical departure from the standard surgical intervention and observational management of VUR [20–22]. VUR was induced in 2–4 weeks old piglets by opening the bladder and slitting the anterior wall of both intravesical ureters and cured by injecting polytetrafluoroethylene (PTFE) paste subureterically. This novel approach created a solid support behind the refluxing intravesical ureter, against which it could be compressed during filling and voiding, recapitulating the effective valve function seen in healthy patients. They called this procedure The STING—that is *s*ubureteric *T*eflon *ing*ection [21]. This innovation brought about a revolution in the surgical management of VUR that has largely stood the test of time with only relatively minor modifications as advances in materials science and our understanding of VUR have progressed [23].

Although the satisfactory long-term results were reported using PTFE for the endoscopic treatment of VUR [24–26], some authors had been concerned by the use of PTFE as the implanted substance because distant migration of PTFE particles after periurethral, periureteral and intravenous injection has been reported in animal studies [27, 28]. Following these reports, Dublin group conducted very detailed studies in dogs and mini-pigs. They reported that there was no distant particle migration following subureteral injection of Teflon on histological examination, polarized light microscopy, scanning electron microscopy and x-ray microanalysis [29, 30]. Despite the convincing long-term outcome, alternatives to PTFE were sought for the endoscopic treatment of VUR because of the possibility of distant particle migration. During the past four decades several other tissue augmenting substances have been used endoscopically to treat VUR including autologous chondrocytes, fat, or heparinised blood, collagen, polydimethylsiloxane (Macroplastique), dextranomer/hyaluronic acid (Dx/HA or Deflux®) and polyacrylate polyalcohol copolymer hydrogel (Vantris) [31].

The greatest paradigm shift in the endoscopic treatment of VUR occurred when the FDA in 2001 approved Deflux® as a biocompatible tissue-augmenting substance for the endoscopic treatment of VUR in children. Now there is a worldwide acceptance that Deflux® is an effective and safe tissue augmenting substance in the endoscopic treatment of VUR. This generated great interest among paediatric urologists, paediatric surgeons and paediatric nephrologists. Currently, Deflux® is the most commonly used tissue augmenting substance for the submucosal injection into the refluxing ureteric orifice. Since the FDA approval of dextranomer/hyaluronic acid (Deflux®) as an acceptable tissue augmenting substance, endoscopic treatment of VUR has gained worldwide popularity and is today an integral part of the American Urological Association guidelines [19] and also the European Association of Urology/European Society of Pediatric Urology guidelines [3, 15] for the management of primary reflux in children. The 15 minute Endoscopic procedure has several advantages. In contrast to long-term antibiotic prophylaxis, it offers immediate cure of reflux, its success does not rely on patient or parent compliance and the procedure is virtually free of complications.

Population-based data from Sweden [23] has shown that the endoscopic treatment has revolutionized the surgical treatment of VUR in recent decades. Currently, almost 90% of the surgical treatment of VUR in Sweden is performed by endoscopic procedures. Furthermore, the number of ureteral reimplantations performed (open or minimally invasive), has decreased to as little as 1/3 the volume performed during the period 1998–2019. At the same time period, the total number of children undergoing endoscopic treatment for VUR was 4 times greater due to the simplicity and lower complication rate of endoscopic procedure. Similar results have been reported from Finland. Ripatti et al. [32] analysed the national trends of surgical treatment of VUR in children in Finland during 2004–2014 and found that 82% of children with VUR were treated by endoscopic procedures and 18% underwent reimplantation of ureters. Endoscopic correction is currently the first-line of treatment for children with grade III–V primary reflux in many institutions worldwide [33–35]. Parental preference has played a major role in the selection of safe and effective outpatient endoscopic procedure compared to long-term antibiotic treatment or ureteral reimplantation [33].

Indications and Contraindications

The indications for endoscopic treatment of VUR are the same as for open, laparoscopic, or robotic-assisted anti-reflux surgery. These include high-grade VUR, breakthrough UTIs on CAP, noncompliance with CAP, and new renal scarring. In recent years we and many other centres have offered endoscopic correction as the first line of treatment to all patients with grade III-V VUR [33–35]. In contrast to continuous antibiotic prophylaxis, this procedure offers immediate cure with resolution rates ranging from 77%–83% after the first injection and is independent of patient or parent compliance [33]. It is an efficient and safe long-term option also for grade IV and V VUR with success rates of 70% after the first injection, which can be easily repeated in cases of failure with a high subsequent resolution rate [33, 36, 37].

In addition to primary reflux, endoscopic injection therapy has been used successfully to treat VUR in duplex renal systems, VUR secondary to neuropathic bladder or posterior urethral valves, VUR in failed reimplanted ureters, VUR following renal transplantation and VUR in refluxing ureteral stumps.

The only accepted contraindications for endoscopic correction of VUR are obstructive refluxing megaureters and VUR with large bladder diverticula measuring greater than 10-15 mm.

Instruments, Equipment, and Materials

All common pediatric cystoscopes, straight or angled working channel, can be used for this procedure. The disposable Puri flexible catheter for injection (STORZ) is a 4F catheter onto which is swaged a 21-gauge needle that protrudes approximately 1 cm from the catheter. Alternatively, a semirigid, metal needle can be used. Since the first description of endoscopic treatment of VUR in the early 1980s, various tissue augmenting substances have been used, but currently only Deflux® is approved by the FDA. Copolymer Deflux®, the most commonly used bulking agent today, is a viscous gel consisting of 80–250 μm dextranomer microspheres (50 mg/mL) in a stabilized hyaluronic acid carrier solution of nonanimal origin (15 mg/mL), which is available in 1-mL prefilled syringes that can be attached to any type of injection catheter. Since 2001, the author has only used Deflux® for the endoscopic correction of VUR. It is easier to inject and, clinically and radiologically, gives better protection against UTIs and a better VUR cure rate compared to other tissue augmenting substances [33, 38, 39].

Injection Techniques

Over the years, several injection techniques have been described for the endoscopic treatment of VUR including subureteric injection (STING) [21, 22], intraureteric hydrodistention implantation technique (HIT) [40], combined HIT/STING, and double HIT (i.e., proximal and distal intraluminal submucosal injections) [41]. Subureteric injection (STING), described by Puri in 1984 is the most adopted technique worldwide, whereas double HIT is the most performed technique for endoscopic correction of VUR in the United States [33, 42].

STING Procedure

Endoscopic correction of VUR is performed under general anesthesia with the patient placed in lithotomy position toward the end of the operating table. After insertion into the urethra, the cystoscope is slowly advanced to allow detailed inspection of bladder wall, trigone, bladder neck, and both ureteric orifices. The bladder should be almost empty before proceeding with the injection, since this helps to keep the refluxing orifice flat rather than away in a lateral part of the field. The injection should not begin until the operator has a clear view all around the affected orifice.

The needle is introduced 2–3 mm below the refluxing orifice at the 6 o'clock position into the bladder mucosa and advanced for approximately 4–5 mm into the submucosal portion of the distal ureter (Fig. 1a). However, in children with grade IV and V reflux with a wide ureteric orifice, the needle should be inserted directly into the affected orifice to increase the length of the intravesical ureter. It is important to introduce the needle with pinpoint accuracy before starting the injection as any perforation of the mucosa or the ureter may allow the injected material to escape, which may result in failure. As the tissue augmenting substance is administrated, a bulge slowly starts to appear at the floor of the submucosal ureter (Fig. 1b). While the injection is in progress, the needle is gradually withdrawn until a "volcanic" bulge of implant is seen (Fig. 1c). Depending on the bulking agent, most refluxing ureters require not more than 0.4–1.0 mL to correct VUR with this technique. In general, a correctly placed injection creates the appearance of a nipple, on top of which sits a slit-like or inverted crescentic orifice (Fig. 2a–c). If the bulge appears in an incorrect place, e.g., at the side of the ureter or proximal to it, the needle should not be withdrawn. Instead, it should be moved so that the point is in a more favourable position. The non-injected ureteric roof usually retains its compliance while preventing reflux.

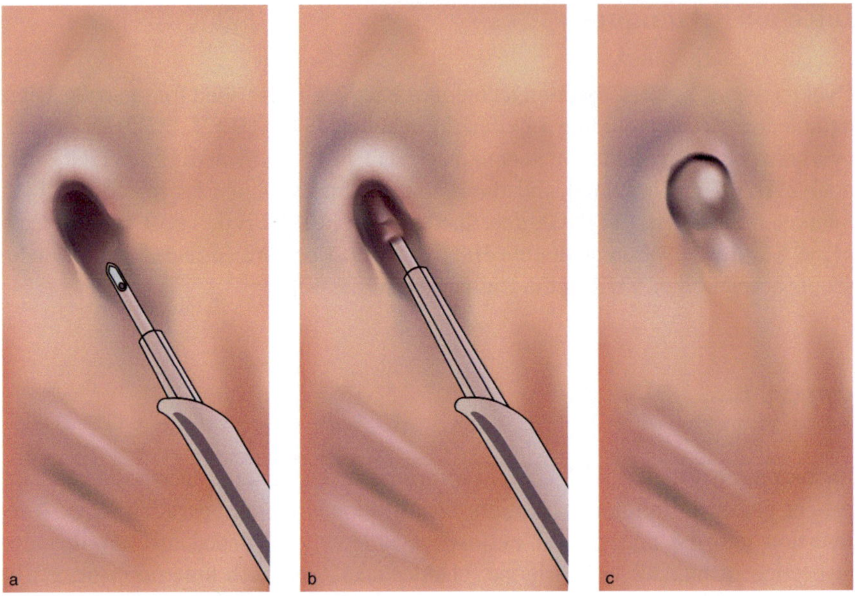

Fig. 1 Technique of STING procedure. (**a**) Site of placement of needle. (**b**) Injection in progress. (c) Slit-like orifice at the completion of injection

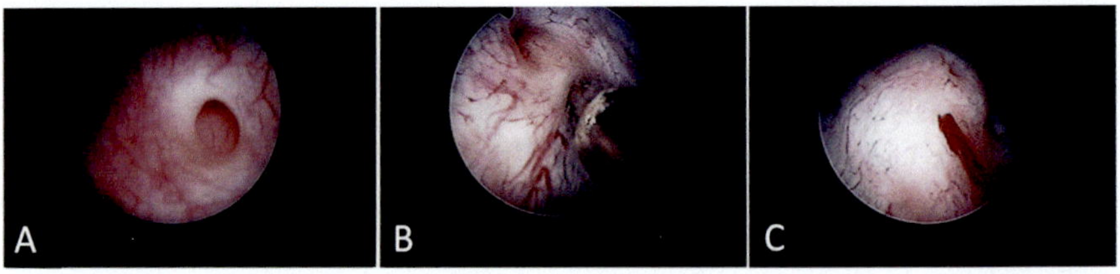

Fig. 2 (**a**) Endoscopic appearance of a grade V refluxing ureteral orifice prior to injection. (**b**) The needle is introduced 2–3 mm below the refluxing ureteral orifice at 6 o'clock position and as the tissue augmenting substance is administered, a bulge starts to appear at the floor of the submucosal ureter. (**c**) A correctly placed injection creates the appearance of a nipple, on the top of which is a slit-like orifice

Ureteric Hydrodistention and Intraluminal Submucosal Injection

For the HIT, the bladder is semi-filled to allow for good visualization of the affected orifice and to avoid tension within the submucosal layer of the ureter secondary to overdistension. Hydrodistention of the refluxing orifice is initiated to define the injection site within the ureteric tunnel. The needle is inserted approximately 4 mm into the submucosa of the intramural ureter at the 6 o'clock position. At this point, irrigation should be stopped while the tissue augmenting substance is injected. Again, only a small volume of 0.5–1.0 mL is needed to create a sufficient bolus, and the ureteric tunnel should coapt with the injection. The cystoscope is then pulled back toward the bladder neck to visualize the full implantation. At end of the procedure, the affected orifice should no longer hydrodistend, indicating complete coaptation of both the ureteric tunnel and orifice. If the latter does not completely coapt with a single intraureteral injection, a second more proximal injection (i.e., double HIT) may be contemplated, or a subureteral implantation (i.e., combined HIT/STING) can be performed.

Although most multivariate analyses have failed to demonstrate a significant difference in outcomes between the STING procedure and HIT [43–45], a meta-analysis showed that the overall resolution of VUR with the STING technique was 71.4%, whereas it was 82.5% with the HIT [46]. However, a large series from Russia including 4898 ureters identified a significantly higher incidence of postoperative obstruction of the ureterovesical junction when comparing HIT (1.6%) to STING procedure (0.5%) [47]. A range of factors have been shown to influence the resolution rate with endoscopic injection including high grade of VUR, injection technique, surgeon's experience, patient age, and the extent of renal scarring at time of treatment [48].

Postoperative Care

The vast majority of infants and children with VUR can be treated as day cases. Postoperatively, patients are usually able to void without any problems after recovery from general anesthesia. Antibiotic prophylaxis should be continued until voiding cystourethrogram (VCUG), and renal ultrasonography is performed 6–12 weeks after the procedure. Antibiotics can be stopped if the VCUG demonstrated resolution of reflux (Fig. 3). Nevertheless, a patient should be considered for further endoscopic treatment if VUR has not resolved. It is recommended that following successful endoscopic correction of VUR, renal and bladder ultrasound is repeated at 1–2 year intervals to monitor the appearance of the urinary tract as well as the site and size of the injected implant.

Traditionally, postoperative VCUG following endoscopic injection for VUR was recommended [34–36]. In recent years, many centres, due to the concern of high ionizing radiation and traumatic experience for the child during VCUG, recommend an ultrasound 2–3 months after endoscopic correction of VUR and stop antibiotic prophylaxis. The VCUG is performed only after recurrent febrile UTIs.

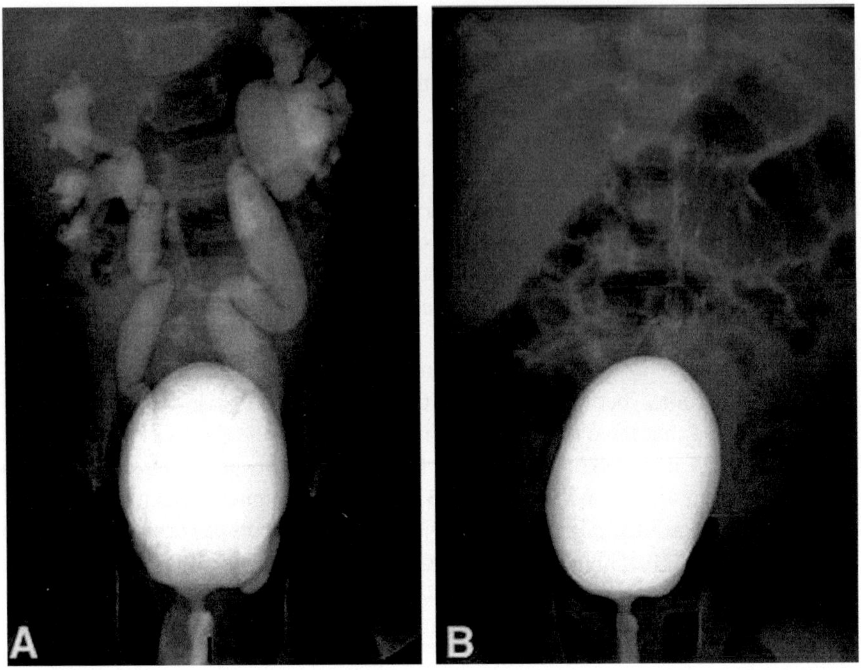

Fig. 3 (**a**) Voiding cystogram showing bilateral high grade VUR. (**b**) Voiding cystogram in the same child showing resolution of VUR 3 months after the procedure

Complications and Outcomes

Clinical data from numerous studies have confirmed long-term safety and efficacy of endoscopic injection. If performed correctly, endoscopic treatment of VUR is a safe procedure, and postoperative complications are rare [34, 36, 49–51].

Persistent or Recurrent Reflux

The only significant problem with endoscopic correction of VUR has been failure in some patients and who needed a repeat injection. A meta-analysis including 5527 patients with VUR calculated resolution rates of 78.5% for grades I and II, 72% for grade III, 63% for grade IV, and 51% for grade V after endoscopic therapy with an aggregate success rate of 85% following one or more injections [52]. Another systematic review of 47 articles reported similar results [53]. Furthermore, a randomized trial, the Swedish reflux trial revealed that outcomes following endoscopic treatment were significantly better than the spontaneous resolution rate or downgrading in the prophylaxis and surveillance groups but recurrent VUR was seen in 20% after 2 years [54]. A single-centre study of 1551 children with intermediate and high-grade reflux that underwent endoscopic Deflux® injection demonstrated that VUR persisted in less than 13% of cases and was subsequently eradicated following a second or third injection [34]. These findings suggest that results can be improved by simply repeating the procedure, thus being as effective as ureteral reimplantation as shown by a randomized clinical trial [55]. The results depend on the grade of VUR, with lower efficiency in grade V and bilateral VUR cases [44, 52]. Recently, Friedmacher and Puri [36] reported results of endoscopic treatment in grade IV and V reflux. VUR resolution rate after the first endoscopic injection was 70.4% for grade IV and 61.9% for grade V cases. Reflux resolved after a second injection in 20.1% and after a third injection in 10.4%.

The success rate of endoscopic treatment is lower for VUR in complete duplex ureters and neurogenic bladder compared to single system primary VUR. However, the simplicity of the endoscopic procedure makes it highly desirable first line of treatment for these complex cases of VUR. A meta-analysis reported a lower overall success rate in ureteral duplication (50%) rather than in single systems (73%) regardless of VUR grade [52]. However, more recent studies reported better success rates. Molitierno et al. [56] reported that VUR resolved in duplex systems after first injection in 73% of cases and in 85% after second injection. Hunziker et al. [57] evaluated the effectiveness of endoscopic injection of dextranomer/hyaluronic acid in intermediate and high grade vesicoureteral reflux in patients with complete duplex collecting systems. Vesicoureteral reflux resolved after the first endoscopic injection in 93 ureters (68.4%), after a second injection in 35 (25.7%) and after a third injection in 8 (5.9%).

Endoscopic treatment is beginning to become more popular in VUR in neurogenic bladder, especially when combined with intravesical botulinum toxin A injections [58]. Success rates with endoscopic subureteral injection of Deflux® in neurogenic bladder patients has been reported at anywhere from 53% to 86% [59, 60].

Urinary Tract Infections After Successful Endoscopic Correction of VUR

The main goals of treatment of children with VUR are to prevent renal parenchymal damage and morbidity associated with recurrent UTIs. Relative few studies have examined the incidence of febrile UTIs after successful resolution of VUR with endoscopic injection. Elder et al. [61] reported reduced number of UTIs per year after endoscopic treatment with Dx/HA vs antibiotic prophylaxis (0.08 vs 0.28), supporting a role for Dx/HA as first-line treatment option for patients with VUR. Swedish trial [62] demonstrated that the rate of febrile UTIs was lower with endoscopic treatment (23%) compared to surveillance (57%) but did not differ between endoscopic treatment (23%) and antibiotic prophylaxis (19%). However, a higher incidence of recurrent febrile UTIs was noted in girls than in boys after successful reflux correction. Hunziker et al. [39] conducted a long-term follow-up (mean follow-up 7.6 years) of incidence of febrile urinary tract infections in 1271 consecutive children after successful endoscopic correction of intermediate and high grade VUR. The authors found that 5.7% of children developed febrile UTIs after correction of VUR and predominantly were girls, all of whom had bladder bowel dysfunction.

Obstruction of the Ureterovesical Junction

Early and delayed ureteral obstructions have been reported following endoscopic correction of VUR. Friedmacher and Puri [51] conducted a literature search to determine the incidence of ureteral obstruction after endoscopic correction of VUR using various different tissue augmenting substances. There were 96 patients (64 females and 32 males) who developed ureteral obstruction (UO) after endoscopic treatment of VUR. The authors found UO to be a rare complication after endoscopic correction of VUR, occurring in less than 1% of treated cases, and appears to be independent of the injected substance, volume, and technique. UO can develop immediately following the procedure or as long as 63 months later [63, 64], emphasizing the need for long-term follow-up as asymptomatic or delayed cases may cause deterioration of renal function. Acute UO may occur due to increased resistance at the ureterovesical junction caused by the implant itself or injection in the wrong tissue plane [65, 66]. Several potential mechanisms, which could explain the occurrence of late-onset or progressive UO, have been suggested: gradual increase of resistance at the ureterovesical junction, ineffective ureteral peristalsis, and coaptation or chronic inflammation [66]. Furthermore, mound calcifications of various tissue augmenting substances at the injection site have been described which may predispose to UO [67–70].

Conclusions

The 40 years' experience with endoscopic correction of VUR has demonstrated that this outpatient procedure is safe, effective, and has had a much less negative impact on patients than any other surgical technique to treat reflux [23]. Endoscopic correction is currently the first-line of treatment for children with grade III–V primary reflux and complex cases of VUR in many institutions worldwide because of the simplicity of the procedure [33–35, 56, 57]. In contrast to CAP, this procedure offers immediate cure with resolution rates ranging from 77 to 83% [19, 53, 71] and is independent of patient or parent compliance. It is an efficient and safe long-term option for grade IV and V VUR with success rates of 70% after the first injection, which can be easily repeated in cases of failure with a high subsequent resolution rate [36, 37]. Endoscopic treatment is also safe and highly effective in eradicating high-grade VUR in infants, a vulnerable group to develop renal parenchymal damage [72–74]. Furthermore, parental preferences, opinion of the nephrologist/pediatric urologist and the treating hospital play a major role in the selection of endoscopic treatment over the traditional methods of CAP or ureteral reimplantation [71, 75–78]. Further studies with standardized outcome reporting and follow-up are needed to evaluate predictors, technical factors, and long-term durability of the success of endoscopic treatment of VUR.

References

1. Smellie JM, Barratt TM, Chantler C, et al. Medical versus surgical treatment in children with severe bilateral vesicoureteric reflux and bilateral nephropathy: a randomised trial. Lancet. 2001;357(9265):1329–33.
2. Hoberman A, Charon M, Hickey RW, et al. Imaging studies after a first febrile urinary tract infection in young children. N Engl J Med. 2003;348(3):195–202.
3. Gnech M, Hoen L, Zachou A, Bogaert G, Castagnetti, O'Kelly F, et al. Update and summary of the European Association of Urology/ European Society of Pediatric Urology Paediatric guidelines on vesicoureteral reflux in children. Eur Urol. 2024;85:433–42.
4. Noe HN. The long-term results of prospective sibling reflux screening. J Urol. 1992;148(5 Pt 2):1739–42.
5. Aggarwal VK, Verrier Jones K. Vesicoureteric reflux: screening of first degree relatives. Arch Dis Child. 1989;64(11):1538–41.
6. Parekh DJ, Pope JCIV, Adams MC, et al. Outcome of sibling vesicoureteral reflux. J Urol. 2002;167(1):283–4.
7. Chertin B, Puri P. Familial vesicoureteral reflux. J Urol. 2003;169:1804–8.
8. Hunziker M, Colhoun E, Puri P. Renal cortical abnormalities in siblings of index patients with vesicoureteral reflux. Pediatrics. 2014;133(4):e933–7.
9. Eccles MR, Bailey RR, Abbott GD, et al. Unravelling the genetics of vesicoureteric reflux: a common familial disorder. Hum Mol Genet. 1996;5 Spec No:1425–9.
10. Noe HN, Wyatt RJ, Peeden JN, et al. The transmission of vesicoureteral reflux from parent to child. J Urol. 1992;148(6):1869–71.
11. Scott JE, Swallow V, Coulthard MG, et al. Screening of newborn babies for familial ureteric reflux. Lancet. 1997;350(9075):396–400.
12. Scoog SJ, Peters CA, Arant BS Jr, et al. Pediatric vesicouretral reflux guidelines panel summary report: clinical practice guidelines for screening siblingsof children with vesicoureteral reflux and neonates/ infants with prenatal hydronephrosis. J Urol. 2010;184:1145–51.
13. Diamond DA, Mattoo TK. Endoscopic treatment of primary vesicoureteral reflux. N Engl J Med. 2012;366(13):1218–26.
14. Brandström P, Nevéus T, Sixt R, Stokland E, Jodal U, Hansson S. The Swedish reflux trial in children: IV. Renal damage. J Urol. 2010a;184(1):292–7.
15. Tekgul S, Riedmiller H, Hoebeke P, Kocvara R, Nijman RJ, Radmayr C, et al. EAU guidelines on vesicoureteral reflux in children. Eur Urol. 2012;62(3):534–42.
16. Knudson MJ, Austin JC, McMillan ZM, Hawtrey CE, Cooper CS. Predictive factors of early spontaneous resolution in children with primary vesicoureteral reflux. J Urol. 2007;178(4 Pt 2):1684–8.
17. Sjöström S, Sillén U, Jodal U, Sameby L, Sixt R, Stokland E. Predictive factors for resolution of congenital high grade vesicoureteral reflux in infants: results of univariate and multivariate analyses. J Urol. 2010;183(3):1177–84.

18. Cara-Fuentes G, Gupta N, Garin EH. The RIVUR study: a review of its findings. Pediatr Nephrol. 2015;30(5):703–6.
19. Peters CA, Skoog SJ, Arant BS Jr, Copp HL, Elder JS, Hudson RG, et al. Summary of the AUA guideline on management of primary vesicoureteral reflux in children. J Urol. 2010;184(3):1134–44.
20. Puri P, O'Donnell B. Correction of experimentally produced vesicoureteric reflux in the piglet by intravesical injection of Teflon. Br Med J (Clin Res Ed). 1984;289:5–7.
21. O'Donnell B, Puri P. Treatment of vesicoureteric reflux by endoscopic injection of Teflon. Br Med J (Clin Res Ed). 1984;289(6436):7–9.
22. Puri P. Endoscopic correction of primary vesicoureteric reflux by subureteric injection of polytetrafluoroethylene. Lancet. 1990;335:1320–2.
23. Kutasy B, Coyle D. History of endoscopic treatment of vesicoureteral reflux. Pediatr Surg Int. 2023;39:187.
24. Puri P. Ten year experience with subureteric Teflon (polytetrafluoroethylene) injection (STING) in the treatment of vesico-ureteric reflux. Br J Urol. 1995;75(2):126–31.
25. Chertin B, Colhoun E, Velayudham M, Puri P. Endoscopic treatment of vesicoureteral reflux: 11 to 17 years of follow-up. J Urol. 2002;167(3):1443–5.
26. Yücel S, Tarcan T, Simşek F. Durability of a single successful endoscopic polytetrafluoroethylene injection for primary vesicoureteral reflux: 14-year follow up results. J Urol. 2007;178(1):265–8.
27. Malizia AA Jr, Reiman HM, Myers RP, Sande JR, Barham SS, Benson RC Jr, et al. Migration and granulomatous reaction after periurethral injection of polytef (Teflon). JAMA. 1984;251(24):3277–81.
28. Aaronson IA, Rames RA, Greene WB, Walsh LG, Hasal UA, Garen PD. Endoscopic treatment of reflux: migration of Teflon to the lungs and brain. Eur Urol. 1993;23(3):394–9.
29. Miyakita H, Puri P. Particles found in lung and brain following subureteral injection of polytetrafluoroethylene paste are not Teflon particles. J Urol. 1994;152(2):636–40.
30. Miyakita H, O'Briain DS, Puri P. Absence of brain parenchymal damage following intravascular injection of polytetrafluoroethylene paste. Eur Urol. 1998;34(3):233–6.
31. Friedmacher F, Puri P. Endoscopic treatment of vesicoureral reflux. In: Puri P, editor. Pediatric surgery. Berlin: Springer Nature; 2023. p. 299–307.
32. Ripatti L, Viljamaa HR, Kauko T, et al. Trends in the surgical management of vesicoureteral reflux in Finland in 2004-2014. Scand J Urol. 2021;55:67–71.
33. Escolino M, Kaffa N, Castagnetti M, et al. Endoscopic injection of bulking agents in pediatric vesicoureteral reflux: a narrative review of literature. Pediatr Surg Int. 2023;39:133.
34. Puri P, Kutasy B, Colhoun E, Hunziker M. Single center experience with endoscopic subureteral dextranomer/hyaluronic acid injection as first line treatment in 1,551 children with intermediate and high grade vesicoureteral reflux. J Urol. 2012;188(4 Suppl):1485–9.
35. Puri P, Pirker M, Mohanan N, Dawrant M, Dass L, Colhoun E. Subureteral dextranomer/hyaluronic acid injection as first line treatment in the management of high grade vesicoureteral reflux. J Urol. 2006;176(4 Pt 2):1856–9.
36. Friedmacher F, Colhoun E, Puri P. Endoscopic injection of Dextranomer/hyaluronic acid as first line treatment in 851 consecutive children with high grade vesicoureteral reflux: efficacy and long-term results. J Urol. 2018;200(3):650–5.
37. Stenbäck A, Olafsdottir T, Sköldenberg E, Barker G, Stenberg A, Läckgren G. Proprietary non-animal stabilized hyaluronic acid/dextranomer gel (NASHA/Dx) for endoscopic treatment of grade IV vesicoureteral reflux: long-term observational study. J Pediatr Urol. 2020;16(3):328.e1–9.
38. Stredele RJ, Dietz HG, Stehr M. Long-term results of endoscopic treatment of vesicoureteral reflux in children: comparison of different bulking agents. J Pediatr Urol. 2013;9(1):71–6.
39. Hunziker M, Mohanan N, D'Asta F, Puri P. Incidence of febrile urinary tract infections in children after successful endoscopic treatment of vesicoureteral reflux: a long-term follow-up. J Pediatr. 2012;160(6):1015–20.

40. Kirsch AJ, Perez-Brayfield M, Smith EA, Scherz HC. The modified sting procedure to correct vesicoureteral reflux: improved results with submucosal implantation within the intramural ureter. J Urol. 2004;171(6 Pt 1):2413–6.
41. Kirsch AJ, Arlen AM. Evaluation of new Deflux administration techniques: intraureteric HIT and double HIT for the endoscopic correction of vesicoureteral reflux. Expert Rev Med Devices. 2014;11(5):439–46.
42. Kirsch AJ, Arlen AM, Lackgren G. Current trends in dextranomer hyaluronic acid copolymer (Deflux) injection technique for endoscopic treatment of vesicoureteral reflux. Urology. 2014;84(2):462–8.
43. Yucel S, Gupta A, Snodgrass W. Multivariate analysis of factors predicting success with dextranomer/hyaluronic acid injection for vesicoureteral reflux. J Urol. 2007;177(4):1505–9.
44. Routh JC, Reinberg Y, Ashley RA, Inman BA, Wolpert JJ, Vandersteen DR, et al. Multivariate comparison of the efficacy of intraureteral versus subtrigonal techniques of dextranomer/hyaluronic acid injection. J Urol. 2007;178(4 Pt 2):1702–5.
45. Watters ST, Sung J, Skoog SJ. Endoscopic treatment for vesicoureteral reflux: how important is technique? J Pediatr Urol. 2013;9(6 Pt B):1192–7.
46. Yap TL, Chen Y, Nah SA, Ong CC, Jacobsen A, Low Y. STING versus HIT technique of endoscopic treatment for vesicoureteral reflux: a systematic review and meta-analysis. J Pediatr Surg. 2016;51(12):2015–20.
47. Baybikov R, Sizonov V, Bondarenko S, Dolgov B, Dubrov V, Kagantsov I, et al. Do the type of bulking agents and injection method have any influence on the incidence of ureteral obstruction by endoscopic treatment of reflux? J Pediatr Urol. 2015;11(Suppl 4)
48. Lackgren G, Cooper CS, Neveus T, Kirsch AJ. Management of vesicoureteral reflux: what have we learned over the last 20 years? Front Pediatr. 2021;9:650326. https://doi.org/10.3389/fped.2021.650326. eCollection 2021. PMID: 33869117
49. Hsieh MH, Madden-Fuentes RJ, Lindsay NE, Roth DR. Treatment of pediatric vesicoureteral reflux using endoscopic injection of hyaluronic acid/dextranomer gel: intermediate-term experience by a single surgeon. Urology. 2010a;76(1):199–203.
50. Läckgren G, Wåhlin N, Sköldenberg E, Stenberg A. Long-term followup of children treated with dextranomer/hyaluronic acid copolymer for vesicoureteral reflux. J Urol. 2001;166(5):1887–92.
51. Friedmacher F, Puri P. Ureteral obstruction after endoscopic treatment of vesicoureteral reflux: does the type of injected bulking agent matter? Curr Urol Rep. 2019;20(9):49.
52. Elder JS, Diaz M, Caldamone AA, Cendron M, Greenfield S, Hurwitz R, et al. Endoscopic therapy for vesicoureteral reflux: a meta-analysis. I. Reflux resolution and urinary tract infection. J Urol. 2006;175(2):716–22.
53. Routh JC, Inman BA, Reinberg Y. Dextranomer/hyaluronic acid for pediatric vesicoureteral reflux: systematic review. Pediatrics. 2010a;125(5):1010–9.
54. Holmdahl G, Brandström P, Läckgren G, Sillén U, Stokland E, Jodal U, et al. The Swedish reflux trial in children: II. Vesicoureteral reflux outcome. J Urol. 2010;184(1):280–5.
55. García-Aparicio L, Rovira J, Blazquez-Gomez E, García-García L, Giménez-Llort A, Rodo J, et al. Randomized clinical trial comparing endoscopic treatment with dextranomer hyaluronic acid copolymer and Cohen's ureteral reimplantation for vesicoureteral reflux: long-term results. J Pediatr Urol. 2013a;9(4):483–7.
56. Molitierno JA Jr, Scherz HC, Kirsch AJ. Endoscopic injection of dextranomer hyaluronic acid copolymer for the treatment of vesicoureteral reflux in duplex ureters. J Pediatr Urol. 2008;4(5):372–6.
57. Hunziker M, Mohanan N, Puri P. Dextranomer/hyaluronic acid endoscopic injection is effective in the treatment of intermediate and high grade vesicoureteral reflux in patients with complete duplex systems. J Urol. 2013;189(5):1876–81.
58. Wu CQ. Franco I management of vesicoureteral reflux in neurogenic bladder. Investig Clin Urol. 2017;58(Suppl 1):S54–8. https://doi.org/10.4111/icu.2017.58.S1.S54. Epub 2017 Jun 2. PMID: 2861206

59. Engel JD, Palmer LS, Cheng EY, Kaplan WE. Surgical versus endoscopic correction of vesicoureteral reflux in children with neurogenic bladder dysfunction. J Urol. 1997;157:2291–4.
60. Perez-Brayfield M, Kirsch AJ, Hensle TW, Koyle MA, Furness P, Scherz HC. Endoscopic treatment with dextranomer/hyaluronic acid for complex cases of vesicoureteral reflux. J Urol. 2004;172(4 Pt 2):1614–6.
61. Elder JS, Shah MB, Batiste LR, Eaddy M. Part 3: endoscopic injection versus antibiotic prophylaxis in the reduction of urinary tract infections in patients with vesicoureteral reflux. Curr Med Res Opin. 2007;23(Suppl 4):S15–20.
62. Brandström P, Esbjörner E, Herthelius M, Swerkersson S, Jodal U, Hansson S. The Swedish reflux trial in children: III urinary tract infection pattern. J Urol. 2010;184(1):286–91.
63. García-Aparicio L, Rodo J, Palazon P, Martín O, Blázquez-Gómez E, Manzanares A, et al. Acute and delayed vesicoureteral obstruction after endoscopic treatment of primary vesicoureteral reflux with dextranomer/hyaluronic acid copolymer: why and how to manage. J Pediatr Urol. 2013b;9(4):493–7.
64. Rubenwolf PC, Ebert AK, Ruemmele P, Rösch WH. Delayed-onset ureteral obstruction after endoscopic dextranomer/hyaluronic acid copolymer (Deflux) injection for treatment of vesicoureteral reflux in children: a case series. Urology. 2013;81(3):659–62.
65. Ben-Meir D, Morgenstern S, Sivan B, Efrat R, Livne PM. Histology proved malpositioning of dextranomer/hyaluronic acid in submucosal ureter in patients after failed endoscopic treatment of vesicoureteral reflux. J Urol. 2012;188(1):258–61.
66. Ben-Meir D, Bahouth Z, Halachmi S. Late-onset Uretero-vesical junction obstruction following endoscopic injection of bulking material for the treatment of Vesico-ureteral reflux. Urology. 2017;101:60–2.
67. Gargollo PC, Paltiel HJ, Rosoklija I, Diamond DA. Mound calcification after endoscopic treatment of vesicoureteral reflux with autologous chondrocytes–a normal variant of mound appearance? J Urol. 2009;181(6):2702–7.
68. Noe HN. Calcification in a Deflux bleb thought to be a ureteral calculus in a child. J Pediatr Urol. 2008;4(1):88–9.
69. Nepple KG, Knudson MJ, Cooper CS, Austin JC. Symptomatic calcification of subureteral collagen ten years after injection. Urology. 2007;69(5):982.e1–2.
70. Palagiri AV, Dangle PP. Distal ureteral calcification secondary to deflux injection: a reality or myth? Urology. 2011;77(5):1217–9.
71. Routh JC, Nelson CP, Graham DA, Lieu TA. Variation in surgical management of vesicoureteral reflux: influence of hospital and patient factors. Pediatrics. 2010b;125(3):e446–51.
72. Puri P, Mohanan N, Menezes M, Colhoun E. Endoscopic treatment of moderate and high grade vesicoureteral reflux in infants using dextranomer/hyaluronic acid. J Urol. 2007;178(4 Pt 2):1714–6. discussion 1717
73. Fuentes S, Gómez-Fraile A, Carrillo-Arroyo I, Tordable-Ojeda C, Cabezalí-Barbancho D. Endoscopic treatment of vesicoureteral reflux in infants. Can we do it and should we do it? Urology. 2017;110:196–200.
74. Al Hindi S, Mubarak M, Al AH. High-grade vesicoureteral reflux in infants: our experience with endoscopicsubureteric injections. Urologia. 2022;89(1):120–5.
75. Ogan K, Pohl HG, Carlson D, Belman AB, Rushton HG. Parental preferences in the management of vesicoureteral reflux. J Urol. 2001;166(1):240–3.
76. Capozza N, Lais A, Matarazzo E, Nappo S, Patricolo M, Caione P. Treatment of vesico-ureteric reflux: a new algorithm based on parental preference. BJU Int. 2003;92(3):285–8.
77. Hsieh MH, Madden-Fuentes RJ, Bayne A, Munch E, Wildenfels P, Alexander SJ, et al. Cross-sectional evaluation of parental decision making factors for vesicoureteral reflux management in children. J Urol. 2010b;184(4 Suppl):1589–93.
78. Puri P, Friedmacher F, Farrugia MK, Sharma S, Esposito C, Mattoo T. Primary vesicoureteral reflux. Nat Rev Dis Primers. 2024;10(1):75.

Endoscopic Treatment for Complex Cases of Vesicoureteral Reflux

Andrew J. Kirsch, Benjamin H. Press, and Angela M. Arlen

Abstract Non-animal stabilized hyaluronic acid/dextranomer gel was developed as a treatment for vesicoureteral reflux (VUR) in the 1990s. Safety and efficacy of endoscopic injection for the management of primary VUR has been well established and well-studied. While endoscopic therapy is highly effective for the treatment of most primary VUR, its efficacy in cases of structural/functional bladder anomalies is not as well established. These "complex cases" of VUR (e.g., high-grade VUR, duplicated systems, the adult population, and kidney transplant ureters) have historically not been deemed suitable candidates for endoscopic therapy. While resolution rates may be lower complex cases when compared to primary VUR, more contemporary evidence suggests that the success rates are high enough to support the use of endoscopic injection in the management of VUR in this patient population.

Keywords Endoscopic injection · Dx/HA · Vesicoureteral reflux · Urinary tract infection · Voiding cystourethrogram

Introduction

As medical technology and surgical techniques have advanced, so too have the broadened indications for minimally invasive approaches within pediatric urology. Today, minimally invasive approaches have become standard practice for many commonly performed pediatric urologic procedures. Within the field of pediatric urology, management of vesicoureteral reflux (VUR) best captures the transition to minimally invasive approaches. Endoscopic injection has reported widespread use in the last two decades for treatment of pediatric VUR, becoming a valid alternative

A. J. Kirsch (✉) · B. H. Press
Department of Pediatric Urology, Emory University and Children's Healthcare of Atlanta, Atlanta, GA, USA

A. M. Arlen
Department of Urology, Yale School of Medicine, Yale University New Haven, CT, USA

P. Puri, A. Yamataka (eds.), *Vesicoureteral Reflux*,
https://doi.org/10.1007/978-3-031-95091-9_17

to open surgery and continuous antibiotic prophylaxis. Endoscopic correction is minimally invasive, well tolerated, and provides cure rates approaching those of open surgery [1]. Based on proven benefits of endoscopic injection, open surgery has been challenged as the "gold standard" for anti-reflux surgery [2, 3]. In fact, the rate of open surgery has consistently decreased over the past 20 years [4]. Despite these trends, open surgery may still be a preferred approach, particularly in young children with complex ureteral anatomy and refluxing megaureter.

Clinical data from numerous studies have confirmed long-term safety and efficacy of endoscopic injection, though there is significant variation depending on surgeons and technique [5, 6] on the ultimate success rates. In a systematic review evaluating dextranomer/hyaluronic acid (Dx/HA) for pediatric VUR, the estimated aggregate success rate for endoscopic therapy, prior to widespread use of the double HIT method, was 72% with 89% success for grade I, 83% for grade II, 71% for grade III, 59% for IV and 62% for grade V reflux [5]. More recently, a meta-analysis, including nine studies and more than 1400 renal units, the authors found no differences in UTIs for patients undergoing endoscopic management than vesicoureteral reimplantation for high grade VUR (grades III-V) [7]. While endoscopic therapy is highly effective for the treatment of most primary VUR using the double HIT method [8], its efficacy in cases of structural/functional bladder anomalies is not as well established. This chapter will outline evidence that endoscopic injection is also effective in specific patient populations that were historically not considered for endoscopic therapy, or complex cases of VUR.

Re-Operation After Failed Ureteral Reimplantation

Technical rates of ureteral reimplantation are exceptionally high, but there are a small subset who do fail. Most cases of persistent VUR following reimplantation resolve spontaneously [9, 10]. In those that do not resolve, reoperation can be technically challenging and it risks ischemic ureteral injury. Endoscopic injection has been shown to be successful in cases of failed ureteral reimplantation, at least in short term follow-up. A multi-institutional cohort of 17 patients with recurrent UTI despite prophylactic antibiotics and persistent VUR following ureteral reimplantation underwent single injection of Dx/HA. Results of this study demonstrated an 88% radiographic success rate, defined as no VUR on post-procedure VCUG at 3 months [11]. Another multi-institutional cohort demonstrated complete VUR resolution in a total of 16 of 20 ureters (80%) in 15 of 18 patients (83%) determined by post-procedure VCUG at 8–12 weeks post-operatively [12]. The type of reimplantation may predict success rates of salvage Dx/Ha in one study [13]. After 1 injection, reflux resolved in 15 patients (71%) or a total of 20 ureteral units (77%), including 12 of 14 (86%) extravesically and 8 of 12 (66%) intravesically reimplanted units. The resolution rate improved to 84% after multiple injections.

Altered Ureteral Anatomy

Ureteral Duplication

In patients with a duplicated collecting system, the altered ureteral anatomy can create technical difficulties that may result in malpositioning of the bulking agent. These technical considerations are highlighted in a meta-analysis of early research where after one treatment, the success rate was significantly lower for duplicated when compared to single systems (50 vs 73%) [14]. More contemporary studies have shown improved success. A single institution study out of Children's Healthcare of Atlanta evaluated 52 children with duplex ureters and VUR treated with endoscopic injection. After initial treatment, 38/52 (73%) patients were cured, defined as complete resolution of reflux on post-operative VCUG at 6–12 weeks. Of the 14 treatment failures, nine children underwent repeat endoscopic treatment with a 67% resolution rate for repeat injection. Overall, 85% were cured after one or two treatments [15]. In a second study out of Ireland investigating endoscopic injection for VUR in 110 patients with duplicated ureters demonstrated resolution of VUR at a rate 68.4% (93 of 136 ureters). VUR resolved after a second injection in 35 ureters (25.7%) and after a third injection in 8 ureters (5.9%) [16]. The HIT and double HIT methods using Dx/HA are safe and effective treatments for VUR in the setting of duplex ureters. This minimally invasive treatment should be considered as an alternative to open ureteral reimplantation or prolonged antibiotic prophylaxis when spontaneous resolution appears unlikely.

Paraureteral Diverticulum and Ureterocele

Paraureteral diverticulum is usually an indication for surgical ureteral reimplantation because of the presumed underlying structural defect of the ureteral hiatus. However, endoscopic injection has been shown to be effective in some cases, with rates of VUR resolution of 79% in one study, [17] and 67% in another [11]. Factors of success included decreased size of diverticulum (<2.6 times the ureteral diameter), late onset of reflux on VCUG, and position of the ureteral orifice [17, 18]. In a third study of 20 ureters with paraureteral diverticulum, VUR resolved in 81% of patients after 1 injection. Multivariate analysis identified higher injected volume (1.1 vs 1.7 ml) and higher PUD index, the ratio of diverticular-to-ureteral diameter, (1.9 vs 4.6) as significant predictors of treatment failure [18].

Endoscopic injection has been proven to be successful in treating persistent VUR despite ureterocele puncture in both the ipsilateral and contralateral refluxing ureter. In a study evaluating 44 persistently refluxing ureters, reflux was corrected in 31 (70%) after a single injection and it resolved after a second injection in another 9 (21%) [19].

Posterior Urethral Valves

Posterior urethral valves are the most common cause of bladder outlet obstruction in boys, occurring in 1–2 in 10,000–25,000 boys and constitutes 10% of urinary obstructions diagnosed in utero [20]. Secondary VUR is present in up to 70% of patients with posterior urethral valves and usually improves and often resolves after valve ablation. However, despite the successful relief of urethral obstruction, VUR may persist and lead to urinary infection and renal dysfunction [21].

Anti-reflux surgery is rarely indicated in cases of secondary VUR. In cases of PUV, open surgery has been associated with a lower cure of VUR and higher risk of ureteral obstruction. Endoscopic injection, however, has been shown in several small studies to be a relatively safe and effective of management of VUR in patients with posterior urethral valves. VUR was eliminated in 17 of 24 (70.8%) ureters after a single injection. Five (20.8%) ureters required 2 (8.4%) injections and two required 3 for the correction of reflux [22]. Follow-up VCUG in the 15 patients (24 ureters) revealed no evidence of recurrence of VUR. In this study no complications were noted related to the procedure. In another retrospective review of 16 patients (19 ureters) with PUV who underwent endoscopic injection to correct persistent VUR after valve ablation, reflux was resolved in 11 (57.9%) or downgraded in 1 (5.2%) ureters after a single injection based on VCUG 3 months post-op.

Renal Transplant Vesicoureteral Reflux

While a refluxing ureteroneocystostomy is often performed in adult patients to avoid the risk of ureteral obstruction, a non-refluxing ureteral reimplantation is generally favored in children to avoid the long-term risks of VUR including recurrent UTIs, and loss of graft function [23]. Despite this, antirefluxing ureteral anastomoses are not routinely performed at pediatric transplantation centers and rates of VUR are as high as 58% in the post-transplant setting [24].

Due to their bladder dome location, short or no ureteral tunnel, and circumferential scarring at the ureteral orifice, transplant ureters present a unique challenge to endoscopic treatment. In a study of 8 patients (9 ureters) who underwent endoscopic injection for febrile UTI in setting of transplant VUR, four ureters demonstrated resolution of VUR and one ureter demonstrated improvement to grade 1 VUR. No patients showed any change in their serum creatinine, and no episodes of transplant pyelonephritis occurred during the 17 month follow-up period [25]. However, in another study, endoscopic injection of Dx/Ha did not prove to be effective with all 11 patients demonstrating either clinical or radiographic failure of treatment [26]. In a long term follow-up (11.2 years) of endoscopic correction of VUR in 117 adult kidney transplant patients, clinical success was achieved in 40 patients (34%) at the first endoscopic procedure, 64 (55%) at a second procedure and 73 (62.4%) at a third procedure, defined as absence of graft pyelonephritis [27]. Overall, despite lower success rates than seen in primary VUR [28], endoscopic injection of Dx/HA remains a safe option for the treatment of symptomatic refluxing transplant ureter in children [29].

Adult Patients

While indications for intervention for VUR are well defined in the pediatric population, in adults, triggers for surgical intervention in adults are not as well defined. While no evidence based guidelines exist, surgery should be considered for the same relative indications as used in children. One study suggests indications to include VUR grade 3 or higher, history of recurrent pyelonephritis, and evidence of nephron loss [30]. With high efficacy of endoscopic injection in the pediatric population, it has been trialed in the adult population as an alternative to a ureteral reimplant which is not as efficacious in adults as it is in children [30]. In one series of 49 patients (81 ureters), reflux was corrected in 63 (77.8%) ureters after a single injection, 9 (10.6%) after a second treatment and 4 (4.8%) after a third. Fourteen (28.6%) patients suffered afebrile UTI. Five (10.2%) developed febrile UTI following successful endoscopic correction, leading to a diagnosis of VUR recurrence in two (4.1%) patients [31]. Another study reports radiographic success of endoscopic injection of 80% in an adult cohort [32]. In a study of 19 women with VUR, the rate of radiographic success was 79% after one treatment, 92% after 5 patients received a second treatment, and 96%, after 2 patients received a third treatment [33].

Conclusion

Historically, the avoidance of endoscopic treatment for complex VUR is due to a paucity of supportive clinical data and the current view that bladder dysfunction and structural defects of the ureterovesical junction necessitate ureteral reimplantation. However, there is now ample evidence suggesting that endoscopic treatment for complex VUR is safe and effective, and should be more frequently utilized as first line therapy for these cases. The growing body of clinical outcomes data will aid in preoperative counseling and patient selection. Success rates of endoscopic VUR treatment will continue to improve with more experience using current bulking agents and modern techniques. As adults with recurrent pyelonephritis are more consistently evaluated for VUR, a patient population with distinct requirements and disease characteristics may emerge. Endoscopic injection should be considered as a safe and viable alternative to open surgery when treating heterogenous patient populations with complex VUR.

References

1. Peters CA, Skoog SJ, Arant BS Jr, Copp HL, Elder JS, Hudson RG, et al. Summary of the AUA guideline on management of primary vesicoureteral reflux in children. J Urol. 2010;184(3):1134–44.
2. Kirsch AJ, Arlen AM. Evolving surgical management of pediatric vesicoureteral reflux: is open ureteral reimplantation still the 'gold standard'? Int Braz J Urol. 2020;46(3):314–21.
3. Kirsch AJ, Cooper CS, Läckgren G. Non-animal stabilized hyaluronic acid/Dextranomer gel (NASHA/dx, Deflux) for endoscopic treatment of vesicoureteral reflux: what have we learned over the last 20 years? Urology. 2021;157:15–28.
4. Garcia-Roig M, Travers C, McCracken CE, Kirsch AJ. National trends in the management of primary vesicoureteral reflux in children. J Urol. 2018;199(1):287–93.
5. Routh JC, Inman BA, Reinberg Y. Dextranomer/hyaluronic acid for pediatric vesicoureteral reflux: systematic review. Pediatrics. 2010;125(5):1010–9.
6. Yap T-L, Chen Y, Nah SA, Ong CCP, Jacobsen A, Low Y. STING versus HIT technique of endoscopic treatment for vesicoureteral reflux: a systematic review and meta-analysis. J Pediatr Surg. 2016;51(12):2015–20.
7. Mina-Riascos SH, Fernández N, García-Perdomo HA. Effectiveness and risks of endoscopic management compared to vesicoureteral reimplantation in patients with high-grade vesicoureteral reflux: systematic review and network meta-analysis. Eur J Pediatr. 2021;180(5):1383–91.
8. Kirsch AJ, Arlen AM. Evaluation of new Deflux administration techniques: intraureteric HIT and double HIT for the endoscopic correction of vesicoureteral reflux. Expert Rev Med Devices. 2014;11(5):439–46.
9. Hendren WH. Complications of megaureter repair in children. J Urol. 1975;113(2):238–54.
10. Hubert KC, Kokorowski PJ, Huang L, Prasad MM, Rosoklija I, Retik AB, et al. Clinical outcomes and long-term resolution in patients with persistent vesicoureteral reflux after open ureteral reimplantation. J Urol. 2012;188(4 Suppl):1474–9.
11. Perez-Brayfield M, Kirsch AJ, Hensle TW, Koyle MA, Furness P, Scherz HC. Endoscopic treatment with DEXTRANOMER/hyaluronic acid for complex cases of vesicoureteral reflux. J Urol. 2004;172(4 Part 2):1614–6.
12. Kitchens D, Minevich E, DeFoor W, Reddy P, Wacksman J, Sheldon C, et al. Endoscopic injection of Dextranomer/hyaluronic acid copolymer to correct vesicoureteral reflux following failed ureteroneocystostomy. J Urol. 2006;176(4S):1861–3.
13. Bar-Yosef Y, Castellan M, Joshi D, Labbie A, Gosalbez R. Salvage dextranomer-hyaluronic acid copolymer for persistent reflux after ureteral reimplantation: early success rates. J Urol. 2011;185(6 Suppl):2531–4.
14. Elder JS, Diaz M, Caldamone AA, Cendron M, Greenfield S, Hurwitz R, et al. Endoscopic therapy for vesicoureteral reflux: a meta-analysis. I. Reflux resolution and urinary tract infection. J Urol. 2006;175(2):716–22.
15. Molitierno JA Jr, Scherz HC, Kirsch AJ. Endoscopic injection of dextranomer hyaluronic acid copolymer for the treatment of vesicoureteral reflux in duplex ureters. J Pediatr Urol. 2008;4(5):372–6.
16. Hunziker M, Mohanan N, Puri P. Dextranomer/hyaluronic acid endoscopic injection is effective in the treatment of intermediate and high grade vesicoureteral reflux in patients with complete duplex systems. J Urol. 2013;189(5):1876–81.
17. Aydogdu O, Burgu B, Soygur T. Predictors of surgical outcome in children with vesicoureteral reflux associated with paraureteral diverticula. Urology. 2010;76(1):209–14.
18. Cerwinka WH, Scherz HC, Kirsch AJ. Endoscopic treatment of vesicoureteral reflux associated with paraureteral diverticula in children. J Urol. 2007;178(4 Pt 1):1469–73.
19. Chertin B, Mohanan N, Farkas A, Puri P. Endoscopic treatment of vesicoureteral reflux associated with ureterocele. J Urol. 2007;178(4 Pt 2):1594–7.
20. Shukla ARSA. Posterior urethral valves. In: Dmochowski RRKL, Partin AW, Peters CA, editors. Campbell-Walsh-Wein urology. 12th ed. Philadelphia: Elsevier; 2021. p. 602–23.

21. Priti K, Rao KL, Menon P, Singh N, Mittal BR, Bhattacharya A, et al. Posterior urethral valves: incidence and progress of vesicoureteric reflux after primary fulguration. Pediatr Surg Int. 2004;20(2):136–9.
22. Puri P, Kumar R. Endoscopic correction of vesicoureteral reflux secondary to posterior urethral valves. J Urol. 1996;156(2 Pt 2):680–2.
23. Vianello A, Pignata G, Caldato C, Di Falco G, Calconi G, Fandella A, et al. Vesicoureteral reflux after kidney transplantation: clinical significance in the medium to long-term. Clin Nephrol. 1997;47(6):356–61.
24. Ranchin B, Chapuis F, Dawhara M, Canterino I, Hadj-Aïssa A, Saïd MH, et al. Vesicoureteral reflux after kidney transplantation in children. Nephrol Dialysis Transpl. 2000;15(11):1852–8.
25. Williams MA, Giel DW, Colleen HM. Endoscopic Deflux injection for pediatric transplant reflux: a feasible alternative to open ureteral reimplant. J Pediatr Urol. 2008;4(5):341–4.
26. Sheth KR, White JT, Stanasel I, Janzen N, Mittal A, Koh CJ, et al. Comparing treatment modalities for transplant kidney vesicoureteral reflux in the pediatric population. J Pediatr Urol. 2018;14(6):554.e1–6.
27. Tadrist A, Morelli M, Gondran-Tellier B, Akiki A, McManus R, Delaporte V, et al. Long-term results of endoscopic treatment in vesicoureteral reflux after kidney transplantation. World J Urol. 2022;40(3):815–21.
28. Rebullar K, O'Kelly F, Koyle MA, Kirsch A, Al-Kutbi R, Zu'bi F. A systematic review of outcomes of Deflux® treatment for vesicoureteral reflux following pediatric renal transplantation. J Pediatr Urol. 2021;17(4):589.e1–6.
29. Vemulakonda VM, Koyle MA, Lendvay TS, Risk MC, Kirsch AJ, Cheng EY, et al. Endoscopic treatment of symptomatic refluxing renal transplant ureteroneocystostomies in children. Pediatr Transplant. 2010;14(2):212–5.
30. Zilberman DE, Mor Y. Has the data efflux regarding the promising outcome following injection of deflux changed the management of adult vesicoureteral reflux? Adv Urol. 2008;2008:361324.
31. Natsheh A, Shenfeld OZ, Farkas A, Chertin B. Endoscopic treatment of vesicoureteral reflux in an adult population: can we teach our adult urology colleagues? J Pediatr Urol. 2010;6(6):600–4.
32. Turk A, Selimoglu A, Demir K, Celik O, Saglam E, Tarhan F. Endoscopic treatment of vesicoureteral reflux with polyacrylate polyalcohol copolymer and dextranomer/hyaluronic acid in adults. Int Braz J Urol. 2014;40(3):379–83.
33. Murphy AM, Ritch CR, Reiley EA, Hensle TW. Endoscopic management of vesicoureteral reflux in adult women. BJU Int. 2011;108(2):252–4.

Tissue Augmenting Substances for the Endoscopic Treatment of Vesicoureteral Reflux

Ciro Esposito, Fulvia Del Conte, and Maria Escolino

Abstract Since in 1984, when VUR induced in piglets was successfully corrected by the subureteric injection of polytetrafluoroethylene (PTFE) paste, the endoscopic subureteric injection has been used successfully to treat primary and secondary VUR in children, radically changed the management of VUR in this large group of patients. Due to the high risk of granuloma formation, new tissues augmenting substances have been appeared: dextranomer/hyaluronic acid (Dx-HA) copolymer and polyacrylate-polyalcohol copolymer (PPC) are the most commonly used bulking agents in the endoscopic treatment of VUR nowdays.

- DEFLUX®: consists of dextranomer microspheres of an average size of 80 to 250 μm in sodium hyaluronic acid solution and it's the only FDA approved.
- DEXELL® VUR**:** is a non-allergic,non-immunogenic and biodegradable Dx/Ha copolymer that consists of cross-linked Dx particles with a size of 80e120 mm
- VANTRIS®: is a biocompatible, non-absorbable, synthetic tissue-bulking substance, and consists of particles of polyacrylate polyalcohol copolymer (PPC) immersed in a carrier.

Keywords VUR · Bulking agents · Tissue augmenting substances · Dextranomer/hyaluronic acid · Polyacrylate-polyalcohol copolymer · Endoscopic injection · Dexell · Deflux · Vantris

Introduction

Since in 1984 when VUR induced in piglets was successfully corrected by the subureteric injection of polytetrafluoroethylene (PTFE) paste, the endoscopic subureteric injection has been used successfully to treat primary and secondary VUR in

C. Esposito (✉) · F. Del Conte · M. Escolino
Pediatric Surgery Unit, "Federico II" University of Naples, Naples, Italy
e-mail: ciroespo@unina.it; fulviadelconte@unina.it; maria.escolino@unina.it

P. Puri, A. Yamataka (eds.), *Vesicoureteral Reflux*,
https://doi.org/10.1007/978-3-031-95091-9_18

children, radically changing the management of VUR in this large group of patients. [13, 26, 27].

Many differnt tissues augmenting substances were used for VUR endoscopic correction in the past 30 years, among these:

- **Polytetrafluoroethylene or Teflon® (PTFE):** It belongs to a family of fluorocarbon polymer, and is probably the most inert of the plastic materials. It presents a high molecular weight, high density (2.15 ± 2.2 g/ml), low tensile strength (17 ± 28 MPa) and low surface tension (18.5 ergs/cm^2). Teflon was already used in medical practice and did not show rejection by the host, and to cause any malignancies in humans. When used for VUR correction PTFE is suspended in glycerin (50%).[26]

- Despite the convincing data regarding the long-term efficacy of PTFE in endoscopic correction of VUR, the data regarding the possibility of PTFE particle migration couldn't be ignored. For this reason, Polytetrafluoroethylene has been set aside and new molecules have emerged.[5]
- **Cross-linked bovine collagen:** Cross-linked bovine collagen is a soluble and purified preparation of bovine collagen that is stabilized by the addition of 0.0075% glutaraldehyde to effect fibril cross-linking. [26]. It was the major alternative to PTFE and as PTFE presented a large use in medicine (cardiac valves, hemostatic agents and sutures, and as a soft tissue substitute).
- Unfortunately after the beginning enthusiasm, many studies demonstrated an high recurrence rate at the long term follow-up [15]
- **Polydimethylsiloxane (Macroplastique ®):** is a silicone paste composed of solid textured polydimethylsiloxane particles (40%) and hydrogel (60%). It is composed in majority by particle of a dimeter equal or superior to 100 μm in diameter, but some 80 μm particles and smaller can be present and may cause distant migration.
- Few report are available, Van Capelle et al. [35]: published a retrospective study with 195 patients who underwent endoscopic correction of VUR utilizing Macroplastique as a bulking agent in two centers. The article cover a period of 10 years. They found an overall success rates ranged between 84% and 77%. The major concern of this study, is that follow-up lasted only 1 year if patient become asymptomatic.
- **Autologous chondrocytes:** Diamond and Caldamone [9] described in 1999 the use of autologous chondrocytes as tissue augmenting substance for endoscopic VUR correction in children. In their preliminary report no significant complications were found and a overall success rate was of 38 on 46 ureters (83%) and 24 on 29 patients (83%).
- The main concern was about the two surgical procedures required: first one for chondrocytes collection and, after 6 months growth of chondrocytes, a second one for the injection. At 1-year followup reflux correction was maintained in 70% of ureters (32 of 46) and 65% of patients (19 of 29). In those patients in whom implantation failed cystoscopy revealed evidence of volume loss and

shifting of subureteral mounds to account for loss of the antireflux effect [3]. No further studies have been published.

- **Bulkamid®:** polyacrylamide hydrogel (PAHG) is a non-absorbable material. It's rarely used in pediatric field so there is a leak in global literature. It has been largely used to correct stress urinary incontinency in women and it received the European conformity mark since 2003 for this. Clautier [7] has published the only prospective study using bulkamid as tissue augmenting substance in pediatric population for VUR endoscopic correctio. He found a success rate for grade I to III vesicoureteral reflux at 3 months after a single treatment of 87%, and the overall success for all grades of 81.2%. Blais in 2015 [2] pulished a comparative study between PAHG and Deflux, demonstrating a similar success rate after one injection in the two groups (73.1% in the PAHG compared with 77.5% in the Dx/HA one). However, the trial has small numbers and long-term data were never pulished.
- **Calcium hydroxyapatite:** supporting by encouraged results in the treatment of stress urinary incontinence in women, FDA approved a a pilot study for VUR in children in 2000. Altought the pilot study showed satisfactory results, during the prospective multicentric study Calcium Hydroxyapatite showed a success rate of only 46% and 40% per ureter treated, at 1 and 2 years, respectively [21].

Despite of the data showing the long-term efficacy of PTFE as a bulking agent, the use of PTFE is drastically decrased due to the possibility of particle migration, granuloma formation (foreign-body reaction), and permanent presence within the body because of their lack of biodegradability [16, 19].

Since 1995 when the first clinical report about Deflux was presented by Stenberg [32], this bulking agent become more and more used in current practices. In 2001, Deflux was approved by the US Food and Drug Administration for VUR correction in pediatric age.

Nowadays, dextranomer/hyaluronic acid (Dx-HA) copolymer and polyacrylate-polyalcohol copolymer (PPC) are the most commonly used bulking agents in the endoscopic treatment of VUR [10].

In current practice three major tissue augmenting substances have been used: Deflux, Dexell and Vantris. All of them are available in pre-filled syringe for immediate use and they present as a sterile and viscous gel.

- **DEFLUX®:** consists of dextranomer microspheres of an average size of 80 to 250 μm in sodium hyaluronic acid solution. In 1995, the first clinical report about using Deflux for grade III and IV VUR was published. The US Food and Drug Administration (FDA) approved the use of Deflux for endoscopic injection in pediatric patients with primary VUR grades II–IV in 2001: it is the only bulking agent FDA approved [38].

- In literature the overall success rate after the endoscopic VUR correction with Deflux, the most widely used bulking agent, ranges between 68% and 92%, depending mainly on the reflux grade, with 50–70% success rate after single injection [5, 6, 37].

- **DEXELL®:** is a non-allergic,non-immunogenic and biodegradable Dx/Ha copolymer that consists of cross-linked Dx particles with a size of 80–120 μm. [31] It's composed of a suspension of microparticles of dextranomers and cross-linked hyaluronic acid of non-animal origin.
- The microparticles of dextranomers form a volume in the connective tissue at the injection site while cross-linked hyaluronic acid (Gel Hyaln) serves primarily as a vehicle for microparticles of dextranomers.
- A retrospective analysis of 240 patients (109 Deflux; 131 Dexell) revealed treatment outcomes and postoperative UTI rates were similar to those obtained when using Deflux [11, 31].
- All of the obstructive complications related to Dexell in the literature are early and transient and usually resolved spontaneously without the need for any intervention. The high recurrence rate of Dexell was attributed to the biodegradable nature of the Dx-HA [10, 20, 25].
- **VANTRIS®:** is a biocompatible, non-absorbable, synthetic tissue-bulking substance, and consists of particles of polyacrylate polyalcohol copolymer (PPC) immersed in a carrier. It was introduced in 2008 and the first clinical experience reported in 2010 by Ormaechea et al. [22–24, 37].
- Vantris injection is described in literature as a procedure to treat primary reflux also in complex cases. The use of PPC to correct grades IV and V is also efficient with an overall success rate achieved of over 80% [6, 18, 30, 33, 36]. However the PPC is associated with high incidence of late VUJO (vesico-ureteral junction obstraction)as reported by Karakus [29] and Kocaoglu [17].

Endoscopic treatment has become a popular minimally invasive choice in VUR treatment: safe and easy. Its advantages include repeatability in cases of failure after the first injection and shorter hospitalization and operation times.

In case of failure after the first application, repeated injections increase success rates [1].

Successful rate is still inferior to traditional surgery: this is why many different bulking agents have been tested and the perfect one has not yet been invented.

Deflux remains the most commonly used bulking agent for the endoscopic treatment of VUR.

Different comparative studies proved that polyacrylate-polyalcohol copolymer and small-size dextranomer/hyaluronic acid copolymer have an efficacy at least as Deflux in correcting VUR [11, 14, 25].

Unfurtunatly the majority of comparative studies are retrospective[5, 10, 11].

Only one of these studies [14] was a prospective, randomized trial; the results showed comparable efficacy of Deflux and polyacrylate-polyalcohol copolymer.

There are other difficulties when comparing different bulking agents. Many different factors can affect the efficacy of VUR correction as the VUR grade, the technique used (STING, HIT or double HIT) or surgeon's experience.

Läckgren suggests that the differences between small-size dextranomer/hyaluronic acid copolymer and Deflux, in the dextranomer microspheres's size and the hyaluronic acid's characteristics, can potentially affect the safety profile, physical properties and ease/controllability of the injection procedure: meaning that clinical results obtained with Deflux are not directly applicable to small-size dextranomer/hyaluronic acid copolymer [19].

Aydogdu [1] in his study compare Dexell and Deflux to evaluate if polymer microsphere diameter affects the success rate in the endoscopic treatment of vesicoureteral reflux. They conclude that the diameter of dextranomer microsphere does not affect the short-term success rate of the procedure. Also, Dogan [11] in his study showed similar results for the two Dx/Ha copolymer.

Warchol [36] in his study compares Deflux and Vantris, reporting a success rate with Deflux in their experience, of 63% after the first injection and 90.7% after the second that is in line with the literature. As for the Vantris they reporte a higher rate success: reflux was resolved in almost 93% after the first procedure, and in 100% after the second procedure.

The biodegradable nature of the dextranomer/hyaluronic acid copolymer is suggested as factor causing reflux recurrence in some cases [4, 18, 22].

Despite his high success rate Vantris is associated with a high incidence of early and delayed ureteral obstruction. Because of its non-absorbable nature a fibrotic capsule can be formed stimulating the surrounding tissue, and can contribute to the formation of VUJO. It can also be supposed that high mass effect can generate a fibrosis of distal ureter by reducing blood supply [10]. This is also associated with higher intraoperative difficulties in cases of reimplantation in patients previously treated by PPC injection [14].

Patients who undergo endoscopic treatment of VUR using Vantris need long-term follow-up because of the possibility of early and delayed ureteral obstruction after PPC injection, which is the main complication encountered [4, 8, 12, 18].

Garcia reported also that the amount of bulking agent used in successful treatment was significantly higher in Dx/HA than in PPC group, this condition could be explained because the biodegradable properties of Dx/HA lead us to inject more substance than PPC. This difference in bulking agent amount did not improve costs, because PPC is 22% more expensive than Dx/HA [14].

As for the differences in costs using different substances there is a lack of studies. Some authors realized observationals study about lower product costs comparing polyacrylamide hydrogel and small size dextranomer/hyaluronic acid copolymer vs. Deflux [2, 28, 34]. Unfortunately bulking agents cost's comparisons do not provide a complete pharmacoeconomic evaluation: further studies including complete long-term costs of patient management (bulking agents' long-term safety and efficacy) are required for valuable pharmacoeconomic data.

Conclusion

Current data suggest PPC confers a higher resolution rate of VUR compared with Dx/HA in the pediatric population. However, the incidence of late-onset VUJO remain high with PPC.

For the dextranomer/hyaluronic acid copolymer the high recurrences rate remains the principal concerns.

New high-quality studies are necessary to make further recommendations.

References

1. Aydogdu O, Ozcan C, Burgu B, et al. Does the diameter of dextranomer microspheres affect the success in endoscopic treatment of vesicoureteral reflux? Urology. 2012;80:703–6. https://doi.org/10.1016/j.urology.2012.05.018.
2. Blais A-S, Morin F, Cloutier J, et al. Efficacy of dextranomer hyaluronic acid and polyacrylamide hydrogel in endoscopic treatment of vesicoureteral reflux: a comparative study. Can Urol Assoc J. 2015;9:202–6. https://doi.org/10.5489/cuaj.2964.
3. Caldamone AA, Diamond DA. Long-term results of the endoscopic correction of vesicoureteral reflux in children using autologous chondrocytes. J Urol. 2001;165:2224–7.
4. Chertin B, Arafeh WA, Zeldin A, et al. Endoscopic correction of VUR using Vantris as a new non-biodegradable tissue-augmenting substance: three years of prospective follow-up. Urology. 2013;82(1):201–4.
5. Chertin B, Kocherov S. Long-term results of endoscopic treatment of vesicoureteric reflux with different tissue-augmenting substances. J Pediatr Urol. 2010;6:251–6.
6. Chertin B, Puri P. Endoscopic Management of Vesicoureteral Reflux: does it stand the test of time? Eur Urol. 2002;42(6):598–606.
7. Cloutier J, Blais AS, Moore K, Bolduc S. A prospective study using a new bulking agent for the treatment of vesicoureteral reflux: polyacrylamide hydrogel. J Urol. 2013;190:1034–7.
8. De Badiola FI, Soria R, Vagni RL, et al. Results of treatment of grades IV and V vesicoureteral reflux with endoscopic injection of polyacrylate polyalcohol copolymer. Front Pediatr. 2013;1:32.
9. Diamond DA, Caldamone AA. Endoscopic correction of vesicoureteral reflux in children using autologous chondrocytes: preliminary results. J Urol. 1999;162:1185–8.
10. Doğan AB, Özkan KU, Güler AG, Karakaya AE. Endoscopic treatment of primary vesicoureteral reflux in children with two different bulking agents, high success and low complication rates: comparison of Dexell and Vantris. Actas Urol Esp. 2021;45:545–51. https://doi.org/10.1016/j.acuro.2020.10.013.
11. Dogan HS, Altan M, Citamak B, et al. Factors affecting the success of endoscopic treatment of vesicoureteral reflux and comparison of two dextranomer based bulking agents: does bulking substance matter? J Pediatr Urol. 2015;11:90.e1–5. https://doi.org/10.1016/j.jpurol.2014.12.009.
12. Esposito C, Yamataka A, Varlet F, et al. Current trends in 2021 in surgical management of vesico-ureteral reflux in pediatric patients: results of a multicenter international survey on 552 patients. Minerva Urol Nephrol. 2023;75:106–15.
13. Farkas A, Moriel EZ, Lupa S. Endoscopic correction of vesicoureteric reflux: our experience with 115 ureters. J Urol. 1990;536:144–531.
14. García-Aparicio L, Blázquez-Gómez E, Martin O, et al. Randomized clinical trial between polyacrylate-polyalcohol copolymer (PPC) and dextranomer-hyaluronic acid copolymer (dx/HA) as bulking agents for endoscopic treatment of primary vesicoureteral reflux (VUR). World J Urol. 2018;36:1651–6. https://doi.org/10.1007/s00345-018-2314-7.
15. Haferkamp A, Contractor H, Mo¨hring K, et al. Failure of subureteral bovine collagen injection for the endoscopic treatment of primary vesicoureteral reflux in longterm follow-up. Urology. 2000;63:55–759.
16. Karakus SC, User İR, Kılıc BD, et al. The comparison of dextranomer/hyaluronic acid and polyacrylate-polyalcohol copolymers in endoscopic treatment of vesicoureteral reflux. J Pediatr Surg. 2016;51:1496–500. https://doi.org/10.1016/j.jpedsurg.2016.02.092.

17. Kocaoglu C. Endoscopic treatment of Grades IV and V vesicoureteral reflux with two bulking substances: dextranomer hyaluronic acid copolymer vs. polyacrylate polyalcohol copolymer in children. J Pediatr Surg. 2016;51(10):1711–5.
18. Kocherov S, Ulman I, Nikolaev S, et al. Multicenter survey of endoscopic treatment of vesicoureteral reflux using polyacrylate polyalcohol bulking copolymer (Vantris). Urology. 2014;84(3):689–93.
19. Läckgren G, Cooper CS, Neveus T, Kirsch AJ. Management of Vesicoureteral Reflux: what have we learned over the last 20 years? Front Pediatr. 2021;9:650326.
20. Mazzone L, Gobet R, González R, et al. Ureteral obstruction following injection of dextranomer/hyaluronic acid copolymer: an infrequent but relevant complication. J Pediatr Urol. 2012;8(5):514–9.
21. Mevorach RA, Hulbert WC, Rabinowitz R, et al. Results of a 2-year multicenter trial of endoscopic treatment of vesicoureteral reflux with synthetic calcium hydroxyapatite. J Urol. 2006;175:288–91. https://doi.org/10.1016/S0022-5347(05)00013-3.
22. Ormaechea M, Paladini M, Pisano R, et al. Vantris, a biocompatible, synthetic, nonbiodegradable, easy-to-inject bulking substance. Evaluation of local tissular reaction, localized migration and long distance migration. Arch Esp Urol. 2008;61(2):263–8.
23. Ormaechea M, Ruiz E, Denes E, et al. New tissue bulking agent (Polyacrylate polyalcohol) for treating vesicoureteral reflux: preliminary results in children. J Urol. 2010a;183:714–8. https://doi.org/10.1016/j.juro.2009.10.047.
24. Ormaechea M, Ruiz E, Denes E, et al. New tissuebulking agent (polyacrylate polyalcohol) for treating vesicoureteral reflux: preliminary results in children. J Urol. 2010b;183:714–8.
25. Oswald J, Riccabona M, Lusuardi L, et al. Prospective comparison and 1-year follow-up of a single endoscopic subureteral polydimethylsiloxane versus dextranomer/hyaluronic acid copolymer injection for treatment of vesicoureteral reflux in children. Urology. 2002;60:894–7.
26. Puri P. Endoscopic correction of vesicoureteral reflux. Curr Opin Urol. 2000;10(6):593–7.
27. Puri P, O'Donnell B. Correction of experimentally produced vesicoureteric reflux in the piglet by the intra-vesical injection of Teflon. Br Med J. 1984;289:5–7.
28. Ramsay S, Blais A-S, Morin F, et al. Polyacrylamide hydrogel as a bulking agent for the endoscopic treatment of vesicoureteral reflux: long-term results and safety. J Urol. 2017;197:963–7. https://doi.org/10.1016/j.juro.2016.08.093.
29. Schemedding A, Zeeh U, Huebner U, et al. Sx IN-prospective multicenter survey of subureteral injection in children. In: Proceedings of the international VUR conference. Goteborg, Sweden; 2009.
30. Sharifiaghdas F, Tajalli F, Otukesh H, Shamsabadi RH. Endoscopic correction of primary VUR by using polyacrylate polyalcohol copolymer (Vantris) in young girls: 2-year follow-up. J Pediatr Urol. 2014;10(6):1032–6.
31. Starmer B, McAndrew F, Corbett H. A review of novel STING bulking agents. J Pediatr Urol. 2019;15:484–90.
32. Stenberg A, Lackgren G. A new bioimplant for the endoscopic treatment of vesicoureteral reflux: experimental and short-term clinical results. 154:800–3. J Urol. 1995;67:168–4.
33. Taşkinlar H, Avlan D, Bahadir GB, et al. The outcomes of two different bulking agents (dextranomer hyaluronic acid copolymer and polyacrylatepolyalcohol copolymer) in the treatment of primary vesico-ureteral reflux. Int Braz J Urol. 2016;42:514–20.
34. Üre I, Gürocak S, Tan Ö, et al. Subureteral injection with small-size Dextranomer/hyaluronic acid copolymer: is it really efficient? Biomed Res Int. 2016;2016:1–6. https://doi.org/10.1155/2016/2168753.
35. van Capelle JW, de Haan T, El Sayed W, Azmy A. The long-term outcome of the endoscopic subureteric implantation of polydimethylsiloxane for treating vesico-ureteric reflux in children: a retrospective analysis of the first 195 consecutive patients in two European centres. BJU Int. 2004;51:94–1348.
36. Warchol S, Krzemien G, Szmigielska A, et al. Comparison of results of endoscopic treatment of vesicoureteral reflux in children using two bulking substances: dextranomer/hyaluronic

acid copolymer (Deflux) versus polyacrylate-polyalcohol copolymer (Vantris). J Pediatr Urol. 2016;12:256.e1–4.
37. Warchoł S, Krzemień G, Szmigielska A, et al. Endoscopic correction of vesicoureteral reflux in children using polyacrylate-polyalcohol copolymer (Vantris): 5-years of prospective follow-up. Cent European J Urol. 2017;70:314–9. https://doi.org/10.5173/ceju.2017.1226.
38. The Japanese Deflux® Injection Therapy Study Group. Deflux® endoscopic treatment of vesicoureteral reflux (VUR) in Japan. Front Pediatr. 2022;10 https://doi.org/10.3389/fped.2022.855378.

Open Ureteral Re-implantation for Vesicoureteral Reflux

Mohamed Sameh Shalaby and Laura Jackson

Abstract Vesicoureteral reflux (VUR) is a well recognised risk factor for pyelonephritis, reflux nephropathy, hypertension and, chronic kidney disease. Open surgical management of VUR with an anti-reflux procedure is undertaken when endoscopic correction with a submucosal injection of bulking agent has been unsuccessful or is not suitable or practicable. Although laparoscopic and robotic-assisted approaches to ureteral re-implantation are gaining popularity, yet the open techniques currently remains the most commonly employed technique with high success rate of >95% of cases and relatively low complication rate.

In this chapter different open procedures are described, both intravesical (Cohen, Politano-Leadbetter, Glenn-Anderson) and extravesical (Lich-Gregoir) techniques. Additional procedures may be required in selected cases as ureteral tailoring and psoas hitch.

Special consideration should be considered in duplex kidneys with a functioning refluxing lower moiety where ureteroureterostomy seems to be an alternative reliable option. Similarly, nephroureterectomy may be employed in the non-functioning kidney.

Different factors may affect the outcome of open ureteral re-implantation especially the grade of VUR or the presence of pre-operative bladder and bowel dysfunction. On the otherhand, the type of the surgical procedure or prior endoscopic injection of bulking agent did not seem to affect the outcome of subsequent surgery.

Keywords Vesico-ureteric reflux · Ureteric re-implantation · Cohen · Politano-Leadbetter · Glenn-Anderson · Lich-Gregoir · Uretrouretrostomy

Vesicoureteric reflux (VUR) is the retrograde flow of urine from the bladder into the ureters and upper renal tract. It is classified as primary or secondary. Primary VUR arises from a congenitally short intravesical submucosal ureter while secondary

M. S. Shalaby (✉) · L. Jackson
Department of Paediatric Surgery and Urology, Bristol Royal Hospital for Children, Bristol, UK
e-mail: mshalaby@doctors.org.uk

P. Puri, A. Yamataka (eds.), *Vesicoureteral Reflux*,
https://doi.org/10.1007/978-3-031-95091-9_19

VUR results from high intravesical pressure associated with conditions such as neuropathic bladder or posterior urethral valves. Initial treatment of primary VUR is non-operative and involves the prevention of urine infection with antibiotic prophylaxis, the management of lower urinary tract dysfunction and active surveillance. Management of secondary VUR is directed towards treating the primary condition as this will usually lead to VUR resolution.

Open Surgical Management of VUR

Indications

The indications for surgical management of VUR include [36]:

- Breakthrough febrile urinary tract infections (UTI) while on antibiotic prophylaxis
- High grade VUR in a single kidney
- Non-compliance with prophylactic antibiotics

Open surgical management of VUR with an anti-reflux procedure is undertaken when endoscopic correction with a submucosal injection of bulking agent (e.g. deflux®) has been unsuccessful or is not suitable or practicable. In infants with severe VUR and breakthrough UTI's a vesicostomy may be beneficial, while circumcision in boys significantly reduces the risk of UTI's [18, 43].

Principles of Management

- Ensure secondary causes of VUR have been excluded or treated.
- Undertake surgery using loupes for optical magnification.
- Ensure a tension free anastomosis by undertaking adequate ureteral mobilisation.
- Perform careful dissection of the ureter, preserving its vascularity and recognising its proximity to extravesical nerve plexi and the vas deferens (boys) which should be protected.
- Aim for an intravesical submucosal tunnel length of 3–4 times the diameter of the ureter. The often recommended 5:1 ratio [37] is often difficult to achieve in a small bladder, risks obstructing the ureter and overestimates what is required [27].
- In the presence of sizeable ureteral dilatation perform distal ureteral refashioning (tapering or plication) in order to achieve the necessary length to diameter ratio of the intravesical submucosal tunnel.
- In cases of VUR affecting a duplicated system a common sheath re-implantation of both ureters in the same submucosal tunnel is recommended [48].
- Routine stenting of the re-implanted ureter is not necessary, but stenting is recommended in the single kidney and in at least one ureter following bilateral

ureteral re-implantation to avoid potential anuria from obstruction secondary to early post-operative oedema. Stenting is also recommended following re-operative re-implantation, when ureteral re-fashioning has been undertaken and if considerable detrusor hypertrophy is present.
- Post-operative continuous bladder drainage using either a urethral or suprapubic catheter is required for 5–7 days, particularly following intravesical procedures.

Open Procedure

Although laparoscopic and robotic-assisted approaches to ureteral re-implantation are described, the open method currently remains the most commonly employed technique. The child receives broad spectrum IV antibiotics at induction of general anaesthesia and is positioned supine on the operating table. The abdomen, genitalia and perineum are prepared leaving access for sterile urethral catheterisation intra-operatively if required. Both intravesical and extravesical techniques for ureteral re-implantation are described and the choice of which to perform will be influenced by the degree of ureteral dilatation, whether the procedure is unilateral or bilateral and by surgeon preference [1].

Intravesical Procedures

Intravesical procedures are undertaken via a Pfannenstiel incision sited approximately 2 cm above the pubic symphysis and reaching to the lateral edge of the rectus muscles. The anterior rectus sheath is incised transversely and released from the underlying rectus muscles, virtually to the umbilicus superiorly, and as far as the pubic symphysis inferiorly. The rectus muscles are split in the midline and the linea alba divided to enter the perivesical space. If the bladder is empty, it is partially filled with saline via a urethral catheter to aid bladder mobilisation, which is undertaken by blunt dissection. The peritoneum is then gently freed from the bladder dome. A Denis-Browne wound retractor, or the pediatric size Balfour retractor in the larger child, is utilised to retract the abdominal wall.

Cautery is used to open the bladder vertically in the midline between stay sutures. The incision extends to within 2 cm of the bladder neck where an interrupted suture is tied to prevent unintentional tearing of the bladder neck. The Denis-Browne retractor is moved to within the bladder to expose the trigone. The dome of the bladder is packed with saline soaked gauze and a narrow blade placed over it for superior retraction. A further narrow blade is sited inferiorly, and 2 wide blades used for lateral retraction of the bladder walls. Alternatively stay sutures may be sited for lateral bladder wall retraction.

Cannulation of the ureteric orifices, usually with a 5 or 6F infant feeding tube is undertaken. The tube is advanced up to the kidney and attached to the ureteric orifice with a 4/0 absorbable suture. Placement of a haemostat across both the tube and the suture enables gentle traction to be employed to assist ureteric mobilisation. Fine needle point cautery is used to circumscribe the urothelium around the ureteric orifice approximately 1–2 mm from the opening. Subsequently the ureter is mobilised by developing a plane outside the ureteral adventitia. This is best achieved by raising the ureteric orifice superiorly and commencing division of the superficial muscle attachments inferiorly and medially. Mobilisation of the ureter continues using bipolar cautery and tenotomy scissors, ensuring dissection remains in the plane outside the adventitia to prevent ureteral devascularistion and consequent ischaemia. Once the peritoneum is reached, it is gently swept away with a pledget. The ureter is fully mobilised into the bladder ensuring there is enough length to permit distal trimming of the ureter and enable a tension free anastomosis. Attention must be paid in boys to the proximity between the vas deferens and the ureter to avoid damage during ureteral dissection.

The remainder of the procedure is determined by the type of intravesical re-implantation to be undertaken. Three commonly used techniques with excellent rates of VUR correction are described below.

Cohen Cross-Trigonal Technique (Fig. 1a–c)

The Cohen cross-trigonal technique is commonly employed as it is a relatively straightforward and versatile procedure which has a low rate of post-operative ureteral obstruction. Furthermore, it can be useful in thick-walled bladders where the trigone is usually relatively spared. The main drawback is that subsequent endoscopic access of the ureteral orifice may be difficult. Several techniques to counteract this are described including flexible ureteroscopy [16], percutaneous retrograde ureteral catheterisation [12] and cystoscopy and ureteral access using curved tip catheters [51].

As the name suggests this technique involves creating transverse submucosal tunnels that cross the trigone of the bladder. A vertical incision is made in the urothelium superolateral to the contralateral ureteral orifice, the precise location depending on the size of the trigone. Employing tenotomy scissors in a cutting and spreading motion a submucosal tunnel is carefully made extending from the incision to the original hiatus ensuring a tunnel of adequate length and width. The ureteral feeding tube is removed and using a right-angled clip passed retrogradely via the submucosal tunnel, the mobilised ureter is pulled through on the attached stay suture. The ureter is then trimmed to length and spatulated on the medial side as required. The tip of the ureter is secured to the bladder urothelium and detrusor at the 5 and 7 o'clock positions with two deep interrupted 4/0 or 5/0 absorbable sutures. The remaining ureteral circumference is then anastomosed to the bladder urothelium using interrupted 5/0 absorbable sutures. At the other side of the tunnel at the site of the original hiatus, an interrupted suture is used to secure the ureter to the detrusor and the urothelium is closed with a 5/0 absorbable suture.

When bilateral ureteral re-implantations are performed the ureter with the more superolateral ureteral orifice is tunnelled superior to the contralateral orifice. The

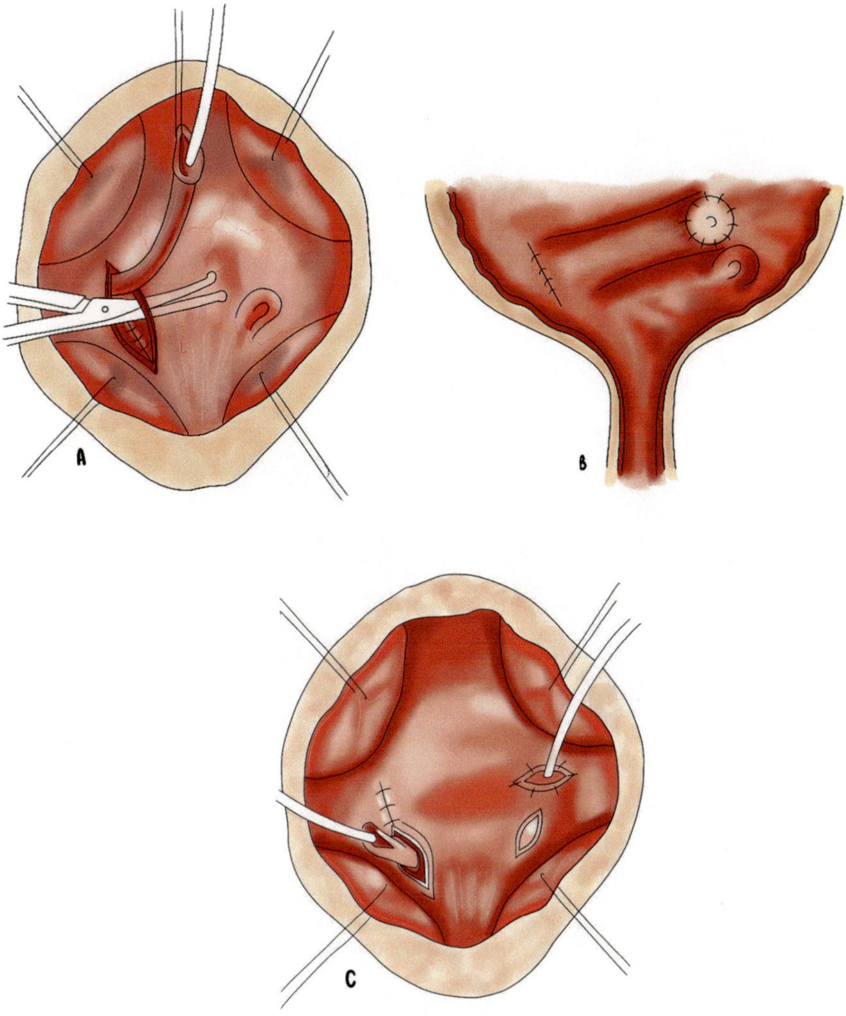

Fig. 1 (**a**–**c**) Cohen cross-trigonal technique. (**a**) Unilateral Cohen. Creating transverse submucosal tunnel which crosses the trigone. (**b**) Unilateral Cohen. New ureteric orifice lies superior to the contralateral ureteric orifice. (**c**) Bilateral Cohen. The ureter whose original hiatus is more superolateral is tunneled superior to the contralateral orifice. The second ureter is then tunneled inferior to the original hiatus of the first ureter

other ureter is then tunnelled inferior to the original hiatus of the first ureter using the same technique as described for the first.

If a feeding tube stent is left in the ureter it should be secured to the ureteral orifice with a 5/0 vicryl rapide and then brought out through the bladder closure. Bladder closure is undertaken in two layers using a 4/0 absorbable suture to the urothelium and the detrusor, bringing a 12F foley balloon catheter through the

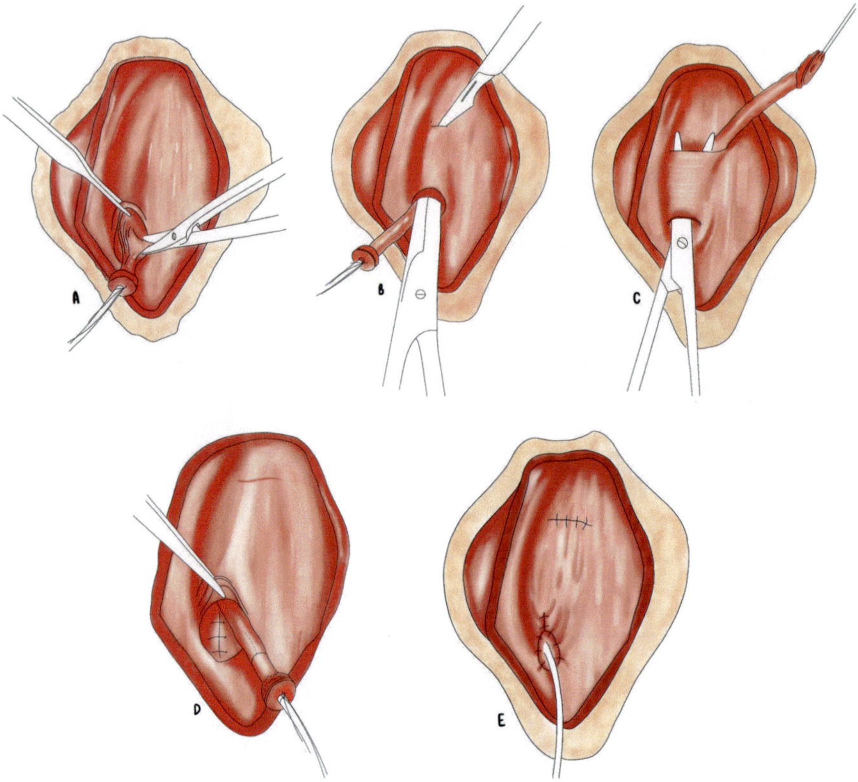

Fig. 2 (**a–e**) Politano-Leadbetter technique. (**a**) The ureteric orifice is dissected. (**b**) A new hiatus superomedial to the original hiatus is dissected. (**c**) The ureter is routed up to the new hiatus. (**d**) The detrusor at the site of the original hiatus is closed. The ureter is passed through the tunnel bringing the distal ureter through from the new hiatus inferiorly. (**e**) The end of the distal ureter is trimmed to length and spatulated if necessary. The anastomosis of ureter to bladder urothelium is completed. The urothelium at the site of the new hiatus is closed vertically over the ureter

closure to provide suprapubic catheter drainage. A perivesical drain is sited and the wound closed in layers.

Politano-Leadbetter Technique (Fig. 2a–e)

This technique produces a long submucosal supra-hiatal tunnel which runs vertically from a new superomedial hiatus down to the original hiatus [39]. Endoscopic access is therefore unaffected post-operatively and a longer submucosal tunnel can be created compared to the Cohen procedure as tunnel length is not limited by the size of the trigone. The Politano-Leadbetter technique is therefore recommended when re-implanting hugely dilated ureters, particularly when combined with a psoas hitch to prevent angulation of the ureter as it inserts into the bladder. This technique, however, is technically more challenging to accomplish than others, with a risk of unintentional angulation or twisting of the ureter and subsequent ureteral obstruction.

Once the ureter has been fully mobilised as described above, the site for the new superomedial hiatus is selected ensuring an adequate length to diameter ratio. A retrovesical pathway for the ureter to be re-routed up to the new hiatus needs to be created by blunt dissection taking care to avoid injury to the peritoneum or bowel. The ureter is drawn up to the new hiatus with a right-angle clip holding the ureteral stay sutures. The new superomedial hiatus is formed by incising through the urothelium and detrusor onto the tips of the right-angle clip. The ureter is then pulled through into the bladder ensuring it is not twisted or kinked. The detrusor at the site of the original hiatus is closed with an interrupted 4/0 absorbable suture. The vertical submucosal tunnel between the new hiatus and original hiatus is created with tenotomy scissors using a spreading and cutting motion. The ureter is drawn through the tunnel, trimmed to length and spatulated as necessary on the medial side. The tip of the ureter is fixed using two deep 4/0 or 5/0 absorbable sutures to the bladder urothelium and detrusor at the 5 and 7 o'clock positions. The remaining circumference of the ureter is secured to the bladder urothelium with 5/0 absorbable interrupted sutures and further interrupted 5/0 absorbable sutures are used to close the urothelium over the new hiatus.

A 5F feeding tube is passed via the new orifice to ensure no angulation of the ureter. If a post-operative stent is required this feeding tube is left in place, secured to the bladder with a 5/0 vicryl rapide suture and then brought out through the bladder closure. Suprapubic catheter insertion, bladder closure, wound closure and post-operative follow-up are undertaken in the same manner as for the Cohen procedure.

Glenn-Anderson Technique (Fig. 3a–c)

The Glenn-Anderson technique involves forming an infra-hiatal tunnel from the original hiatus onto the trigone. This technique enables easy endoscopic access to the ureteric orifice post-operatively and avoids retrovesical dissection. However, the applicability of this technique is somewhat limited by the shorter length of tunnel that can be created.

Following full mobilisation of the ureter into the bladder as described above, the urothelium is incised on the trigone inferomedial to the original hiatus and a submucosal tunnel between the two is created with tenotomy scissors. The full thickness of the bladder wall superior to the original hiatus is incised and the ureter is moved superiorly within this incision in order to relocate the hiatus cranially thus increasing the tunnel length. The detrusor is then closed inferior to the ureter with interrupted 4/0 absorbable sutures ensuring it is not closed too tightly. Pass a right-angle clip retrogradely via the submucosal tunnel, grasp the stay suture attached to the ureter and draw the ureter through the submucosal tunnel. Trim the distal ureter to length and spatulate on the medial aspect if required. Anastomose the distal ureter to the bladder urothelium and detrusor with 2 deep interrupted 4/0 or 5/0 absorbable sutures at the 5 and 7 o'clock positions. Complete the circumferential anastomosis

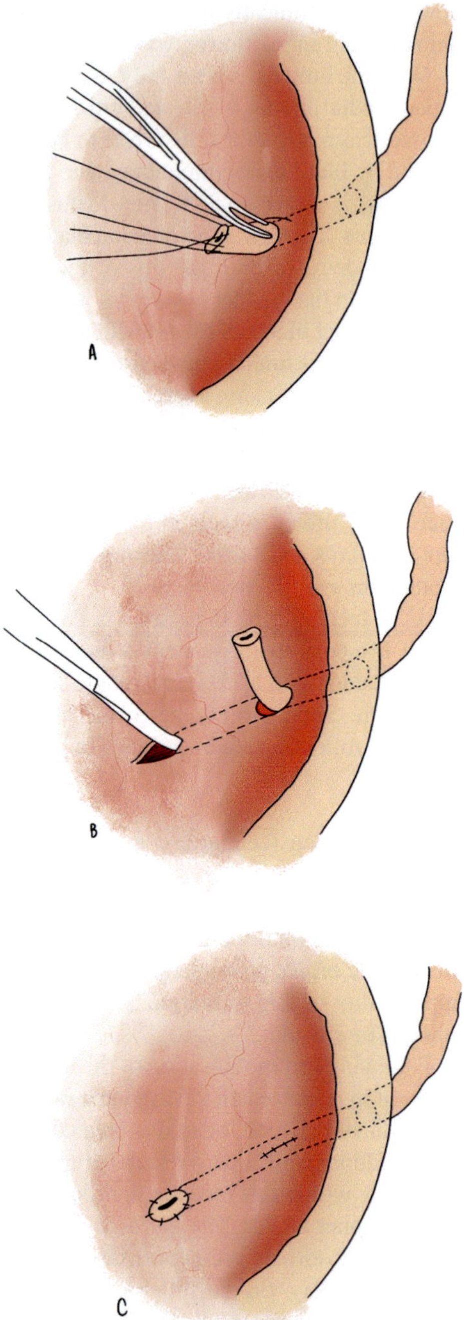

Fig. 3 (**a**–**c**) Glenn-Anderson technique. (**a**) The ureter is mobilized into the bladder. (**b**) A submucosal tunnel extending inferomedial onto the trigone from the original hiatus is created. (**c**) Appearance at the end

of ureter to bladder urothelium with 5/0 absorbable interrupted sutures. Close the urothelium vertically over the original hiatus with 5/0 absorbable interrupted sutures.

Suprapubic catheter insertion, ureteric stenting, bladder closure, wound closure and post-operative management are undertaken in the same manner as for the Cohen procedure.

Extravesical Procedures as Lich-Gregoir Technique (Fig. 4a–c)

The benefit of extravesical procedures is their association with fewer post-operative symptoms such as haematuria and bladder spasms [3] because this technique avoids opening the bladder. Furthermore, the risk of contralateral VUR is reported to be lower (<5%) following a unilateral extravesical compared to a unilateral cross-trigonal procedure [14].

Extravesical techniques carry a small increased risk of post-operative voiding problems, particularly after bilateral procedures. Urinary retention is likely related to neuropraxia resulting from extensive retrovesical dissection. Rarely, intermittent urethral catheterisation may be required long-term. Consequently, many urologists will perform the Lich-Gregoir technique for unilateral procedures only.

Ureteral dissection may be facilitated by initial cystoscopy and insertion of a ureteral stent. Subsequently patient positioning and preparation is similar to the intravesical techniques. A urethral catheter is inserted for intra-operative bladder filling to assist dissection. Access to the bladder is achieved via a Pfannenstiel incision (performed in the same manner as for the intravesical technique). For unilateral procedures, an inguinal incision is another option [24].

Blunt dissection is utilised to mobilise the bladder. The peritoneum is cleared from the bladder dome. The obliterated umbilical artery on the side to be re-implanted is identified, ligated and divided, thus improving access to the adjacent ureter positioned deeply. Subsequently the distal ureter is mobilised. The bladder is rotated medially and the peritoneum on the anterior surface of the distal ureter is swept away. The ureter is dissected circumferentially and controlled with a vessel loop. The ureter is carefully mobilised distally down to the VUJ ensuring the ureteric vasculature is preserved. However, dissection should stay close to the ureter to avoid damage to the detrusor nerves and trigone, which are primarily located dorso-medial to the VUJ [32]. Damage to the vesical nerve plexi likely contributes to the incidence of post-operative voiding difficulties. Circumferential dissection at the VUJ and distal mobilisation beyond the VUJ is therefore not advised.

The bladder is returned to the anatomical position. Using needle point diathermy, a vertical incision few centimetres long is made on the bladder extending superiorly from the VUJ in the line of the mobilised ureter. This incision is extended in a small, inverted v shape around the superior aspect of the VUJ. A traction suture placed at the superior limit of the intended incision facilitates this dissection. The detrusor is then divided carefully with diathermy until the urothelium bulges through. Using a pledget, detrusor muscle flaps are raised to permit tension free closure over the

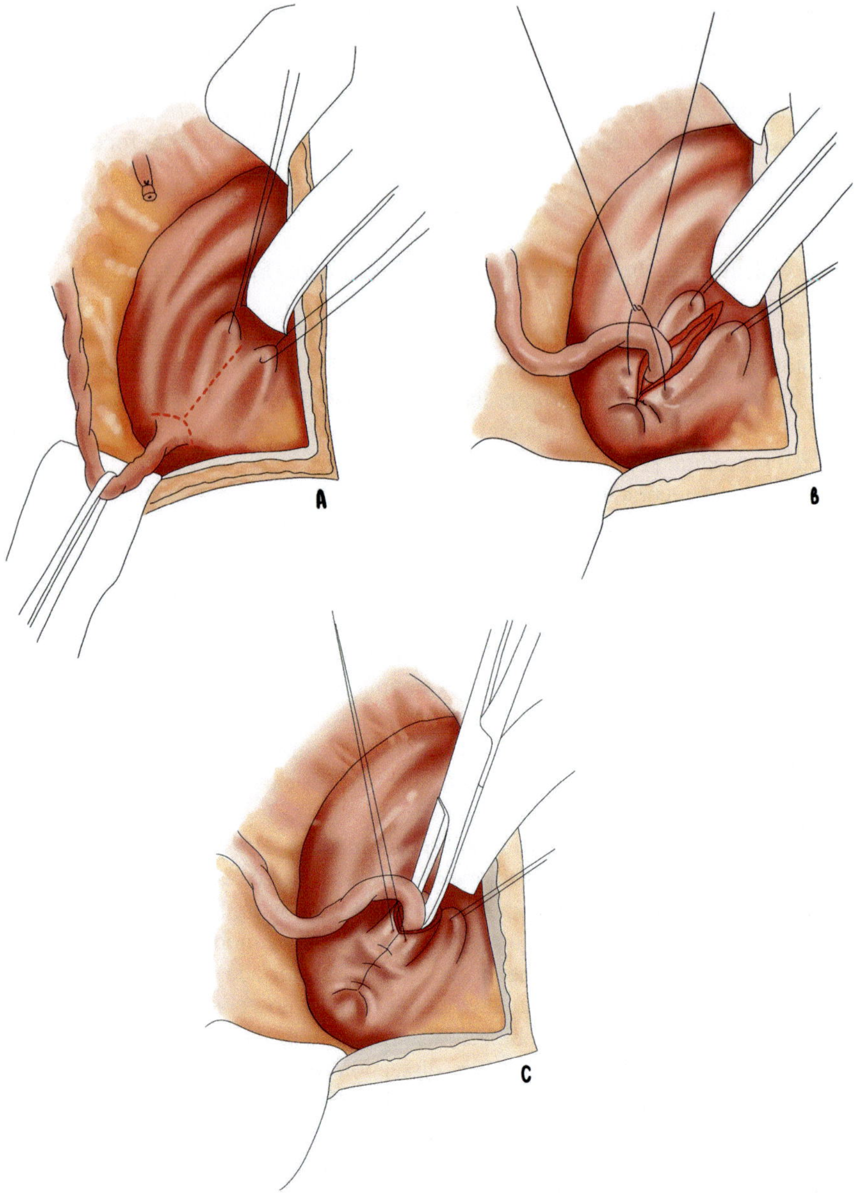

Fig. 4 (**a**–**c**) Lich-Gregoir technique. (**a**) A vertical incision a few centimeters long is marked superiorly on the bladder wall from the VUJ in the line of the mobilized ureter. The marked incision includes a small, inverted v shape at the VUJ. (**b**, **c**) The detrusor flaps are brought over the ureter ensuring that the channel is sufficiently wide, and the ureter is not twisted or constricted

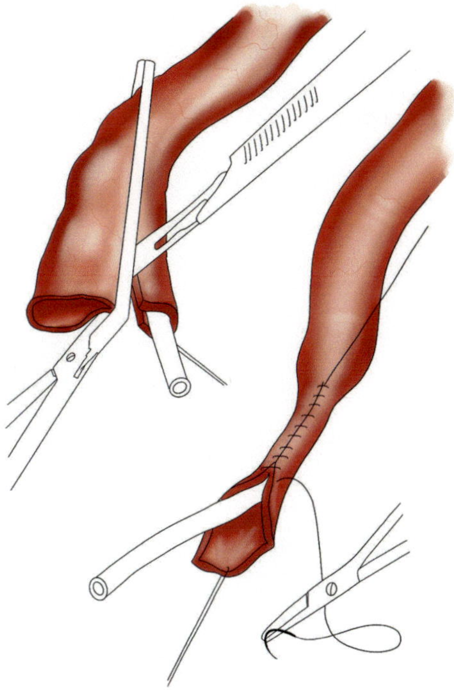

Fig. 5 Ureteric tapering. The ureter is tapered along its lateral aspect. The tapered ureter is closed with running suture up to the proximal 2/3 of its length. The remaining closure is completed with interrupted sutures

ureter. The bladder is partially emptied, and the ureteric stent is removed. The ureter is laid into the detrusorotomy ensuring the length of the tunnel is approximately 4 times the width of the ureter. The detrusor flaps are closed over the ureter with interrupted 3/0 or 4/0 absorbable sutures ensuring the ureter is not twisted or constricted. To prevent movement of the ureter within the tunnel, a number of the sutures should include the ureteric adventitia. Additionally, a single 4/0 absorbable suture is sited at the superior end of the tunnel to attach the muscle wall of the ureter to the detrusor. Urethral catheterisation is required for 24–48 hours post-operatively.

Additional Procedures

Ureteral Remodelling/Tapering/Tailoring (Fig. 5)

In the presence of large megaureters, the ureteral width may prohibit the formation of a sub-mucosal tunnel of adequate length to prevent reflux. In this situation ureteral remodelling is required. The most common technique used is tapering although ureteral plication is also undertaken.

Tapering is performed on the lateral side of the ureter on order to preserve the vascular supply on the medial aspect. A feeding tube (10F) is passed into the medial aspect of the ureter and a tapered lateral portion of ureter is excised with a blade or scissors. Excision may be assisted by use of Hendron clamps to mark out the

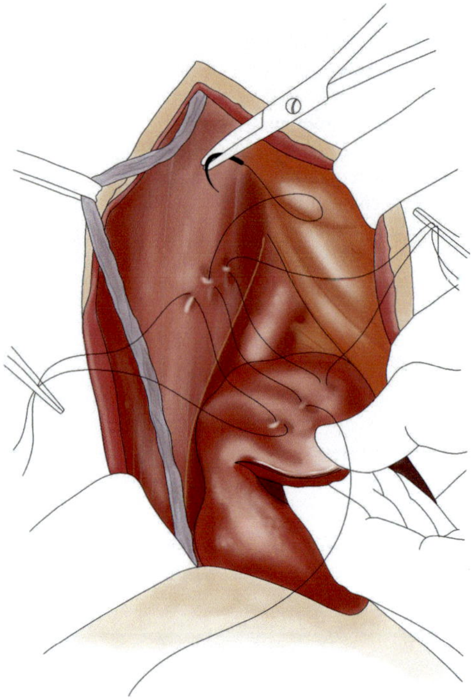

Fig. 6 Psoas hitch. The superolateral corner of the bladder is fixed to the psoas muscle to facilitate a straight ureter

intended line of excision. It is important to avoid excising too much ureter as this risks the vascularity of the remaining tissue and may lead to subsequent ureteral stricture. The proximal two-thirds of the remaining ureter is then closed with a continuous 4/0 or 5/0 absorbable suture. The distal one-third of the ureter is closed with interrupted sutures to enable subsequent trimming of the distal ureter if required. To reduce the risk of ureterovesical fistula the re-implanted ureter should be sited in the submucosal tunnel with the suture line laid posteriorly against the detrusor.

Psoas Hitch (Fig. 6)

A psoas hitch may be employed in re-operative cases where there is a short length of ureter. It is also advantageous, particularly when combined with a Leadbetter-Politano procedure, for children with an extremely dilated megaureter to prevent kinking of the re-implanted ureter. A psoas hitch involves anchoring the superolateral bladder with several interrupted 2/0 or 3/0 absorbable sutures to the psoas minor tendon (if present) and the psoas muscle superior and lateral to the iliac vessels. Sutures are tied loosely to prevent detrusor injury. Care should be taken to avoid the genitofemoral nerve trunk when placing sutures.

Post-operative Care

Following intravesical procedures, oral treatment dose antibiotics are continued for 1 week until the catheter and ureteral stents (when present) are removed. The urethral catheter is removed 24–48 hours following extra-vesical procedures. Following all techniques, the child takes prophylactic dose oral antibiotics until clinic review with a renal ultrasound scan performed 2–3 months post-operatively. If, at review, the child has not had any UTI's and the ultrasound scan is satisfactory, the antibiotics can be discontinued. Due to the reliable and successful nature of open ureteral re-implantation, routine post-operative voiding cystourethrogram is not required but is considered in those with recurrent febrile UTI's.

Outcome

Open techniques for ureteral re-implantation are extremely reliable with a general success rate for VUR correction of >95% [14]. The success rate of an open Cohen cross-trigonal ureteral re-implantation in completely resolving VUR varies between 96% and 100% [2, 28, 42], while the success rate with the Politano-Leadbetter ureteral re-implantation is 93–96% [21, 28]. Similarly, excellent results are reported following the Lich-Gregoir technique with a success rate of between 92% and 98% of ureters treated [6, 21, 23, 33, 34, 42].

The incidence of new renal scars following re-implantation is affected by the pre-operative grade of VUR [38] and is traditionally reported at 10–15% [21], however, others report a much lower incidence of ≤2% [50]. Despite successful VUR correction 5–10% of children will experience febrile UTI's during the first ten post-operative years [14].

Factors Affecting Outcome

Grade of VUR

Overall, the outcome of open ureteral re-implantation is less successful in higher grade VUR with a pooled success rate of 99% for grades I–IV and 81% for grade V VUR [47]. The Leadbetter-Politano technique has a success rate of 99% for grades I–II, 95% for grades III–IV and 80% for grade V [21]. Similarly, the success rates 1 year following extravesical re-implantation are significantly better in grade I–III VUR (99%) versus grades IV–V (96%) [6].

Prior Endoscopic Surgery

Some patients may have had endoscopic injection of a bulking agent such as Deflux® prior to ureteral re-implantation. Evidence suggests this does not affect the outcome of subsequent surgery with no difference in mean operative time, length of hospital stay, success rate and complication rate [11, 19, 31, 42].

Age and Gender

Barrieras et al. demonstrated that age had no significant effect on the success of extravesical ureteral re-implantation but that males had a lower success rate than females (93.2% vs 98.1%) [6]. Similarly, Hubert et al. when reviewing both intra and extravesical techniques of open re-implantation reported that children with persistent VUR following surgery were more likely to be male than those with successful correction but contrary to the former group, children with persistent VUR were significantly younger [25]. Younger age at initial diagnosis also impacts the subsequent incidence of development of new renal scars and/or reduction in differential function post-operatively [38].

Bladder and Bowel Dysfunction

Third of children with VUR have dysfunctional voiding. Pre-operative bladder and bowel dysfunction increases the risk of post-operative complications and surgical failure following VUR correction. It is therefore imperative that bladder and bowel dysfunction is appropriately managed before undertaking ureteral re-implantation [21, 22].

Type of Surgery

A systematic review and meta-analysis have not shown any significant difference in success rate for correcting VUR between intravesical and extravesical techniques. Neither is there any significant difference in the rate of post-operative hydronephrosis or the rate of post-operative febrile urinary tract infections [42].

Compared to intravesical re-implantations, extravesical techniques are associated with shorter operative time, fewer post-operative bladder spams, reduced pain scores, less analgesic requirement, less haematuria and reduced post-operative length of stay [3, 41, 42, 44] (Law et al. 2022). Bilateral extravesical re-implantations have a significantly higher rate of post-operative urinary retention compared to bilateral intravesical procedures (8.1% vs 1.7% respectively).

Urinary retention is not, however, reported in patients following unilateral extravesical or unilateral intravesical ureteral re-implantation (Law et al. 2022).

Complications

Persistent Ipsilateral VUR

Children with persistent VUR following open re-implantation are younger at the time of operation, more often antenatally diagnosed and have a higher rate of ureteral tapering compared to those with resolution of VUR on post-operative voiding cystourethrogram (VCUG). The surgical technique (extravesical vs intravesical) does not affect the likelihood of post-operative persistent VUR [25].

VUR noted in the early post-operative period on VCUG is often low-grade and frequently resolves spontaneously within 1–2 years post-operatively. This phenomenon may be related to bladder dysfunction secondary to bladder irritation in the early post-operative period which subsequently resolves [6]. Following extravesical ureteric re-implantation, success on VCUG was noted in 93% of ureters (91% patients) at 3 months, which increased to 98% of ureters (95% patients) at 12 months [6]. Similarly, following either extravesical or intravesical re-implantation 6% (59/965) of patients had persistent VUR on post-operative VCUG. Thirty-seven patients had serial cystography and VUR resolved in 72% at a median of 20.4 months post-operatively. One patient out of 965 required further re-implantation.

No association between age, gender, surgical method, ureteral tapering, pre or post-operative VUR grade and time to resolution was noted [25]. Conversely, following extravesical re-implantation, post-operative VUR has been reported to be less likely to resolve in children with pre-operative high-grade VUR [6].

Contralateral VUR

Following unilateral open re-implantation up to 1 in 5 children develop contralateral VUR [14, 21, 26]. There is conflicting evidence as to whether the type of procedure affects the risk of contralateral VUR. Some authors suggest no difference between extra and intravesical techniques [13, 26] while others suggest the risk appears to be lower (<5%) following the extravesical Lich-Gregoir technique [14].

In almost 80% of children, contralateral VUR resolves spontaneously within 2–3 years [21, 26]. The risk of contralateral VUR is increased in the presence of a bladder capacity <50% predicted and in children ≤6 years of age [26]. Furthermore, contralateral VUR is more likely if there was a duplex system or high grade VUR on the operated side or if the contralateral ureter itself previously refluxed but resolved pre-operatively [13, 14, 26].

Obstruction

Following open ureteral re-implantation up to 7% of children will have minor self-resolving hydroureteronephrosis [6, 40]. A small number of children present post-operatively with acute ureteral obstruction and symptomatic hydronephrosis, with abdominal pain, nausea, vomiting and fatigue. A fever indicates concomitant infection.

Acute ureteral obstruction has multiple causes including mechanical obstruction secondary to a kink/twist of the distal ureter and ureteral compression by hematoma or oedema. Management involves urgent decompression of the upper tract which may be achieved by cystoscopy and double J stent insertion or by ultrasound-guided insertion of a percutaneous nephrostomy.

Post-operative hydroureteronephrosis should be monitored with serial ultrasonography. If there is persistence beyond 12 weeks post-operatively then assessment for new or ongoing bladder dysfunction should be undertaken. Additionally, diuretic renography should be considered. Obstruction secondary to ureteric stricture is reported in 1% of children following Politano-Leadbetter re-implantation and 2–4% of children following the Lich-Gregoir technique [21, 45]. Stricture likely arises due to ureteral devascularisation during mobilisation. Surgical management depends on the length of the stricture. Short strictures at the vesicoureteral junction may respond to either balloon dilatation and/or ureteral stenting. Longer strictures may necessitate re-do ureteral re-implantation. Overall <1% of ureteral re-implantations require revision for ureteral obstruction [40].

Urinary Retention

Temporary urinary retention is reported following bilateral extravesical ureteral re-implantation in 4–16% of children [5, 23, 34]. It is likely secondary to vesical nerve plexus injury.

Boys, children <3 years of age and children with grade IV/V VUR have a greater rate of post-operative urinary retention (20%, 36% and 25% respectively). Post-operative retention resolves in the majority at around 7 days post-operatively [5, 33] however a small number (4%) require longer-term intermittent catheterisation over a period of months [5].

Bowel Injury

Bowel injury is a rare complication of all ureteral re-implantations but is reported in 0.5% of Politano-Leadbetter procedures. This complication is likely to be secondary to the retrovesical dissection undertaken to re-direct the ureter to the new superiorly sited hiatus [21].

Re-operative Reimplantation

Re-operative surgery may be indicated for children who present with recurrent febrile UTI's following previous ureteral re-implantation and have confirmation of either ongoing VUR or ureteral obstruction on imaging. It is important to have excluded bladder dysfunction as a cause of ongoing VUR prior to undertaking re-operation.

Evidence suggests that successful correction of recurrent or persistent VUR can be achieved in 77–100% of ureters with endoscopic submucosal injection of a bulking agent such as Deflux® [9, 35]. Kumar and Puri demonstrated increasing success with repeated injections. Out of 40 refluxing ureters, 27 (68%) were corrected after a single injection of Teflon. Seven ureters required 2 injections and 4 ureters required 3 injections to fully correct VUR. Only 2 out 40 ureters required a re-do re-implantation [29].

Re-do re-implantations, when required, are more challenging than primary procedures and techniques to deal with a short ureter may need to be employed. Both intra and extravesical dissection should be carefully utilised to fully mobilise the ureter and enable a sufficient submucosal tunnel. The refluxing ureter is approached transvesically. The ureteral meatus is circumscribed and then the intact ureter is dissected from the submucosal tunnel which is completely opened. The ureter is mobilised cranial to the hiatus to enable enough length for a tension free repair. A Leadbetter-Politano re-implantation is then undertaken.

If the ureter is too short, a Boari flap may be useful. To create a Boari flap, the bladder is filled with saline and mobilised extraperitoneally and the strictured portion of the ureter is excised. A broad-based flap that will reach and overlap the distal end of the ureter by about 3 cm is marked out with stay sutures from the dome of the bladder onto the anterior bladder wall. The distal flap needs to be 3 times the diameter of the ureter to avoid ureteral constriction. The flap is incised and rotated cranially to meet the ureter. A submucosal tunnel is created with scissors at the cranial end of the flap and the ureter drawn through, trimmed and spatulated. The Boari flap may be fixed to the psoas minor tendon avoiding the ilioinguinal and genitofemoral nerves as described above in the psoas hitch procedure. A 5F feeding tube is inserted via the ureter into the renal pelvis. The distal ureter is anastomosed circumferentially to the urothelium and detrusor of the flap in the same manner as a standard re-implantation. The tube and bladder are closed in 2 continuous layers.

Special Considerations

Duplex Kidneys with a Functioning Refluxing Lower Moiety

VUR is commonly present in the duplex system, affecting the ipsilateral lower moiety ureter (50%) and also the contralateral ureter (25%) [49]. When undertaking an anti-reflux procedure for a duplex system both upper and lower moiety ureters should be re-implanted in their common sheath to avoid disruption to their shared vascular supply. Overall, the success of common sheath ureteral re-implantation by extravesical or intravesical techniques is comparable to that of single systems. The success rate is approximately 96%, with failure generally due to ongoing VUR [4, 7, 15] although post-operative vesicoureteral obstruction is also reported in up to 4% [20].

Despite an excellent success rate, common sheath ureteral re-implantation in the duplex system is a predictor of an increased risk of post-operative complications [46]. It is also associated with a higher risk of new contralateral VUR compared to single system re-implantation (26% vs 12%) [13].

When the upper moiety ureter opens into the bladder and is non-obstructed, an alternative to common sheath re-implantation is ipsilateral ureteroureterostomy. Ureteroureterostomy may be undertaken open or laparoscopically. Compared to common sheath re-implantation ureteroureterostomy avoids the morbidity of opening the bladder, avoids the risk of iatrogenic vesicoureteral reflux or vesicoureteral obstruction of the associated ureter, avoids the technical difficulties of common sheath re-implantation in a large, dilated ureter and has a shorter hospital stay. The success rate of correcting VUR in a duplex system with ureteroureterostomy is reported between 96% and 100%. Complications of ureteroureterostomy for all indications (obstruction and VUR) include anastomotic leak (12.5%), donor ureteral obstruction (3%), persistent reflux in a concomitantly re-implanted recipient ureter (2%) and a non-draining ureteral stump (1%) [20, 30].

Indications for Nephrectomy

Nephroureterectomy should be considered in patients who have a poorly functioning (<10% on DMSA) refluxing kidney, a normal contralateral kidney, and recurrent febrile UTI's or ongoing hypertension. Nephrectomy normalises blood pressure in 88% of patients with renal parenchymal scarring and hypertension [45]. Furthermore, in the symptomatic patient with a poorly functioning refluxing lower moiety of a duplex kidney, a lower moiety heminephroureterectomy should be considered. Laparoscopic nephroureterectomy or heminephroureterectomy can be performed retroperitoneally or transperitoneally.

The retroperitoneal approach avoids traversing the peritoneal cavity and mobilising the colon, but, because the ureter cannot be excised all the way to the hiatus it leaves a longer distal ureteral stump into which reflux can occur [17]. There is conflicting evidence as to how problematic this is but some children (2.6–10%) may need a further procedure to remove the distal ureteral stump if they remain symptomatic with UTI's [8, 10, 17]. Consequently, some urologists recommend the transperitoneal approach only for poorly functioning refluxing ureters to enable initial excision of the ureter all the way down to the hiatus.

Conclusions

Open ureteral re-implantation for vesicoureteral reflux is indicated when non-operative management with chemoprophylaxis or endoscopic management of VUR has not been successful. Excellent and reproducible results are obtained from open ureteral re-implantation in both single and duplicated systems. Ureteroureterostomy is an alternative reliable option in the duplicated system while nephroureterectomy may be employed in the non-functioning kidney.

References

1. Shalaby MS, Jackson L. Surgical treatment of vesicoureteric reflux. In: Puri P, editor. Pedaitric surgery. Springer, Berlin, Heidelberg; 2023.
2. Ansari MS, Banthia R, Jain S, Kaushik VN, Danish N, Yadav P. Long term outcomes of Cohen's cross trigonal reimplantation for primary vesicoureteral reflux in poorly functioning kidney. World J Clin Cases. 2023;11(16):3750–5.
3. Aydin C, Akkoc A, Topaktas R, Senturk AB, Aydin ZB, Ürkmez A, Yaytokgil M. Comparison of Cohen and Lich-Gregoir ureteral reimplantation in the surgical management of primary unilateral vesicoureteral reflux in children. Rev Assoc Med Bras (1992). 2020;66(4):424–9.
4. Barrett DM, Malek RS, Kelalis PP. Problems and solutions in surgical treatment of 100 consecutive ureteral duplications in children. J Urol. 1975;114(1):126–30.
5. Barrieras D, Lapointe S, Reddy PP, Williot P, McLorie GA, Bägli D, Khoury AE, Merguerian PA. Urinary retention after bilateral extravesical ureteral reimplantation: does dissection distal to the ureteral orifice have a role? J Urol. 1999;162(3 Pt 2):1197–200.
6. Barrieras D, Lapointe S, Reddy PP, Williot P, McLorie GA, Bagli D, Khoury AE, Merguerian PA. Are postoperative studies justified after extravesical ureteral reimplantation? J Urol. 2000;164(3Pt2):1064–6.
7. Barrieras D, Lapointe S, Houle H. Is common sheath extravesical reimplantation an effective technique to correct reflux in duplicated collecting systems? J Urol. 2003;170(4 Pt 2):1545–7; discussion 1547.
8. De Caluwé D, Chertin B, Puri P. Long-term outcome of the retained ureteral stump after lower pole heminephrectomy in duplex kidneys. Eur Urol. 2002;42(1):63–6.
9. Capozza N, Nappo S, Caione P. Endoscopic treatment of vesicoureteral reflux in the previously reimplanted ureter: technical aspects and results. Arch Esp Urol. 2008;61:249–53.
10. Casale P, Grady RW, Lee RS, Joyner BD, Mitchell ME. Symptomatic refluxing distal ureteral stumps after nephroureterectomy and heminephroureterectomy. What should we do? J Urol. 2005;173(1):204–6; discussion 206.
11. Chertin B, Prosolovich K, Aharon S, Nativ O, Halachmi S. Surgical reimplantation for the correction of vesicoureteral reflux following failed endoscopic injection. Adv Urol. 2011:352716.

12. De Castro R, Hubert KC, Palmer JS. Retrograde ureteral access after cross-trigonal ureteral re-implantation: a straightforward technique. J Pediatr Urol. 2011;7(1):57–60.
13. Diamond DA, Rabinowitz R, Hoenig D, Caldamone AA. The mechanism of new onset contralateral reflux following unilateral ureteroneocystostomy. J Urol. 1996;156(2 Pt 2):665–7.
14. Elder JS. Vesicoureteral reflux – surgical treatment. In: Puri P, Höllwarth M, editors. Pediatric surgery. 2nd ed. Heidelberg: Springer; 2019.
15. Ellsworth PI, Lim DJ, Walker RD, Stevens PS, Barraza MA, Mesrobian HG. Common sheath reimplantation yields excellent results in the treatment of vesicoureteral reflux in duplicated collecting systems. J Urol. 1996;155(4):1407–9.
16. Emiliani E, Talso M, Audouin M, Traxer O. Modern flexible ureteroscopy in Cohen cross-trigonal ureteral re-implantations. J Pediatr Urol. 2017;13(3):329–31.
17. Escolino M, Farina A, Turrà F, Cerulo M, Esposito R, Savanelli A, Settimi A, Esposito C. Evaluation and outcome of the distal ureteral stump after nephro-ureterectomy in children. A comparison between laparoscopy and retroperitoneoscopy. J Pediatr Urol. 2016;12(2):119.e1–8.
18. Evans K, et al. What is the risk of urinary tract infection in children with antenatally presenting dilating vesico-ureteric reflux? J Pediatr Urol. 2015;11(2):93 e1–6.
19. Friedlander DA, Ludwig WW, Jayman JR, Akhavan A. The effect of prior endoscopic correction of vesicoureteral reflux on open ureteral reimplantation: surgical outcomes and costs. J Pediatr Urol. 2018;14(3):268 e261–5.
20. Gerwinn T, Gnannt R, Weber DM, Gobet R, Mazzone L. Laparoscopic ureteroureterostomy vs. common sheath ureteral reimplantation in children with duplex kidney anomalies. Front Pediatr. 2021;9:637544.
21. Heidenreich A, Ozgur E, Becker T, Haupt G. Surgical management of vesicoureteral reflux in pediatric patients. World J Urol. 2004;22(2):96–106.
22. Herz D, Fuchs M, Todd A, McLeod D, Smith J. Robot-assisted laparoscopic extravesical ureteral reimplant: a critical look at surgical outcomes. J Pediatr Urol. 2016;12(6):402 e401–9.
23. Houle AM, McLorie GA, Heritz DM, McKenna PH, Churchill BM, Khoury AE. Extravesical nondismembered ureteroplasty with detrusorrhaphy: a renewed technique to correct vesicoureteral reflux in children. J Urol. 1992;148(2 Pt 2):704–7.
24. Howe AS, Palmer LS. An inguinal approach to complex extravesical ureteral re-implantation. Urology. 2017;106:178–82.
25. Hubert KC, Kokorowski PJ, Huang L, Prasad MM, Rosoklija I, Retik AB, Nelson CP. Clinical outcomes and long-term resolution in patients with persistent vesicoureteral reflux after open ureteral reimplantation. J Urol. 2012;188(4 Suppl):1474–9.
26. Hubert KC, Kokorowski PJ, Huang L, Prasad MM, Rosoklija I, Retik AB, Nelson CP. New contralateral vesicoureteral reflux after unilateral ureteral reimplantation: predictive factors and clinical outcomes. J Urol. 2014 Feb;191(2):451–7.
27. Kalayeh K, Fowlkes JB, Schultz WW, Sack BS. The 5:1 rule overestimates the needed tunnel length during ureteral re-implantation. Neurourol Urodyn. 2021;40:85–94.
28. Kruppa C, Wilke A, Hörz C, Kosk T, Hörz T, Fitze G, Schuchardt K, Vesicoscopic vs. Open ureteral reimplantation according to Cohen and Leadbetter-Politano for vesicoureteral reflux. J Clin Med. 2023;12(17):5686.
29. Kumar R, Puri P. Endoscopic correction of vesicoureteric reflux in failed reimplanted ureters. Eur Urol. 1998;33:98–100.
30. Lashley DB, McAleer IM, Kaplan GW. Ipsilateral ureteroureterostomy for the treatment of vesicoureteral reflux or obstruction associated with complete ureteral duplication. J Urol. 2001;165(2):552–4.
31. Lee S, Jeong SC, Chung JM, Lee SD. Secondary surgery for vesicoureteral reflux after failed endoscopic injection: comparison to primary surgery. Investig Clin Urol. 2016;57(1):58–62.
32. Leissner J, Allhof EP, Wolff W, Feja C, Hockel M, Black P, Hohenfellner R. The pelvic plexus and antireflux surgery: topographical findings and clinical consequences. J Urol. 2001;165(5):1652–5.

33. Lipski BA, Mitchell ME, Burns MW. Voiding dysfunction after bilateral extravesical ureteral reimplantation. J Urol. 1998;159(3):1019–21.
34. Minevich E, Aronoff D, Wacksman J, Sheldon CA. Voiding dysfunction after bilateral extravesical detrusorrhaphy. J Urol. 1998;160(3 Pt 2):1004–6; discussion 1038.
35. Nerli RB, Pujar SV, Ghagane SC, Hiremath MB, Dixit NS. Persistence and appearance of vesicoureteral reflux/obstruction following open reimplantation for vesicoureteral reflux. J Sci Soc. 2019;46(3):90–4.
36. NICE. Urinary tract infection in children; diagnosis, treatment and long-term management. 2018.
37. Paquin AJ Jr. Ureterovescial anastomosis: the description and evaluation of a technique. J Urol. 1959;82:573–83.
38. Piepsz A, Tamminen-Möbius T, Reiners C, Heikkilä J, Kivisaari A, Nilsson NJ, Sixt R, Risdon RA, Smellie JM, Söderborg B. Five-year study of medical or surgical treatment in children with severe vesico-ureteral reflux dimercaptosuccinic acid findings. International Reflux Study Group in Europe. Eur J Pediatr. 1998;157(9):753–8.
39. Politano VA, Leadbetter WF. An operative technique for the correction of vesicoureteral reflux. J Urol. 1958;79(6):932–41.
40. Riddell J, Franc-Guimond J. Learning from history or the rationale for considering surgical correction of vesicoureteral reflux. Can Urol Assoc J. 2010;4(4):280–3.
41. Schwentner C, Oswald J, Lunacek A, Deibl M, Koerner I, Bartsch G, Radmayr C. Lich-Gregoir reimplantation causes less discomfort than Politano-Leadbetter technique: results of a prospective, randomized, pain scale-oriented study in a pediatric population. Eur Urol. 2006;49(2):388–95.
42. Silay MS, Turan T, Kayali Y, Basibuyuk I, Gunaydin B, Caskurlu T, Karaman MI. Comparison of intravesical (Cohen) and extravesical (Lich-Gregoir) ureteroneo-cystotomy in the treatment of unilateral primary vescioureteric reflux in children. J Pediatr Urol. 2018;14(1):65 e61–4.
43. Singh-Grewal D, et al. Circumcision for the prevention of urinary tract infection in boys: a systematic review of randomised trials and observational studies. Arch Dis Child. 2005;90(8):853–8.
44. Sriram K, Babu R. Extravesical (modified Gregoir Lich) versus intravesical (Cohen's) ureteric reimplantation for vesicoureteral reflux in children: a single center experience. Indian J Urol. 2016;32(4):306–9.
45. Steffens J, Langen PH, Haben B, Hiebl R, Steffens L, Polsky MS, Politano-leadbetter ureteroneocystostomy. A 30-year experience. Urol Int. 2000;65(1):9–14.
46. Suer E, Ozcan C, Mermerkaya M, Gokce MI, Gulpinar O, Telli O, Soygur T, Burgu B. Can factors affecting complication rates for ureteric re-implantation be predicted? Use of the modified Clavien classification system in a paediatric population. BJU Int. 2014;114(4):595–600.
47. Tejwani R, Routh J. Vesicoureteral reflux. In: Wilcox DT, Thomas DFM, editors. Essentials of paediatric urology. 3rd ed. Abingdon: Taylor and Francis; 2021.
48. Thomas JC. Vesicoureteral reflux and duplex systems. Adv Urol. 2008;2008:651891. https://doi.org/10.1155/2008/651891.
49. Timberlake MD, Corbett ST. Minimally invasive techniques for management of the ureterocele and ectopic ureter: upper tract versus lower tract approach. Urol Clin North Am. 2015;42(1):61–76.
50. Webster RI, Smith G, Farnsworth RH, Rossleigh MA, Rosenberg AR, Kainer G. Low incidence of new renal scars after ureteral reimplantation for vesicoureteral reflux in children: a prospective study. J Urol. 2000;163(6):1915–8.
51. Wallis MC, Brown DH, Jayanthi VR, Koff SA. A novel technique for ureteral catheterisation and/or retrograde ureteroscopy after cross-trigonal ureteral re-implantation. J Urol. 2003;170(4Pt2):1664–6; Discussion 1666.

Laparoscopic and Robotic Ureteral Reimplantation for Vesicoureteral Reflux

Leon Chertin and Boris Chertin

Abstract The development of laparoscopy is an important advance in surgery. Since the beginning of this century, it has evolved to become the standard approach to several operations, replacing open procedures because of its less invasive nature. Following successful animal laparoscopic reimplantation several studies utilizing different modifications of laparoscopic reimplantation in humans were published showing results similar to the open reimplantation.

However, the main drawback has been the relatively steep learning curve for this procedure because of technical difficulties in suturing and anastomosis. With Robot Assisted-Surgery (RAS) it is possible to overcome many impediments of conventional laparoscopic surgery and to reduce the learning curve for Minimally Invasive Surgery (MIS), especially for pediatric reconstructive procedures.

An ergonomic advantage to the surgeon and extra freedom in suturing deep within the pelvic cavity, make RAS very attractive for reconstructive surgery. Relatively easier learning curve with robotic surgery and similar to laparoscopic surgery manual skills with speed increase of robotic platforms in medical centers around the world together with similar to laparoscopic and open surgery complications rate will make this approach a gold standard for pediatric reimplantation in VUR patients.

Keywords Vesicoureteral reflux · Open ureteral reimplantation · Laparoscopic ureteral reimplantation · Robotic assisted laparoscopic reimplantation of ureters · Pneumovesicoscopic cross-trigonal ureteral reimplantation

---

L. Chertin
Department of Urology, Shamir Medical Center, Faculty of Medicine Tel Aviv University, Zerifin, Israel

B. Chertin (✉)
Departments of Urology & Pediatric Urology, Shaare Zedek Medical Center, Faculty of Medicine, Hebrew University, Jerusalem, Israel
e-mail: chertinb@szmc.org.il

P. Puri, A. Yamataka (eds.), *Vesicoureteral Reflux*,
https://doi.org/10.1007/978-3-031-95091-9_20

Introduction

Vesicoureteral reflux (VUR) is associated with increased risk of urinary tract infection, renal scarring and reflux nephropathy. Numerous studies have examined the links between VUR, UTIs, pyelonephritis, renal scarring and impaired renal function. Hidas et al. developed an instrument for predicting the risk of breakthrough UTI in children with VUR [1]. They provided data that clearly showed that VUR grade, gender, circumcision status, presence of bladder/bowel dysfunction (BBD) and cause of presentation of VUR enable stratification of children into different risk groups. At practice, when the instrument was applied to a studied cohort, the predicted 2-year incidence of breakthrough UTI was 19.5%, compared with an actual rate of 21%.

The EAU and AUA guidelines recommend VCUG in infants with prenatally diagnosed hydronephrosis, and siblings and offspring of VUR patients [2, 3].

EAU guidelines also recommend VCUG examination in children with a febrile UTI or lower urinary tract dysfunction. For infants diagnosed in the first year of life, antibiotic prophylaxis is recommended as first-line treatment, with ureteral reimplantation or endoscopic treatment for those with breakthrough infections [4]. Antibiotic prophylaxis is also recommended in the EAU guidelines as initial treatment for children aged 1–5 years with grade III–V VUR, although ureteral reimplantation should be considered as an alternative in those with high-grade VUR [3].

We have published our data on renal function in patients with VUR who underwent successful endoscopic correction of VUR [5].

Over two decades we have treated almost 700 renal refluxing units (RRU) utilizing endoscopic approach to correct VUR. The majority of patients have had Grade III and IV VUR, while 73% of RRU demonstrated presence of renal scarring on radionuclide scan. During maximum of 20 years of follow up the majority of RRU have demonstrated an insignificant 2.3% change in relative function after successful reflux correction, while renal deterioration was noted only in 11 of 26 RRU with initially severe renal scarring (less than 20% uptake on [99m] technetium-dimercaptosuccinic acid scan). Moreover, patients with corrected VUR or those who showed vesicoureteral reflux downgrading did not show new renal scars. We have concluded that successful endoscopic correction of vesicoureteral reflux is accompanied by a low incidence of new renal scarring and febrile urinary tract infection. AUA has amended published in 2010 guidelines on VUR stated as an expert opinion that surgical intervention for VUR, including both open and endoscopic methods, might be used [2]. Prospective randomized, controlled trials have shown a reduction in the occurrence of febrile urinary tract infections in patients who have undergone open surgical correction of VUR as compared to those receiving continued antibiotic prophylaxis [4].

Furthermore, the guidelines recommend open or endoscopic surgery, in order to treat recurrent infections, new renal abnormalities determined by DMSA scanning, or if there is a parental preference to see a definitive treatment. Success rates for open surgery are 98%, with few complications, compared to rates of 83% for endoscopic surgery; however, the higher success rates for open surgery are offset by the greater expense and the need for in-patient hospitalization. The guidelines did not mention neither laparoscopic nor robotic assisted approach for the treatment of VUR.

In all patients with VUR, there is a need to balance risks, benefits and costs of treatment vs. risks (particularly to the kidneys) of not treating the condition [6–9].

Some authors believe that first-line endoscopic injection is preferable for many VUR patients requiring intervention, while reserving ureteral reimplantation for patients not responding to endoscopic injection, for those with primary obstructive refluxing megaureter, and those with grade V VUR and concomitant narrowing of the vesicoureteral junction [4, 10].

Open ureteral reimplantation (OUR) remains the gold standard surgical treatment of VUR, with success rates of 95–100% [11]. However, the success rate following open reimplantation might be different and reported to be only 80% in patents with bilateral Grade V VUR [12]. Moreover, longer recovery, high demand for painkillers, patients unsatisfaction with incisional scars could not to be brushed aside. Although it has been shown that open renal and bladder surgeries such as nephrectomy, pyeloplasty and ureteral reimplantation can also be done in an outpatient setting whilst open ureteral reimplantation demonstrated higher incidence of readmission and ER visits [13]. The introduction and advancement of laparoscopic and later robot-assisted surgical systems have revolutionized minimally invasive surgery in pediatric urology.

The development of laparoscopy is an important advance in surgery. In the beginning of this century, it has evolved to become the standard approach to several operations, replacing laparotomy procedures because of its less invasive nature. Conventional laparoscopic procedures for urological diseases such as nephrectomy, pyeloplasty, and radical prostatectomy have also proved to be safe and effective with outcome comparable with the open procedure. Laparoscopic approach allows excellent view of the pelvic anatomy and easier access to most pelvic structures. However, the main drawback has been the relatively steep learning curve for this procedure because of technical difficulties in suturing and anastomosis. By utilizing this surgical platform, surgeons maintain the benefits of laparoscopic surgery while having the additional advantages of added dexterity, greater range of movement, enhanced three-dimensional visualization, and increased control of high-resolution cameras.

With the advancement of robotic-assisted laparoscopic surgery (RALS), minimally invasive techniques for urologic surgeries have evolved greatly over the last decade.

Laparoscopic Extravesical Ureteral Reimplantation (LEVUR)

Extravesical ureteral reimplantation (EVUR) was described by Willy Gregoir [14].

This technique had demonstrated similar successful rates to the intravesical approach especially when it is combined with some modifications described in the literature [15, 16].

However, this operation gained poor acceptance in some regions due to the risk of denervation of the bladder, especially in bilateral cases [17].

After successful animal experiment in 1993 first human cases of laparoscopic extravesical ureteral reimplantation were reported [18, 19]. Since then, several series were reported comparing LEVUR to outcomes after open reimplantation (Table 1).

Technique of LEVUR

The technical steps of LEVUR resemble and preserve the principle of open reimplantation according to Lich Gregoir [20, 21].

Following general anesthesia with caudal block or quadrates lumborum blocks as we have previously demonstrated, urinary catheter is inserted and the patient is placed in a supine position [20, 22, 23]. Surgeon is behind patient head and the first

Table 1 Laparoscopic ureteral reimplantation publications

Author; Year	No of units	Mean age (years)	Duration of surgery (minutes)	Time to discharge (days)	Success rate %	No of Clavien-Dindo I–IV complications
Capolicchio 2008	31	7.3	NA	NA	96	2
Tsai 2008	14	3.4	170 U 218 B	1.4	93	1
Lopez 2010	43	4.4	70 U 124 B	1	100	2
Bayne 2012	144	6.7	NA	1.7	95	6
Javali 2015	98	9.5	102 U 95 B	1.5	98	3
Esposito 2012	38	4.8	95 U 128B	2.4	89	2
Soulier 2017	159	3.9	96 U 128 B	1.2	99	3
Badawy 2017	17	5	90 U	2	100	3
Bustangi 2018	57	4.2	127 U 184 B	1.6	98	4

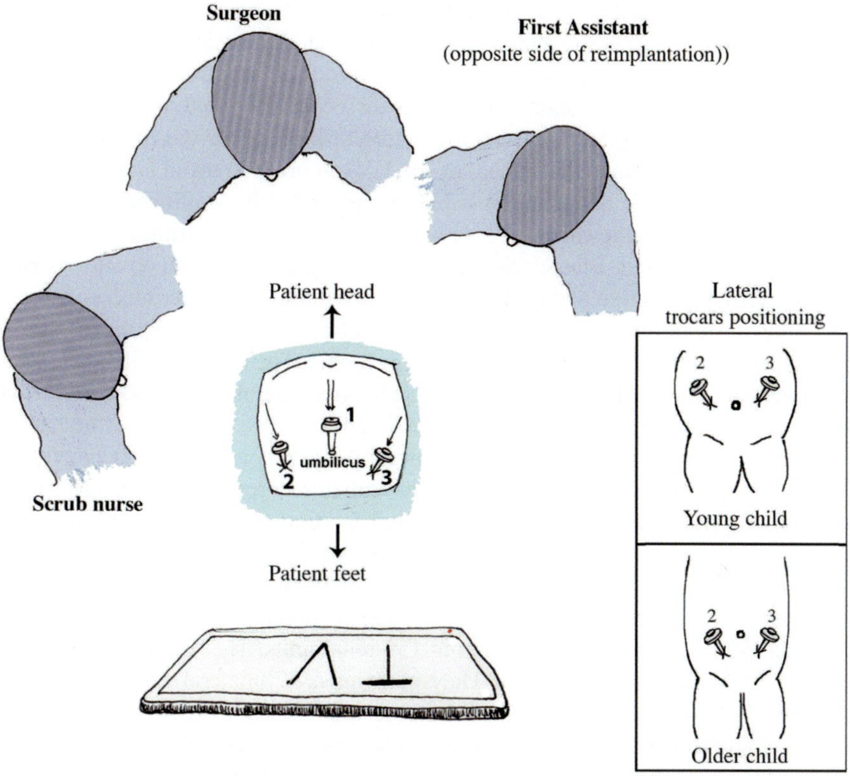

Fig. 1 Surgeon, first-assistant, scrub nurse and trocars positioning: example of an extra-vesical laparoscopic right reimplantation utilizing Lich–Gregoir approach. (Adapted from Soulier et al. [21])

assistant to his right (Fig. 1). Pneumoperitoneum might be obtained with Veress technique or via trans-umbilical incision and first trocar is placed in an open fashion utilizing carbon dioxide with a pressure ranging from 8 to 12 mm Hg. The rest of the trocars are placed under direct vision using a 5-mm scope with a 30° or 45° angle. The laparoscopic instruments used are 3 or 5 mm according to patient's age and size. Trocar disposition was a 5-mm trocar on the umbilicus, a 3–5-mm trocar on the right flank, and a 3- or 5-mm trocar on the left flank. Dissection can be carried using different forms of energy such as monopolar scissors on one hand and bipolar current diathermy on the other via 3 mm trocar or Harmonic Scalpel (Ethicon EndoSurgery, Cincinnati, Ohio, United States) or our preference 5 mm LigaSure with Curved Tip (Covidien, Mansfield, MA, USA) through a 5-mm trocar. The distal end of the ureter was dissected up to the ureterovesical junction through the posterior surface of the broad ligament in women finally cutting the round ligament. In the first cases, dissection was performed through the anterior edge of the broad ligament without cutting the round ligament. However, it was found that by cutting the broad ligament, a greater space was created and instruments mobility was improved. In male patients maximum attention should be paid to avoid any injury to the vas deference during dissection. We do recommend to avoid any devascularization of the vas trying to stay away of the vas and to avoid any use of cautery during and near vas dissection. Proximal ureter was dissected as needed to gain 2–3 cm of distal ureter inside the tunnel in a tension-free fashion. We avoid performing any dissection on the dorsomedial aspect of the UVJ in order to avoid an injury to the branches of the pelvic nerve and possible urinary difficulties following surgery. A lateral detrusor tunnel towards UVJ with a length of four to five times the diameter of the ureter is created. Bladder filling and emptying during tunnel creation is very helpful during dissection and observation of the bulging of bladder mucosa.

Following exposure of bladder mucosa blunt-tip scissors of Hook monopolar diathermia is utilized to complete the detrusor tunnel. The ureter was then placed in the tunnel and the edges of the detrusor were sutured over the ureter. The first stitch was placed in the superior apex of the tunnel and had to be precise to avoid having it too tight. If the first knot was too tight, ureteral dilation was immediately evident. We do use Maxon 4/0 monofilament stitches with intracorporeal knotting. Recently, to close the tunnel a V-Loc 4/0 stich is used facilitating intracorporeal suturing. Finally, port site incisions were closed with subcuticular absorbable suture.

Soulier et al. [21] published their result of over 10 years of experience with laparoscopic reimplantation utilizing Lich Gregoir technique. They have treated 117 children (92 girls, 25 boys) representing 159 renal units. The mean age at surgery was 47.1 months (±32.7 months). They performed 49 bilateral and 61 unilateral reimplantations and achieved 98% of reflux resolution. They experienced Clavien–Dindo Grade IIIa and b complications in 5 patients [21]. Also, Riquelme et al. [20] reported their results in 81 patients (95 refluxing units) also in this series the success rate was around 96%, while only 4 patients demonstrated VUR after surgery. However, in this series only 8% were patients with Gr IV VUR and none presented with Gr V. It is important to mention that the authors have performed 14 bilateral cases with none of the patients presented in the follow up with dysfunctional voiding [20]. Lakshmanan and Fung refined the laparoscopic technique and reported 71 cases in children with high grade VUR, and concluded that the laparoscopic technique was comparable to open reimplantation techniques and could be first choice in children with high grade of VUR and concomitant pathology. Addition technical refreshments such as utilization of Psoas Hitch, intracorporeal tapering when indicated might increase the successes rate and achieve an outcome comparable with open surgery.

Although LEVUR has been practiced for almost two decades, there have been no notable increase in the number of pediatric urologists and pediatric surgeons, who have adapted this technique in their routine practice [24].

Moreover, the number of GR V VUR treated with LEVUR is significantly lower than with open reimplantation or other minimally invasive technique [25].

It could be related to the necessity of ureteral tapering for majority of the cases of high grade VUR and subsequent intracorporeal suturing or creation of the long tunnel which is not always possible in small children. In order to overcome this problem laparoscopic extravesical transverse ureteral reimplantation originally proposed for primary obstructive megaureter was suggested [26].

In this approach, the anti-reflux tunnel is created on the lower aspect of the posterior bladder wall in the transverse fashion allowing creation of a long tunnel even in severe dilated ureters. The tunnel is created just above the vas deferens and starts just from the level of the umbilical artery and ending at the contralateral side. One could be argued that transverse position of the ureter might cause a problem with endoscopic manipulation on the ureter in these kids grow into adulthood, however the variety of flexible endoscopic and single use equipment now days will help to overcome this problem. In fact, we have treated so far 3 patients with De Novo reflux following extravesical dismembered laparoscopic robotic assisted reimplantation due to primary obstructive megaureter with great success and did not experience any problems with needle positioning for bulking agent injection [27].

Pneumovesicoscopic Cross-Trigonal Ureteral Reimplantation for Vesicoureteral Reflux

Maintenance of the peritoneal cavity pressure, manipulation in the pelvic area in small children could be very challenging, as a result of that Young et al. following successful animal study have proposed another minimally invasive approach to correct VUR named vesicoscopic reimplantation [28, 29].

Transvesicoscopic approach using pneumovesicum has some advantages. First, the transvesicoscopic approach using pneumovesicum provides excellent visualization, especially around the bladder neck. Second, since CO_2 insufflation is limited to the bladder, the transvesicoscopic approach using pneumovesicum is free from the intra-abdominal pressure that causes oliguria. Last, CO_2 pneumovesicum does not appear to affect the renal arterial or venous flow, nor does it introduce a CO_2 embolism.

Young et al. have treated ten boys and six girls with mean age of 4.1 years old who have had persistent dilating primary VUR (7 bilateral; 23 refluxing ureters) associated with recurrent urinary-tract infections and/or multiple pyelonephritic renal scars. All studied patients underwent endoscopic Cohen's cross-trigonal ureteral reimplantation with CO_2 pneumovesicum. Of those, 14 patients had grade V, 10 grade IV, 4 grade III, and 1 grade II refluxing ureters subsequently.

The technique consisted of placing the patient in supine or lithotomy position with the legs separated so the surgeons have accessibility to the bladder. For small infants, the surgeon stands above the patient's head, whereas for older children, the surgeon usually stood on the patient's left side. The video tower is placed between the patients' legs.

The first 5 mm camera port under is placed inside the bladder under the cystoscopic guidance following filling with saline and bladder wall is fixed to the anterior abdominal wall in order to avoid slipping away of the camera trocar. We do recommend as others to fix also a camera port in order to avoid its dislodgement during the procedure which in fact is a major cause of technical failure of this type of reimplantation. The bladder is drained via urethral catheter and insufflated with CO_2 insufflation to 10–12 mm Hg pressure. The balloon of the urethral catheter occludes the bladder neck in order to secure CO_2 pneumovesicum and it could also serve as an additional suction irrigation device during subsequent dissection and ureteral reimplantation. A 5-mm 30° endoscope is used during the entire procedure. Two additional 3 or to 5-mm working ports were then inserted along the interspinous skin crease on either side of the lower lateral wall of the distended bladder under vesicoscopic guidance. A 3–4-cm-long segment of 4F or 6F catheter was inserted into the respective ureter as a stent to facilitate ureteral mobilization and dissection. Intravesical mobilization of the ureter, dissection of the submucosal tunnel, and a Cohen's type of ureteral reimplantation was performed under endoscopic guidance in a manner similar to the open procedure. The ureter is mobilized by first circumscribing it around its orifice using hook electrocautery. With traction on the ureteral stent using a blunt grasper, the fibrovascular tissue surrounding the lower ureter could be seen and divided using fine 3-mm endoscopic scissors and a diathermy hook while preserving the main ureteral blood supply. Mobilization of the ureter was continued for 2.5–3 cm to the extravesical space. Once adequate ureteral length had been obtained, the muscular defect in the ureteral hiatus was repaired using 4-0 absorbable sutures, a submucosal tunnel was then created as in an open Cohen's procedure. Ureteroneocystostomy was performed under endoscopic guidance with intracorporeal suturing using interrupted 4-0 or 5-0 monofilament Maxon sutures. Most of the surgeons do not leave routinely JJ stents at the end of procedure except tapered ureters or some bilateral cases. The port sites are closed, and urethral catheter is left indwelling for 24–48 hours postoperatively. The authors have mentioned that that there is a steep learning curve with this procedure and special attention should be paid to anchoring and securing the trocars in order to avoid their dislodgement during the operation. Their results were outstanding in terms of reflux resolution, while all patients, but one demonstrated absence of reflux on 3–4 month VCUG examination. Only one patient with initial Gr V showed Gr I VUR postoperatively.

Most vesicoscopic procedures are performed using the transtrigonal Cohen technique, as in the case of open surgery. One of the disadvantages of the Cohen technique, whether under an open or vesicoscopic approach, is that postoperative transureteral treatment may be difficult. On the other hand, as a non-transtrigonal technique, the Politano-Leadbetter technique has been performed under both open and vesicoscopic approaches. This technique may allow postoperative transureteral treatment because the ureter is not crossed but requires extravesical manipulation and may incur injury to other organs, particularly to the vas deferens in boys.

Nishi et al. have proposed Glenn Anderson modification of vesicoscopic reimplantation. During this technique following ureter mobilization and ureteral hiatus closing below the ureter in the vertical fashion a submucosal tunnel was then made toward the internal urethral orifice and ureteral advancement was performed as per the Glenn-Anderson technique to make the total length of the tunnel combined with the closed section of hiatus 5 times the ureteral diameter. Out of 18 patients who underwent this procedure, 17 have had postoperative VCUG showing no reflux [30].

Striking evidence of vesicoscopic technique is limited cases studies, which were performed till today, with up to the 30 patients in some series only. Most of the studies reported on an average number of patients around 16–19 cases. Almost all studies reported an experience of the single experienced laparoscopic surgeon and did not provide any evidence of the possibility to replicate this technique in the routine practice. Kruppa et al. published the largest series of 229 ureters which were treated with vesicoscopic Cohen technique. Although the authors results showing 96% success rates of reflux resolution are impressive, also in this study all cases were done by single surgeon and only some parts of the surgery were performed by the trainees, which again raise the question of reproducibility of this technique in the routine surgical armamentarium [31].

While comparing with LEVUR technique a recent meta-analysis by Baby and Chandrasekharam demonstrated that vesicoscopic technique has lower success rate, takes more time to complete and has longer hospital stay. However more GR V cases were treated with this approach as well as more bilateral cases. Finally, both techniques have comparable complications rate [25] (Table 2).

Table 2 Vesicoscopic ureteral reimplantation publications

Author; Year	No of units	Mean age (years)	Duration of surgery (minutes)	Time to discharge (days)	Success rate %	No of Clavien-Dindo I–IV complications
Yeung 2005	23	4.1	112 U 178 B	1.9	96	2
Kutikov 2006	46	5	168 B	1.9	93	3
Valla 2009	113	4.2	82 U 130 B	2.8	92	8
Kawauchi 2009	29	5	145 U 230 B	2.5	96	1
Marte 2010	19	7.6	112 U 178 B	3	94	1
Abraham 2011	32	2.2	166 U 189 B	3	93	1
Chung 2012	90	3.7	155 B	1.6	96	3
Emir 2012	17	6.9	217 U 306 B	3.8	94	2
Soh 2015	19	15	235 U 268 B	3.4	95	1
Ansari 2017	34	4.6	135 B	4	94	3
Lau 2017	42	6.1	221	7.4	87	4
Chung 2018	92	3.3	147	4.4	98	0
Jayanthi 2018	317	7	169 U 197 B	1.6	93	10

Robotic Assisted Laparoscopic Ureteral Reimplantation

Robot-assisted surgeries have gained popularity in complex reconstruction in pediatric urology due to their proven effectiveness, particularly in surgeries such as pyeloplasty even in small children, uretero-ureteral anastomosis in children with duplex anomalies effectively replacing partial nephrectomy and in lower tract reconstruction in adult patients following gynecological injury [32, 33]. Robotic reconstruction has several significant advantages compared with pure laparoscopic technique such possibility to work in small spaces and providing excellent three-dimensional vision, intracorporeal suturing and tailoring of the ureter if indicated, fewer postoperative narcotics needed, and shorter hospital stays. However, it is important to consider the disadvantages, such as long learning curves, costs, and longer operative times in the beginning and preferably previous robotic experience in pediatric population in surgeries such as pyeloplasty [34–36]. Since first introduced in 2004 robot-assisted laparoscopic ureteral reimplantation (RALUR) it has been increasingly adopted and described in several clinical series [37, 38] (Table 3).

Similar to conventional laparoscopic technique during robot assisted surgery proximal ureter was dissected as needed to gain 2–3 cm of distal ureter inside the tunnel in a tension-free fashion and a lateral detrusor tunnel towards UVJ with a length of four to five times the diameter of the ureter is created Fig. 2a. The ureter was then placed in the tunnel and the edges of the detrusor were sutured over the ureter Fig. 2b.

In 2011, Smith et al. compared surgical outcomes of 25 extravesical Robotic Assisted laparoscopic ureteric reimplantation (RALUR) patients with those of 25 open cross-trigonal ureteral reimplantation patients. The overall success rate was 97% for RALUR compared to 100% for open reimplantation, but with a reduced mean length of stay (33 hours vs. 53 hours) and reduced pain medication usage in the RALUR group [39]. Several other studies published demonstrated feasibility and efficacy of RALUR in different pediatric population utilizing not only extravesical but also trans vesical approach [40].

In order to standardize the robotic approach to the ureteral reimplantation and to equalize the surgical outcome to one after open reimplantation Gundeti et al. published RALUR-EV outcomes [41].

They have renamed the technique of RALUR-EV, which was termed LUAA to represent the length of detrusor tunnel (L), use of a U stitch (U), placement of permanent ureteral alignment suture (A), and inclusion of ureteral adventitia (A) in detrusorrhaphy. The authors suggested to keep the length of the detrusor tunnel 4–5 cm, to put a U shape stich between the distal part of the ureter and bladder following creation of the new orifice and also the placement a permanent alignment stich preventing sliding to the ureter from detrusor tunnel therefore decreasing the rate of the VUR recurrence and finally inclusion of the ureteral adventitia into the closure of detrusor. In spite the fact that the authors demonstrated good results almost identical to the open reimplantation results we felt that the sufficient length of the tunnel is not always possible with this technique specially in the small

Table 3 Robot assisted laparoscopic ureteral reimplantation publications

Author; Year	No of units	Mean age (years)	Duration of surgery (minutes)	Time to discharge (days)	Success rate %	No of Clavien-Dindo I–IV complications
Peters 2004	27	5.8	NA	NA	88	3
Casale 2008	82	3.2	153	1.1	97.6	0
Smith 2011	33	5.9	235 U 262 B	1.4	97	4
Marchini 2011	27	8.6	209 U 233 B	1.3	85	6
Kasturi 2012	300	3.6	110	1	99.3	0
Chalmers 2012	22	6.3	237 U 285 B	1.3	91	0
Dangle 2014	40	5.4	NA	1.8	80	NA
Schomburg 2014	35	6.2	165 U 227 B	1	100	3
Akhavan 2014	78	7.2	NA	2	92.3	6
Hayashi 2014	15	7.6	217 U 298 B	7.4	93	0
Grimsby 2015	93	6.7	NA	NA	77	6
Herz 2016	72	5.2	206 U 306 B	1.6	85.2	10
Arlen 2016	13	9.3	169.3	1	100	1
Gundeti 2016	83	5.3	NA	2	82	1
Boysen 2017	363	6.4	152 U 198 B	1.6	87.9	11
Boysen 2018	199	6.6	174 U 218 B	1.5	93.8	10
Sachdev 2019	230	5.9	161 U 208 B	NA	97	14
Kim 2019	101	5	161 U 205 B	1.3	96	6

children or following failure of previous surgery. Furthermore, extensive dissection around UVJ even in unilateral case might cause voiding disfunction with special attention in bilateral cases. Therefore, we have suggested a different technique when a new anti-reflux tunnel is created in the transverse fashion at the posterior wall of the bladder at the level of two orifices. We have called this technique dismembered extravesical cross-trigonal ureteral reimplantation (RADECUR) [42]. The operation is performed under general anesthesia with caudal Morphine block as we have

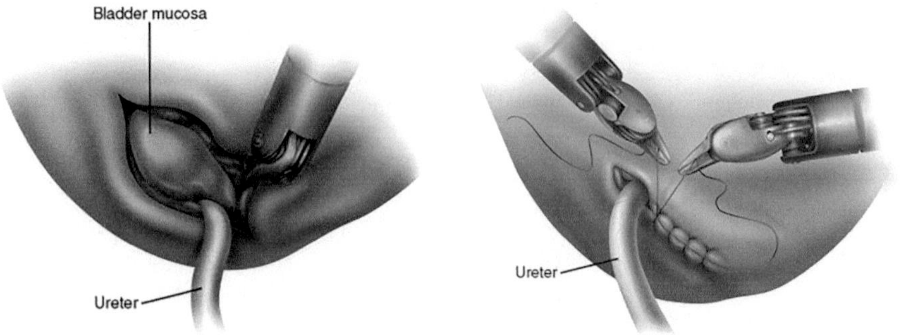

Fig. 2 (**a**) creation of the antireflux tunnel (**b**) suturing the detrusor over the ureter

published or Quadratum Lumborum block in older children as have also previously demonstrated [43, 44]. Patients were positioned in a low lithotomy position. A urethral catheter was inserted at the beginning of the operation. Pneumoperitoneum was achieved using the Hasson technique through the umbilicus. We have used a standard port configuration including a camera port inserted in the umbilicus, two 8 mm robotic ports, and a 5 or 10 mm assistant port usually on the contralateral side from the operated ureter. During entire procedure the bladder is filled and emptied with saline in order to facilitate bladder and ureter exposure, to improve visualization and to plan detrusorrhaphy and anastomosis.

A transverse detrusorrhaphy approximately 5 cm in length was made ipsilateral to contralateral ureter in the posterior-inferior aspect of the bladder. Mucosa opening in the contralateral end was performed without cautery. Ureteral tailoring is performed when indicated intracorporeally over an 8F or 10F ureteral catheter inserted through a trocar.

Ureter-bladder anastomosis is performed using interrupted 4/0 monofilament sutures such as Maxon over the Double J stent which is inserted through the assistant port. The Stent length is calculated according the formula Age +10. An anchoring suture at the lateral most point of the anti-reflux tunnel is placed between detrusor and ureteral adventitia in order to avoid kinking of the ureter and sliding from the tunnel Detrusorrhaphy was closed over the ureter incorporated ureteral adventitia in the first two sutures with a running 4-0 V-Lock suture (Fig. 3).

We do not use any drains. The patient is discharged on the following day with catheter removed at the day of discharge. Stents are removed under short general anesthesia 2–6 weeks after surgery.

We have recently summarized our experience with this technique in the low ureteral pathology compared this technique with pure laparoscopic approach in a large multicenter study of 13 center and 17 pediatric surgeons/urologists which took part in the study world wide [27].

Over all 1343 patients with VUR underwent RADECUR. Of those 861 had Grade III–V VUR. 118 (8%) required incisional ureteral tapering. All surgeries were completed utilizing robotic assisted approach. All tailoring cases were

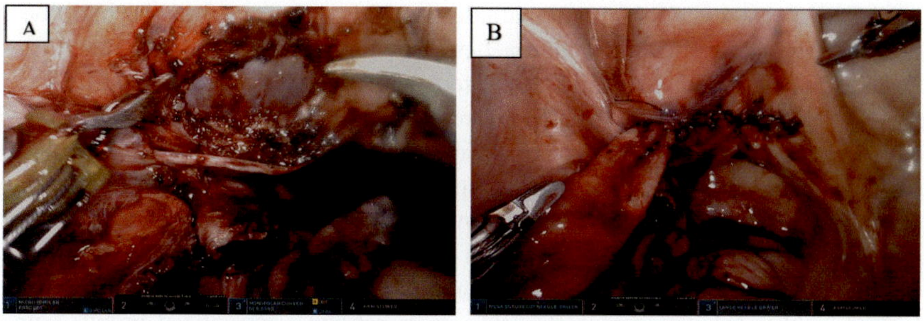

Fig. 3 (**a**) Submucosal tunnel. (**b**) Completion of detrusor closure

completed intracorporeally. The success rate was 96%. All cases with reflux recurrence have had primary Grade V VUR. Residual reflux was cured with endoscopic correction. The RADECUR patients did better than classical laparoscopic cases in terms of reflux correction rate, length of the hospital stay and complications. Also, none of the patients in the robotic arm needed open surgery.

One of the worrying issues with extravesical approach is voiding dysfunction and urinary retention following surgery. In order to avoid it the surgeon should keep in mind to avoid extensive dissection of the ureter at UVJ area in the dorsal medial aspect in order to avoid injury to the brunches of the pelvic nerve. The use of cautery should also be diminished maximally. Philadelphia group published their observations with urinary retention following RALUR cases showing 8–9% rate of urinary retention [45]. Majority were bilateral cases and univariant analysis showed male gender and longer operative times as predictive factors for urinary retention. Laterality did not appear as an independent predictive factor for development of complications.

There is still a debate over the cost of robotic surgeries and its application in the pediatric practice. Kurtz et al. published a cost and complication comparison of robotic versus open pediatric ureteral reimplantation and reported higher median operative times, incidence of any 90-day complications and median hospital cost for RALUR ($9128 vs. $7273) compared to open ureteral reimplantation [46]. However, this manuscript reported an experience with robotic assisted reimplantation during an initial learning curve. Furthermore, the cohort of open surgery was significantly larger than the robotic, and the cost of surgery is different among centers of excellence around the world, therefore further studies on financial outcomes are necessary.

Conclusions

Utilization of minimally invasive techniques has shown many benefits in postoperative outcomes such as improved cosmetics, shorter hospitalizations, and decreased postoperative pain. In addition, there is a growing evidence that robotic procedures in pediatric urology result in comparable or better outcomes than the traditional open or classical laparoscopic approaches. However, prospective randomized controlled trials are needed to validate the reported outcomes. RALUR and LEVUR seem to be good alternatives to open ureteral reimplantation. It seems that wide employment of the robotic platforms around the word will lead robotic assisted surgery to become a preferable surgical approach. Employing a new technique such as RADECUR might lead to the improved rate of reflux resolution and shorter learning curve with the robotic approach.

Robotic-assisted technology for minimally invasive surgery is becoming popular among the pediatric urologists. With more robotic - specialized brands being introduced to the market, the overall costs of these procedures will eventually decrease and the desire for more miniaturized instruments adopted for VUR surgery in infants and children could be addressed [47].

References

1. Hidas G, Billimek J, Nam A, et al. Predicting the risk of breakthrough urinary tract infections: primary vesicoureteral reflux. J Urol. 2015;194(5):1396–401. https://doi.org/10.1016/j.juro.2015.06.019.
2. Peters CA, Skoog SJ, Arant BS, et al. Summary of the AUA guideline on management of primary vesicoureteral reflux in children. J Urol. 2010;184(3):1134–44. https://doi.org/10.1016/j.juro.2010.05.065.
3. Tekgül S, Riedmiller H, Hoebeke P, et al. EAU guidelines on vesicoureteral reflux in children. Eur Urol. 2012;62(3):534–42. https://doi.org/10.1016/j.eururo.2012.05.059.
4. Läckgren G, Cooper CS, Neveus T, et al. Management of vesicoureteral reflux: what have we learned over the last 20 years? Front Pediatr. 2021;9:650326. https://doi.org/10.3389/fped.2021.650326.
5. Chertin B, Natsheh A, Fridmans A, et al. Renal scarring and urinary tract infection after successful endoscopic correction of vesicoureteral reflux. J Urol. 2009;182(4 Suppl):1703–6. https://doi.org/10.1016/j.juro.2009.03.011.
6. Kirsch AJ, Arlen AM. Evolving surgical management of pediatric vesicoureteral reflux: is open ureteral reimplantation still the "Gold Standard"? Int Braz J Urol. 2020;46(3):314–21. https://doi.org/10.1590/S1677-5538.IBJU.2020.99.05.
7. Subcommittee on Urinary Tract Infection. Reaffirmation of AAP clinical practice guideline: the diagnosis and management of the initial urinary tract infection in febrile infants and young children 2–24 months of age. Pediatrics. 2016;138(6):e20163026. https://doi.org/10.1542/peds.2016-3026.
8. Anonymous. Urinary tract infection in under 16s: diagnosis and management | Guidance | NICE. NICE; 2007. Available from: https://www.nice.org.uk/guidance/cg54. Last accessed: 10/28/2023.
9. Cooper CS. Diagnosis and management of vesicoureteral reflux in children. Nat Rev Urol. 2009;6(9):481–9. https://doi.org/10.1038/nrurol.2009.150.
10. Chertin B, Mele E, Kocherov S, et al. What are the predictive factors leading to ureteral obstruction following endoscopic correction of VUR in the pediatric population? J Pediatr Urol. 2018;14(6):538.e1–7. https://doi.org/10.1016/j.jpurol.2018.04.021.
11. Elder JS, Peters CA, Arant BS, et al. Pediatric Vesicoureteral Reflux Guidelines Panel summary report on the management of primary vesicoureteral reflux in children. J Urol. 1997;157(5):1846–51.

12. Chertin B, De Caluwé D, Puri P. Endoscopic treatment of primary grades IV and V vesicoureteral reflux in children with subureteral injection of polytetrafluoroethylene. J Urol. 2003;169(5):1847–9; discussion 1849. https://doi.org/10.1097/01.ju.0000062300.71507.3a.
13. Crute W, Wofford A, Powers J, et al. Comprehensive review of a large cohort of outpatient versus inpatient open renal and bladder surgery in children. J Pediatr Urol. 2023;19(4):432.e1–8. https://doi.org/10.1016/j.jpurol.2023.04.033.
14. Gregoir W. Congenital vesico-ureteral reflux. Acta Urol Belg. 1962;30:286–300.
15. Lich R, Howerton LW, Davis LA. Recurrent urosepsis in children. J Urol. 1961;86(5):554–8. https://doi.org/10.1016/S0022-5347(17)65219-4.
16. Riedmiller H, Gerharz EW. Antireflux surgery: Lich-Gregoir extravesical ureteric tunnelling. BJU Int. 2008;101(11):1467–82. https://doi.org/10.1111/j.1464-410X.2008.07683.x.
17. Minevich E, Aronoff D, Wacksman J, et al. Voiding dysfunction after bilateral extravesical detrusorrhaphy. J Urol. 1998;160(3 Pt 2):1004–6; discussion 1038. https://doi.org/10.1097/00005392-199809020-00010.
18. Atala A, Kavoussi LR, Goldstein DS, et al. Laparoscopic correction of vesicoureteral reflux. J Urol. 1993;150(2 Pt 2):748–51. https://doi.org/10.1016/s0022-5347(17)35604-5.
19. Ehrlich RM, Gershman A, Fuchs G. Laparoscopic vesicoureteroplasty in children: initial case reports. Urology. 1994;43(2):255–61. https://doi.org/10.1016/0090-4295(94)90058-2.
20. Riquelme M, Lopez M, Landa S, et al. Laparoscopic extravesical ureteral reimplantation (LEVUR): a multicenter experience with 95 cases. Eur J Pediatr Surg. 2013;23(2):143–7. https://doi.org/10.1055/s-0032-1329708.
21. Soulier V, Scalabre AL, Lopez M, et al. Laparoscopic vesico-ureteral reimplantation with Lich-Gregoir approach in children: medium term results of 159 renal units in 117 children. World J Urol. 2017;35(11):1791–8. https://doi.org/10.1007/s00345-017-2064-y.
22. Capolicchio J-P. Laparoscopic extravesical ureteral reimplantation: technique. Adv Urol. 2008;2008:567980. https://doi.org/10.1155/2008/567980.
23. Farina A, Esposito C, Escolino M, et al. Laparoscopic extravesical ureteral reimplantation (LEVUR): a systematic review. Transl Pediatr. 2016;5(4):291–4. https://doi.org/10.21037/tp.2016.10.01.
24. Bowen DK, Faasse MA, Liu DB, et al. Use of pediatric open, laparoscopic and robot-assisted laparoscopic ureteral reimplantation in the United States: 2000 to 2012. J Urol. 2016;196(1):207–12. https://doi.org/10.1016/j.juro.2016.02.065.
25. Babu R, Chandrasekharam VVS. A systematic review and meta-analysis comparing outcomes of laparoscopic extravesical versus trans vesicoscopic ureteric reimplantation. J Pediatr Urol. 2020;16(6):783–9. https://doi.org/10.1016/j.jpurol.2020.09.006.
26. Bondarenko S. Laparoscopic extravesical transverse ureteral reimplantation in children with obstructive megaureter. J Pediatr Urol. 2013;9(4):437–41. https://doi.org/10.1016/j.jpurol.2013.01.001.
27. Chertin L, Kocherov S, Bakaleyshchik P, et al. Laparoscopic and robotic assisted laparoscopic reimplantation for lower ureter pathology: multi-institutional comparative study in 1343 patients. Houston, Texas: Presented at SPU Fall meeting in pediatric urology; 2023.
28. Olsen LH, Deding D, Yeung CK, et al. Computer assisted laparoscopic pneumovesical ureter reimplantation A.M. Cohen: initial experience in a pig model. APMIS Suppl. 2003;109:23–5.
29. Yeung CK, Sihoe JDY, Borzi PA. Endoscopic cross-trigonal ureteral reimplantation under carbon dioxide bladder insufflation: a novel technique. J Endourol. 2005;19(3):295–9. https://doi.org/10.1089/end.2005.19.295.
30. Nishi M, Eura R, Hayashi C, et al. Vesicoscopic ureteral reimplantation with a modified Glenn-Anderson technique for vesicoureteral reflux. J Pediatr Urol. 2023;19(3):322.e1–7. https://doi.org/10.1016/j.jpurol.2023.02.018.
31. Kruppa C, Fitze G, Schuchardt K. Vesicoscopic cross-trigonal ureteral reimplantation for vesicoureteral reflux: intermediate results. Children (Basel). 2022;9(2):298. https://doi.org/10.3390/children9020298.

32. Chertin L, Neeman BB, Stav K, et al. Robotic versus laparoscopic ipsilateral uretero-ureterostomy for upper urinary tract duplications in the pediatric population: a multi-institutional review of outcomes and complications. J Pediatr Surg. 2021;56(12):2377–80. https://doi.org/10.1016/j.jpedsurg.2020.12.022.
33. Kumar S, Modi P, Mishra A, et al. Robot-assisted laparoscopic repair of injuries to bladder and ureter following gynecological surgery and obstetric injury: a single-center experience. Urol Ann. 2021;13(4):405–11. https://doi.org/10.4103/UA.UA_69_20.
34. Neeman BB, Kocherov S, Jaber J, et al. Long term results of non-refluxing ureteral reimplantation in the pediatric population. Pediatr Surg Int. 2023;39(1):173. https://doi.org/10.1007/s00383-023-05466-2.
35. Rappaport YH, Kord E, Noh PH, et al. Minimally invasive dismembered extravesical cross-trigonal ureteral reimplantation for obstructed megaureter: a multi-institutional study comparing robotic and laparoscopic approaches. Urology. 2021;149:211–5. https://doi.org/10.1016/j.urology.2020.10.018.
36. Neheman A, Kord E, Koucherov S, et al. A novel surgical technique for obstructed megaureter: robot-assisted laparoscopic dismembered extravesical cross-trigonal ureteral reimplantation-short-term assessment. J Endourol. 2020;34(3):249–54. https://doi.org/10.1089/end.2019.0192.
37. Peters CA. Robotically assisted surgery in pediatric urology. Urol Clin North Am. 2004;31(4):743–52. https://doi.org/10.1016/j.ucl.2004.06.007.
38. Peters CA, Woo R. Intravesical robotically assisted bilateral ureteral reimplantation. J Endourol. 2005;19(6):618–21; discussion 621–622. https://doi.org/10.1089/end.2005.19.618.
39. Smith RP, Oliver JL, Peters CA. Pediatric robotic extravesical ureteral reimplantation: comparison with open surgery. J Urol. 2011;185(5):1876–81. https://doi.org/10.1016/j.juro.2010.12.072.
40. Esposito C, Castagnetti M, Autorino G, et al. Robot-assisted laparoscopic extra-vesical ureteral reimplantation (Ralur/Revur) for pediatric vesicoureteral reflux: a systematic review of literature. Urology. 2021;156:e1–e11. https://doi.org/10.1016/j.urology.2021.06.043.
41. Gundeti MS, Boysen WR, Shah A. Robot-assisted laparoscopic extravesical ureteral reimplantation: technique modifications contribute to optimized outcomes. Eur Urol. 2016;70(5):818–23. https://doi.org/10.1016/j.eururo.2016.02.065.
42. Neheman A, Shumaker A, Gal J, et al. Robot-assisted laparoscopic extravesical cross-trigonal ureteral reimplantation with tailoring for primary obstructive megaureter. Urology. 2019;134:243–5. https://doi.org/10.1016/j.urology.2019.09.003.
43. Chertin B, Zeldin A, Kocherov S, et al. Use of caudal analgesia supplemented with low dose of morphine in children who undergo renal surgery. Curr Urol. 2016;9(3):132–7. https://doi.org/10.1159/000442867.
44. Rotem S, Raisin G, Ostrovsky IA, et al. Is ultrasound-guided single-shot quadratus lumborum block a viable alternative to a caudal block in pediatric urological surgery? Eur J Pediatr Surg. 2022;32(3):263–7. https://doi.org/10.1055/s-0040-1722223.
45. Kawal T, Srinivasan AK, Chang J, Long C, Chu D, Shukla AR. Robotic-assisted laparoscopic ureteral re-implant (RALUR): can post-operative urinary retention be predicted? J Pediatr Urol. 2018;14(4):323.e1–5. https://doi.org/10.1016/j.jpurol.2018.05.010. Epub 2018 Jun 7.
46. Kurtz MP, Leow JJ, Varda BK, et al. Robotic versus open pediatric ureteral reimplantation: costs and complications from a nationwide sample. J Pediatr Urol. 2016;12(6):408.e1–6. https://doi.org/10.1016/j.jpurol.2016.06.016.
47. Puri P, Friedmacher F, Farrugia MK, Sharma S, Esposito C, Matto TK. Primary vesicoureteral reflux. Nat Rev Dis Primers. 2024;10:75.

Vesicoureteral Reflux in Infants

Atsuyuki Yamataka and Soichi Shibuya

Abstract Vesicoureteral reflux (VUR) is commonly diagnosed in infancy during investigation of infants with urinary tract infection (UTI) or following demonstration of prenatal urinary tract dilatation. High grade reflux in infancy is mainly seen in males, in contrast to older children when it is less severe and affects females more commonly. Associated renal parenchymal damage in infants can be congenital renal dysplasia or acquired segmental scarring that results after a combination of UTI and intrarenal reflux. Whether it is congenital damage or infection related damage, these infants need early identification and protection from further damage to ongoing high grade VUR and/or UTIs. Endoscopic correction is a safe, effective, minimally invasive procedure for high grade VUR in infants. Early correction of VUR may provide protection from reflux associated renal damage and prolonged antibiotic use.

Keywords Vesicoureteral reflux · Urinary tract infections · Infant · Renal scarring · Congenital renal dysplasia · Continuous antibiotic prophylaxis · Endoscopic treatment

Introduction

Vesicoureteral reflux (VUR) is the most common urinary tract anomaly in children. The association of VUR, urinary tract infection (UTI) and renal scarring is well recognized. Reflux associated nephropathy is an important cause of hypertension and chronic renal failure. Renal parenchymal injury in VUR occurs early, and in most patients before the age of 3 years [1]. It has been reported that infants with high grade VUR and febrile UTIs are most vulnerable to renal parenchymal damage

A. Yamataka (✉) · S. Shibuya
Department of Pediatric General and Urogenital Surgery, Juntendo University School of Medicine, Tokyo, Japan
e-mail: yama@juntendo.ac.jp

P. Puri, A. Yamataka (eds.), *Vesicoureteral Reflux*,
https://doi.org/10.1007/978-3-031-95091-9_21

[2–4]. Various studies have shown renal parenchymal damage in 26–65% of infants with high grade VUR [2, 5–7]. Early detection and treatment of VUR is of paramount importance in infants to provide protection from exposure to febrile UTIs and reflux related renal damage. Whether it is congenital damage or infection related damage, these infants need early identification and protection from further damage due to ongoing high-grade reflux and/or UTIs. Congenital renal dysplasia, which occurs because of abnormal embryological development, currently cannot be prevented. However, in these infants it is mandatory to discover VUR at early stages to prevent exposure to UTIs and avoid the possible progression of renal damage.

Characteristics

Vesicoureteral reflux has been reported in 24–70% of infants presenting with febrile UTIs [7–9]. Neonates and premature infants represent a special group with regard to UTIs, with a male predominance of two to sixfold, which is in striking contrast to the prevalence rate of UTI among females in the over 6-month age group [10]. Bahat et al. reported that 10% of infants less than 2 months of age admitted for a first febrile infection were found to have grade III–V VUR on voiding cystourethrography (VCUG) [11]. Vachharajani et al. reported VUR in 14% of premature infants hospitalized with first UTI [12]. Although VUR is reported to be more common in girls for children of all ages, VUR is overwhelmingly male dominant in infancy possibly related to boys having a longer urethra and thus higher urinary pressure, as well as the foreskin acting as a source of retrograde infection [13–15]. High grade VUR is common with around 70% of VUR in infant boys being grades IV or V, and therefore at high risk for reflux nephropathy. Grade V VUR is almost exclusively seen in male infants, and in one-third of cases occurring with a generalized small kidney, whereas in females, high-grade reflux is uncommon and kidney damage almost always less severe and of the focal type, as in older children [13].

Although, prenatal hydronephrosis is generally considered to represent an obstructive lesion, VUR is not an uncommon cause. Among infants in whom hydronephrosis is prenatally identified on ultrasound, the VUR prevalence is reported to be 16.2% (7–35%) [16]. A meta-analysis performed by Skoog et al. reported that VUR in infants diagnosed by screening after prenatally detected hydronephrosis was significantly associated with renal parenchymal damage. Renal abnormalities occurred in a mean of 6.2% versus 48% of those with grade I–III versus grade IV–V reflux [17]. Yeung et al. observed renal parenchymal damage in 42% of the infants with prenatally hydronephrosis and postnatally diagnosed VUR, with 75% in males [18]. Similarly, Nguyen et al. reported renal parenchymal damage 65% of the predominantly male infants with sterile high-grade VUR [5].

Natural Course of VUR in Infants

Spontaneous resolution of vesicoureteral reflux has been shown to be dependent on age at presentation, gender, grade, laterality, mode of clinical presentation and ureteral anatomy. Estrada et al. reported that infants less than 1 year at presentation, lower reflux grade, reflux diagnosed on postnatal evaluation for prenatal hydronephrosis, or sibling screening and single ureter were associated with significantly earlier resolution of reflux [19]. The natural history of VUR in infant boys differs from that of infant girls. Male infants with grade IV and V VUR initially have 29% rate of spontaneous resolution in year 1 but then in males and females the yearly resolution rate is only 9% [20]. Anatomic immaturity of the ureterovesical junction has long been noted in neonates and infants, and it is thought that VUR occurs when there is further stress from infection of the lower immature urinary tract [3, 21]. In recent years, from detailed studies of the lower urinary tract function, it has become clear that functional immaturity of the lower urinary tract is involved in the pathogenesis of VUR in young infants [13, 18, 22]. Abnormal urodynamic patterns have been observed in infants with high grade VUR. Sjostrom S et al. studied urodynamic patterns in infants and showed that the urodynamic patterns changed between the first and second year of life in patients with dilating reflux, from an immature pattern with high pressure levels to high-capacity bladder with incomplete voiding [20]. This may explain the high-resolution rates observed in infants with grade IV and V VUR.

Spontaneous resolution of VUR as a child grows is expected as the ureterovesical junction and lower urinary tract function mature. The rate of spontaneous VUR resolution in neonates and infants appears to be higher than in older children [19, 23]. There is also evidence that resolution of high grade VUR (grades IV and V) in neonates and infants is less than 30% and bilateral VUR even lower at less than 10% [3, 21, 24]. Furthermore, a prospective study on infantile VUR managed conservatively showed there was no spontaneous resolution in 70% of infants with grade III and IV VUR, suggesting that grade IV and grade V VUR have even lower rates of spontaneous resolution [3]. Low-grade VUR in infants can be expected to resolve spontaneously and to this end, observation with continuous antibiotic prophylactic (CAP) is a viable option although evidence for CAP reducing the incidence of febrile UTI in infants with VUR is controversial [25].

Recently distal ureteral diameter ratio (UDR) has been reported to be an objective measure reflective of ureterovesical junction anatomy that has been shown to independently predict both spontaneous resolution and breakthrough febrile UTI in children with primary reflux [26]. The authors reported that children with primary VUR and a UDR of greater than 0.30 are significantly less likely to spontaneously resolve regardless of length of follow-up.

Renal Scarring

The association of VUR, febrile UTIs and renal parenchymal damage is well recognized. Essentially there are two different mechanisms in the pathogenesis of renal scarring in patients with VUR, including the commonly acquired renal scarring associated with the reflux of infected urine and congenital reflux nephropathy, which is characterized by the morphological features of renal dysplasia. With the widespread use of prenatal ultrasound and therefore the possibility of detecting hydronephrosis and renal damage before the onset of UTIs it has become evident that a substantial number of infants with VUR show congenital renal dysplasia. Anderson and Rickwood found that 71% of uninfected neonates with grade III to V had renal scarring on 99mTc-dimercaptosuccinic acid (DMSA) scintigraphy, suggesting a congenital cause [27].

Intrarenal reflux (IRR) is often observed in infants with high grade VUR and usually associated with renal scarring. Klien et al. evaluated the prevalence of intrarenal reflux identified on contrast-enhanced voiding urosonography (ceVUS) and found that Intrarenal reflux was often seen on ceVUS, with the highest frequency occurring in infants with grades 4 and 5 VUR and during voiding [28]. Cvitkovic-Roic et al. used ceVUS to detect IRR as well as its association with age, and grade of VUR. The majority of VUR with IRR were found in children <12 months of age, with VUR grades IV and V (170/285 renal units; 60%) [29]. Boubnova et al. evaluated the prognostic significance of IRR in relation to renal scarring and found moderate to severe scarring in 60% of the renal units with IRR [30].

Impact of the Foreskin, Labial Fusion, and UTI on VUR

Controversy surrounds correlation between the foreskin of the penis and UTI/VUR in male infants. One large study showed a tenfold increase in UTIs in uncircumcised male infants: 1.12% versus 0.11% [31]. Of note was the large number of infant males requiring hospital admission for management of clinical pyelonephritis. In contrast, another large study found an increased risk for UTI and hospitalization in uncircumcised boys that was much less than previously published, questioning the mythical belief that routine circumcision protects boys from infections, i.e., UTI [32].

Labial adhesions in infantile girls have posed similar concerns with respect to UTIs. The concern is scientifically sound in theory because promotion of abnormal perineal bacterial growth is possible, but no data is available to prove or disprove this hypothesis. Labial adhesions are extremely rare in neonatal and young infant girls but if UTI has developed, the UTI should be treated promptly, and the labial adhesions treated with estrogen cream or rarely by surgical separation. The authors have experience 41 cases of congenital labial adhesions in infants; none had UTI.

Presentation

The health care professionals will encounter infants with VUR typically with two presentations. Asymptomatic cases for assessment of abnormal prenatal ultrasonography (US) showing hydroureteronephrosis suggestive of the presence of VUR, or symptomatic cases with UTI [33].

Presence of VUR in infants may be suggested by urinary tract dilatation on prenatal US or by investigation of UTI after birth. However, symptoms and signs of UTI in neonates and infants can be non-specific and may not be associated with fever, so a thorough work-up is recommended whenever caregivers seek medical attention for a neonate or infant. All concerns expressed by caregivers require careful consideration especially if non-specific, such as failure to thrive or simple irritability in the first weeks of life as neonates and infants may not exhibit overt clinical signs of infection as clearly as older children, because of immune response immaturity placing them at increased risk for developing serious complications such as severe pyelonephritis. UTI must always be excluded when a neonate or infant has a fever of unexplained origin or is suspected of sepsis and should be assessed comprehensively, investigated promptly, and treated without any delay. During the first few months of life, several studies have shown that boys have a higher incidence of UTI at up to 14% compared to girls at 7% [34]. The reported prevalence of UTI in febrile infants without an identifiable source ranges from 7.0% to 15% [10, 34–36].

Imaging

Accurate imaging of the urinary tract is essential in a patient suspected to have VUR in order to plan treatment, whether medical or surgical. The various imaging modalities for evaluating an infant with febrile UTI or prenatally detected hydronephrosis include renal and bladder ultrasound, VCUG, and nuclear renography. NICE, AAP, and EAU/ESPU have developed guidelines providing imaging recommendations for evaluating patients with UTIs or prenatally diagnosed hydronephrosis [37].

US is invaluable for evaluating neonates and infants presenting with febrile UTIs. It provides information on renal architecture, size, urinary tract dilatation and renal scarring. It is not reliable for predicting VUR.

In asymptomatic cases with abnormal prenatal US, urinary tract dilatation is dynamic and even gross dilatation can appear to be intermittent, related to pressure changes in the urinary tract and the upper urinary tracts can at times appear normal on postnatal US. What constitutes significant renal dilatation on prenatal ultrasound is still debated. Some authors advocate evaluating all infants whose renal pelvic diameter is greater than 7–10 mm [33]. The American Urologic Association (AUA) published a meta-analysis of screening studies of infants with prenatally detected hydronephrosis [17]. The incidence of VUR ranged from 9% in low-grade hydronephrosis to 25% in high-grade hydronephrosis [17, 38].

VCUG is the gold standard for the diagnosis of VUR (Fig. 1). A carefully performed and interpreted VCUG documents if VUR is present and its grade, whether it is unilateral or bilateral, and identify any associated ureterovesical junction anomalies such as diverticulum or ureterocele as well as the internal renal anatomy on the affected side, and bladder function to a certain extent. Ureteral tortuosity associated with high-grade VUR, also referred to as refluxing megaureter, may appear as a cause for obstruction but is not associated with functional obstruction. Presence of any residual urine after voiding, trabeculation, dysfunctional sphincter closure, or obstruction from posterior urethral valves could influence management. It should be noted that VCUG is less reliable in neonates and infants because voiding is involuntary and some cases of VUR may be missed because VUR may only appear during voiding.

Other useful diagnostic imaging modalities include radionuclide renal scintigraphy with DMSA or Mercaptoacetyltriglycine (MAG3) scan for confirming renal status such as size, scarring, drainage status as obstructive, static, or normal, and differential renal function. Care is required as refluxed contrast or tracer can simulate activity, leading to a scan result suggesting renal function is active. Thus, all renal function tests should be performed with a bladder catheter *in situ*, otherwise, results are at risk for misinterpretation.

Urodynamic evaluation and magnetic resonance imaging are required if there is risk for a neurologic indication for urinary tract anomalies. Of note are myelomeningocele and spina bifida. Urodynamic studies are a valuable adjunct for assessing

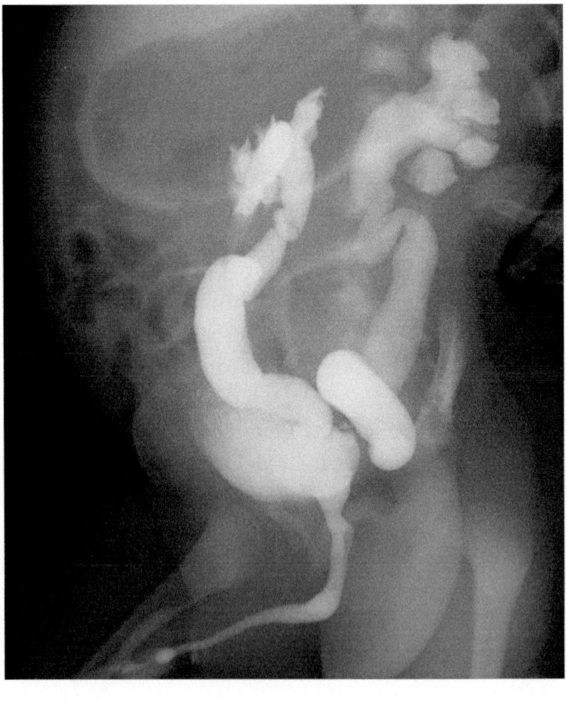

Fig. 1 Bilateral grade V vesicoureteral reflux in 2-month-old boy. The urethra is normal

bladder function, with abnormal patterns of bladder dysfunction reported in over half of the infants with VUR, most of whom are male [18]. Other indications include trabeculation identified on other modes of evaluation, especially if associated with obstruction, or VCUG irregularities associated with sphincter activity, however, this may be difficult to assess accurately in neonates and infants.

Management

Management of VUR in infants is intimately related to UTI but can be problematic because of a broad spectrum of signs and symptoms contributing to a variety of clinical presentations arising from urologic and non-urologic conditions.

Acute UTI

Acute UTI in neonates and infants is generally treated empirically with oral antibiotics but requires hospitalization for intravenous antibiotics with or without vesical decompression using an indwelling bladder catheter if clinically severe. There is an ever-present risk that renal scarring and potential deterioration in kidney function associated with VUR can stress renal glomerular function, especially if UTI persist or become recurrent because of immature immunity and organ function in neonates and infants. Initial blood studies should include an assessment of renal function, glomerular filtration, electrolytes, acid-base status, and general biochemistry, and a sepsis workup should be considered.

Detection of bacteria or evidence of infection in a urine sample, coupled with elevated serum white blood cell counts and inflammatory markers, are pathognomonic for UTI. Various pathogens, including Escherichia coli, Enterococcus, Klebsiella pneumoniae, Klebsiella oxytoca, and Enterobacter cloacae, can be identified in the urine cultures of infants with UTI. Although Escherichia coli is the most common bacterium, the presence of other species, such as Klebsiella, is more indicative of VUR [10, 36]. Broad spectrum antibiotics are generally prescribed and commenced before urine culture results are available and antibiotic prophylaxis is often recommended. More aggressive metabolic therapy for correction of hydration, acidosis, and hyperkalemia may also be required. Sepsis may induce ureteral atony and hydronephrosis although they can be treatable [39]. The authors believe that placing an indwelling bladder catheter decompresses the upper urinary tract when VUR or hydroureteronephrosis are present allowing stagnated potentially infected urine in the upper urinary tract to be drained from the bladder. Thus, all severely ill infants suspected of UTI presenting to the author's institute have their bladders drained by *in situ* catheterization as an initial procedure. Post-catheterization diuresis may occur as a physiological response to release of a function obstruction and antibiotic administration and could induce secondary loss of electrolytes.

VUR After UTI

After successfully managing an acute UTI, observation with CAP is an option, however, extensive caregiver motivation, compliance, and diligence are required. Thus, the management of VUR in infants must be customized according to VUR status and likelihood of effectiveness requiring a choice between conservative or surgical management. Surgical intervention, i.e., ureteric implantation, is much more technically challenging in infants compared with older children, although it should be considered, if needed to prevent recurrent UTI. Endoscopic treatment is currently well accepted, internationally as first line treatment for primary severe VUR to prevent renal damage [40, 41].

Primary VUR

CAP has been recommended for infants diagnosed with VUR following a febrile UTI aiming to prevent renal scarring from recurrent febrile pyelonephritis, however, recent studies reported that CAP in children with VUR is useful to prevent UTI, but does not prevent occurrence of renal scarring [7, 42–45]. When VUR is low-grade without a history of a febrile UTI, CAP may not be indicated because of low risk for renal scarring [7, 45]. On the other hand, infants with grades III to V at higher risk for UTIs, should be commenced on CAP without delay because the risk for renal scarring is so high. Once CAP is commenced, careful monitoring of type of antibiotic, dosage, and duration are required to prevent antibiotic resistance. The occurrence of breakthrough UTI in infants on CAP is relatively high at 20–38% and is of concern [8, 25, 46].

In any case, outpatient management requires exceptional caregiver compliance requiring regular urine cultures, renal function assessment, VCUG, and imaging to monitor structural changes, including scarring. No consistent guidelines for the duration of CAP or the optimal timing for surgery have been established, but when high-grade VUR exists, there seems to be no obvious benefit of CAP associated with prolonged observation because the chance of spontaneous resolution of VUR is low and endoscopic intervention is readily available [16]. Some authors suggest 2 years is reasonable for observation and CAP [45, 47], but factors such as break through UTI can challenge even the most motivated caregivers and any deterioration in renal function requires more urgent specific attention.

Surgical intervention for high-grade VUR in infants is controversial. Ureteral reimplantation, can be performed at any age and is highly successful for treating VUR. However, surgical intervention for VUR must be considered carefully, especially in small infants, because it is invasive and has potential for complications. Ureteral reimplantation in infants does not appear to have the same prognosis as in older children although this can vary between treating surgeons based on experience. Procedural risks must be weighed against risks associated with conservative management, but overtreating must be avoided, particularly in neonates. Procedurally, ureteral reimplantation in infants is more difficult technically as tissues in infants are more delicate and structures are smaller. Thus, some surgeons prefer diversion such as vesicostomy for early intervention in severe cases of VUR to correct serious metabolic derangement caused by renal dysfunction, or chronic UTI, but the authors regard bladder catheterization as a less invasive, effective alternative allowing time for the patient to grow to a suitable weight and size to perform ureteric implantation safely.

Surgical intervention is indicated when anatomic anomalies likely to hinder any spontaneous improvement in VUR are present. Such anomalies would include ureteral duplication, single ectopic ureter, and ureterocele. Ureterocele can be associated with functional obstruction to urine flow and may have priority over VUR for treatment. Ipsilateral ureteropelvic junction obstruction falls into the same category. In other words, any anomaly present with risk for obstruction has priority over VUR if surgical intervention is planned.

Open or pneumovesicoscopic ureteric reimplantation in infants can only be performed confidently by expert surgeons because it is too technically demanding [48]. As a result, there has been an almost universal trend for open intervention to be replaced by endoscopic intervention, notably with Deflux® [40]. Minimally invasive techniques are increasingly being favored for treating high-grade VUR overtaking open ureteric reimplantation, the definitive treatment for high-grade VUR for decades. Endoscopic correction is currently the first line of treatment for children with grade IV–V primary reflux and complex cases of VUR in many institutions worldwide because of the simplicity of the procedure. While endoscopic treatment offers a less invasive alternative, suitable for infants as young as 2 months [40, 49, 50], endoscopic treatment has disadvantages compared with open surgery such as treatment failure in some patients that later needed a repeat injection [24, 51].

Interestingly, research has shown that UTI rates and renal scaring are similar for CAP and endoscopically treated cases and risk of overtreating, particularly in very young patients, must be considered carefully [51]. A Swedish study supports this outcome, by comparing outcomes of grade IV and V reflux in 77 infants less than 8 months old treated by endoscopic intervention using Deflux (n = 39) versus CAP alone (n = 38): There were 27 febrile UTI in 16 patients during the study overall, with no difference between the incidence of UTI compared between Deflux (n = 6) and CAP alone (n = 10) [46, 52]. At 1-year follow-up, there was worsening of scarring in 5/39 (12.8%) patients in the Deflux group and in 3/38 (7.9%) patients in the CAP group, which was not statistically significant (p = NS). However, successful down grade of VUR (improvement to grades 0–II) was observed in 22/38 (59%) of endoscopically treated patients, which was higher than 8/39 (21%) of patients treated by CAP alone ($p < 0.01$).

The authors' technique for confirming endoscopic Deflux injection has not caused obstruction.

Ureteral obstruction (UO) is a rare but well-known complication after endoscopic treatment of VUR. Incidence rates of postoperative UO are generally about 1% of treated patients, which appears to be independent of bulking agent, volume, and injection technique [53] UO can develop immediately following the procedure or as far as 63 months [41, 53–55]. The senior author (A.Y.) devised a technique for confirming post-Deflux ureteral patency and urine flow, intraoperatively [56–58].

For infants indicated for endoscopic treatment, an 8.0 Fr cystoscope with an offset lens (Karl Storz, Inc., Tuttlingen, Germany) is used. The offset lens of this type of scope permits direct passage of a 3.7 Fr needle in line with the ureter without needing to bend the needle. The bladder is filled to three-quarters of its full capacity, which allows for clear visualization of the ureteric orifices and applies moderate tension to the mucosal layer, facilitating needle puncture. It is critical to avoid over-distending the bladder, as excessive intravesical pressure can flatten the submucosal layer and cause the injected material to disperse rather than remain localized.

An epidural catheter is inserted into the ureter through the side channel of the cystoscope, and once the catheter is positioned in the ureter, the cystoscope is withdrawn leaving the epidural catheter *in situ*. Following placement of the catheter, the cystoscope is carefully re-inserted into the bladder, and a Deflux needle is introduced through the scope's side channel. After Deflux is injected, the needle used for injection is withdrawn and 1–3 mL of a 20% indigo carmine solution is administered into the ureter through the intra-ureteric epidural catheter to verify that no obstruction had been caused by injecting Deflux. If dye flow from the orifice treated by Deflux to the bladder is observed (Fig. 2), the epidural catheter is removed to complete the procedure. If dye flow is not observed after 15 minutes, the epidural catheter is clamped *in situ* and the patient returned to the ward. The patient is observed overnight, during which time, dye typically appears in the urine, signifying patency. US is also performed to exclude hydroureteronephrosis. If no signs of obstruction are present, the epidural catheter is removed, and the patient is discharged.

From 2011 to 2023, 9 cases (2.8%) of ureteral obstruction were identified using this technique during 319 endoscopic treatments with Deflux. Of the 9 cases, 6 resolved spontaneously after the epidural catheter was left *in situ* overnight. The remaining 3 cases had a double-J stent placed for 1 month with no evidence of obstruction after their removal. It is worth mentioning that one of the abovementioned 3 patients who had Deflux for bilateral grade V VUR and a double-J stent in the left ureter inserted for a month was continuously asymptomatic with the left VUR downgrading to Grade I and the right VUR resolving, eventually underwent ureteric reimplantation of the left ureter due to left hydroureteronephrosis, ipsilateral back pain and recurrent UTI, 3 years 8 months after Deflux treatment.

Conclusions

Management of VUR in infants has been controversial. In the case of infants diagnosed during the first year of life, the initial approach typically involves antibiotic prophylaxis primarily due to the heightened susceptibility of infants to

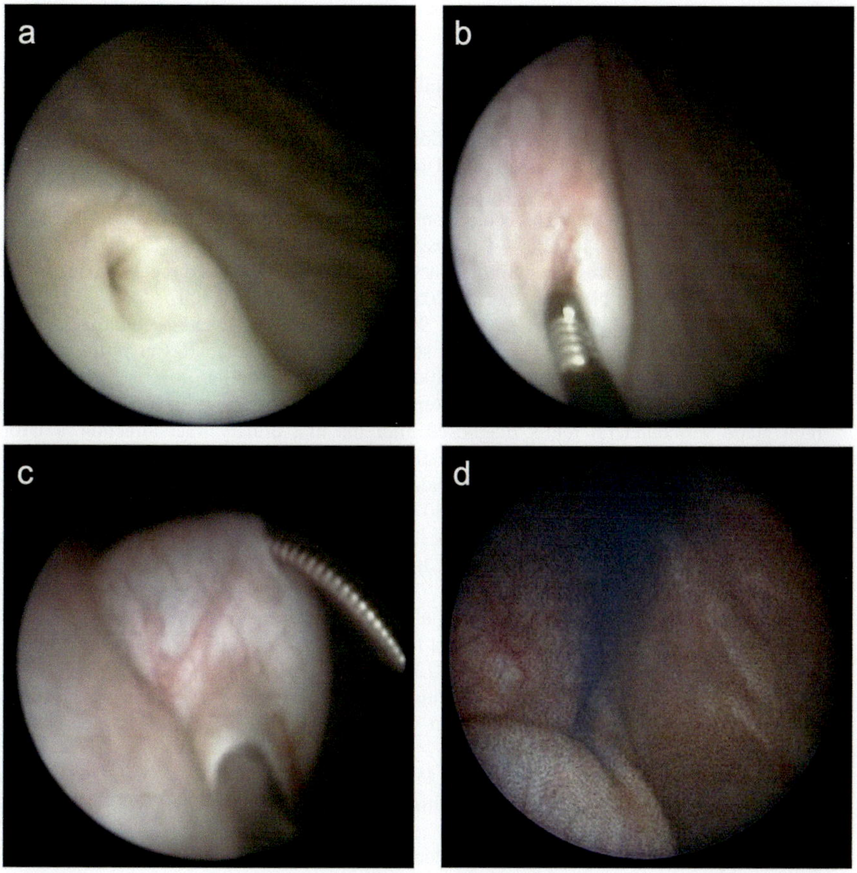

Fig. 2 The authors' technique for confirming no obstruction after endoscopic Deflux injection. (**a**) Left ureteric orifice; note it is large and not slit-like. (**b**) Epidural catheter being inserted in the left ureter. (**c**) Bulging under the left ureteric orifice after injecting Deflux. Note the epidural catheter in the left ureteric orifice. (**d**) Indigo carmine solution instilled via the epidural catheter flowing into the bladder verifies that Deflux has not caused any obstruction

infection-related complications. For those with high grade VUR or those who experience breakthrough UTIs despite prophylaxis, interventions such as endoscopic treatment or ureteral reimplantation are recommended. Early endoscopic treatment is a viable option, particularly in male infants with high grade reflux, when they are most vulnerable to renal parenchymal damage. The authors' technique of inserting an epidural catheter into the ureteral orifice during endoscopic injection is recommended to prevent ureteral obstruction.

References

1. Risdon RA. The small scarred kidney in childhood. Pediatr Nephrol. 1993;7:361–4. https://doi.org/10.1007/BF00857538.
2. Swerkersson S, Jodal U, Sixt R, et al. Relationship among vesicoureteral reflux, urinary tract infection and renal damage in children. J Urol. 2007;178:647–51. https://doi.org/10.1016/J.JURO.2007.04.004.
3. Sjöström S, Sillén U, Bachelard M, et al. Spontaneous resolution of high grade infantile vesicoureteral reflux. J Urol. 2004;172:694–9. https://doi.org/10.1097/01.JU.0000130747.89561.CF.
4. Lama G, Russo M, De Rosa E, et al. Primary vesicoureteric reflux and renal damage in the first year of life. Pediatr Nephrol. 2000;15:205–10. https://doi.org/10.1007/s004670000455.
5. Nguyen HT, Bauer SB, Peters CA, et al. 99mTechnetium dimercapto-succinic acid renal scintigraphy abnormalities in infants with sterile high grade vesicoureteral reflux. J Urol. 2000;164:1674–9. https://doi.org/10.1016/S0022-5347(05)67081-4.
6. Cascio S, Chertin B, Colhoun E, et al. Renal parenchymal damage in male infants with high grade vesicoureteral reflux diagnosed after the first urinary tract infection. J Urol. 2002;168:1708–10. https://doi.org/10.1016/s0022-5347(05)64394-7.
7. Miyakita H, Hayashi Y, Mitsui T, et al. Guidelines for the medical management of pediatric vesicoureteral reflux. Int J Urol. 2020;27:480–90. https://doi.org/10.1111/iju.14223.
8. Nakai H, Kakizaki H, Konda R, et al. Clinical characteristics of primary vesicoureteral reflux in infants: multicenter retrospective study in Japan. J Urol. 2003;169:309–12. https://doi.org/10.1016/S0022-5347(05)64113-4.
9. Juliano TM, Stephany HA, Clayton DB, et al. Incidence of abnormal imaging and recurrent pyelonephritis after first febrile urinary tract infection in children 2 to 24 months old. J Urol. 2013;190:1505–10. https://doi.org/10.1016/J.JURO.2013.01.049.
10. Cleper R, Krause I, Eisenstein B, Davidovits M. Prevalence of vesicoureteral reflux in neonatal urinary tract infection. Clin Pediatr (Phila). 2004;43:619–25. https://doi.org/10.1177/000992280404300706.
11. Bahat H, Ben-Ari M, Ziv-Baran T, et al. Predictors of grade 3–5 vesicoureteral reflux in infants ≤ 2 months of age with pyelonephritis. Pediatr Nephrol. 2019;34:907–15. https://doi.org/10.1007/s00467-018-4167-0.
12. Vachharajani A, Vricella GJ, Najaf T, Coplen DE. Prevalence of upper urinary tract anomalies in hospitalized premature infants with urinary tract infection. J Perinatol. 2015;35:362–6. https://doi.org/10.1038/jp.2014.209.
13. Sillén U. Vesicoureteral reflux in infants. Pediatr Nephrol. 1999;13:355–61. https://doi.org/10.1007/S004670050625/METRICS.
14. Jang HC, Lee KH, Park JS. Primary vesico-ureteral reflux: comparison of factors between infants and children. Korean J Urol. 2011;52:206–9. https://doi.org/10.4111/kju.2011.52.3.206.
15. Ishikawa N, Ohama K. Management strategies for vesicoureteral reflux (in Japanese). Jpn J Pediatr Nephrol. 2005;18:67–71. https://doi.org/10.3165/jjpn.18.147.
16. Gnech M, 't Hoen L, Zachou A, et al. Update and summary of the European Association of Urology/European Society of Paediatric Urology paediatric guidelines on vesicoureteral reflux in children. Eur Urol. 2024;85:433–42. https://doi.org/10.1016/j.eururo.2023.12.005.
17. Skoog SJ, Peters CA, Arant BS, et al. Pediatric vesicoureteral reflux guidelines panel summary report: clinical practice guidelines for screening siblings of children with vesicoureteral reflux and neonates/infants with prenatal hydronephrosis. J Urol. 2010;184:1145–51. https://doi.org/10.1016/j.juro.2010.05.066.
18. Yeung CK, Godley ML, Dhillon HK, et al. Urodynamic patterns in infants with normal lower urinary tracts or primary vesico-ureteric reflux. Br J Urol. 1998;81:461–7. https://doi.org/10.1046/j.1464-410X.1998.00567.x.
19. Estrada CR, Passerotti CC, Graham DA, et al. Nomograms for predicting annual resolution rate of primary vesicoureteral reflux: results from 2,462 children. J Urol. 2009;182:1535–41. https://doi.org/10.1016/j.juro.2009.06.053.

20. Sjöström S, Bachelard M, Sixt R, Sillén U. Change of urodynamic patterns in infants with dilating vesicoureteral reflux: 3-year followup. J Urol. 2009;182:2446–54. https://doi.org/10.1016/j.juro.2009.07.057.
21. Tamminen-Mobius T, Brunier E, Ebel KD, et al. Cessation of vesicoureteral reflux for 5 years in infants and children allocated to medical treatment. J Urol. 1992;148:1662–6. https://doi.org/10.1016/s0022-5347(17)36997-5.
22. Chandra M, Maddix H. Urodynamic dysfunction in infants with vesicoureteral reflux. J Pediatr. 2000;136:754–9. https://doi.org/10.1016/S0022-3476(00)64048-9.
23. Tekgül S, Riedmiller H, Hoebeke P, et al. EAU guidelines on vesicoureteral reflux in children. Eur Urol. 2012;62:534–42. https://doi.org/10.1016/j.eururo.2012.05.059.
24. Elder JS, Peters CA, Arant BSJ, et al. Pediatric Vesicoureteral Reflux Guidelines Panel summary report on the management of primary vesicoureteral reflux in children. J Urol. 1997;157:1846–51.
25. Morello W, Baskin E, Jankauskiene A, et al. Antibiotic prophylaxis in infants with grade III, IV, or V vesicoureteral reflux. N Engl J Med. 2023;389:987–97. https://doi.org/10.1056/nejmoa2300161.
26. Arlen AM, Leong T, Kirsch AJ, Cooper CS. Spontaneous vesicoureteral reflux resolution curves based on ureteral diameter ratio. J Pediatr Urol. 2023;19:468.e1–6. https://doi.org/10.1016/j.jpurol.2023.04.028.
27. Anderson PAM, Rickwood AMK. Features of primary vesicoureteric reflux detected by prenatal sonography. Br J Urol. 1991;67:267–71. https://doi.org/10.1111/j.1464-410X.1991.tb15132.x.
28. Klein EL, Wyers MR, Prendergast FM, et al. Prevalence of intrarenal reflux in pediatric patients on contrast-enhanced voiding urosonography. Pediatr Radiol. 2023;53:387–93. https://doi.org/10.1007/s00247-022-05548-8.
29. Cvitkovic-Roic A, Turudic D, Milosevic D, et al. Contrast-enhanced voiding urosonography in the diagnosis of intrarenal reflux. J Ultrasound. 2022;25:89–95. https://doi.org/10.1007/s40477-021-00568-w.
30. Boubnova J, Sergent-Alaoui A, Deschênes G, Audry G. Evolution and prognosis value of intrarenal reflux. J Pediatr Urol. 2011;7:638–43. https://doi.org/10.1016/j.jpurol.2010.09.015.
31. Wiswell TE, Roscelli JD. Corroborative evidence for the decreased incidence of urinary tract infections in circumcised male infants. Pediatrics. 1986;78:96–9. https://doi.org/10.1542/peds.78.1.96.
32. To T, Agha M, Dick PT, Feldman W. Cohort study on circumcision of newborn boys and subsequent risk of urinary-tract infection. Lancet. 1998;352:1813–6. https://doi.org/10.1016/S0140-6736(98)02392-7.
33. Grazioli S, Parvex P, Merlini L, et al. Antenatal and postnatal ultrasound in the evaluation of the risk of vesicoureteral reflux. Pediatr Nephrol. 2010;25:1687–92. https://doi.org/10.1007/s00467-010-1543-9.
34. Shaikh N, Morone NE, Bost JE, Farrell MH. Prevalence of urinary tract infection in childhood: a meta-analysis. Pediatr Infect Dis J. 2008;27:302–8. https://doi.org/10.1097/INF.0b013e31815e4122.
35. Ismaili K, Lolin K, Damry N, et al. Febrile urinary tract infections in 0- to 3-month-old infants: a prospective follow-up study. J Pediatr. 2011;158:91–4. https://doi.org/10.1016/j.jpeds.2010.06.053.
36. Bonadio W, Maida G. Urinary tract infection in outpatient febrile infants younger than 30 days of age: a 10-year evaluation. Pediatr Infect Dis J. 2014;33:342–4. https://doi.org/10.1097/INF.0000000000000110.
37. Greenfield SP. The diagnosis and medical management of vesicoureteral reflux: an update and current controversies. Pediatr Surg. 2022:1–22. https://doi.org/10.1007/978-3-642-38482-0_178-1.

38. Szymanski KM, Al-Said AN, Pippi Salle JL, Capolicchio JP. Do infants with mild prenatal hydronephrosis benefit from screening for vesicoureteral reflux? J Urol. 2012;188:576–81. https://doi.org/10.1016/j.juro.2012.04.017.
39. Pais VM, Retik AB. Reversible hydronephrosis in the neonate with urinary sepsis. N Engl J Med. 1975;292:465–7. https://doi.org/10.1056/NEJM197502272920907.
40. Puri P, Mohanan N, Menezes M, Colhoun E. Endoscopic treatment of moderate and high grade vesicoureteral reflux in infants using dextranomer/hyaluronic acid. J Urol. 2007;178:1714–7. https://doi.org/10.1016/j.juro.2007.03.172.
41. Garcia-Aparicio L, Rovira J, Blazquez-Gomez E, et al. Randomized clinical trial comparing endoscopic treatment with dextranomer hyaluronic acid copolymer and Cohen's ureteral reimplantation for vesicoureteral reflux: long-term results. J Pediatr Urol. 2013;9:483–7. https://doi.org/10.1016/j.jpurol.2013.03.003.
42. Wang HHS, Gbadegesin RA, Foreman JW, et al. Efficacy of antibiotic prophylaxis in children with vesicoureteral reflux: systematic review and meta-analysis. J Urol. 2015;193:963–9. https://doi.org/10.1016/j.juro.2014.08.112.
43. Craig JC, Simpson JM, Williams GJ, et al. Antibiotic prophylaxis and recurrent urinary tract infection in children. N Engl J Med. 2009;361:1748–59. https://doi.org/10.1056/NEJMoa0902295.
44. Hoberman A, Charron M, Hickey RW, et al. Imaging studies after a first febrile urinary tract infection in young children. N Engl J Med. 2003;348:195–202. https://doi.org/10.1056/nejmoa021698.
45. Khoury AE, Wehbi E. Management strategies for vesicoureteral reflux. In: Partin AW, Dmochowski RR, Kavoussi LR, Peters CA, editors. Campbell-Walsh-Wein urology. 12th ed. Philadelphia: Elsevier Inc.; 2021. p. 489–571.
46. Nordenström J, Sjöström S, Sillén U, et al. The Swedish infant high-grade reflux trial: UTI and renal damage. J Pediatr Urol. 2017;13:146–54. https://doi.org/10.1016/j.jpurol.2016.12.023.
47. Craig PA, Alan RB. Massive vesicoureteral reflux in the newborn. In: Gonzales Jr E, Roth D, editors. Common problems in pediatric urology. Missouri: Mosby-Year Book Inc.; 1991. p. 259–65.
48. Cui X, Huang WH, Wang YJ, et al. Effect of pneumovesicoscopic Cohen surgery with adjustable suspension technique through the urethra on the treatment of primary vesicoureteral reflux disease in infants. BMC Surg. 2023;23:1–7. https://doi.org/10.1186/s12893-023-01996-7.
49. Dawrant MJ, Mohanan N, Puri P. Endoscopic treatment for high grade vesicoureteral reflux in infants. J Urol. 2006;176:1847–50. https://doi.org/10.1016/S0022-5347(06)00621-5.
50. Hunziker M, Mohanan N, D'Asta F, Puri P. Endoscopic treatment of primary grade V vesicoureteral reflux using hyaluronic acid copolymer (DX/HA). Pediatr Surg Int. 2010;26:977–9. https://doi.org/10.1007/s00383-010-2650-1.
51. Brandström P, Esbjörner E, Herthelius M, et al. The Swedish reflux trial in children: III. Urinary tract infection pattern. J Urol. 2010;184:286–91. https://doi.org/10.1016/j.juro.2010.01.061.
52. Nordenström J, Holmdahl G, Brandström P, et al. The Swedish infant high-grade reflux trial: study presentation and vesicoureteral reflux outcome. J Pediatr Urol. 2017;13:130–8. https://doi.org/10.1016/j.jpurol.2016.08.026.
53. Friedmacher F, Puri P. Ureteral obstruction after endoscopic treatment of vesicoureteral reflux: does the type of injected bulking agent matter? Curr Urol Rep. 2019;20:49. https://doi.org/10.1007/S11934-019-0913-5.
54. Rubenwolf PC, Ebert AK, Ruemmele P, Rösch WH. Delayed-onset ureteral obstruction after endoscopic dextranomer/hyaluronic acid copolymer (Deflux) injection for treatment of vesicoureteral reflux in children: a case series. Urology. 2013;81:659–62. https://doi.org/10.1016/j.urology.2012.11.044.
55. Chung JM, Park CS, Lee SD. Postoperative ureteral obstruction after endoscopic treatment for vesicoureteral reflux. Korean J Urol. 2015;56:533–9. https://doi.org/10.4111/kju.2015.56.7.533.

56. Okawada M, Esposito C, Escolino M, et al. Treatment of vesico-ureteral reflux in infants and children using endoscopic approaches. Transl Pediatr. 2016;5:282–90. https://doi.org/10.21037/tp.2016.10.04.
57. Okawada M, Shibuya S, Doi T, et al. Ureteric patency after Deflux®injection for the treatment of vesicoureteric reflux in children confirmed by a novel epidural catheter-assisted endoscopic technique. Pediatr Surg Int. 2015;31:977–82. https://doi.org/10.1007/s00383-015-3778-9.
58. Okawada M, Murakami H, Tanaka N, et al. Incidence of ureterovesical obstruction and Cohen antireflux surgery after Deflux® treatment for vesicoureteric reflux. J Pediatr Surg. 2018;53:310–2. https://doi.org/10.1016/j.jpedsurg.2017.11.027.

Duplex System and Vesicoureteral Reflux

Andrew J. Kirsch, Benjamin H. Press, and Angela M. Arlen

Abstract Ureteral duplication is one of the most common malformations of the urinary tract, affecting 1 in 125 children (0.8%). Duplication can be complete or partial. A bifid renal pelvis includes only a single ureter, but confluence of the upper and lower ureters below the ureteropelvic junction (UPJ) and above the bladder constitutes partial duplication of the ureter or bifid ureter. Partial duplication does not predispose to vesicoureteral reflux (VUR), and surgical correction is based on the same indications as a single refluxing ureter. In contrast, complete ureteric duplication may be associated with UPJ obstruction, VUR, ureteral ectopia and/or ureterocele. This chapter will focus on management of vesicoureteral reflux in the setting of complete ureteral duplication.

Keywords Vesicoureteral reflux (VUR) · Ureteral duplication · Hydroureteronephrosis · Ureteral reimplantation · Ureteroureterostomy · Endoscopic injection

Introduction

Ureteral duplication anomaly occurs in approximately 0.8% of the general population and is more common in females. Vesicoureteral reflux, typically involving the lower pole ureter, is the most common abnormality associated with ureteral duplication [1]. Multiple operative possibilities exist for reflux in ureteric duplication,

A. J. Kirsch (✉) · B. H. Press
Department of Pediatric Urology, Emory University and Children's Healthcare of Atlanta, Atlanta, GA, USA

A. M. Arlen
Department of Urology, Yale School of Medicine, Yale University, New Haven, CT, USA
e-mail: angela.arlen@yale.edu

P. Puri, A. Yamataka (eds.), *Vesicoureteral Reflux*,
https://doi.org/10.1007/978-3-031-95091-9_22

depending on associated anomalies and whether the VUR affects the lower pole ureter or both ureters. Need for surgical correction is dictated by a child's risk for further infections, potential for renal scarring, and likelihood of spontaneous resolution, along with parental preferences. Therapeutic considerations for surgical correction of VUR associated with duplication are similar to those for a single refluxing ureter, though spontaneous resolution is less likely to occur [2, 3]. Nuclear scintigraphy or magnetic resonance urography (MRU) with differential function of the upper and lower pole moieties may be performed to assist with operative planning [4, 5].

Pathogenesis

The caudal part of the Wolffian duct forms the common excretory duct which connects via a ureteric bud with the adjacent nephrogenic cord. Migration of these tissues leads to a single ureter draining the kidney and opening into the trigone of the bladder. Incomplete duplication arises from early branching of a single ureteric bud. Complete duplication is the result of an extra ureteric bud [6]. Primary vesicoureteral reflux is caused by the failure of the vesicoureteric junction to develop properly. Frequently, the ratio of the length of the ureter within the bladder wall to its diameter is reduced in refluxing ureters [7]; given that in duplex systems the lower pole ureters are laterally displaced, this results in shorter intramural tunnels contributing to VUR.

Diagnosis

Duplicated collecting system is a commonly encountered congenital anomaly of the urinary tract and is easily diagnosed on ultrasound when associated with hydroureteronephrosis (Fig. 1). A 2014 consensus statement suggests that a VCUG (Fig. 2) is an option for all children with antenatal dilation of the urinary tract and is indicated in children with more severe dilation or other abnormalities such as duplication [8]. As is the case with VCUG obtained for any indication, the American Academy of Pediatrics Sections on Urology and Radiology standardized VCUG protocol which should be adhered to. During cyclic filling (at least two voiding cycles are recommended), multiple spot images and urethral images are obtained during voiding [9]. In cases of duplex systems where additional information may be desired for surgical planning, functional MRU (Fig. 3) provides comprehensive morphological and functional evaluation including anatomic details such as ureteral ectopia and differentiation of functioning from barely or non-functioning renal moieties [4].

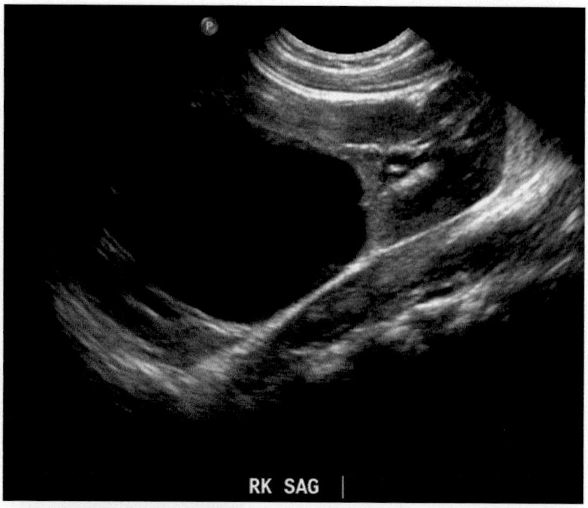

Fig. 1 Infant with severe right upper pole hydronephrosis and normal lower pole consistent with complete duplication

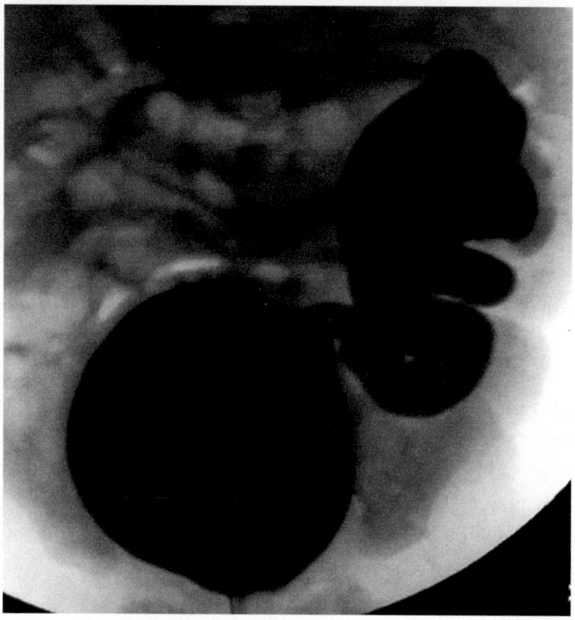

Fig. 2 Voiding cystourethrogram demonstrating left lower pole high grade vesicoureteral reflux. Note the "drooping lily" sign (inferolateral displacement of the opacified lower pole moiety)

Management

The natural tendency of primary reflux is to resolve over time, however spontaneous resolution is less likely to occur in duplex systems [2, 3]. The key focus in selecting patients for surgical correction is on identifying those with VUR unlikely to resolve *and* at greatest risk for recurrent pyelonephritis along with its sequela of renal injury. Surgical indications for correction of VUR associated with duplication are

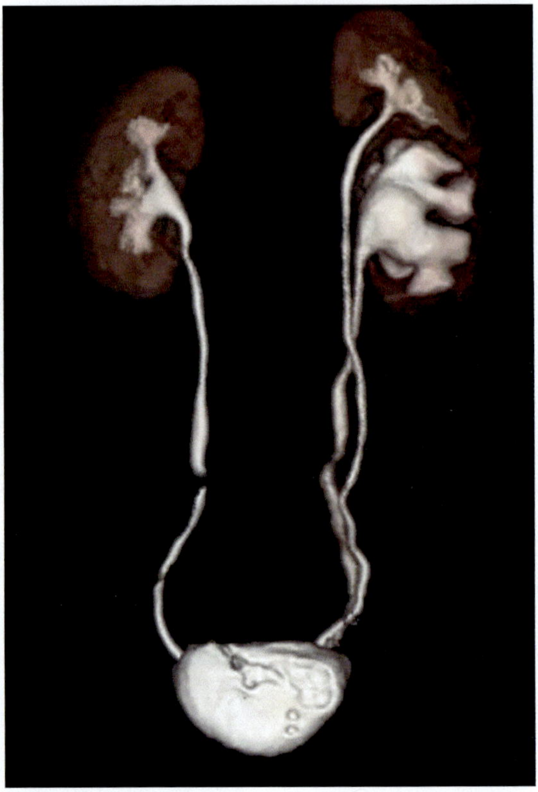

Fig. 3 MRU demonstrating complete left duplication with lower pole dilation but no obstruction

similar to those for a single refluxing ureter, however associated anomalies and whether reflux affects one or both moieties must also be considered when determining the optimal surgical approach for a given child. In addition to endoscopic repair and ureteral implantation (both open and robot-assisted approaches), ureteroureterostomy (UU) is also an option in select duplex cases with reflux into a single moiety. Compared to open surgery, minimally invasive approaches offer several advantages including smaller incisions and more rapid convalescence. However, this must be balanced with increased operative times and cost, particularly when a robotic approach is employed.

Endoscopic Injection

Endoscopic VUR correction using an injectable bulking agent was initially described decades ago. O'Donnell and Puri popularized endoscopic repair with subureteric injections using Teflon paste, i.e. the "STING" (subureteric teflon injection) procedure [10]. Double hydrodistention implantation technique (Double HIT), the

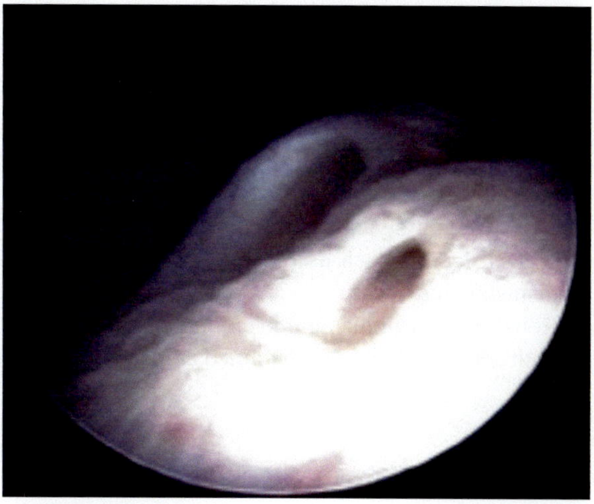

Fig. 4 Complete ureteral duplication, note that medial upper pole ureteral orifice appears patulous

hallmark of which is ureteral hydrodistention, allows for direct visualization and injection into the intraluminal ureteral submucosal plane and improved success rates [11].

Aggregate literature suggests that endoscopic therapy is relatively effective for the treatment of most *primary* VUR, while stressing the importance of reflux grade and structural/functional bladder anomalies on ultimate success rates [12]. Complete duplication (Fig. 4) is known to impact the success rate of endoscopic injection, though acceptable outcomes have been reported [13, 14]. Proponents of the endoscopic approach highlight benefits including its performance as an outpatient procedure and decreased patient morbidity, while opponents note both higher initial failure and recurrence rates compared to ureteral reimplantation—this ongoing debate underscores the importance of individualized care for children with VUR.

Ureteral Reimplantation

Open ureteroneocystostomy prevents VUR by increasing the intravesical ureteral length, facilitating compression of the ureter(s) against the detrusor muscle. Various open reimplantation techniques have been described including both intravesical and extravesical approaches. Cohen cross-trigonal reimplant is the most widely utilized intravesical ureteroneocystostomy technique, due to reliable results and broad applicability including in duplex systems with one or both moieties refluxing [15, 16]. Robot-assisted laparoscopic approaches have increasingly gained favor, with robust evidence demonstrating safe and effective outcomes [17]. Robotic common sheath ureteral reimplantation for duplex collecting systems is typically performed in an extravesical fashion with outcomes approaching that of open reimplantation [17, 18].

General Surgical Principles for Ureteral Reimplantation

- As both ureters are bound together distally in a common sheath, they are treated en bloc as a single unit in order to prevent devascularization
- Adequate length should be achieved to allow for 5:1 tunnel-to-ureteral diameter ratio
- Ureteral stenting and need for postoperative bladder drainage is dependent upon clinical factors such as patient age, ureteral tapering, or whether the ureter is dismembered
- Renal-bladder ultrasound is obtained approximately 4–8 weeks postoperatively, with additional imaging obtained as clinically indicated

Ureteroureterostomy

Advantages of UU include the ability to remain extravesical, thus avoiding the potential morbidity inherent with a transvesical approach. The successful outcome and the relatively low morbidity of UU for treating obstruction and/or reflux in duplex kidneys have been demonstrated by several groups even with massive ureteral dilation or poorly functioning renal moieties [17–22]. UU and UP can be performed via an open, laparoscopic, or robot-assisted approach (Figs. 5 and 6).

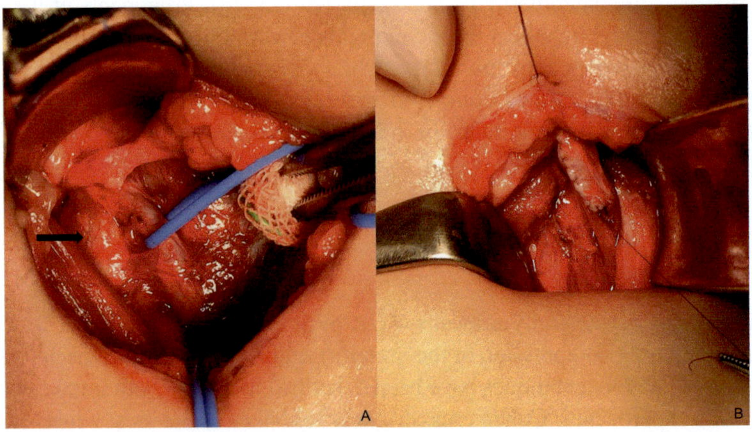

Fig. 5 Open distal ureteroureterostomy can be performed via Pfannenstiel, Gibson or inguinal incision. Upper vessel loop encircling a normal caliber lower pole ureter; the dilated upper pole ureter is denoted with an arrow (**a**). The upper pole ureter is anastomosed to the lower pole in a running, water-tight fashion using monofilament suture (**b**)

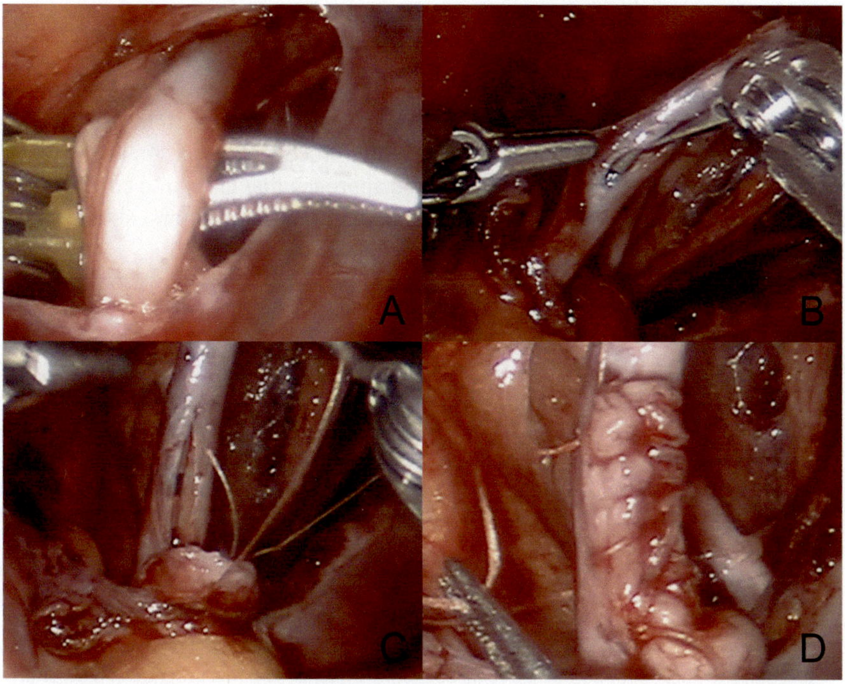

Fig. 6 Robotic distal ureteroureterostomy. Both ureters are identified in the pelvis (**a**). After transection of the refluxing ureter, the receipt non-refluxing ureter (with temporary stent in place) is incised (**b**). An end-to-side anastomosis is then performed in a running, water-tight fashion (**c**, **d**)

General Surgical Principles for Ureteroureterostomy

- Cystoscopy with stent or ureteral catheter placement to distinguish upper from lower pole ureters can be considered in cases where ureteral size discrepancy is lacking
- Dissection kept to a minimum with limited direct handling of ureters; mobilization of recipient ureter should be limited with care taken to preserve ureteral adventitia
- Anastomosis may be performed in a running or interrupted fashion; the authors prefer a small absorbable monofilament suture in running fashion with the knots placed extraluminally
- After the posterior anastomosis is complete, a double J stent is placed in the lower pole system if not previously done, and the anterior anastomosis performed; the authors leave an indwelling stent for 4–6 weeks postoperatively
- Anastomosis should be tension-free and watertight
- Placement of a closed suction or penrose drain is at the surgeon's discretion; the authors do not routinely leave a drain
- Renal-bladder ultrasound is obtained approximately 4–6 weeks after stent removal, with additional imaging obtained as clinically indicated

Conclusion

Ureteral duplication is a common anomaly and is often an incidental finding on prenatal sonography. Vesicoureteral reflux in duplex collecting systems is less likely to resolve spontaneously and multiple antireflux procedures exist. As is always the case with VUR, an individualized risk-based approach that takes into consideration a multitude of demographic, radiographic, and clinical factors should guide management.

References

1. Kaplan WE, Nasrallah P, King LR. Reflux in complete duplication in children. J Urol. 1978;120(2):220–2.
2. Afshar K, Papanikolaou F, Malek R, Bagli D, Pippi-Salle JL, Khoury A. Vesicoureteral reflux and complete ureteral duplication. Conservative or surgical management? J Urol. 2005;173(5):1725–7.
3. Kirsch AJ, Arlen AM, Leong T, Merriman LS, Herrel LA, Scherz HC, et al. Vesicoureteral reflux index (VURx): a novel tool to predict primary reflux improvement and resolution in children less than 2 years of age. J Pediatr Urol. 2014;10(6):1249–54.
4. Calle-Toro JS, Maya CL, Emad-Eldin S, Adeb MS, Back SJ, Darge K, et al. Morphologic and functional evaluation of duplicated renal collecting systems with MR urography: a descriptive analysis. Clin Imaging. 2019;57:69–76.
5. Sheth KR, White JT, Janzen N, Koh CJ, Austin PF, Roth DR, et al. Evaluating outcomes of differential surgical management of nonfunctioning upper pole renal moieties in duplex collecting systems. Urology. 2019;123:198–203.
6. Smith P, Dunn M. Duplication of the upper urinary tract. Ann R Coll Surg Engl. 1979;61(4):281–6.
7. Lopez PJ, Celis S, Reed F, Zubieta R. Vesicoureteral reflux: current management in children. Curr Urol Rep. 2014;15:447.
8. Nguyen HT, Benson CB, Bromley B, et al. Multidisciplinary consensus on the classification of prenatal and postnatal urinary tract dilation (UTD classification system). J Pediatr Urol. 2014;10:982–98.
9. Frimberger D, Mercado-Deane MF, AAP Section on Urology, AAP Section on Radiology. Establishing a standard protocol for the voiding cystourethrography. Pediatrics. 2016;138(5):e20162590.
10. O'Donnell B, Puri P. Treatment of vesicoureteral reflux by endoscopic injection of Teflon. Br Med J. 1984;289:7.
11. Kirsch AJ, Kaye JD, Cerwinka WH, et al. Dynamic hydrodistention of the ureteral orifice: a novel grading system with high interobserver concordance and correction with vesicoureteral reflux grade. J Urol. 2009;182:1688.
12. Routh JC, Inman BA, Reinberg Y. Dextranomer/hyaluronic acid for pediatric vesicoureteral reflux: systemic review. Pediatrics. 2010;125:1010–9.
13. Cerwinka WH, Scherz HC, Kirsch AJ. Dynamic hydrodistention classification of the ureter and the double hit method to correct vesicoureteral reflux. Arch Esp Urol. 2008;61(8):882–7.
14. Chertin B, Arafeh WA, Kocherov S. Endoscopic correction of complex cases of vesicoureteral reflux utilizing Vantris as a new non-biodegradable tissue-augmenting substance. Pediatr Surg Int. 2014;30:445–8.
15. Cohen SJ. Ureterozystoneostomie: Eine neue antireflux Technik. Aktuelle Urol. 1975;6:1.

16. Sung J, Skoog S. Surgical management of vesicoureteral reflux in children. Pediatr Nephrol. 2012;27:551–61.
17. Hou SW, Xing MH, Gundeti MS. Pediatric robotic urologic procedures: indications and outcomes. Indian J Urol. 2023;39(2):107–20.
18. Arlen AM, Broderick KM, Travers C, et al. Outcomes of complex robot-assisted extravesical ureteral reimplantation in the pediatric population. J Pediatr Urol. 2016;12(3):169e1–6.
19. Lashley DB, McAleer IM, Kaplan GW. Ipsilateral ureteroureterostomy for the treatment of vesicoureteral reflux or obstruction associated with complete ureteral duplication. J Urol. 2001;165:552–4.
20. McLeod DJ, Alpert SA, Ural Z, et al. Ureteroureterostomy irrespective of ureteral size or upper pole function: a single center experience. J Pediatr. 2014;10:616–9.
21. Abdelhalim A, Chamberlin JD, Truong H, et al. Ipsilateral ureteroureterostomy for ureteral duplication anomalies: predictors of adverse outcomes. J Pediatr Urol. 2019;15(5):468.e1–6.
22. Ellison JS, Lendvay TS. Robot-assisted ureteroureterostomy in pediatric patients: current perspectives. Robot Surg. 2017;4:45–55.

Coincidental Reflux and Upper Urinary Tract Obstruction

Balazs Kutasy and Gundela Holmdahl

Abstract The prevalence of vesicoureteral reflux (VUR) among patients with ureteropelvic junction (UPJ) obstruction patients is 8.2%, where one-third of the concomitant VUR are dilated VUR, and two-thirds are cases with non-dilated, low grade VUR with no need for surgical intervention. The etiology for coincidental VUR and UPJ obstruction is a primary ureteral abnormality affecting both ends of the ureter. Children with reflux and true blockage at the ureteropelvic junction have distinct cystographic patterns and the original grading system is not valid when dilatation is also due to obstruction. In the presence of concomitant disease, it is only possible to grade reflux accurately as high or low based on ureteral appearance. For evaluation of the upper urinary tract, technetium-99m (99mTc) mercaptoacetyltriglycine (MAG3) should be used. Once, the decision for UPJ obstruction is made, the child requires surgical correction with pyeloplasty. The choice of treatment can be challenging with refluxing megaureter.

Keywords Vesicoureteral reflux (VUR) · Ureteropelvic junction (UPJ) obstruction · Coincidental VUR and UPJ obstruction

B. Kutasy
Division of Pediatric Urology, Astrid Lindgren's Children's Hospital, Karolinska University Hospital, Stockholm, Sweden
e-mail: balazs.kutasy@regionstockholm.se

G. Holmdahl (✉)
Division of Pediatric Urology, Astrid Lindgren's Children's Hospital, Karolinska University Hospital, Stockholm, Sweden

Department of Women's and Children's Health, Karolinska Institutet, Stockholm, Sweden
e-mail: gundela.holmdahl@regionstockholm.se

P. Puri, A. Yamataka (eds.), *Vesicoureteral Reflux*,
https://doi.org/10.1007/978-3-031-95091-9_23

Introduction

Ureteropelvic junction (UPJ) obstruction is defined as impaired urinary flow from the renal pelvis into proximal ureter with subsequent dilatation of the collecting system and with the potential to damage the kidney [1]. It is the most common abnormality of the upper urinary tract [1]. It has an overall incidence of 1:1500 birth and a ratio of males to females of 2:1 in newborns [1].

The coincidental appearance of VUR in the case of UPJ obstruction was described first by Hutch et al. in 1962 [2]. More than a decade later Williams [3] described 2 categories of cases which was modified into 3 clinical categories in 1989 by Hollowell et al. [4]: Group1, primary UPJ obstruction with incidental low grade VUR into ureters without dilatation, kinking or tortuosity; Group2, secondary UPJ obstruction to massive high grade VUR where the ureters are dilated, tortuous and have a fixed kink at the UPJ; Group3, pseudo-UPJ obstruction defined as VUR into a distended pelvis with a kink at the UPJ radiographically mimicking an obstruction, however drainage films or a renal scan documents good drainage.

The tortuous, dilated refluxing ureter with a diameter greater than 10 mm in a newborn with or without secondary obstruction by kinking, is called a refluxing megaureter [1, 5]. Megaureters are generally classified as refluxing, obstructed or non-refluxing/non-obstructed [5]. The current book and chapter are not focusing on the megaureters in general. However, briefly we must discuss this as well to see the difference in etiology and its consequences in the treatment and results of the treatment.

Incidence

Concomitant VUR and UPJ obstruction are uncommon [6]. In a large clinical study, Mami et al. [7] screened 11,801 healthy newborns for severe renal dilatation. They detected 46 cases with a relevant obstruction, however none had concomitant VUR. Masson et al. [8] investigated 10,677 newborns who had moderate to severe hydronephrosis prenatally. They found that only 3 infants developed VUR and UPJ obstruction together, and none of them required surgery.

Recent systematic review [9] with 20 included studies demonstrated that the pooled prevalence of VUR among UPJ obstruction patients is 8.2% (range 0–21.3%). However, this might be overestimated since routinely not every study performed VCUG, sampling can occur selectively according to clinical presentation and some studies included pseudo-UPJ obstruction cases as well. An analysis of subgroups showed the pooled prevalence of VUR among UPJ obstruction patients with less than 2 years of age to be 11.1%. Stratification according to the side of VUR in relation to the kidney with UPJ obstruction showed that both kidneys, or only contralateral kidney were affected by VUR in 5.7% of cases. The approximate general prevalence of VUR is 1.6–2.6%, (which is likely an underestimation and verification by screening for VUR in otherwise healthy children cannot be justified). Based on this assumption, the prevalence for VUR in UPJ obstruction patients detected in that review represents about threefold increase compared to the general pediatric population.

Hubertus et al. [6] investigated 266 patients with UPJ obstruction. Concomitant VUR was observed in 7.3%. There was an equal distribution of VUR in both genders. Thus, the percentage of female patients with VUR and UPJ obstruction was 10.1%, whereas this percentage was only 3% in male patients. Regarding the preponderance of males with UPJ obstruction, females might be at higher risk to have a concomitant VUR. They also demonstrated that one-third of the concomitant VUR was dilated VUR, and two-thirds were cases with non-dilated, low grade VUR with no need for any surgical intervention for VUR.

Etiopathogenesis

The etiology for coincidental VUR and UPJ obstruction is a primary ureteral abnormality affecting both ends of the ureter [10]. Contact of the ureteral bud with metanephric blastema at week 4 of gestation induces branching to form the renal pelvis, calices and papillary collecting ducts [10]. The importance of this relationship is manifested by the observation that abnormal ureteral orifice configuration is directly related to an upper tract pathological condition [10]. It has been shown that patients with ectopic orifices have abnormal ureteral budding and renal dysplasia [10]. Multicystic dysplastic kidneys are associated with contralateral UPJ obstruction and VUR [10, 11].

Traditionally, it has been assumed in refluxing megaureter that over distension of the renal pelvis due to high grade VUR leads to kinking of the UPJ, which then becomes fixed secondary to inflammation [10]. While this process seems logical, it has not been provided clinical or experimental evidence for this mechanism [10]. Many studies have investigated the structure and ultrastructure of the normal and dilated ureter [12, 13]. Patients with primary refluxing megaureters demonstrated a twofold increase in the ratio of collagen to smooth muscle compared with obstructed megaureters and controls [12]. This twofold increase was due not only to markedly increases in collagen (type I, III and IV) but also to significant decrease in smooth muscle [12]. There is a disparity between the reported success rates in the reimplantation of obstructive versus refluxing megaureters [12]. The poor peristalsis and "floppy nature" of the refluxing megaureter of childhood is due to an abnormal accumulation of one or more collagen types and an overall decrease in smooth muscle (causing lesser chance for surgical success even with a technically sound reimplant), whereas the normal and obstructed megaureter have many similar architectural and collagen/smooth muscle ratios and distribution of collagen types (causing better chance for surgical success) [13].

Pirker et al. [14] studied bladder specimens from porcine fetuses and piglets. They found that the intravesical ureter did not mature until after birth. The time-course of muscular development in this study correlates with findings in humans, in whom smooth muscle bundles of the extramural ureter first appear in week 17–22 of gestation, and ureteral muscle development proceeds in a craniocaudal direction [5]. Tanagho [15] also observed that the distal ureter is the last portion to develop its muscular coat, and that early muscular differentiation is primarily of the circular muscles. The process whereby the circular muscle pattern, which is typical of the fetal ureter, changes progressively into double muscle layers of the full-term infant, may last up to 2 years, and may explain the transient functional disturbances of vesico-ureteral junction during this period [5].

C-kit-positive interstitial cells of Cajal (ICCs) are known to play an important role in the peristalsis and pacemaker activity of smooth muscle contraction; and to form a network between the smooth muscle and neurons [16]. Although traditional ICCs have been found in the gastrointestinal tract, ICCs have also been demonstrated outside the gut in various organs, such as the ureter and the bladder [16]. Kang et al. [16] investigated the number of apoptotic and ICCS cells. They found an increased apoptotic and decreased ICCs cell numbers in the obstructed megaureters, and dramatically increased apoptotic and ICCs cell numbers in the refluxing megaureters. It has been suggested that an insufficient blood supply causes ischemia and ischemic injury of the ureter leads up to increased apoptosis, which is later replaced by fibrotic tissue [16]. Therefore, Kim et al. [17] suggested that cell proliferation and apoptosis might play an important role in the pathogenesis of the obstructive megaureter. Studies of mice with mutations of ICCs leading to defects in the development of ICCs populations have shown that without pacemakers, the contraction of smooth muscle contractions is lost [18]. Several studies have shown that ICCs disappear from the intestines when the c-kit receptors are blocked during development [16, 19]. The blockage of c-kit signaling during development might be an explanation for the decrease of ICCs in the refluxing megaureter [16]. This can be congenital, or even acquired since Oberritter et al. [20] demonstrated investigating surgically created VUR in pigs that the ICCs are markedly decreased in the refluxing ureter in the vesicoureteral junction compared to controls. Interestingly several studies showed similar results investigating human UPJ, the expression of ICCs in primary or seconder UPJ obstruction are also markedly decreased compared to controls [21, 22].

Diagnostic Evaluation

Renal ultrasound (US) is the cornerstone in the diagnostic pathway of children with hydronephrosis [23]. The widespread use of US during pregnancy has resulted in a higher detection rate for antenatal hydronephrosis [1]. The most sensitive time for fetal urinary tract evaluation is the 28th week [1]. If dilatation is detected, the grade defined by the Society for Fetal Urology, which grade the renal pelvic dilatation, the number of calyces seen and parenchymal atrophy within five grades of increasing severity [23]. Since transitory neonatal dehydration lasts about 48 hours after birth, postnatal imaging should be performed after this period of postnatal oliguria [1]. However, in severe cases (bilateral dilatation, solitary kidney, oligohydramnios), immediate postnatal sonography is recommended [1]. Ultrasound should assess the anteroposterior diameter of the renal pelvis, calyceal dilatation, kidney size, thickness of the parenchyma, cortical echogenicity, ureters (including retrovesical part), bladder wall and residual urine [1, 6].

In newborns with identified upper urinary tract dilatation, the primary or important associated factors that must be detected include vesicoureteral reflux; urethral valves; ureteroceles; diverticula; and neurogenic bladder [1]. Therefore, conventional VCUG (see Chap. 11) is the next step, the method of choice for primary diagnostic procedures [1]. Children with reflux and true blockage at the ureteropelvic junction have distinct cystographic patterns [10]. The usual grading system for primary reflux is based on upper tract dilatation secondary to reflux alone [10]. This grading system is not valid when dilatation is also due to obstruction. In the presence of concomitant disease, it is only possible to grade reflux accurately as high or low based on ureteral appearance [10]. Contrast medium may be unable to traverse the ureteropelvic junction and there will be a dilated, possibly tortuous ureter with an abrupt cutoff of contrast material at the ureteropelvic junction [10]. If contrast medium spills into an upper tract already distended with urine, it will visualize the renal pelvis [10]. A drainage film is crucial whenever upper tract dilatation is seen on VCUG [10]. Contrast material remaining in the renal pelvis after the ureter and bladder are empty suggests UPJ obstruction [10].

Diuretic renography is the most commonly used diagnostic tool to detect the severity and functional significance of problems with urine transport [1]. Technetium-99m (99mTc) mercaptoacetyltriglycine (MAG3) is the radionuclide of choice [1]. It is important to perform the study under standardised circumstances (hydration, ensure good drainage of the bladder, using transurethral catheter with suspicion of VUR) at the earliest after the fourth and sixth weeks of life [1]. Oral fluid intake is encouraged prior to the examination. At 15 minutes before the injection of the radionuclide, it is mandatory to administer normal saline intravenous infusion at a rate of 15 mL/kg over 30 minutes, with a subsequent maintenance rate of 4 mL/kg/h throughout the entire time of the investigation [1]. The recommended dose of furosemide is 1 mg/kg for infants during the first year of life, while 0.5 mg/kg should be given to children aged 1–16 years, up to a maximum dose of 40 mg [1].

The diagnosis of UPJ obstruction can be made when the impaired split renal function comprise (<40%), a decrease of split renal function of >10% in subsequent studies, poor drainage function after the administration of furosemide, increased anteroposterior diameter on US, and grade III and IV dilatation as defined by the Society for Fetal Urology [1].

The diagnostic workup for a symptomatic hydronephrosis (recurrent flank/abdominal pain, febrile UTI, symptomatic stones) would include US, and MAG3 [23]. VCUG should be performed when hydroureter detected on the US [23]. CT or MR urography can be considered when the anatomic situation is not clear (for example a crossing vessel), or there is a high suspicion for kidney stone [23].

Historically the excretory urogram (IVP) has been the classic modality for evaluation of the upper urinary tract. This imaging procedure maybe a useful and appropriate method for diagnosis UPJ obstruction when nuclear scintigraphy is not accessible [24]. However, it has significant limitations: less sensitivity for diagnosis than MAG3; allergic reactions, aggravation of pain and acute renal failure induced by contrast media have been reported; and it has more radiation than nuclear scintigraphy [24, 25]. In this method it is important to give a proper bowel preparation for better visualization; to use delayed films, even up to 24 hours; and to insert a transurethral catheter especially when coexisting VUR is suspected [10, 24, 25].

For the clinical decision making on screening for VUR patients with UPJ obstruction, the benefit-harms-concept has to be taken into account [9]. The diagnosis with VCUG itself is an invasive, time-consuming, expensive, and unpleasant test with radiation exposure and may even cause UTI [9, 26]. Weitz and Schmidt [9] calculated that a total of 287 or 207 children with UPJ obstruction would need to undergo systematic screening with VCUG to prevent one case of febrile UTI or one case of new abnormality on a DMSA scan. Moreover, two thirds of coincidental VUR are low grade reflux [6]. Therefore, screening for VUR in children with UPJ obstruction should be restricted to risk groups, such as patients with recurrent febrile UTIs, or ureteral dilatation detected by US [6, 9].

Management

The benefits and harms of starting continous antibiotic prophylaxis (CAP) immediately after birth versus observation in patients with antenatal hydronephrosis are controversial [1]. Key findings of the recent systematic review are that CAP may or may not be superior to observation in children with antenatal hydronephrosis in terms of decreasing UTI [1]. However, noncircumcised male infants, children diagnosed with high-grade hydronephrosis and hydroureteronephrosis were shown to be at higher risk of developing a UTI [1]. Continuous antibiotic prophylaxis should be reserved for this sub-group of children who are proven to be at high risk [1].

It is most important that management decisions are made on the basis of serial investigations that have used the same technique and have been performed by the same institution under standardised circumstances [1]. Once, the decision for UPJ obstruction was made, the child requires surgical correction using a pyeloplasty, according to the standardised open technique of Hynes and Anderson (OP) [1]. In experienced hands, laparoscopic or retroperitoneoscopic techniques and robot-assisted techniques have the same success rates as standard open procedures [1]. A recent meta-analysis [27] in children has shown that laparoscopic pyeloplasty (LP) was associated with decreased length of hospital stay and complication rates but prolonged operative time when compared to OP. Additionally, both LP and OP had equal success rates [27]. Laparoscopic pyeloplasty can also be performed for re-do cases with the same advantages of the primary cases. Robotic-assisted laparoscopic pyeloplasty has all the same advantages as LP plus better manoeuvrability, improved vision, ease in suturing and increased ergonomics but at a higher costs [1].

When VUR was confirmed and the child has low grade reflux, the conservative therapy should start since resolution is nearly 80% in VUR grades I and II within 4–5 years of follow-up [1]. The conservative approach includes watchful waiting, intermittent or continuous antibiotic prophylaxis (CAP), and bladder and bowel rehabilitation in those with lower urinary tract dysfunction (LUTD) [1]. Although the literature does not provide any reliable information about the CAP and the duration of CAP in coexisting VUR and UPJ obstruction patients, our practical recommendation would be to use CAP until after children have been toilet-trained and ensuring that there is no LUTD. Circumcision during early infancy may be considered as part of the conservative approach since circumcision reduces the incidence of UTIs in boys with antenatal detected hydronephrosis and VUR [1, 28].

The choice of treatment can be challenging with refluxing megaureter. Unfortunately, there are no or not enough data on the treatment choice specifically in refluxing megaureter. Most of our data on the treatment of megaureter are coming from primary obstructive megaureter (POM) or megaureters in general. Studies with POM demonstrated a spontaneous remission rate of up to 85%, therefor surgical management is no longer recommended [5, 29]. Low-dose prophylactic antibiotics within the first year of life are recommended for the prevention of UTIs; and surgery (open or minimal invasive anti-reflux surgery) is indicated for symptomatic children, if there is a drop in split renal function in conservative follow-up, hydroureteronephrosis is increasing, or recurrent UTI [1, 5]. This treatment strategy seems reasonable even for refluxing megaureter patients. However, we have to keep in mind that true obstruction cannot be expected to resolve after ureteral reimplantation and therefore the obstructive uropathy should be treated first [4]; and the poor peristalsis and "floppy nature" of the refluxing megaureter of childhood may cause lesser chance for surgical success even with a technically sound reimplant [12].

Conclusion

The prevalence for VUR in UPJ obstruction patients represents about threefold increase compared to the general pediatric population. However, it seems that two-thirds of the coincidental cases were cases with non-dilated, low grade VUR. Screening for VUR in children with UPJ obstruction should be restricted to risk groups, such as patients with recurrent febrile UTIs, or ureteral dilatation detected by US. When VUR was confirmed and the child has low grade reflux, the resolution of VUR is high. The clinical challenge is to determine when UPJ obstruction is in fact clinically significant. Once, the decision for UPJ obstruction was made, the child requires surgical correction using a pyeloplasty.

Case

A 5-day old healthy boy born after uncomplicated gravidity and delivery, presented with pyelonephritis. After iv antibiotic treatment investigation started with US, VCUG and DMSA. The US revealed that he had a hydronephrosis (AP diameter 17 mm) on the right side. The VCUG showed Grade III reflux on the same side (Fig. 1). Right sided renal damage was detected on DMSA scan with 35% split function on the right (Fig. 2). Initial conservative treatment with CAP was started. He had break-through febrile UTI at 11 months of age. The re-evaluation showed right sided hydronephrosis on US, right sided Grade III VUR on VCUG with delay of the contrast from pyelon on the post miction picture (Fig. 3), and stable split kidney function on MAG3 but delayed wash out, without obstruction (Fig. 4). He was booked for cystoscopy and endoscopic treatment of VUR (with Deflux). The postop control demonstrated persisting Grade III–IV VUR on the right side, and he was scheduled for a second endoscopic treatment. The new postop control showed no VUR on VCUG (Fig. 5), and no hydroureter on either side, but still hydronephrosis on right side with 15 mm AP diameter (Figs. 6 and 7). After 4 asymptomatic years the child came back with right sided abdominal/flank pain. The new US showed increased right sided hydronephrosis with 22 mm on AP diameter. The new MAG3 demonstrated right sided UPJ obstruction with 33% function on the right side (Fig. 8).

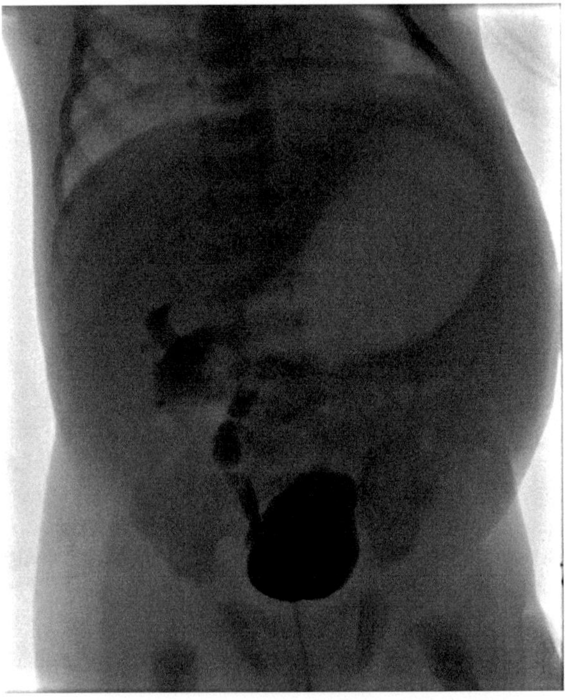

Fig. 1 Initial VCUG showed a Grade III VUR on the right side. (Special thanks for the pictures to Dr. Jacob Strömgren, Department of Pediatric Radiology, Karolinska University Hospital)

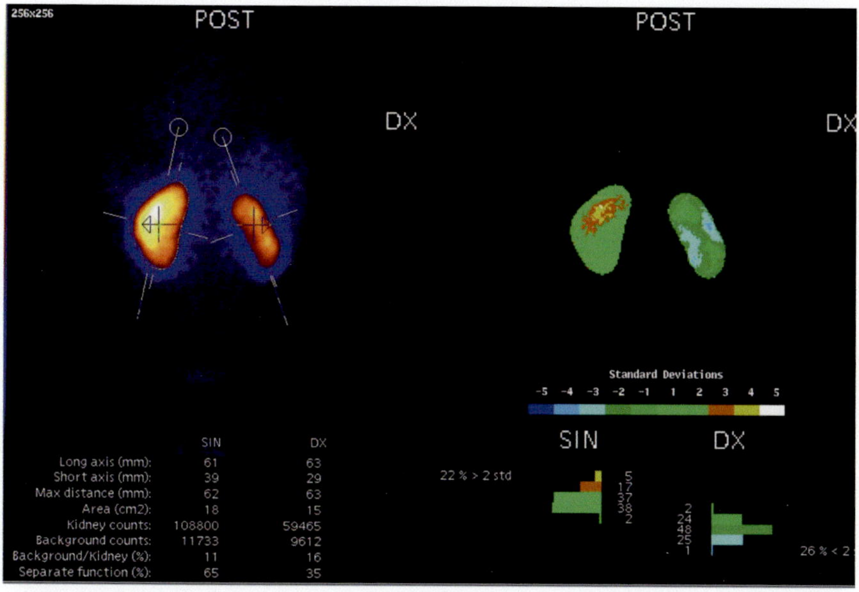

Fig. 2 Initial DMSA demonstrated a right sided nephropathy with a generalized kidney damage and a split function of 35%

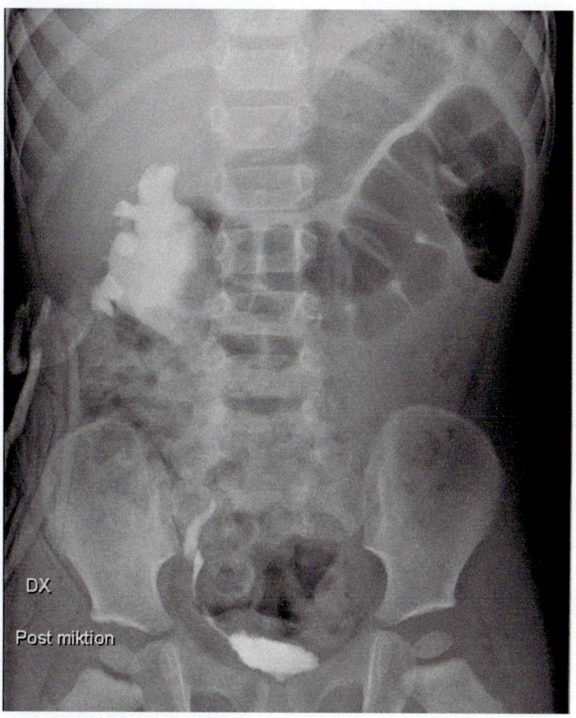

Fig. 3 Incomplete emptying of the renal pelvis on VCUG on post miction picture

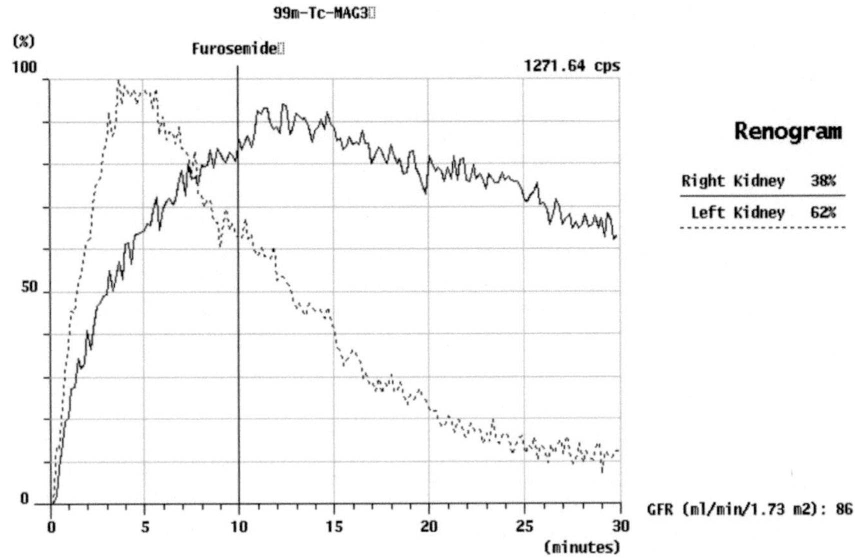

Fig. 4 First MAG3 with delayed washout but with a with a non-obststructed curve and stable split function of 38%

Fig. 5 No VUR on postop VCUG after the second endoscopic injection

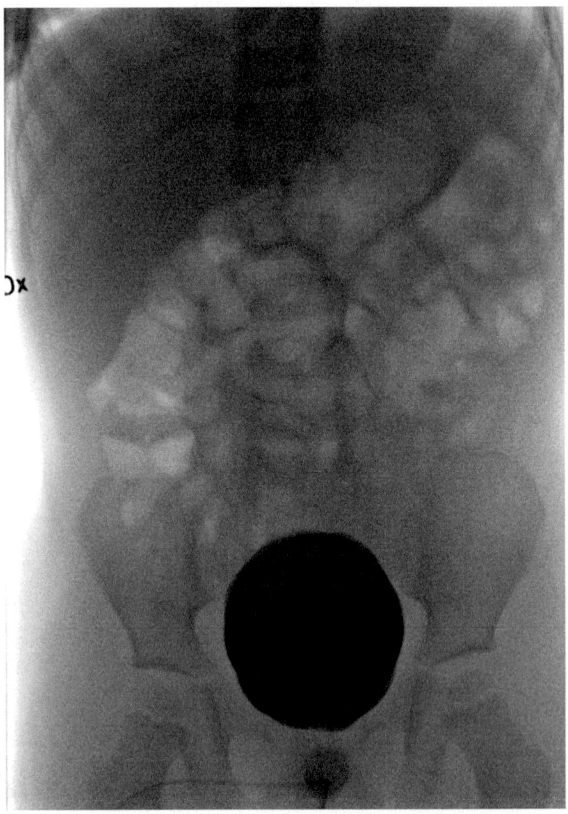

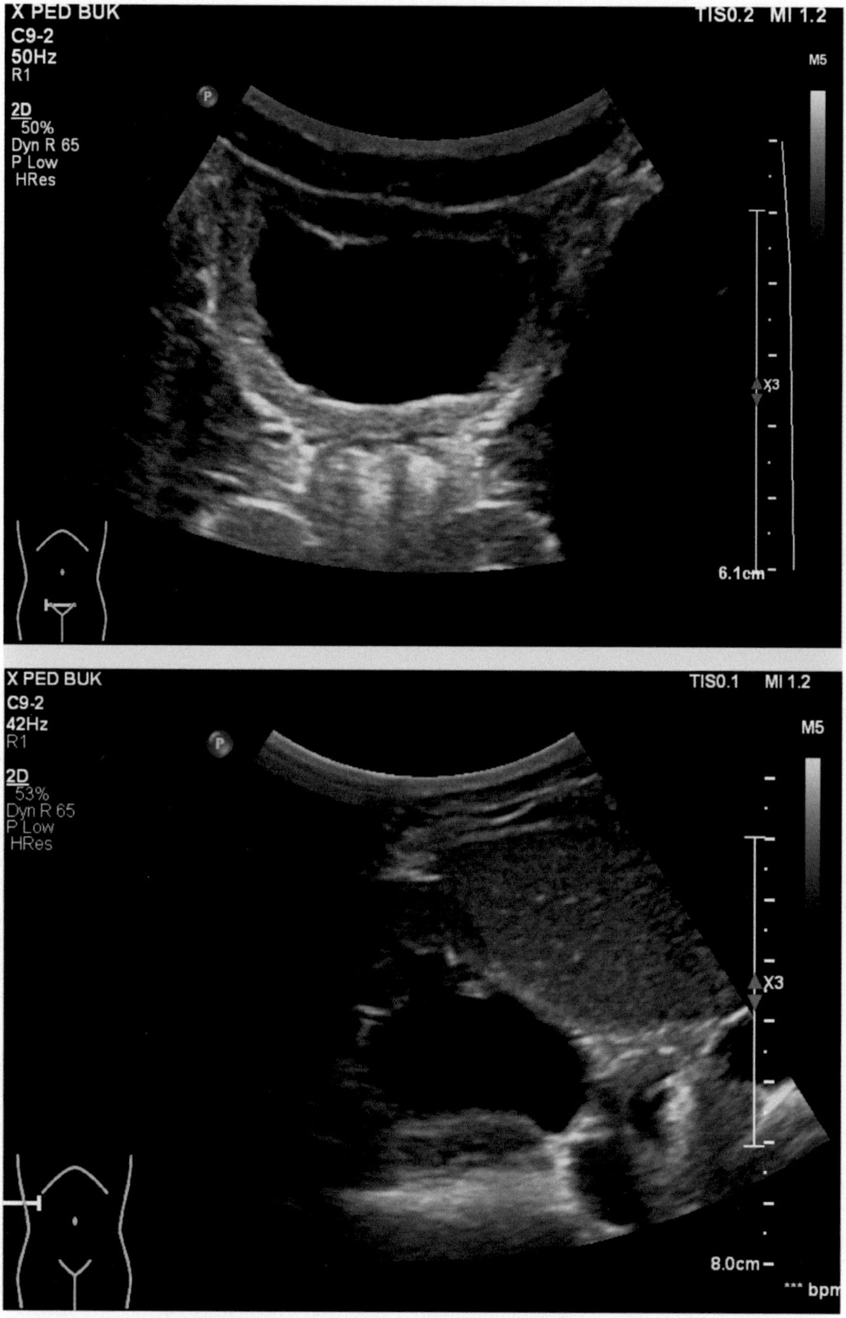

Figs. 6 and 7 Postop US after the second endoscopic injection revealed no hydroureter, but hydronephrosis on the right side, with an AP diameter of 15mm

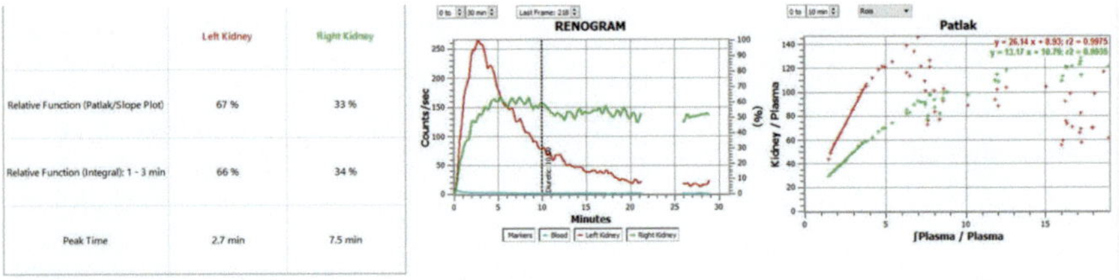

Fig. 8 Follow up MAG-3 due to flank pain and recurrent UTI, showing an obstructed washout curve on the right side and decreasing split function to 33%

Conclusion of this case 1. Keep in mind, that obstruction can develop even a few years after successful reflux treatment. 2. After successful endoscopic treatment, postop US control for hydronephrosis control would be beneficial, especially in those cases where delay of the contrast was noticed on the post micturition picture.

References

1. Rademayr CBG, Dogan HS, Nijman JM, Rawashdeh YFH, Silay MS, Stein R, Tekgul S. EAU guidelines on paediatric urology. Arnhem: EAU Guidelines Office; 2023.
2. Hutch JA, Hinman F Jr, Miller ER. Reflux as a cause of hydronephrosis and chronic pyelonephritis. J Urol. 1962;88:169–75.
3. Williams DI, editor. Vesico-ureteric reflux. New York: Springer; 1974.
4. Hollowell JG, Altman HG, Snyder HM 3rd, Duckett JW. Coexisting ureteropelvic junction obstruction and vesicoureteral reflux: diagnostic and therapeutic implications. J Urol. 1989;142(2 Pt 2):490–3; discussion 501.
5. Farrugia MK, Hitchcock R, Radford A, Burki T, Robb A, Murphy F, et al. British Association of Paediatric Urologists consensus statement on the management of the primary obstructive megaureter. J Pediatr Urol. 2014;10(1):26–33.
6. Hubertus J, Plieninger S, Martinovic V, Heinrich M, Schuster T, Burst M, et al. Children and adolescents with ureteropelvic junction obstruction: is an additional voiding cystourethrogram necessary? Results of a multicenter study. World J Urol. 2013;31(3):683–7.
7. Mami C, Paolata A, Palmara A, Marrone T, Berte LF, Marseglia L, et al. Outcome and management of isolated moderate renal pelvis dilatation detected at postnatal screening. Pediatr Nephrol. 2009;24(10):2005–8.
8. Masson P, De Luca G, Tapia N, Le Pommelet C, Es Sathi A, Touati K, et al. Postnatal investigation and outcome of isolated fetal renal pelvis dilatation. Arch Pediatr. 2009;16(8):1103–10.
9. Weitz M, Schmidt M. To screen or not to screen for vesicoureteral reflux in children with ureteropelvic junction obstruction: a systematic review. Eur J Pediatr. 2017;176(1):1–9.
10. Bomalaski MD, Hirschl RB, Bloom DA. Vesicoureteral reflux and ureteropelvic junction obstruction: association, treatment options and outcome. J Urol. 1997;157(3):969–74.
11. Heikkinen ES, Herva R, Lanning P. Multicystic kidney. A clinical and histological study of 13 patients. Ann Chir Gynaecol. 1980;69(1):15–22.
12. Lee BR, Partin AW, Epstein JI, Quinlan DM, Gosling JA, Gearhart JP. A quantitative histological analysis of the dilated ureter of childhood. J Urol. 1992;148(5):1482–6.
13. Lee BR, Silver RI, Partin AW, Epstein JI, Gearhart JP. A quantitative histologic analysis of collagen subtypes: the primary obstructed and refluxing megaureter of childhood. Urology. 1998;51(5):820–3.

14. Pirker ME, Rolle U, Shinkai T, Shinkai M, Puri P. Prenatal and postnatal neuromuscular development of the ureterovesical junction. J Urol. 2007;177(4):1546–51.
15. Tanagho EA. Intrauterine fetal ureteral obstruction. J Urol. 1973;109(2):196–203.
16. Kang HJ, Lee HY, Jin MH, Jeong HJ, Han SW. Decreased interstitial cells of Cajal-like cells, possible cause of congenital refluxing megaureters: histopathologic differences in refluxing and obstructive megaureters. Urology. 2009;74(2):318–23.
17. Kim HG, Paick SH, Kwak C, Kim HH, Lho YS. Serial microscopic changes in cell proliferation and apoptosis in obstructed ureter of rat. J Endourol. 2006;20(8):590–7.
18. Brading AF, McCloskey KD. Mechanisms of disease: specialized interstitial cells of the urinary tract--an assessment of current knowledge. Nat Clin Pract Urol. 2005;2(11):546–54.
19. Burns AJ. Disorders of interstitial cells of Cajal. J Pediatr Gastroenterol Nutr. 2007;45(Suppl 2):S103–6.
20. Oberritter Z, Rolle U, Juhasz Z, Cserni T, Puri P. Altered expression of c-kit-positive cells in the ureterovesical junction after surgically created vesicoureteral reflux. Pediatr Surg Int. 2009;25(12):1103–7.
21. Yang X, Zhang Y, Hu J. The expression of Cajal cells at the obstruction site of congenital pelviureteric junction obstruction and quantitative image analysis. J Pediatr Surg. 2009;44(12):2339–42.
22. Nandan R, Jain V, Agarwala S, Das P, Goel P, Kalaivani M, et al. Evaluation of interstitial cells of Cajal-like cells at the pelviureteric junction in children with pelviureteric junction obstruction: a prospective study and review of literature. J Indian Assoc Pediatr Surg. 2022;27(4):395–401.
23. ESPU. Paediatric Urology Web book 2015. Available from: www.espu.org.
24. Esmaeili M, Esmaeili M, Ghane F, Alamdaran A. Comparison between diuretic urography (IVP) and diuretic renography for diagnosis of ureteropelvic junction obstruction in children. Iran J Pediatr. 2016;26(1):e4293.
25. Shokeir AA. The diagnosis of upper urinary tract obstruction. BJU Int. 1999;83(8):893–900; quiz -1.
26. Stratton KL, Pope JC, Adams MC, Brock JW 3rd, Thomas JC. Implications of ionizing radiation in the pediatric urology patient. J Urol. 2010;183(6):2137–42.
27. Huang Y, Wu Y, Shan W, Zeng L, Huang L. An updated meta-analysis of laparoscopic versus open pyeloplasty for ureteropelvic junction obstruction in children. Int J Clin Exp Med. 2015;8(4):4922–31.
28. Chan JY, Khondker A, Lee MJ, Kim JK, Chancy M, Chua ME, et al. The role of circumcision in preventing urinary tract infections in children with antenatal hydronephrosis: systematic review and meta-analysis. J Pediatr Urol. 2023;19(6):766–77.
29. Peters CA, Mandell J, Lebowitz RL, Colodny AH, Bauer SB, Hendren WH, et al. Congenital obstructed megaureters in early infancy: diagnosis and treatment. J Urol. 1989;142(2 Pt 2):641–5; discussion 67–8.

Vesicoureteral Reflux Secondary to Neurogenic Bladder

Salvatore Cascio

Abstract This chapter deals with Vesicoureteral Reflux (VUR) in neurogenic bladder (NB), which is a specific type of reflux that compared to primary VUR is less likely to resolve spontaneously, has a unique underlying pathophysiological mechanism and whose management is still controversial. VUR can be detected in up to a third of children with NB. When VUR is detected at first video urodynamic (VUD), resolves in up to 30–50% of children within 2–3 years after commencing clean intermittent catheterization and anticholinergic medication. Endoscopic Treatment or Total Endoscopic Treatment should be reserved to children with NB who fail conservative management and demonstrate a smooth bladder wall, good compliance and a bladder capacity >75% of the Expected Bladder Capacity on VUD. Bladder augmentation should be recommended for children with VUR in a poorly compliant trabeculated bladder. High pressure VUR is likely to resolve in 50–97% of these patients with an isolated bladder augmentation while low pressure VUR, detected in the early filling phase of the VUD, in trabeculated bladders has a low-resolution rate and should be dealt with ureteric reimplantation associated to bladder augmentation. It is of greatest importance that the treatment of VUR in children with NB is discussed at multidisciplinary meeting and individualized according to the patients' symptoms, patients/parents' compliance to treatment, comorbidity, renal investigations (US, DMSA), renal function (estimated GFR) and most importantly video urodynamics.

Keywords Neurogenic bladder · Neuropathic bladder · Endoscopic management · Total endoscopic management · Bladder augmentation · Ureteric reimplantation · Clean intermittent catheterization · Anticholinergic · Video-urodynamic

S. Cascio (✉)
School of Medicine, University College Dublin and Children's Health Ireland, Dublin, Ireland
e-mail: salvatorecascio@doctors.org.uk

P. Puri, A. Yamataka (eds.), *Vesicoureteral Reflux*,
https://doi.org/10.1007/978-3-031-95091-9_24

Introduction and Classification

Vesicoureteral reflux (VUR) in neurogenic bladder (NB) is a specific type of reflux that, compared to primary VUR, is less likely to resolve spontaneously, has a unique underlying pathophysiological mechanism and whose management is still controversial despite having gone through significant changes over the last 40 years. VUR can be detected in up to a third of children with neurogenic or neuropathic bladder [33], with 16% of patients with spina bifida showing reflux at their first video urodynamic (VUD) study, with unilateral reflux more common than bilateral (3:1) [4]. The relevance of VUR lies upon the retrograde flow of urine from the bladder into the upper urinary tract which may lead to dilatation of the urinary tract increasing the risk of pyelonephritis, hypertension and progressive renal damage (Fig. 1a–d). Historically, vesicoureteral reflux has been classified in primary, due to a congenital anatomical defect of the ureterovesical junction, and secondary due to an abnormal bladder function or obstruction to the urinary flow. However, in recent years this rigid dichotomous classification of primary and secondary, has been challenged and VUR is now seen more as a continuous disease spectrum where different anatomical and physiological factors may play a significant role and may even coexist in the same patient. Important anatomical factors responsible for VUR are represented by a short intramural length of the ureter, a lateral and superior displacement of the ureteric orifice as it occurs in lower pole ureters of duplex kidney, the apperance of the ureteric orifice with the horseshoe and golf hole configuration being associated with higher rates of VUR. In addition, VUR is closely related to ectopic ureter and bladder diverticula specifically the para ureteral type (Hutch diverticulum). Similarly, physiology of the bladder also has a major role in the development of VUR with high bladder pressures generated by, either detrusor overactivity or detrusor sphincter dyssynergia, thought to overpower the ureterovesical junction to drive VUR. Children with VUR in NB represent the perfect example of the complexity of the VUR spectrum; in these children reflux can be detected in the early filling phase of a VUD in the presence of a quiet detrusor trace due to a short intramural ureteric length or can be detected during the filling phase due to high-pressure detrusor contractions or finally at the end of the VUD due to the high voiding pressures (>75 cm H_2O) in children with detrusor sphincter dyssynergia. A detailed VUD in the first 3 month of life remain, together with an ultrasound of the urinary tract, the most important investigations that can help to clarify the underlying cause of VUR in children with NB. Neurogenic bladders can be divided into three groups: primary, secondary and idiopathic. **Primary neurogenic** bladder develops because of a lesion at any level in the central nervous system, cerebral cortex and spinal cord, or in the peripheral nervous system. The most common causes are congenital such as open or closed neural tube defects (spinal dysraphism). **Secondary neurogenic bladder**, also called **neuropathic bladder**, occurs when the bladder acts like a neurogenic bladder but is not caused by a neurological defect. Causes in a neonate include imperforate anus, Prune Belly Syndrome, bladder exstrophy, cloacal exstrophy and posterior urethral valves. **Idiopathic neuropathic bladder** is very rare, causes include the Urofacial Syndrome and the Hinman Syndrome [5].

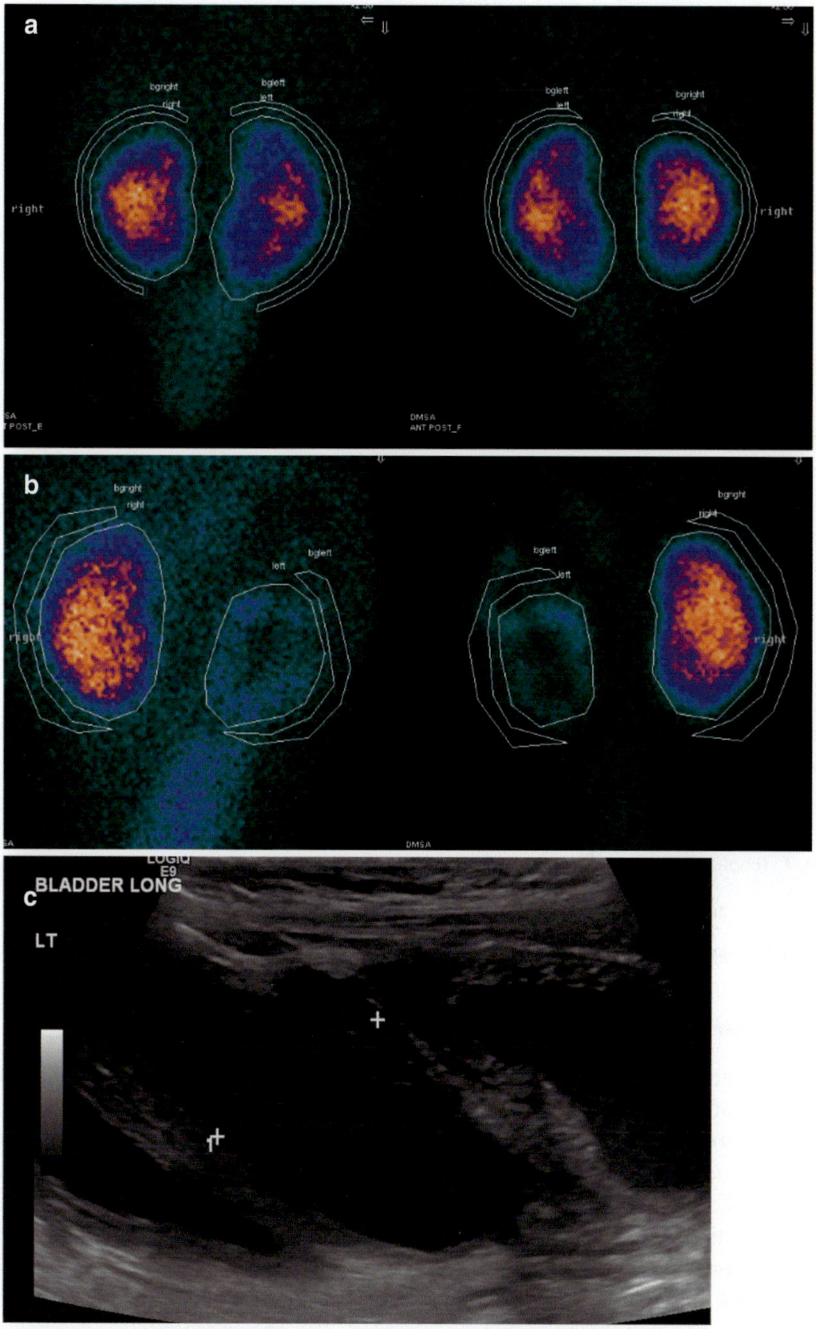

Fig. 1 (**a**) DMSA in a 9-month-old patient with neurogenic bladder (**b**) DMSA in the same patient lost to follow up at the age of 6 years. Uptake in the left kidney has dropped to 13%, right kidney 87% (**c**) An ultrasound in the same patient demonstrates a dilated, tortuous left ureter while a micturating cystourethrogram (**d**) shows high grade reflux in the left duplex kidney and a " Christmas tree" bladder, vertically oriented, with a wide base, which tapers superiorly towards the dome and has irregular walls from associated trabeculations

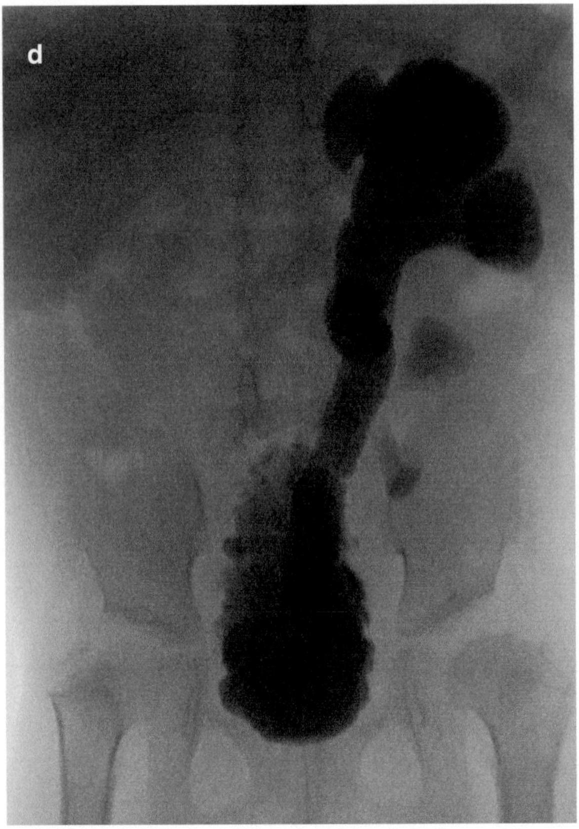

Fig. 1 (continued)

Management

(a) **Conservative Management**

The treatment of VUR in neurogenic bladder relies on the optimization of the management of the underlying bladder dysfunction and includes a combination of *clean intermittent catheterization* (CIC) to allow regular bladder emptying and *bladder relaxant (anticholinergic medication)* to try to maintain low intravesical pressure. Catheterization is usually undertaken 4–6 times daily in conjunction with feeds and diaper changes while oxybutynin is administered at a dose of 0.3–0.6 mg/kg in two or three divided doses [5]. With conservative management, VUR resolves in 30–50% of children after commencing clean intermittent catheterization and anticholinergic medication within 2–3 years [2, 19]. In our prospective database of children with neurogenic bladders secondary to myelomeningocele at Children's

Health Ireland, VUR resolved in 4 of 12 patients (33%) after commencing CIC and anticholinergic medication following initial video-urodynamics at 3–6 months (Fig. 2). Regular urinary surveillance and prophylactic antibiotic are usually recommended in the first year of life at discretion of the managing multidisciplinary team. When conservative management fails surgical options should be considered, these include endoscopic treatment (STING or HIT), total endoscopic management (TEM), ureteric reimplantation, isolated bladder augmentation, bladder augmentation with concomitant ureteric reimplantation and formation of a diverting vesicostomy.

(b) **Endoscopic treatment**

In 1984, the concept of *endoscopic treatment* was introduced by Puri and O'Donnell as a minimally invasive treatment for VUR, following a successful experimental study in piglets [16, 17]. In the following years, many studies have confirmed that the endoscopic treatment is a simple, safe and effective 15-min outpatient procedure to correct all grades of VUR. In 2006 Elder et al. published a meta-analysis of the existing literature relative to endoscopic treatment. A total of 63 articles were reviewed, including 5527 patients and 8101 renal units. The authors showed that reflux resolution, following a single endoscopic treatment, was significantly lower for patients with a neuropathic bladder compared to those with a normal bladder (61.64% vs 74.24%) [7]. The lower success rates of endoscopic treatment in NB have been confirmed by long term study showing a 90% immediate success rate which decreased to 15% at 2 years follow up [10]. Similarly, Polackwich et al., retrospectively reviewed 12 patients with associated neurogenic bladder, and demonstrated that after an initial improvement, vesico ureteral reflux recurred with a success rate of only 25% at a median follow up of 4.5 years [25]. Additional procedures were required in 41% of patients including bladder augmentation with ureteral reimplantation in 3, bladder augmentation alone in 1 and nephroureterectomy in 1. Analysis of patients' outcome for the presence of risk factors for failure or success did not show any significant statistical difference. However, a detailed review of the VUDs of the patients who failed endoscopic treatment with recurrence of high grade VUR (3–5), showed that 5 of 6 patients had a trabeculated bladder wall and 2 of the 6 had a poorly compliant (<7 ml/cm H_2O) small capacity bladder (<60% EBC) suggesting an underlying bladder dysfunction. In addition, trabeculated bladders from an endoscopic point of view, are particularly challenging because the ureteral orifices may be either not easily identifiable or can be wide and patulous from bladder distortion [33]. The presence of trabeculations may also explain why complications such as obstruction at the uretero- vesical junction have been reported more commonly in NBs compared to non-NBs [30]. Therefore, if endoscopic treatment is utilized in NBs, it should be confined to those bladders with a normal compliance, preserved bladder capacity and no trabeculations on VUD.

(c) **Ureteric reimplantation**

For nearly 50 years *ureteric reimplantation* has been shown to be a successful surgical option to treat VUR in NB with resolution rate ranging from 82% to 100% (Table 1). Comparison between the studies may be difficult as the success rate reported by some investigators is the result of a combination of different surgical techniques (Politano-Leadbetter, Cohen, Glen-Anderson, Paquin) [9]. The Cohen ureteric reimplantation is the most popular and reliable technique

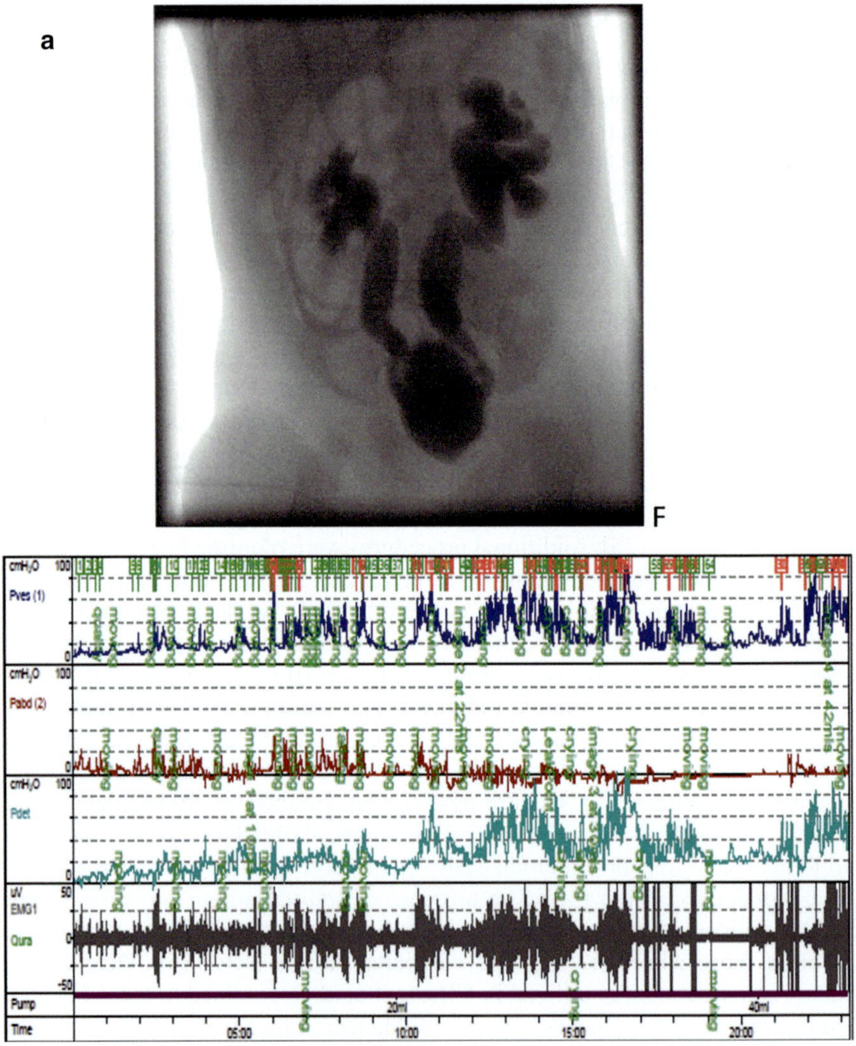

Fig. 2 (**a**) First video urodynamic in a patient with spina bifida at 3 month (**b**) Repeat video urodynamic at 6 month in the same patient showing resolution of VUR after starting clean intermittent catheterization and anticholinergic medication

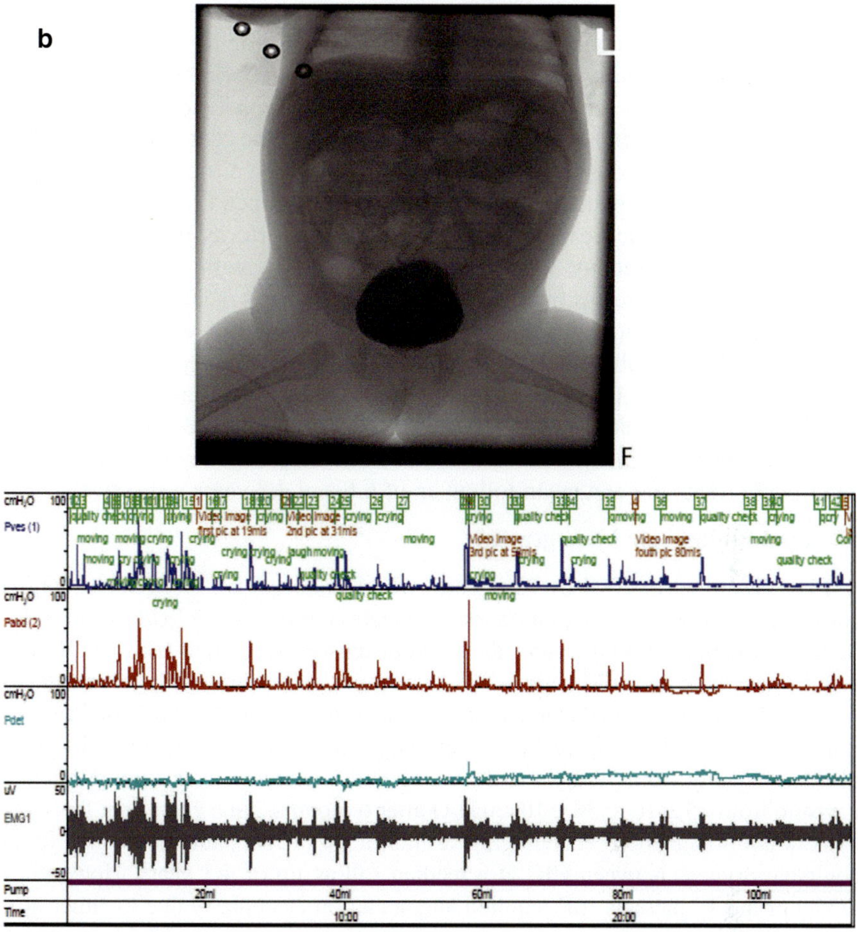

Fig. 2 (continued)

Table 1 Resolution rate of VUR after ureteric reimplantation

Study	Year	N	Success rate (%)
Jeffs et al [13]	1976	23	87
Belloli et al [3]	1979	26	85
Kaplan et al [14]	1983	25	96
Sidi et al [26]	1986	12	100
Kondo et al [15]	1987	18	89
Merlini et al [19]	1993	36	82
Engel et al [8]	1997	49	83.7

performed in the United States and Europe in patients with NB. The widespread use of the Cohen technique is due to its simplicity avoiding any extravesical dissection of the ureter with preservation of the original ureteric hiatus. The procedure is performed by creating a new submucosal tunnel across the trigone bringing the new ureteral orifice superior and closer to the contralateral one. The main disadvantage of the technique is represented by the difficulty to access the ureter in a retrograde manner. Few studies comparing open ureteric reimplantation versus endoscopic treatment have showed the superiority of the open surgical approach in correcting VUR in children with NB, with a success rate of 84.3% versus 56.7% respectively [8]. The greater success rate of ureteroneocystostomy seems to be not related to patient sex, reflux grade, laterality or bilateral versus unilateral; finally endoscopic treatment was more likely to fail in higher grades of reflux [8]. These results were confirmed 2 years later by an Italian study showing a success rate of 95.5% in children with NB who underwent Cohen ureteric reimplantation versus 72.5% in those who were treated with endoscopic treatment at a mean follow up of 6.6 and 4.8 years respectively [9].

(d) **Total Endoscopic Management**

First described in 2008 by Neel et al., *Total Endoscopic Management* (TEM) consisted of the association of intravesical injection of BTX-A (12 U/kg) and endoscopic correction of VUR using the hydrodistension technique (HIT) [23]. The authors described the TEM approach in 10 patients (8 female) with myelomeningocele (MM) who had failed standard conservative treatment. They reported resolution of VUR in 15 (93%) of the 16 refluxing ureters, a 100% increase in mean bladder capacity from 79 ± 49 to 149 ± 51 and a decrease in maximum bladder pressure from 55 ± 16 to 38 ± 10 cm H_2O after 6 months. Nine years later the same authors confirmed these encouraging results in 10 (72%) patients who achieved complete dryness between CIC at a median follow up of 4.3 years. However, 4 (28%) of the 14 patients still required augmentation cystoplasty due to either progressive hydronephrosis and/or persistent UTIs (3 patients) or a wide bladder neck (1 patient) [1]. In 2009, Mosiello et al. described the results of TEM in 7 patients with neurogenic bladder and VUR who had failed conservative treatment. VUR disappeared in all patients. In one patient with severe bilateral VUR, who refused a second Botulinum Toxin A injection, VUR recurred at 15.6 months follow up. The authors noted an increase in maximum cystometric capacity (mean 79 mls) and a decrease in maximum detrusor pressure (mean = 23 H_2O) [21] (Fig. 3).

(e) **Bladder Augmentation**

Since the early 90s different studies have demonstrated that *bladder augmentation* alone can abolish the need for ureteral reimplantation with resolution rate of reflux ranging from 50% to 97% of the patients (Table 2). It is controversial whether the resolution rate after bladder augmentation is correlated to the severity of the preoperative VUR, with some studies showing that low-grade reflux had a higher resolution rate (90%) than high grade reflux (53%) [11, 27]. On the contrary Pereira et al. have reported the opposite findings with greater resolution rates in high grade reflux (81%) than in low grade reflux (50%) [24]. The authors hypothesized that low grade reflux may be related to a congenital anomaly of the ureterovesical junction while high grade reflux is secondary to increased intravesical pressures. These conclusions were strengthened by a study showing that when reflux occurs in the early stage of the bladder filling phase, augmentation alone may not be enough to correct VUR [28]. The requirement for a concomitant ureteric reimplantation at the same time of the bladder augmentation has been challenged by few other studies. Wan et al. compared the resolution of VUR in children who underwent augmentation cystoplasty alone versus children who received augmentation with simultaneous ureteral reimplantation demonstrating an incidence of residual VUR of 57% in the former group compared to 0% in the latter [31]. These findings were confirmed by a recent larger study of 160 patients with neurogenic and neuropathic bladders who underwent augmentation cystoplasty and concomitant anti reflux procedure for either VUR or uretero vesical junction stenosis. The authors showed a 92%

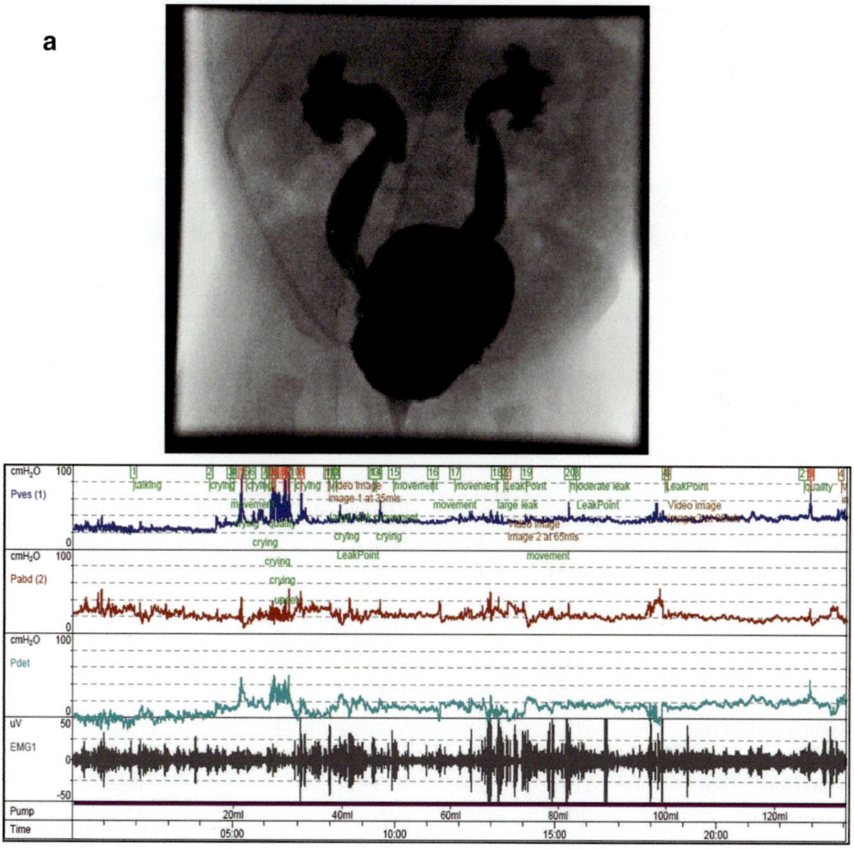

Fig. 3 (**a**) Total Endoscopic Management: pre-operative video urodynamic (**b**) Total Endoscopic Management: post-operative video urodynamic

b

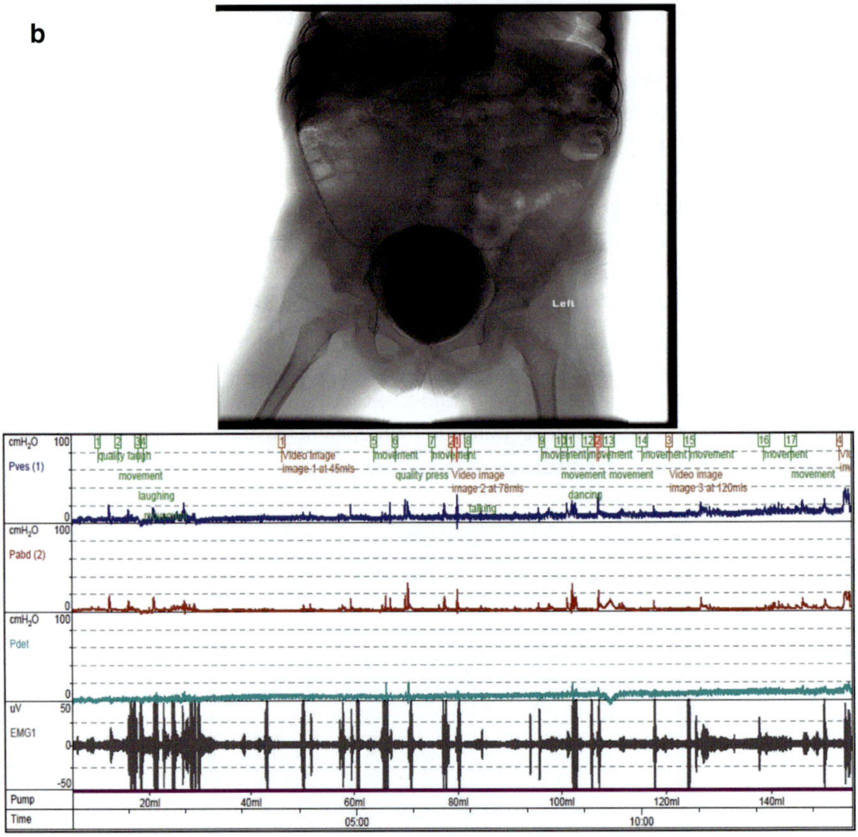

Fig. 3 (continued)

Table 2 Resolution rate of vesicoureteral reflux after bladder augmentation without ureteric reimplantation [6]

Authors	Year	N	Resolution Rate of VUR	Downgraded
Nasrallah and Aliabadi [22]	1991	14	86%	
Soylet et al. [29]	1994	15	97%	
Lopez-Pereira et al.	2001	16	81% high grade 50% low grade	12%
Simforoosh et al.	2002	130	85%	11%
Soygur et al.	2010	19	53%	
Helmy and Hafez	2013	32	Unilateral 82%, Bilateral 38%	
Zhang et al. [34]	2016	29	83%	10%
Chiba et al.	2022	19	85%	11%

resolution rate in all type of VUR, low and high pressure [32]. Hence both studies concluded recommending bladder augmentation with simultaneous ureteral reimplantation in children with VUR and NB.

(f) **Vesicostomy**

In a small, selected group of patients with neurogenic bladder and high grade VUR, in whom conservative management has failed, the formation of vesicostomy should be considered. It is a simple, well tolerated, easily reversible procedure which is highly effective in reversing upper tract dilatation. Vesicostomy is only a temporising measure for draining the bladder and has been shown to reverse or improve upper tract dilatation associated with neurogenic bladder in 86%–100% of patients [12, 18, 20]. It should only be considered when there is no evidence of uretero vesical junction obstruction to allow the upper urinary tract to drain safely and promptly. Indications for formation of vesicostomy include worsening dilatation of the urinary tract, impaired renal function, progression of renal scarring or recurrent urinary tract infections in a patient with neurogenic bladder who has failed conservative management (CIC + anticholinergic) and is not suitable for any other surgical intervention. Complications are encountered in 17–43% of patients, and include peristomal dermatitis followed by stomal stenosis, bladder prolapse, bladder calculi and recurrent urinary tract infections [20].

Conclusion

Vesicoureteral reflux in Neurogenic Bladder is a specific type of reflux that compared to primary VUR has a unique underlying pathophysiological mechanism, different outcome and its management is complex and still controversial. When VUR is present, resolves in 30–50% of children after commencing clean intermittent catheterization and anticholinergic medication within 2–3 years. In the remaining patients VUR is less likely to resolve spontaneously. Endoscopic Treatment or Total Endoscopic Treatment should be reserved to those children with NB who demonstrate a smooth bladder wall, good compliance and a bladder capacity >75% of the Expected Bladder Capacity on VUD. Bladder augmentation should be recommended for children with VUR in a poorly compliant trabeculated bladder. High pressure VUR is likely to resolve in 50–97% of these patients with an isolated bladder augmentation. Low pressure VUR detected in the early filling phase of the VUD in trabeculated poorly compliant bladders has a low-resolution rate and should be dealt with a ureteric reimplantation associated to a bladder augmentation. It is of greatest importance that the treatment of VUR in children with NB is discussed at multidisciplinary meetings and individualized according to the patients' symptoms, patients/parents' compliance, comorbidity, renal investigations (US, DMSA), renal function (estimated GFR) and most importantly video urodynamics.

References

1. Alqarni N, Alhazmi H, Alsowayan O, Eweda T, Neel KF. Total endoscopic and anal irrigation management approach to noncompliant neuropathic bladder and bowel in children: a long-term follow-up. Urol Ann. 2017;9(4):362–5.
2. Bauer SB. Neurogenic bladder: etiology and assessment. Pediatr Nephrol. 2008;23:541–51.
3. Belloli GP, Musi L, Campobasso P, Cattaneo A. Ureteral reimplantation in children with neurogenic bladder. J Pediatr Surg. 1979;14(2):119–27.
4. Cascio S, Doyle M, Mc Mahon O, Kelly G. Urinary tract imaging in infants with spina bifida: a selective approach to a baseline DMSA. J Pediatr Urol. 2021;17(3):396–e1.
5. Cascio S, O'Toole S, Lewis MA. Neurogenic bladder, Chapter 29. In: Puri P, editor. Pediatric surgery: pediatric urology. Springer Nature; 2023.
6. Chiba H, Kitta T, Higuchi M, Kusakabe N, Kon M, Nakamura M, Shinohara N. Ureteral reimplantation during augmentation cystoplasty is not needed for vesicoureteral reflux in patients with neurogenic bladder: a long-term retrospective study. BMC Urol. 2022;22(1):48.
7. Elder JS, Diaz M, Caldamone AA, Cendron M, Greenfield S, Hurwitz R, Kirsch A, Koyle MA, Pope J, Shapiro E. Endoscopic therapy for vesicoureteral reflux: a meta-analysis. I. Reflux resolution and urinary tract infection. J Urol. 2006;175(2):716–22.
8. Engel JD, Palmer LS, Cheng EY, Kaplan WE. Surgical versus endoscopic correction of vesicoureteral reflux in children with neurogenic bladder dysfunction. J Urol. 1997;157(6):2291–4.
9. Granata C, Buffa P, Di Rovasenda E, Mattioli G, Scarsi PL, Podesta E, Dodero P, Jasonni V. Treatment of vesico-ureteric reflux in children with neuropathic bladder: a comparison of surgical and endoscopic correction. J Pediatr Surg. 1999;34(12):1836–8.
10. Haferkamp A, Möhring K, Staehler G, Gerner HJ, Dörsam J. Long-term efficacy of subureteral collagen injection for endoscopic treatment of vesicoureteral reflux in neurogenic bladder cases. J Urol. 2000;163(1):274–7.
11. Helmy TE, Hafez AT. Vesicouretral reflux with neuropathic bladder: studying the resolution rate after ileocystoplasty. Urology. 2013;82(2):425–9.
12. Hutcheson JC, Cooper CS, Canningm DA, Zderic SA, Snyder HM III. The use of vesicostomy as permanent urinary diversion in the child with myelomeningocele. J Urol. 2001;166:2351–3.
13. Jeffs RD, Jonas P, Schillinger JF. Surgical correction of vesicoureteral reflux in children with neurogenic bladder. J Urol. 1976;115(4):449–51.
14. Kaplan WE, Firlit CF. Management of reflux in the myelodysplastic child. J Urol. 1983;129(6):1195–7.
15. Kondo A, Otani T. Correction of reflux with the ureteric crossover method clinical experience in 50 patients. Br J Urol. 1987;60(1):36–8.
16. O'Donnell BA, Puri P. Treatment of vesicoureteric reflux by endoscopic injection of Teflon. Br Med J (Clin Res Ed). 1984;289(6436):7–9.
17. O'Donnell BA, Puri P. Endoscopic correction of primary vesicoureteric reflux. Br J Urol. 1986;58(6):601–4.
18. Mandell J, Bauer SB, Colodny AH, Retik AB. Cutaneous vesicostomy in infancy. J Urol. 1981;126:92–3.
19. Merlini E, Beseghi U, De Castro R, Perlasca E, Podesta E, Riccipetitoni G. Treatment of vesicoureteric reflux in the neurogenic bladder. Br J Urol. 1993;72(6):969–71.
20. Morrisroe SN, O'Connor RC, Nanigian DK, et al. Vesicostomy revisited: the best treatment for the hostile bladder in the myelodysplastic children. Br J Urol. 2005;96:397–400.
21. Mosiello G, Salsano ML, Pascali MP, Camanni D, De Gennaro M. A minimally invasive approach in the treatment of vesicoureteral reflux in neurogenic bladder in children. Eur Urol. 2009;55(1):254–6.
22. Nasrallah PF, Aliabadi HA. Bladder augmentation in patients with neurogenic bladder and vesicoureteral reflux. J Urol. 1991;146(2):563–6.
23. Neel KF, Salem M, Soliman S. Total endoscopic management (TEM approach) of children with non-compliant neuropathic bladder: a preliminary report. J Pediatr Urol. 2008;4(2):124–6.

24. Pereira PL, Urrutia MM, Romera RL, Jaureguizar E. Should we treat vesicoureteral reflux in patients who simultaneously undergo bladder augmentation for neuropathic bladder? J Urol. 2001;165(6):2259–61.
25. Polackwich AS, Skoog SJ, Austin JC. Long-term followup after endoscopic treatment of vesicoureteral reflux with dextranomer/hyaluronic acid copolymer in patients with neurogenic bladder. J Urol. 2012;188(4):1511–5.
26. Sidi AA, Peng W, Gonzalez R. Vesicoureteral reflux in children with myelodysplasia: natural history and results of treatment. J Urol. 1986;136(1):329–31.
27. Simforoosh N, Tabibi A, Basiri A, Noorbala MH, Danesh AD, Ijadi A. Is ureteral reimplantation necessary during augmentation cystoplasty in patients with neurogenic bladder and vesicoureteral reflux? J Urol. 2002;168(4):1439–41.
28. Soygur T, Burgu B, Zümrütbas A, Süer E. The need for ureteric re-implantation during augmentation cystoplasty: video-urodynamic evaluation. BJU Int. 2010;105(4):530–2.
29. Soylet Y, Emir H, Ilce Z, Yesildag E, Buyukunal SN, Danismend N. Quo vadis? Ureteric reimplantation or ignoring reflux during augmentation cystoplasty. BJU Int. 2004;94(3):379–80.
30. Vandersteen DR, Routh JC, Kirsch AJ, Scherz HC, Ritchey ML, Shapiro E, Wolpert JJ, Pfefferle H, Reinberg Y. Postoperative ureteral obstruction after subureteral injection of dextranomer/hyaluronic acid copolymer. J Urol. 2006;176(4):1593–5.
31. Wang JB, Liu CS, Tsai SL, Wei CF, Chin TW. Augmentation cystoplasty and simultaneous ureteral reimplantation reduce high-grade vesicoureteral reflux in children with neurogenic bladder. J Chin Med Assoc. 2011;74(7):294–7.
32. Wang Z, Liao L. Effectiveness and complications of augmentation cystoplasty with or without nonrefluxing ureteral reimplantation in patients with bladder dysfunction: a single center 11-year experience. J Urol. 2018;199(1):200–5.
33. Wu CQ, Franco I. Management of vesicoureteral reflux in neurogenic bladder. Investig Clin Urol. 2017;58(Suppl 1):S54–8.
34. Zhang HC, Yang J, Ye X, Hu HF. Augmentation enterocystoplasty without reimplantation for patients with neurogenic bladder and vesicoureteral reflux. Kaohsiung J Med Sci. 2016;32(6):323–6.

Vesicoureteral Reflux Secondary to Posterior Urethral Valves

Armando Lorenzo and Priyank Yadav

Abstract Vesicoureteral reflux (VUR) is commonly seen in patients with posterior urethral valves (PUV). The high intravesical pressures and bladder dysfunction associated with PUV predispose these patients to secondary VUR. Early detection through investigations like voiding cystourethrography, radionuclide cystography, and renal cortical scintigraphy is crucial for timely intervention and prevention of complications such as recurrent urinary tract infections, pyelonephritis, renal scarring, and deterioration of renal function. Management strategies involve a multidisciplinary approach, including antibiotic prophylaxis, urotherapy, clean intermittent catheterization, and surgical options like endoscopic injection or ureteral reimplantation. Bladder dysfunction plays a pivotal role in influencing clinical outcomes and treatment success. Urodynamic studies, combined with fluoroscopy, provide valuable insights into bladder function and guide tailored treatment decisions. Further research is needed to identify predictive factors, evaluate long-term outcomes, and explore innovative diagnostic and therapeutic approaches for optimizing the management of VUR in PUV patients.

Keywords Bladder dysfunction · Clean intermittent catheterization · Posterior urethral valves · Urodynamics · Vesicoureteral reflux

A. Lorenzo (✉)
Division of Urology, The Hospital for Sick Children, University of Toronto, Toronto, ON, Canada
e-mail: armando.lorenzo@sickkids.ca

P. Yadav
Department of Urology and Renal Transplantation, Sanjay Gandhi Postgraduate Institute of Medical Sciences, Lucknow, India

P. Puri, A. Yamataka (eds.), *Vesicoureteral Reflux*,
https://doi.org/10.1007/978-3-031-95091-9_25

Introduction

Vesicoureteral reflux (VUR) is a condition characterized by the abnormal flow of urine from the bladder back into the ureters and potentially up to the kidneys. The prevalence of VUR in general population is 1–2 per 100 [1]. Untreated VUR can lead to progressive deterioration of renal function, leading to chronic kidney disease (CKD) and end stage renal disease (ESRD), particularly in bilateral cases or in patients with a solitary kidney. VUR can be primary (due to an incompetent uretero-vesical junction) or secondary (due to functional or anatomical lower urinary tract obstruction leading to high intravesical pressure overwhelming the ureterovesical junction). Posterior urethral valves (PUV) are the leading cause of lower urinary tract obstruction in the male babies and have a wide range of presentation ranging from asymptomatic antenatal hydronephrosis and/or megacystis to lower urinary tract symptoms and/or urinary tract infection (UTI) and renal deterioration. Around one third of the patients with PUV develop ESRD [2].

Understanding VUR in patients with PUV is crucial due to the high prevalence of VUR in this population. Studies have shown that nearly 40%–70% of patients with PUV also have VUR, which significantly increases the risk of renal damage and long-term complications [3–5]. The incidence of unilateral reflux is similar to bilateral reflux but the latter is associated with a greater incidence of End Stage Kidney Disease [6]. Therefore, accurate diagnosis and appropriate management of VUR in PUV patients are essential to optimize outcomes and prevent renal deterioration.

This chapter will provide a comprehensive guide on VUR in patients with PUV, including the pathophysiology, clinical presentation, diagnosis, and management strategies in this specific patient population. Understanding and management of VUR in PUV patients is critical for improving patient outcomes and prevent long-term renal complications.

Pathophysiology of VUR in Patients with PUV

VUR in patients with PUV is typically secondary in nature and occurs due to a combination of different pathophysiological factors (Fig. 1). The main underlying feature is obstruction at the bladder outlet which leads to high intravesical pressure and incomplete bladder emptying. The bladder tries to overcome this obstruction by increasing its contractility resulting in detrusor hypertrophy. Sustained high bladder pressures can also overwhelm the ureterovesical junction leading to retrograde flow of urine from bladder to ureters. In the long term, bladder remodelling takes place which is associated with deposition of collagen in the bladder wall resulting in worsening of bladder compliance and capacity. Detrusor hypertrophy along with collagen deposition and bladder remodelling gives such bladder its typical

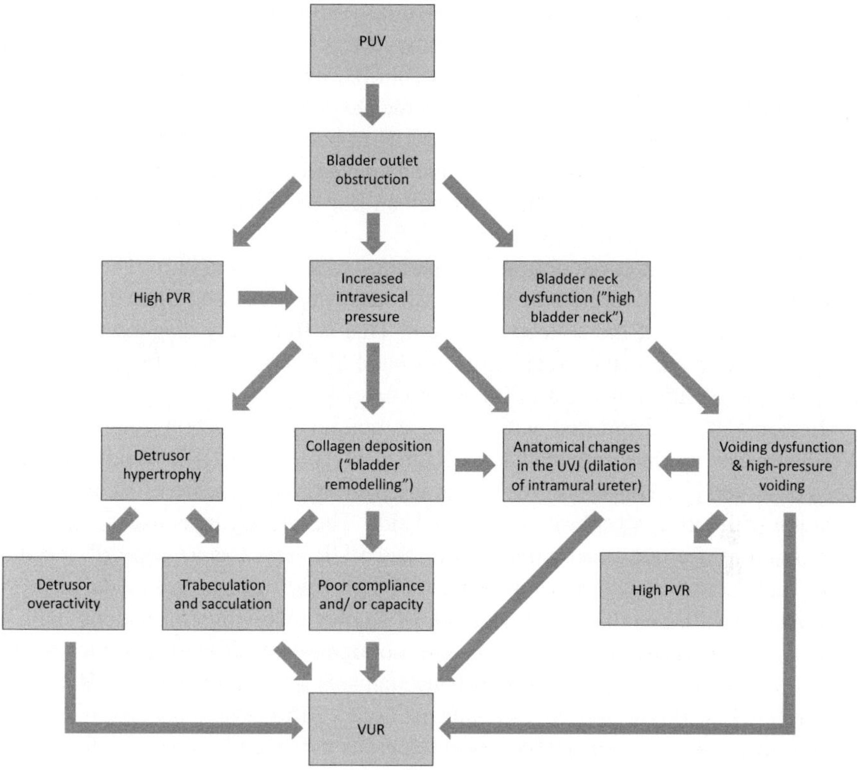

Fig. 1 Schematic showing pathophysiological changes in patients with PUV leading to VUR

trabeculated appearance. These anatomical changes along with detrusor overactivity predispose the patient to VUR.

Another factor that contributes to high intravesical pressure particularly during voiding is bladder neck dysfunction that frequently accompanies PUV and may represent another consequence of bladder outlet obstruction. These bladder neck typically appear "high" on cystoscopy and lead to voiding dysfunction by failing to relax completely during micturition [7]. Such high voiding pressure during voiding also leads to VUR. The average incidence of voiding dysfunction after PUV ablation is 21% [8].

Clinical Features

VUR in patients with PUV can present with a variety of symptoms and signs. These can include UTIs, pyelonephritis, renal scarring, hydronephrosis, and even renal failure. UTIs are a common presentation in patients with VUR and occur due to a combination of incomplete bladder emptying and retrograde flow of infected urine from the bladder into the ureters and potentially up to the kidneys. Symptoms of UTIs can include fever, dysuria, frequency, urgency, and fowl smelling urine. In severe cases, UTIs can progress to pyelonephritis, which is characterized by fever, chills, flank pain, and systemic symptoms such as malaise and fatigue. Renal scarring is another potential consequence of VUR in patients with PUV. The reflux of infected urine can lead to inflammation and damage to the renal parenchyma, resulting in scar tissue formation. This scarring can impair kidney function and predispose to renal failure in the long term.

Hydronephrosis is commonly seen in patients with VUR and PUV. The backflow of urine from the bladder into the ureters can cause pressure build-up in the kidneys, leading to dilation of the collecting system. This is frequently diagnosed incidentally such as on antenatal screening or postnatal ultrasound done after first UTI or during the evaluation of a child with abdominal pain.

In some boys diagnosed with PUV, a unique phenomenon referred to as Vesicoureteral Reflux and Ipsilateral Kidney Dysplasia (VURD syndrome) has been observed [9]. This syndrome is characterized by the presence of VUR in combination with kidney dysplasia on the same side. The underlying concept is that this combination of a non-functioning kidney and VUR serves as a "pop-off" mechanism, which effectively reduces the impact of high voiding pressures on the healthy, contralateral kidney [10]. In a review of 15 studies involving 185 patients with a median follow-up of 6.8 years, there was no significant difference in the risk of ESRD between patients with pop-off mechanisms and those without (RR 0.34, $p = 0.07$) [11]. While pop-off mechanisms appeared to reduce the risk of kidney insufficiency (RR 0.57, $p = 0.04$), this effect was not consistent across all studies, and the certainty of the evidence was low.

The role of "pop-off" mechanism in preventing pressure induced bladder dysfunction is also not well understood. However, recent data suggests that the presence of VURD syndrome may not significantly alter long-term bladder outcomes, voiding efficiency, or the rates of CIC in patients with PUV [12]. High-grade VUR and the "pop-off" mechanism associated with VURD syndrome were associated with a similar time to initiation of CIC in this study.

Investigations and Diagnosis

Early detection and diagnosis of VUR in patients with PUV are crucial for several reasons. Firstly, prompt identification allows for timely intervention and management to prevent complications such as recurrent UTIs, pyelonephritis, renal scarring, and renal failure. Secondly, early diagnosis enables the implementation of preventive measures like antibiotic prophylaxis to minimize the risk of complications. Additionally, close monitoring of renal function and imaging studies can be initiated to assess the severity of VUR and guide treatment decisions. Early detection allows for appropriate counselling and education of patients and their families regarding the condition. This can help them understand the importance of compliance with treatment and follow-up recommendations, as well as recognize signs and symptoms that may indicate worsening or complications of VUR. Following investigations are useful in the evaluation of patients with PUV who may have VUR:

1. Voiding cystourethrography (VCUG)

VCUG is considered the gold standard for the diagnosis of VUR. This procedure involves the instillation of contrast material into the bladder via a catheter, followed by fluoroscopic imaging during voiding. VCUG is the first investigation after ultrasound for suspected PUV and the standard VCUG film contains the following views: scout, early filling, oblique voiding images to assess UVJ, and postvoid images. The diagnosis of PUV as well as VUR can be made at the same time on a VCUG (Fig. 2). The retrograde flow of contrast material into the ureters and kidneys indicates the presence of VUR which is graded from 1 to 5 as proposed by the International Reflux Study (IRS) [13]. However, this grading system is not without limitations. Firstly, there is lack of consensus regarding the clinical significance and long-term implications of different VUR grades. The IRS grading system primarily focuses on anatomical findings and does not adequately capture the functional consequences of VUR. As a result, there is a need for a classification system that incorporates both anatomical and functional parameters to better predict outcomes and guide management decisions.

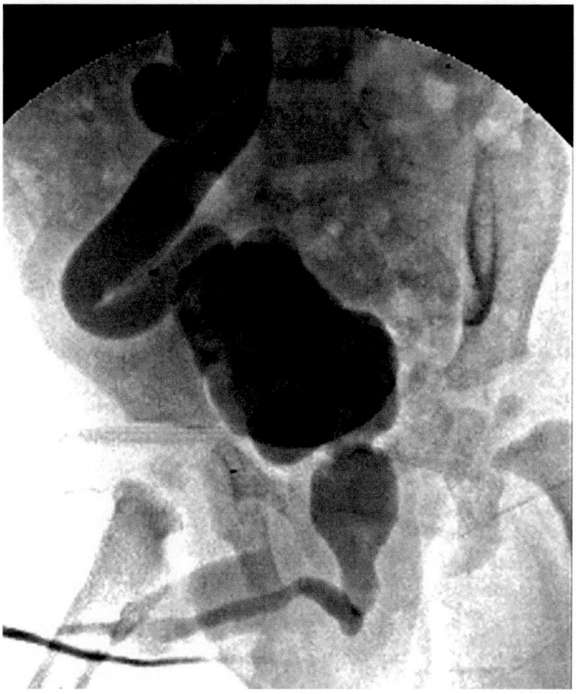

Fig. 2 VCUG of a 2-month-old boy with PUV and unilateral VUR

2. Radionuclide cystography (RNC)

RNC is an alternative imaging modality for the evaluation of VUR. This procedure involves the injection of a radioactive tracer into the bladder, followed by imaging with a gamma camera during voiding. The tracer is excreted in the urine, allowing visualization of any reflux into the ureters and kidneys. It can detect even subtle cases of reflux and typically involves a 3-point grading system. It can reveal delayed voiding and the accumulation of tracer in the renal collecting system after voiding, suggesting possible ureteral blockage. Additionally, the procedure allows for the measurement of bladder volumes and pressures. However, it provides very limited anatomical detail compared to VCUG and thus not preferred for evaluation of PUV related VCUG.

3. Renal Cortical Scintigraphy

It uses 99mTc–dimercaptosuccinic acid (DMSA) and generates functional images of the renal cortex (Fig. 3). It does not visualize the ureters or the bladder. It is used to assess the gross morphology of the renal cortex, especially in the context of scarring and helps in identifying renal scars caused by recurrent infections or other underlying conditions like renal dysplasia. Imaging during acute pyelonephritis due to VUR will reveal cortical defect which will be indistinguishable from renal scar and a follow up scan after around 6 months is necessary to diagnose renal scar. It also yields the percentage function of the kidney with VUR.

4. Urodynamic studies: Bladder dysfunction plays a crucial role in the context of VUR associated with PUV, significantly impacting the clinical course and outcomes of surgical interventions like ureteric reimplantation. Hypertrophy of the bladder wall, a consequence of PUV, becomes evident during the filling phase, leading to reduced compliance, often accompanied by detrusor overactivity (Fig. 4). In the voiding phase, high detrusor pressures can signal the presence of residual valves, a raised bladder neck, or sphincter contraction due to coexisting

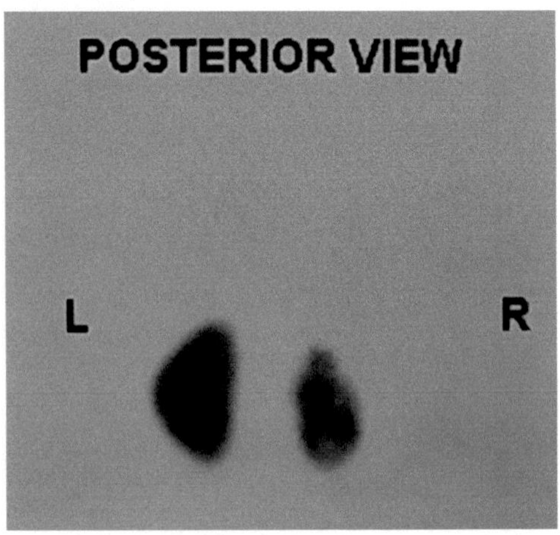

Fig. 3 DMSA of patient in Fig. 2 showing small right kidney with photopenic areas suggestive of renal scars

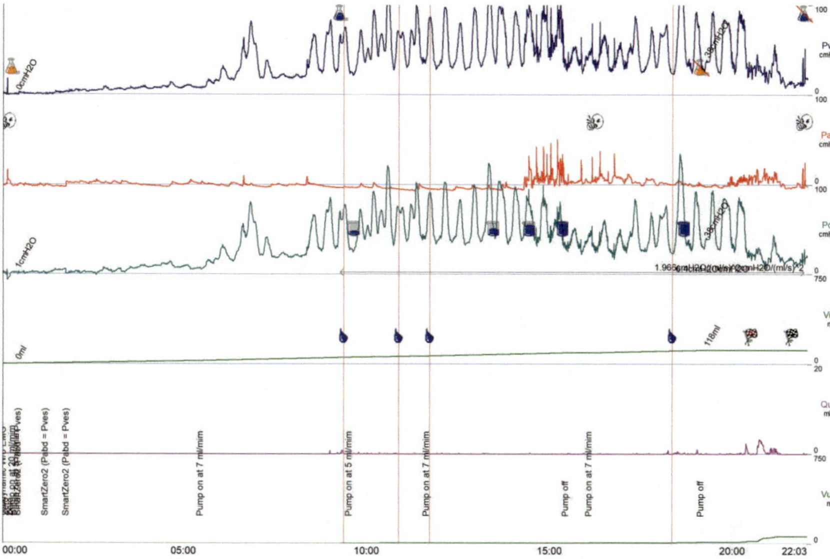

Fig. 4 Urodynamic study showing detrusor overactivity with leak in a patient with PUV

dysfunctional voiding. Conversely, bladder pressures may be low during voiding in case of myogenic failure. When VUR is present, interpreting urodynamic data benefits from combining it with fluoroscopy (videourodynamics), which can identify the bladder volume at which VUR first occurs. This is crucial as VUR can falsely inflate bladder compliance. Although VUR-related factors may affect urodynamic measurements, boys with reflux continue to present with uniform abnormal urodynamic results [14]. Treating persistent bladder outlet obstructions, lowering intravesical pressures through anticholinergic treatment, and addressing underlying bladder dysfunction constitute the core of the management plan for patients with PUV. Urodynamic studies serve as a vital tool in guiding this comprehensive approach.

Management Strategies for VUR in Patients with PUV

The management of VUR in patients with PUV involves both non-surgical and surgical options, which are chosen based on the severity of VUR, the presence of associated renal abnormalities, and individual patient factors. In infancy, the initial surgical management of PUV is guided by individualized response to bladder decompression measured by improvement in serum creatinine levels and the degree of hydroureteronephrosis [15].

Once valve fulguration/ablation has been performed and there is no anatomical lower urinary tract obstruction, the indications of treatment of VUR are no different in patients with PUV than those without PUV. VUR is typically managed conservatively and surgery, if deemed necessary, involves urinary diversion for recurrent UTIs or worsening renal function. Patients with functional lower urinary tract obstruction (dysfunctional voiding or bowel and bladder dysfunction) will require Urotherapy, pelvic floor exercises and CIC as per usual indications. For persistent hydronephrosis in a stable patient, selective alpha blockers can be initiated [15]. After valve ablation, rates of resolution of VUR vary between 25% to around 80% and mostly early after ablation, typically within 6 months [3, 4], although resolution can also occur later, up to 15 years of age [5]. Lower grades of reflux resolve sooner.

A. Non-surgical management options

1. Antibiotic prophylaxis: The goal of antibiotic prophylaxis is to prevent UTIs in patients with VUR and low-dose, long-term antibiotics, such as trimethoprim-sulfamethoxazole or nitrofurantoin, are often prescribed to reduce the risk of UTIs. Patients with PUV have a greater risk of febrile UTIs compared to the normal population [16, 17]. Data from the CIRCUP randomized controlled trial shows that high grade VUR is associated with a higher chance of febrile UTI which decreases after 9 months of age [17, 18]. EAU-ESPU guidelines recommend use of antibiotic prophylaxis in boys with PUV and high grade VUR [19]. Circumcision decreases the risk of febrile UTI in these patients [18].
2. Urotherapy: Non-surgical management also involves implementing voiding and behavioral modifications to reduce the risk of UTIs and improve bladder emptying. Timed voiding, where the patient is encouraged to empty their bladder at regular intervals, can help prevent urine stagnation and reduce the likelihood of reflux. Double voiding, where the patient empties their bladder twice during each visit to the bathroom, can also be effective in promoting complete bladder emptying [6]. Additionally, ensuring adequate fluid intake can help maintain good hydration and reduce the risk of UTIs, especially with concomitant timed and regular voiding.
3. Alpha blockers: Selective alpha blockers like Terazosin and Tamsulosin have been used for improving voiding efficiency in patients with PUV. They relax the smooth muscles at the trigone and proximal urethra. By decreasing the outlet resistance, they decrease the post void residual urine in the bladder by 85%–88% and improve hydronephrosis [20, 21]. Alpha blockers may also improve VUR although their primary indication for use is to improve bladder emptying [6].
4. Anticholinergics: Anticholinergics reduce detrusor overactivity and improve bladder compliance in patients with PUV by reducing stretch induced smooth muscle proliferation collagen deposition [22]. They are first line drugs prescribed to improve functional bladder capacity and reduce incontinence episodes. They also decrease the intravesical pressure and help in reducing secondary VUR, bringing about resolution in up to 50% [23]. However, the patients who progress to myogenic failure may worsen with anticholinergics and will require their cessation along with initiation of CIC [6].

5. Clean intermittent catheterization (CIC): Approximately one-third of patients who undergo PUV ablation continue to experience bladder dysfunction that necessitates ongoing intervention. This residual bladder dysfunction can manifest as various issues, including urinary retention, urinary incontinence, or an inability to empty the bladder effectively. In such cases, the use of CIC becomes indispensable [6]. Bilateral VUR is associated with rapid deterioration of renal function in PUV. CIC not only facilitates bladder emptying when the normal mechanism is compromised but also contributes to improving bladder dysfunction thereby reducing the impact of VUR on the kidneys. Limited data is available regarding the incidence of CIC in patients with PUV. A recent multi-institutional study reported that 13%–26% of the patients with PUV require CIC [24]. In boys with PUV, CIC also reduces the need for bladder augmentation [24].

B. Surgical management options

1. Endoscopic treatment: Endoscopic injection of bulking agents, such as Dextranomer/hyaluronic acid copolymer, is a minimally invasive surgical option for correcting VUR. This procedure involves injecting the bulking agent into the submucosal tissue at the ureterovesical junction, creating a bulge that acts as a valve to prevent reflux (Fig. 5). Endoscopic injection is the preferred technique for management of VUR in patients with PUV especially for bilateral cases as overzealous treatment with ureteric reimplantation can aggravate myogenic failure [25]. Endoscopic injections can be performed on a day care basis with minimal morbidity and can be repeated if necessary. Success rate is high, around 86% for single injection and reaches up to 94% after three sessions but is lower compared to that for patients with primary VUR [25, 26].

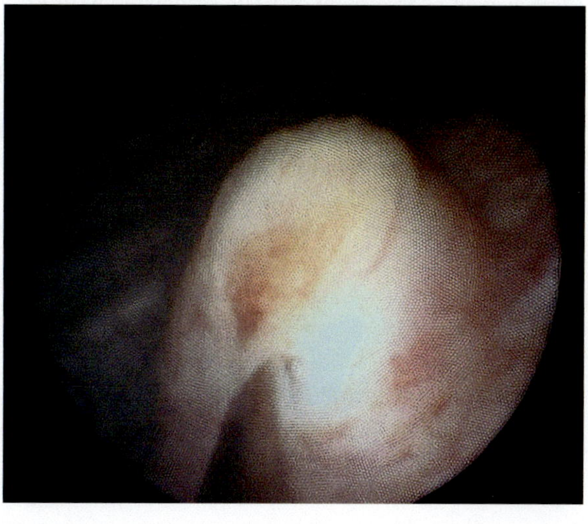

Fig. 5 Endoscopic correction of VUR: Dextranomer/hyaluronic acid copolymer injection creating a bulge to prevent reflux

2. Open/laparoscopic/robotic surgical procedures: Ureteral reimplantation is a well-established surgical procedure for correcting VUR. In this procedure, the ureter is repositioned in the bladder at a different angle to create an anti-reflux mechanism with or without detachment from the native opening. Success rate is high, usually >95% [25, 27]. Open surgical procedures are typically reserved for higher-grade VUR (grades IV-V) or cases where endoscopic techniques have failed. However, they have a higher incidence of bladder spasms [28]. Laparoscopic and robotic-assisted techniques offer advantages such as reduced postoperative pain, shorter hospital stays, and faster recovery compared to open surgery [27]. Nevertheless, reimplantation of ureters in the bladder of a boy with PUV is inherently associated with more complications such as strictures and persistent reflux owing to thick-walled bladder and dilated (and/or tortuous) ureters [29, 30].

Future Directions

An essential area for future research in the management of VUR associated with PUV is the identification of predictive factors. Understanding these factors holds significant importance as they can guide treatment decisions and enhance patient outcomes. Parameters such as age, VUR severity, the presence of renal scarring, and the extent of bladder dysfunction need thorough examination to discern their impact on treatment success. By elucidating these predictive factors, clinicians can tailor their management strategies more precisely, ensuring the best possible care for PUV patients with VUR.

Furthermore, exploring the long-term effects of various surgical techniques applied to PUV patients is another crucial avenue of research. A comprehensive study is necessary to assess the durability of the techniques for primary treatment of PUV as well as treatment of VUR associated with PUV and their impact on patient outcomes. Comparing endoscopic injection techniques with open ureteral reimplantation can provide valuable insights into the optimal approach to managing VUR in this specific patient population. Additionally, the field may benefit from the exploration of innovative diagnostic and therapeutic approaches, leveraging advances in imaging and minimally invasive interventions to further enhance VUR management in the context of PUV.

Conclusion

In conclusion, the prevalence of VUR in PUV patients is substantial, emphasizing the need for accurate diagnosis and effective management to prevent renal complications. The optimal management approach for VUR in PUV patients remains a topic of debate, and individualized decision-making is crucial. Understanding the pathophysiology, clinical presentation, and diagnostic methods related to VUR in PUV patients is vital for improving patient outcomes. Bladder dysfunction, often associated with PUV, plays a pivotal role in influencing clinical outcomes, impacting treatment decisions and the success of surgical interventions. Urodynamic studies, combined with fluoroscopy when necessary, serve as essential tools for comprehensively managing VUR in this context, allowing for tailored treatment strategies. Further research is needed to evaluate the long-term outcomes, cost-effectiveness, and safety of different surgical techniques and emerging technologies.

References

1. Sargent MA. What is the normal prevalence of vesicoureteral reflux? Pediatr Radiol. 2000;30(9):587–93. https://doi.org/10.1007/s002470000263.
2. Heikkilä J, Holmberg C, Kyllönen L, Rintala R, Taskinen S. Long-term risk of end stage renal disease in patients with posterior urethral valves. J Urol. 2011;186(6):2392–6. https://doi.org/10.1016/j.juro.2011.07.109.
3. Priti K, Rao KLN, Menon P, Singh N, Mittal BR, Bhattacharya A, Mitra SK. Posterior urethral valves: incidence and progress of vesicoureteric reflux after primary fulguration. Pediatr Surg Int. 2004;20(2):136–9. https://doi.org/10.1007/s00383-003-1107-1.
4. Hassan JM, Pope JC 4th, Brock JW 3rd, Adams MC. Vesicoureteral reflux in patients with posterior urethral valves. J Urol. 2003;170(4 Pt 2):1677–80. discussion 1680. https://doi.org/10.1097/01.ju.0000087491.16553.0d.
5. Heikkilä J, Rintala R, Taskinen S. Vesicoureteral reflux in conjunction with posterior urethral valves. J Urol. 2009;182(4):1555–60. https://doi.org/10.1016/j.juro.2009.06.057.
6. Sharma S, Joshi M, Gupta DK, Abraham M, Mathur P, Mahajan JK, et al. Consensus on the management of posterior urethral valves from antenatal period to puberty. J Indian Assoc Pediatr Surg. 2019;24(1):4–14. https://doi.org/10.4103/jiaps.JIAPS_148_18.
7. Androulakakis PA, Karamanolakis DK, Tsahouridis G, Stefanidis AA, Palaeodimos I. Myogenic bladder decompensation in boys with a history of posterior urethral valves is caused by secondary bladder neck obstruction? BJU Int. 2005;96(1):140–3. https://doi.org/10.1111/j.1464-410X.2005.05583.x.
8. Peters CA, Bauer SB. Evaluation and management of urinary incontinence after surgery for posterior urethral valves. Urol Clin North Am. 1990;17(2):379–87.
9. Hoover DL, Duckett JW Jr. Posterior urethral valves, unilateral reflux and renal dysplasia: a syndrome. J Urol. 1982;128(5):994–7. https://doi.org/10.1016/s0022-5347(17)53313-3.
10. Donnelly LF, Gylys-Morin VM, Wacksman J, Gelfand MJ. Unilateral vesicoureteral reflux: association with protected renal function in patients with posterior urethral valves. AJR Am J Roentgenol. 1997;168(3):823–6. https://doi.org/10.2214/ajr.168.3.10.
11. Khondker A, Kim K, Najafabadi BT, Nguyen D-D, Kim JK, Yadav P, et al. Posterior urethral valves, pressure pop-offs, and kidney function: systematic review and meta-analysis. World J Urol. 2023;41(7):1803–11. https://doi.org/10.1007/s00345-023-04451-7.
12. Khondker A, Yadav P, Kim JK, Chua ME, Brownrigg N, Richter J, et al. Does VURD syndrome impact voiding efficiency in posterior urethral valves? J Pediatr Urol. 2023;19(4):424.e1–7. https://doi.org/10.1016/j.jpurol.2023.03.022.
13. Lebowitz RL, Olbing H, Parkkulainen KV, Smellie JM, Tamminen-Möbius TE. International system of radiographic grading of vesicoureteric reflux. International reflux study in children. Pediatr Radiol. 1985;15(2):105–9. https://doi.org/10.1007/bf02388714.

14. Kim YH, Horowitz M, Combs AJ, Nitti VW, Borer J, Glassberg KI. Management of posterior urethral valves on the basis of urodynamic findings. J Urol. 1997;158(3 Pt 2):1011–6. https://doi.org/10.1097/00005392-199709000-00085.
15. Rickard M, Lorenzo AJ, Richter J, Brownrigg N, Kim JK, Chua M, et al. Implementation of a standardized clinical pathway in a dedicated posterior urethral valves clinic: short-term outcomes. Pediatr Nephrol. 2023;38(11):3735–44. https://doi.org/10.1007/s00467-023-06040-7.
16. Hutton KAR. Management of posterior urethral valves. Curr Paediatr. 2004;14(7):568–75.
17. Harper L, Botto N, Peycelon M, Michel J-L, Leclair M-D, Garnier S, et al. Risk factors for febrile urinary tract infection in boys with posterior urethral valves. Front Pediatr. 2022;10:971662. https://doi.org/10.3389/fped.2022.971662.
18. Harper L, Blanc T, Peycelon M, Michel JL, Leclair MD, Garnier S, et al. Circumcision and risk of febrile urinary tract infection in boys with posterior urethral valves: result of the CIRCUP randomized trial. Eur Urol. 2022;81(1):64–72. https://doi.org/10.1016/j.eururo.2021.08.024.
19. EAU Guidelines. Edn. presented at the EAU Annual Congress Amsterdam 2022. ISBN 978-94-92671-16-5.
20. Cain MP, Wu SD, Austin PF, Herndon CDA, Rink RC. Alpha blocker therapy for children with dysfunctional voiding and urinary retention. J Urol. 2003;170(4 Pt 2):1514–5. discussion 1516–7. https://doi.org/10.1097/01.ju.0000085961.27403.4a.
21. Abraham MK, Nasir ARA, Sudarsanan B, Puzhankara R, Kedari PM, Unnithan GR, et al. Role of alpha adrenergic blocker in the management of posterior urethral valves. Pediatr Surg Int. 2009;25(12):1113–5. https://doi.org/10.1007/s00383-009-2469-9.
22. Scheepe JR, de Jong BWD, Wolffenbuttel KP, Arentshorst ME, Lodder P, Kok DJ. The effect of oxybutynin on structural changes of the obstructed Guinea pig bladder. J Urol. 2007;178(4 Pt 2):1807–12. https://doi.org/10.1016/j.juro.2007.03.187.
23. Norris JJ, Raj JP, Thomas TT, Maleperambil TT, Shubha AM. Effects of oxybutynin in children with posterior urethral valves post fulguration: report in a select cohort of children. J Family Med Prim Care. 2021;10(10):3706–11. https://doi.org/10.4103/jfmpc.jfmpc_2554_20.
24. Yadav P, Rickard M, Weaver J, Chua M, Kim JK, Khondker A, et al. Pre-versus postnatal presentation of posterior urethral valves: a multi-institutional experience. BJU Int. 2022;130(3):350–6. https://doi.org/10.1111/bju.15708.
25. Tourchi A, Kajbafzadeh A-M, Aryan Z, Ebadi M. The management of vesicoureteral reflux in the setting of posterior urethral valve with emphasis on bladder function and renal outcome: a single center cohort study. Urology. 2014;83(1):199–205. https://doi.org/10.1016/j.urology.2013.07.033.
26. Bajpai M, Verma A, Panda SS. Endoscopic treatment of vesico-ureteral reflux: experience of 99 ureteric moieties. J Indian Assoc Pediatr Surg. 2013;18(4):133–5. https://doi.org/10.4103/0971-9261.121112.
27. Smith RP, Oliver JL, Peters CA. Pediatric robotic extravesical ureteral reimplantation: comparison with open surgery. J Urol. 2011;185(5):1876–81. https://doi.org/10.1016/j.juro.2010.12.072.
28. Marchini GS, Hong YK, Minnillo BJ, Diamond DA, Houck CS, Meier PM, et al. Robotic assisted laparoscopic ureteral reimplantation in children: case matched comparative study with open surgical approach. J Urol. 2011;185(5):1870–5. https://doi.org/10.1016/j.juro.2010.12.069.
29. Atwell JD. Posterior urethral valves in the British Isles: a multicenter B.A.P.S. review. J Pediatr Surg. 1983;18(1):70–4. https://doi.org/10.1016/s0022-3468(83)80276-0.
30. Coleman JW, McGovern JH. Ureterovesical reimplantation in children. Surgical results in 491 children. Urology. 1978;12(5):514–8. https://doi.org/10.1016/0090-4295(78)90463-6.

Parental Preferences in the Management of Vesicoureteral Reflux

Nicola Capozza and Ermelinda Mele

Abstract Pediatricians, pediatric nephrologists, pediatric surgeons, and pediatric urologists often have different approaches, but parental preferences are rarely considered when discussing the management of vesicoureteral reflux (VUR). The main goal of treating VUR is prevention of recurrent febrile urinary tract infections (UTIs) and renal scarring. The choice of management of VUR is dependent on patient age, gender, grade of VUR, bilaterality, clinical course, presence of renal scars, ipsilateral renal function, bladder function, patient compliance, adverse effects of antibacterial therapy and anti-microbial resistance. Definitive endoscopic or surgical correction is the preferred treatment in patients with recurrent febrile UTIs, persistent high-grade VUR, non-compliance with continuous antibiotic prophylaxis and new renal scarring. Data from numerous studies have confirmed the long-term safety and efficacy of endoscopic treatment and therefore endoscopic correction is currently the first-line treatment for children with grade III–V primary VUR in many institutions worldwide because of the simplicity of the day care procedure. In this chapter we discuss the parental preferences which have a major role in the selection of endoscopic treatment over the traditional methods of continuous antibiotic prophylaxis or ureteral reimplantation. Parental preferences play a critical role in determining the most suitable approach, as parents weigh the risks, benefits, and potential impacts of each option on their child's health and well-being. In recent years, social media has become an influential platform in healthcare decision-making, significantly shaping how parents perceive and choose management options for their children with vesicoureteral reflux (VUR). While it offers opportunities for information-sharing and support, it also introduces challenges related to misinformation and biased perspectives. By prioritizing clear communication, empathy, and shared decision-making, healthcare providers can support parents in selecting the most appropriate treatment option, ensuring both the child's well-being and the family's peace of mind.

N. Capozza (✉)
Department of Surgery, Luigi Maria Monti Foundation, Rome, Italy

E. Mele
Department of Pediatric Urology, Bambino Gesù Children's Hospital, Rome, Italy

P. Puri, A. Yamataka (eds.), *Vesicoureteral Reflux*,
https://doi.org/10.1007/978-3-031-95091-9_26

Keywords Vesicoureteral reflux · Endoscopic treatment · Parental preference · Antibiotic prophylaxis · Ureteral reimplantation

Introduction

Vesicoureteral reflux (VUR) is the main cause of urinary tract infections in children and represents a risk for permanent kidney damage, arterial hypertension and chronic renal failure in the most severe cases. Despite the interest of clinicians and researchers from all over the world, the enormous amount of data and the attempts to express shared guidelines, vesicoureteral reflux is still the subject of controversy.

Pediatricians, pediatric surgeons, and pediatric urologists often have different approaches, but parental preferences are rarely considered when discussing the management of vesicoureteral reflux. Of course, the choice of VUR management is influenced by age, gender, degree of reflux, presence of nephropathy, and symptoms. In the last two decades, attention has focused on this last aspect, which is prevalent over the others; In the presence of reflux "complicated" by febrile urinary infections, an "active" management is recommended, rather than watchful waiting, associated with antibiotic prophylaxis or occasional antibiotic treatment.

Active treatment of vesicoureteral reflux can be surgical or endoscopic; according to some authors there would be no difference between open and endoscopic surgery, but for others there is no doubt that these are non-equivalent options, especially in terms of invasiveness and according to some, efficacy [1–3]. Evidently, the invasiveness, efficacy, advantages and disadvantages of each option are the crucial elements of discussion when they are presented to the family of the child with vesicoureteral reflux.

The family must receive as much information as possible, with the obvious limitations of the objectivity of the specialist who takes care of the child with vesicoureteral reflux. Often the guidance of the specialist ends up greatly influencing the opinion of the parents. These suggestions are not unfounded, as they depend on the child's clinical situation; no one would propose a form of surgery for asymptomatic and low-grade reflux, found more or less by chance; on the other hand, it might be imprudent to suggest simple observation, with occasional antibiotic treatment, in an infant with reflux complicated by febrile urinary tract infections.

These are two situations at the extremes of a range and recommendations must be expressed, but in most cases these are patients in which the various options can be considered equivalent. In these cases our opinion has always been that parents can and should be involved in the management decision. Once parents, properly informed about the various options, express a preference, it must be considered and possibly honoured [3].

From 1997 to 1999, our team conducted a double-blind randomized controlled study, aimed at evaluating the differences between endoscopic treatment of reflux and antibiotic prophylaxis [4]. One of the major challenges of the study was patient enrollment. The randomization required a prior consent of the family to participate in the study without knowing the patient's allocation in one of the two protocols, endoscopic treatment or antibiotic prophylaxis. By the end of the 1990s, endoscopic treatment had become so popular that many parents refused to participate in the study for fear of being allocated to the antibiotic prophylaxis group. The decision we made in those years, once the randomized study was completed, was to adapt whenever possible to parental preferences. To investigate this aspect further, a questionnaire was prepared to be administered to families; the questionnaire was developed in collaboration with pediatricians and pediatric nephrologists, trying to offer the most balanced point of view possible, highlighting the advantages and disadvantages of each method; moreover, it was decided to have the questionnaire illustrated by a group of nurses not directly involved in the management of the patient with reflux, to avoid influencing the decision even with facial expressions or tone of voice (non-verbal communication).

The results of this study were later published in the British Journal of Urology in 2003 [5]. In this chapter, we will briefly outline the results of the study and then provide an overview of the current situation. Surprisingly, nothing has substantially changed over the course of the last 20 years with respect to parental preferences. On the contrary, the increasing preference of families, with the improvement of techniques, tissue augmenting substances and ultimately the effectiveness of the method, has allowed endoscopic treatment to spread throughout the world as the first choice treatment of vesicoureteral reflux.

The Word to the Parents? Results of a Questionnaire

In 2003, we published a study based on a questionnaire administered to the parents of 100 patients with grade 3 reflux [5]. The choice of an intermediate degree of reflux was made to focus the study on those patients in whom the major reflux treatment options are by almost unanimous opinion equivalent; in accordance with the main guidelines, antibiotic prophylaxis was currently recommended in low-grade reflux, at least in the first phase; in high-grade reflux, open surgery was recommended, especially when recurrent urinary infections were associated in spite of antibiotic prophylaxis and the reflux did not tend to heal. Occasional antibiotic therapy was at the time considered a management method under investigation, however reserved for children with mild or moderate reflux [6]. Endoscopic treatment, although increasingly widespread in Europe, was not yet recommended by the main scientific societies (AUA, ESPU) due to insufficient data on the safety of tissue augmenting substances and long-term efficacy [3, 7].

In reflux grade 3, endoscopic treatment, although considered an option still awaiting definitive confirmations, represented a useful compromise between the other two current management methods, both in terms of invasiveness and efficacy. Endoscopic treatment was then presented to parents as an option equivalent to antibiotic prophylaxis and ureter reimplantation surgery, effectively allowing a free decision under equal conditions and after having been fully informed.

Given the absence of definitive data on the various management methods, especially in moderate reflux, the opinion of the parents (and of the patient of the right age) becomes important if not even crucial in the orientation of the specialist. The 1997 AUA guidelines had already recommended that parents be informed in detail about the treatment options available and that their preferences be honored when making the decision [3]. Few data had been published on this precise topic, but as will be seen later with very different results [8].

The study included 100 consecutive patients who attended our clinic with a diagnosis of primary vesicoureteral reflux of the grade III. Other degrees of reflux and secondary reflux were excluded from the study. The patients were examined in the Pediatric Urology and Pediatric Nephrology clinic; undergoing voiding cystourethrography, ultrasound and renal scintigraphy with DMSA; patients with grade III reflux were enrolled in the study, asking the parents to complete dedicated questionnaire. To avoid that the parents' answers were influenced by the subjective orientation of the authors, the questionnaire was administered by outpatient nurses not directly involved in the urological management of vesicoureteral reflux. The three options compared, antibiotic prophylaxis, open surgery and endoscopic treatment, were illustrated in all their aspects, in relation to the success rate, complications and ultimately the advantages and disadvantages of each.

The parents were informed that antibiotic prophylaxis does not treat reflux but prevents urinary infections by reducing the risk of kidney damage, pending spontaneous resolution; the greatest advantage is the absence of invasiveness of the daily administration of the antibiotic, signaling a risk (however low) of allergies and the occurrence of resistance with consequent intercurrent infections; these occurrences do not represent a contraindication, since prophylaxis can be continued with another antibiotic; the success rate (no reflux or grade 1) was quoted as 33% in 1 year (after 1 year of prophylaxis, watchful waiting is possible). The planned follow-up, in accordance with international guidelines [3], included a 1-year voiding cystourethrography or an indirect radioisotope cystography in children over 3 years of age (to avoid the use of the catheter and reduce the radiation dose).

Open surgery was best defined as reimplantation of the ureter. The most common intravesical and extravesical reimplantation techniques have been illustrated. The short-term and medium-term complications, including the risk of postoperative ureteral obstruction of 1–2%; the invasiveness associated with surgery lasting an average of 90 min, with an incision in the lower abdomen, the need for general anesthesia, analgesics, the presence of a ureteral and bladder stent for some days, a hospital stay of around 7 days; the success rate provided was 95–98%. The follow-up used at the time of the study was VCUG or radioisotope cystography after 6 months.

Endoscopic treatment was explained as subureteral injection of tissue augmenting substance. Information relating to the material used and the instruments was provided; the procedure, lasting a few minutes, is performed under general anesthesia and does not require a post-operative catheter; the discharge is on the same day or the morning following the procedure; analgesics are usually not needed and complications are rare; the main advantage is the low invasiveness and the easy repetitiveness in case of failure; the success rate, at the time of the study, was listed as 70% in the mean of all grades of reflux, 80% in the grade 3.

Parents were asked to confirm that they understood all the information and were given the opportunity to ask questions. Furthermore, they were informed of the possibility of requesting a second opinion in accordance with our hospital policy. Finally they were asked to express their preference.

In total, the parents of 100 patients with grade III reflux participated in the study. Of these, 38 were male and 62 female, with an average age of 4 years. In detail, 78 families declared that they fully understood the information given, and 22 families requested further clarifications.

Eighty percent of families favoured endoscopic treatment. The second preference went to antibiotic prophylaxis (5%) and only 2% expressed a preference for open surgery. Thirteen families declared that they had no preferences and entrusted themselves to the advice of the authors; in these cases endoscopic treatment has been recommended. In all other cases, the chosen treatment was actually honoured.

Endoscopic treatment was the treatment of choice for most of the families interviewed, already at a time when this treatment was being criticized in many centres, especially outside Europe.

A study performed just 2 years earlier had come to different conclusions, indicating antibiotic prophylaxis as the treatment of choice by the parents if the prediction of recovery was expected to last less than 3–4 years; while a corrective treatment was preferred when the prediction was greater; it is interesting to note that in the case of corrective treatment, 60% still expressed themselves in favor of endoscopic treatment, even though it was not widespread at the time in the USA [8]. Actually, the study design was very different from ours, including patients with varying degrees of reflux. In particular, 65% of refluxes were grade 1 and 2, where the possibility of spontaneous resolution associated with prophylaxis is very high; on the other hand, 9% of refluxes were grade IV and V, a condition in which open surgery is considered to offer greater guarantees of success.

Returning to our study, the favourable response towards endoscopic treatment that emerged from the interview has strongly influenced the policy of our center. Endoscopic treatment has been proposed as a first line treatment for symptomatic and persistent vesicoureteral reflux after a suitable period of observation. Open surgery has been recommended in case of failure of at least two endoscopic treatments when urinary infections persist, in the presence of high-grade reflux.

Reassessment of Study Results 20 Years Later

Endoscopic treatment of reflux has gained increasing popularity since its introduction in the early 1980s [9, 10]. The reason for this success is certainly linked to the simplicity of the procedure, effectiveness of the treatment and the comparison with alternative procedures. Antibiotic prophylaxis, in addition to the long times of administration, has often proved to be ineffective due to non-compliance of families and due to the occurrrance of bacterial resistance (individuals and the general population) with consequent intercurrent infections. On the other hand, open surgery is a major procedure, with its intrinsic invasiveness, even if associated with a low risk of complications [11].

In the last two decades, little or nothing has changed in the area of antibiotic prophylaxis and open surgery, while advances have taken place in endoscopic treatment. These cover all aspects of treatment, including injectable materials, injection techniques, instrumentation, follow-up. This evolution has led on the one hand to a widespread increase in efficacy and on the other to a new awareness of possible complications, although rare but worthy of being discussed with parents when choosing treatment.

Injectable Materials

The search for injectable materials to carry out the endoscopic treatment of vesicoureteral reflux has been continuous. The main aspects related to the materials concern efficacy and safety. The ideal material should have characteristics of biocompatibility, durability at the injection site, ease of injection and absence of distant migration. Polytetrafluoethylene (Teflon, Polytef) was the first material used, soon abandoned after the demonstration of migration of some particles to distant organs [9, 10, 12]. Subsequently bovine collagen was used [13–16], abandoned due to its relatively too rapid degradability, the need for preliminary verification of individual tolerability (allergies?) and the doubts advanced on the possible cross-reaction with human collagen. In the years 1996–2013, our center used the copolymer of dextranomer and hyaluronic acid (Deflux) with good results in terms of efficacy and safety [17–20]. However, starting from 2013, after a period of comparison, our preference went to the polyacrylate/polyalcohol copolymer (Vantris) [21–23]. The main reason for switching materials is evidence of better long-term results with the latter. The biophysical characteristics of the polyacrylate/polyalcohol copolymer are very different from those of the dextranomer. Polyacrylate, unlike dextranomer, is not reabsorbable and persists indefinitely at the injection site, reducing only minimally in volume over time. The greater stability of the implant volume is an advantage for efficacy, even if it must be taken into account by using a smaller amount of material, to reduce the risk of secondary ureteral obstruction [24–26].

Injection Technique

The standard technique for the endoscopic treatment of reflux is the subureteral injection, initially described by Puri with the use of Teflon and known as STING (subureteral teflon injection) [9]. In the following years, some technical modifications were described, such as intraureteral injection, possibly preceded by hydrodistension [27] and the technique defined as "ureteral repositioning and injection (URI) [28].

In our experience the intraureteral technique has not produced a significant increase in the success rate. The adoption of a rigid metal needle would instead seem to be associated with a significant improvement in efficacy, because it allows the operator to manipulate the needle and at the same time inject the material without the help of an assistant. The use of the rigid needle is essential for the realization of the URI modification; this consists in bringing the uretero-vesical junction back inside the bladder, with a lever maneuver of the needle tip, thus injecting the material which would also make a sort of welding of the junction in the ideal position [28]. In our experience, the use of this technique has achieved success rates close to 100% in grade 2 reflux and over 90% overall for all grades.

These success rates, reported to the parents during the interview to decide on the management of the reflux, have certainly had a further influence in favor of the endoscopic treatment. This increase in success rate near 100% resulted in less use of post-treatment follow-up cystography; in many centers VCUG is currently performed only in selected cases, in the presence of recurrent febrile urinary infections, while in the majority of cases the evaluation of success is based on a clinical basis.

Complications

While on the one hand it is right to inform parents about the improvement in efficacy, on the other it is equally necessary to illustrate the possible complications of endoscopic treatment.

The only complication usually considered is secondary obstruction of the ureterovesical junction. The problem has long been underestimated until about 10 years ago. For many years, after the decline of Teflon, the preference of most authors went to the use of biodegradable materials, initially bovine collagen and subsequently dextranomer/hyaluronic acid copolymer; the obstructive complication was neglected because a progressive degradation of the injected material was supposed. In reality, the material is not completely replaced by newly formed collagen by the body, except in minimal quantities on the periphery of the implant; the formation of a pseudo-capsule interrupts the degradation process and the original material can be found even many years after the injection [20]. However, there is no doubt that the aforementioned materials undergo a reduction in volume, just a few days after implantation. Several authors have confirmed a non-negligible incidence of long-term treatment failure; for this reason, many centers have re-evaluated the use of a non-biodegradable material, such as the polyacrylate/polyalcohol copolymer [25]. At the same time, awareness of the risk of ureteral obstruction secondary to endoscopic treatment has increased. It was therefore hypothesized that the increased incidence of obstruction was associated with the change in material used [24, 29]. However, numerous studies seem to exclude a relationship between the type of material used and the risk of ureteral obstruction [26, 30, 31], even if it is advisable to use a smaller volume of material when choosing the non-biodegradable one [32]. Other risk factors, such as a pre-existing dilatation of the ureter and an inflammatory state of the bladder, would appear to play a role in the obstructive complication [26].

Correct Information

Having examined all the aspects that can determine a parental choice, in the light of the experience of recent years, a fundamental point remains to be discussed: what is "correct information"? Who informs the parents? In other words, how much parental choice is influenced by the beliefs of the interviewing doctor and what can be done to avoid this bias. In accordance with the main guidelines, the type of reflux management does not directly depend on the degree of reflux, but rather on the symptoms, age and the presence of nephropathy. Antibiotic prophylaxis is recommended in the first year of life, in the presence of "complicated" vesicoureteral reflux (febrile urinary infections). After the first year of life, endoscopic treatment is recommended in complicated reflux and is also an option in uncomplicated reflux, as the parents' free choice with respect to antibiotic prophylaxis.

Let's imagine a scenario where the parents of a child with vesicoureteral reflux go to the medical specialists to discuss the type of management of the reflux. These are often equivalent options with respect to the ultimate goal which is to avoid kidney damage, but with implications of a family and social nature (compliance with antibiotic prophylaxis, fear of major surgery, fear of anesthesia…). The decision will still be influenced by the professional figure that the parents are faced with. The pediatric surgeon and the pediatric urologist are experts in surgery and will also unconsciously or out of conviction tend to favor surgical/endoscopic treatment. The pediatric nephrologist and the pediatrician will tend to emphasize the superiority of antibiotic prophylaxis. Some, indeed skeptical about the real danger of vesicoureteral reflux, will suggest a simple watchful waiting, relying on the tendency of the reflux to regress.

This problem does not exclusively concern vesicoureteral reflux, but concerns all areas in which the decision-making process is conditioned by several possible choices, more or less equivalent in terms of results.

In recent decades, the internet has been added to the professional figures mentioned as a powerful new means of communication, increasingly used in the decision process. There are some very interesting studies that have investigated the influence of the internet and social media on decision process in the medical field [33]. These studies also revealed differences between people (parents in our case) of different ages. Everyone knows that parents, even when they turn to a medical specialist, are already informed via the internet of the options, guidelines, endoscopic and surgical techniques. Very often social media provides reviews of individual specialists, with scores similar to those used to choose a restaurant or go shopping. In particular, the young parents follow this path, as soon as they know the diagnosis and are preparing to evaluate possible solutions.

Finally, some authors have found that socioeconomic factors could play a fundamental role in the choice of management of vesicoureteral reflux, through the different trust that families place in the opinions of the pediatric urologist [34, 35]. By admission of the authors, this hypothesis needs further confirmation; moreover, in our Italian and European experience these factors do not seem to have any relevance.

Conclusions

Parental preferences greatly influence the choice of management of vesicoureteral reflux. The variability of the type of management lies in the possibility of choosing between options considered equivalent with regard to the ultimate goal, which is the prevention of renal damage related to reflux. It has been known for many years that kidney damage is in most cases only associated with reflux and not caused by reflux. Congenital nephropathy associated with reflux cannot be modified in any way, while acquired nephropathy is a result of pyelonephritis and its prevention is desirable to avoid further damage and the onset of arterial hypertension.

In 2003, the results of our study showed a strong parental preference for endoscopic treatment of vesicoureteral reflux, compared to antibiotic prophylaxis and surgical treatment, allowing us to propose a new management algorithm. In the following two decades there have been significant changes regarding indications, materials and techniques which have determined a further favor towards endoscopic treatment. The possibility of treating reflux quickly and with minimal invasiveness certainly represents the key to the success of endoscopic treatment, generally allowing a great advantage also in the quality of life of the child and his family. A fundamental role, which in part escapes our responsibility, is represented by the means of communication. Parents' choices are increasingly influenced by social media. This phenomenon is not negative in itself and represents an evolution of society in general, which is more aware of health problems. The responsibility of us medical specialists is to offer correct and transparent information, as much as possible based on the evidence of clinical data.

References

1. Elder JS. Guidelines for consideration for surgical repair of vesicoureteral reflux. Curr Opin Urol. 2000;10(6):579–85.
2. International Reflux Study Committee. Medical versus surgical treatment of primary vesicoureteral reflux: report of the International Reflux Study Committee. Paediatrics. 1981;67:392–400.
3. Elder JS, Peters CA, Arant BS Jr, et al. Pediatric Vesicoureteral Reflux Guidelines Panel summary report on the management of primary vesicoureteral reflux in children. J Urol. 1997;157(5):1846–51.
4. Capozza N, Caione P. Dextranomer/hyaluronic acid copolymer implantation for vesico-ureteral reflux: a randomized comparison with antibiotic prophylaxis. J Pediatr. 2002;140(2):230–4.
5. Capozza N, Lais A, Matarazzo E. Treatment of vesico-ureteric reflux: a new algorithm based on parental preference. BJU Int. 2003;92(3):285–8.
6. Garin EH, Campos A, Homsy Y. Primary vesicoureteral reflux: review of current concepts. Pediatr Nephrol. 1998;12:249–56.
7. Riedmiller H, Androulakakis P, Beurton D, et al. EAU guidelines on paediatric urology. Eur Urol. 2001;40(5):589–99.
8. Ogan K, Pohl HG, Carlson D, et al. Parental preferences in the management of vesicoureteral reflux. J Urol. 2001;166(1):240–3.
9. Puri P, O'Donnel B. Correction of experimentally produced vesicoureteric reflux in the piglet by intravesical injection of Teflon. Br Med J. 1984;289:5–7.
10. O'Donnel B, Puri P. Endoscopic correction of primary vesicoureteric reflux. Br J Urol. 1986;58:601–4.
11. Ellsworth PI, et al. Surgical management of vesicoureteral reflux. AORN J. 2000;71:498–505.508–13, [quiz] 517–20, 523–4.
12. Malizia AA Jr, Reiman HM, Myers RP, et al. Migration and granulomatous reaction after periurethral injection of polytef (Teflon). JAMA. 1984;251(24):3277–81.
13. Peters CA, Jeffs RD. Endoscopic correction of vescicoureteral reflux with bovine collagen injected submucosally at the ureteral orifice. J Urol. 1987;137:122A.
14. Frey P, Jenny P, Herzog B. Endoscopic subureteric collagen injection (SCIN): a new alternative treatment of vesico-ureteric reflux in children: experience in 82 refluxing ureters. Pediatr Surg Int. 1991;6:287–94.
15. Frey P, Berger D, Jenny P, et al. Subureteral collagen injection for the endoscopic treatment of vesico-ureteral reflux in children: follow-up study of 93 treated ureters and histological analysis of collagen implants. J Urol. 1992;148:718–23.
16. Capozza N, Caione P, De Gennaro M, et al. Endoscopic treatment of vesico-ureteric reflux and urinary incontinence: technical problems in the paediatric patient. Br J Urol. 1995;75(4):538–42.
17. Stenberg AM, Sundin A, Larsson BS, et al. Lack of distant migration after injection of a 125iodine labeled dextranomer based implant into the rabbit bladder. J Urol. 1997;158(5):1937–41.
18. Stenberg AM, Larsson E, Lindholm A, et al. Experimental studies of an injectable dextranomer-based implant. Histopathology, volume changes and DNA analysis. Postmenopausal disorders with special reference to urinary incontinence. Acta Univ Ups. 1998;1:1–15.
19. Lackgren G, Stenberg A, Wahlin N, et al. Long-term follow-up of children treated with dextranomer/hyaluronic acid copolymer for vesico-ureteral reflux. J Urol. 2001;166:1887–92.
20. Capozza N, Lais A, Nappo S, et al. The role of endoscopic treatment of vesicoureteral reflux: a 17-year experience. J Urol. 2004;172(4 Pt 2):1626–8. discussion 1629.
21. Ormaechea M, Ruiz E, Denes E, et al. New tissue bulking agent (polyacrylate polyalcohol) for treating vesicoureteral reflux: preliminary results in children. J Urol. 2010;183(2):714–7.
22. Chertin B, Arafeh WA, Zeldin A, et al. Preliminary data on endoscopic treatment of vesicoureteric reflux with polyacrylate polyalcohol copolymer (Vantris): surgical outcome following single injection. J Pediatr Urol. 2011;7:654–6.

23. Kocherov S, Ulman I, Nikolaev S, et al. Multicenter survey of endoscopic treatment of vesicoureteral reflux using polyacrylate-polyalcohol bulking copolymer (Vantris). Urology. 2014;84(3):689–93.
24. Alizadeh F, Mazdak H, Khorrami MH, et al. Postoperative ureteral obstruction after endoscopic treatment of vesicoureteral reflux with polyacrylate polyalcohol copolymer (Vantris). J Pediatr Urol. 2013;9:488–92.
25. Chertin B, Kocherov S. Long-term results of endoscopic treatment of vesicoureteric reflux with different tissue-augmenting substances. J Pediatr Urol. 2010;6(3):251–3.
26. Chertin B, Mele E, Kocherov S, et al. What are the predictive factors leading to ureteral obstruction following endoscopic correction of VUR in the pediatric population? J Pediatr Urol. 2018;14(6):538.e1–7.
27. Kirsch AJ, Perez-Brayfield MR, Scherz HC. Minimally invasive treatment of vesicoureteral reflux with endoscopic injection of dextranomer/hyaluronic acid copolymer: the Children's Hospitals of Atlanta experience. J Urol. 2003;170:211–5.
28. Capozza N, Caione P. Modification of the STING procedure for vesicoureteral reflux: ureteral repositioning and injection. Arch Esp Urol. 2008;61(2):254–7.
29. Sencan A, Yildirim H, Ozkan KU. Late ureteral obstruction after endoscopic treatment of vesicoureteral reflux with polyacrylate polyalcohol copolymer. Urology. 2014;84:1188–91.
30. Friedmacher F, Puri P. Ureteral obstruction after endoscopic treatment of vesicoureterl reflux: does the type of iniected bulkin agent matter? Curr Urol Rep. 2019;20:40–9.
31. Kocherov S, Nikolaev S, Gaber G, et al. Incidence of UVJ obstruction during long-term follow-up after endoscopic correction of VUR utilizing polyacrylate polyalcohol copolymer (PPC). J Pediatr Endosc Surg. 2020;2:183–7.
32. Tekin A, Yagmur I, Tiryaki S. Changing bulking agent may require change in injection volume for endoscopic treatment of vesicoureteral reflux. Int Braz J Urol. 2018;44(6):1194–9.
33. Lewis T. Seeking health information on the internet: lifestyle choice or bad attack of cyberchondria? Media Cult Soc. © 2006 SAGE Publications (London, Thousand Oaks and New Delhi). 28(4):521–39.
34. Hsieh MH, Madden-Fuentes RJ, Bayne A, et al. Cross-sectional evaluation of parental decision making factors for vesicoureteral reflux management in children. J Urol. 2010;184:1589–93.
35. Puri P, Friedmacher F, Farrugia MK, Sharma S, Esposito C, Mattoo TK. Primary vesicoureteral reflux. Nat Rev Dis Primers. 2024;10:75.

Cost-Utility Analysis of Treatment Algorithms for Vesicoureteral Reflux

Jonathan C. Routh, Diana A. Aponte-Colon, and David L. Barquin

Abstract Vesicoureteral Reflux (VUR) is a common pediatric urologic condition that affects approximately 1% of children in the United States (Pohl et al. J Urol 177:1659–1666. https://doi.org/10.1016/j.juro.2007.01.059, 2007). There are a variety of management options and surrounding discourse regarding the optimal treatment course. Based on the 2017 American Urological Association guidelines, treatment options include surveillance with or without antibiotic prophylaxis, surgical reimplantation (open, laparoscopic, or robotic), and minimally invasive endoscopic correction with injectable ureteral bulking agents. The best treatment option depends on several factors including age, reflux grade, breakthrough urinary tract infections, and the presence of renal scarring, bowel/bladder dysfunction, or other congenital abnormalities. The economic impact of these treatment options varies widely, so standardized comparisons that evaluate both costs and outcomes is appropriate.

Keywords Utility · Cost-utility analysis (CUA) · Vesicoureteral reflux (VUR) Continuous antibiotic prophylaxis (CAP) · Quality adjusted life year (QALY)

J. C. Routh (✉) · D. A. Aponte-Colon · D. L. Barquin
Department of Urology, Duke University School of Medicine, Durham, NC, USA
e-mail: jonathan.routh@duke.edu

P. Puri, A. Yamataka (eds.), *Vesicoureteral Reflux*,
https://doi.org/10.1007/978-3-031-95091-9_27

Introduction: Overview of Health Economic Analyses

Health economic analyses can be used to study the utility of an intervention in relation to cost. This can highlight the impact of an outcome in relation to the investment/cost and help guide decision-making. There are different types of health economic analyses, including cost-effectiveness analysis (CEA), cost-utility analysis (CUA), cost-benefit analysis, cost-minimization analysis, and cost-consequence analysis [9]. This chapter will focus on summarizing the existing literature regarding CUA of VUR treatment algorithms.

CUA is a specific form of CEA in which different interventions are compared based on their relative costs and outcomes, with outcomes being expressed as "utility values" [6]. A utility is a numerical score (usually between 0 and 1) that quantifies the impact of a health state on a person's well-being, with 1 representing perfect health and 0 representing death. Thus, a very severe condition that negatively impacts all aspects of daily living might have a utility value near 0, while a minor condition that does not result in significant impairment might have a utility value very close to 1. Utility values have a linear relationship, so the quality of life of someone with a utility of 0.5 is assumed to be exactly half of the quality of life of someone with a utility of 1. Importantly, utility assessments of health states can be combined in a multiplicative manner, meaning that if a patient is affected by two different disease processes, the values of each can be multiplied to give the overall estimated health utility for that particular patient. For example, if a patient has Disease A with a utility value of 0.8 and Disease B with a utility value of 0.5, then their overall health state utility for that time period would be $0.8 \times 0.5 = 0.4$. For reference, utility scores for known pediatric conditions include otitis media with pain (0.97), severe ADHD (0.90), monocular blindness (0.89), severe hearing loss (0.86), severe seizure disorder (0.71), and severe cerebral palsy (0.55) [1].

Typically, utility values are estimated via in-person interviews with the community, during which the interviewer describes the health state and the respondent states how they value the health state compared to perfect health. More recently, online methods have been used to perform these estimations more quickly and at a lower cost, with overall good results compared to traditional in-person methods. There are multiple valid methods for estimating utility, including direct estimation methods such as the standard gamble (SG), time trade-off (TTO), and visual analogue scale (VAS) methods. Of these, the TTO method is the most commonly used, as it is relatively easy for respondents to comprehend and gives a middle-of-the-road estimation compared to the more conservative SG and more liberal VAS.

Indirect estimation methods can also be used. These methods involve indirectly converting a respondent's answers on a generic health related quality of life questionnaire (most commonly the European quality of life five dimensions (EQ-5D), short form six dimensions (SF-6D), or health utilities index (HUI)). Questionnaire responses are then mathematically weighted in order to convert to utilities. These weights are typically derived or calibrated by means of a TTO method from a surveyed sample of the general population.

"Disutility" values also exist, and are often used to describe the decrement to perfect health associated with a particular intervention or health state. Dysutilities can be mathematically described as 1—utility value.

Utility Values for VUR

A necessary component of CUA is an accurate estimation of the utility value for the health state. For VUR, previous analyses have demonstrated mean utility values ranging from 0.82 to 0.87 for VUR [3, 4]. In both studies the utility scores did not differ significantly based on inclusion of continuous antibiotic prophylaxis or the occurrence of febrile urinary tract infections.

Lloyd and colleagues used Amazon's 'Mechanical Turk' (MTurk) online platform to conduct a cross-sectional survey and study utility values for VUR using a TTO method. They found a mean utility score of 0.87 for VUR, with higher values noted among respondents who had children on statistical analysis. Furthermore, they also calculated utility value for the 6-week post-operative period after open ureteroneocystostomy, which was found to be 0.45. When averaging these values over a year, the net utility value for patients with VUR undergoing open surgical correction was 0.93 (assuming the patients had perfect health during the rest of the year).

By contrast, Nelson et al. used a national cross-sectional survey that included adults who are or had previously been parents in order to obtain utility scores for vesicoureteral reflux and anti-reflux surgery, which were similarly elicited using the TTO method. Their results demonstrated a mean utility score of 0.82 for VUR. A multivariate regression model associated higher scores for VUR health state with female patients, those living in a single-family household, and those who had at least one child living at home as compared to having no children at home. Utility scores were also obtained for the 6-week period after anti-reflux surgery, with an overall score of 0.71. Higher scores for anti-reflux surgery were associated with higher education (having a high school or bachelor's degree vs education less than high school), White race (compared to Black race or Hispanic ethnicity), and single-family home in the multivariate regression model.

Tejwani et al. [8] also used Amazon's MTurk online platform to determine whether utilities can be affected by disease point of view. Their multivariate analysis demonstrated that VUR utility was reduced by 34% when estimated from a parent's perspective and by 13% when estimated from a dyad perspective (vs a child's perspective). Contrarily, they found higher utilities among single and older respondents. These studies demonstrate the complexities of calculating utility scores and highlight how VUR is seen by patients and families as a condition with significant burden. The impact on the health state is more prominent in the 6-week period following surgical interventions for VUR.

Cost-Utility Analysis for VUR Treatment Options

Vesicoureteral Reflux (VUR) is a common pediatric urologic condition that affects approximately 1% of children in the United States [5]. There are a variety of management options and surrounding discourse regarding the optimal treatment course. Based on the 2017 American Urological Association guidelines, treatment options include surveillance with or without antibiotic prophylaxis, surgical reimplantation (open, laparoscopic, or robotic), and minimally invasive endoscopic correction with injectable ureteral bulking agents. The best treatment option depends on several factors including age, reflux grade, breakthrough urinary tract infections, and the presence of renal scarring, bowel/bladder dysfunction, or other congenital abnormalities. The economic impact of these treatment options varies widely, so standardized comparisons that evaluate both costs and outcomes is appropriate.

Once utility scores have been established, CUA can be performed to help guide treatment options based on cost and patient preference. Shaikh et al. performed a cost-utility analysis on the risk/benefit ratio of using CAP for patients <6 years old with varying grades of VUR [7]. They analyzed four different treatment strategies: (i) CAP for all children with VUR, (ii) CAP for children with Grade III or Grade IV VUR, (iii) CAP for children with Grade IV VUR, and (iv) no prophylaxis. The threshold to determine a treatment strategy as cost-effective was $100,000/quality adjusted life year (QALY), which is a broadly accepted threshold value. This was calculated by multiplying the time spent in the specific health state by the disutility value of that particular health state. When looking at strict costs and effectiveness, the results were as follows, from most expensive and effective to least expensive and effective: i > ii > iii > iv. Thereby, CAP for all children was both the most expensive and most effective, while CAP for no children was the least expensive and least effective. After cost-utility analysis, CAP for Grade IV VUR was determined to be cost effective while CAP for children with Grade I-III was not. The incremental cost-utility ratio for VUR Grade IV only was $37,903/QALY, while prophylaxis for VUR Grades III or IV only was $303,024/QALY and prophylaxis for all grades was $339,740/QALY. Using a willingness-to-pay threshold of $40,000/QALY gained or more, it was determined that CAP for Grade IV VUR was cost effective while CAP for children with Grade I-III was not.

Hsieh and colleagues [2] also performed CUA using Markov modeling, which is a method of modeling population-level cohorts based on measured and/or estimated values, to determine what treatment algorithm minimized cost and morbidity utilizing the perspective of parents whose children have grades II and III VUR. Of note, Markov modeling uses hypothetical patients that progress through health states based on predetermined probabilities. The protocols included five arms: (1) without antibiotics or follow up imaging (antibiotics were only given for acute pyelonephritis, no surgical procedures or CAP), (2) early surgery protocol (patients are on CAP until the second year of presentation, at that point they are stopped if VUR resolves or otherwise the patients undergo open surgery without postoperative imaging, unless they develop pyelonephritis), (3) immediate surgery protocol (identical to early surgery protocol except that open surgery is performed during the year of presentation), (4) Okeke-Katz (OK) protocol (Patients receive CAP 1 year after presentation, at that point if VUR persists the patients undergo endoscopy and repeat imaging. A second endoscopic procedure/imaging is repeated if VUR persists after the first one. Open surgery is performed if VUR persists after two endoscopic procedures without postoperative imaging, unless the patient presents with pyelonephritis), and (5) immediate endoscopy protocol (identical to early OK protocol except that endoscopy is performed during the year of presentation). They began the simulation with a perfect utility score that was decreased by interventions, adverse events, or lack of VUR resolution. The model tracked outcomes such as time to VUR resolution, number of imaging studies and procedures, years of antibiotics, and pyelonephritis episodes that were used in utility calculations. Their results demonstrated that the protocol without antibiotics or follow up imaging resulted in the best cost-utility for VUR grades II and III.

Conclusions

There are multiple treatment options for VUR, and determining the optimal management pathway can be challenging for physicians and their families. In this setting, CUA can help by mathematically comparing the relative costs and health effects of each treatment and assist in the decision-making process. The extant literature on CUA for VUR shows a mean utility value of 0.85, thereby demonstrating how VUR is seen as a condition with significant burden on par with hearing loss, blindness, and other severe congenital or acquired conditions. There is a relatively small number of rigorous studies regarding CUA and VUR treatment algorithms, but the studies currently published suggest the highest utility and least costly treatment pathways result from limiting surgical interventions to symptomatic patients and restricting CAP to patients with high-grade VUR.

References

1. Carroll AE, Downs SM. Improving decision analyses: parent preferences (utility values) for pediatric health outcomes. J Pediatr. 2009;155:21–5.e5. https://doi.org/10.1016/j.jpeds.2009.01.040.
2. Hsieh MH, Swana HS, Baskin LS, Meng MV. Cost-utility analysis of treatment algorithms for moderate grade vesicoureteral reflux using Markov models. J Urol. 2007;177:703–9. https://doi.org/10.1016/j.juro.2006.10.002.
3. Lloyd JC, Yen T, Pietrobon R, Wiener JS, Ross SS, Kokorowski PJ, Nelson CP, Routh JC. Estimating utility values for vesicoureteral reflux in the general public using an online tool. J Pediatr Urol. 2014;10(6):1026–31.
4. Nelson CP, Routh JC, Logvinenko T, Rosoklija I, Kokorowski PJ, Prosser LA, Schuster MA. Utility scores for vesicoureteral reflux and anti-reflux surgery. J Pediatr Urol. 2015;11:177–82. https://doi.org/10.1016/j.jpurol.2015.03.008.

5. Pohl HG, Joyce GF, Wise M, Cilento BG. Vesicoureteral reflux and ureteroceles. J Urol. 2007;177:1659–66. https://doi.org/10.1016/j.juro.2007.01.059.
6. Prosser LA, Hammitt JK, Keren R. Measuring health preferences for use in cost-utility and cost-benefit analyses of interventions in children: theoretical and methodological considerations. PharmacoEconomics. 2007;25:713–26. https://doi.org/10.2165/00019053-200725090-00001.
7. Shaikh N, Rajakumar V, Peterson CG, Gorski J, Ivanova A, Gravens Muller L, Miyashita Y, Smith KJ, Mattoo T, Pohl HG, Mathews R, Greenfield SP, Docimo SG, Hoberman A. Cost-utility of antimicrobial prophylaxis for treatment of children with vesicoureteral reflux. Front Pediatr. 2020;7:530. https://doi.org/10.3389/fped.2019.00530.
8. Tejwani R, Wang H-HS, Lloyd JC, Kokorowski PJ, Nelson CP, Routh JC. Utility estimation for pediatric vesicoureteral reflux: methodological considerations using an online survey platform. J Urol. 2017;197:805–10. https://doi.org/10.1016/j.juro.2016.09.119.
9. Turner HC, Archer RA, Downey LE, Isaranuwatchai W, Chalkidou K, Jit M, Teerawattananon Y. An introduction to the main types of economic evaluations used for informing priority setting and resource allocation in healthcare: key features, uses, and limitations. Front Public Health. 2021;9:722927. https://doi.org/10.3389/fpubh.2021.722927.

Vesicoureteral Reflux, Hypertension and Chronic Renal Failure

Dunya Mohammad and Tej K. Mattoo

Abstract Vesicoureteral reflux (VUR) is the most common congenital urinary tract anomaly in children. Most cases of VUR are diagnosed after urinary tract infection (UTI) or during follow-up for antenatally diagnosed renal anomalies. Patients with VUR are at high risk for UTI recurrence and renal scarring, which is also called reflux nephropathy (RN). RN can occur at any age and the important risk factors for renal scarring are a high-grade VUR, recurrent UTI, and delayed antibiotic treatment for acute pyelonephritis. Hypertension is the most common complication of RN seen in pediatric patients. Other complications that occur mostly in adults include proteinuria, recurrent UTI, and chronic kidney disease. Pregnancy-related complications have also been reported. Appropriate follow-up of patients with VUR, particularly in those with high-grade VUR, is recommended. Patients with renal scarring should be monitored for hypertension and those with significant scarring, particularly bilateral, should also be monitored for proteinuria and chronic kidney disease.

Keywords Vesicoureteral reflux (VUR) · Urinary tract infection (UTI) · Bladder-bowel dysfunction (BBD) · Renal scarring · Reflux nephropathy · Chronic kidney disease · Hypertension · Proteinuria

D. Mohammad
Division of Pediatric Nephrology, Department of Pediatrics, University of South Alabama, Mobile, AL, USA

T. K. Mattoo (✉)
Division of Pediatric Nephrology, Wayne Pediatrics, Departments of Pediatrics and Urology, Wayne State University School of Medicine, Detroit, MI, USA
e-mail: Tmattoo@med.wayne.edu

P. Puri, A. Yamataka (eds.), *Vesicoureteral Reflux*,
https://doi.org/10.1007/978-3-031-95091-9_28

Introduction

Vesicoureteral reflux (VUR) is the most common congenital anomaly of the urinary tract (CAKUT) in children. The reported prevalence of VUR varies from 1.3% of healthy children to 8–50% of children evaluated after a urinary tract infection UTI [1]. The highest prevalence (36–49%) is in newborn and young infants diagnosed with UTI [1]. Most cases of VUR are diagnosed after a UTI or during follow-up for renal anomalies diagnosed during routine antenatal ultrasound examination. A few cases are also diagnosed during family screening, evaluation for renal scarring or renal transplant work-up. VUR diagnosed after UTI is more common in females whereas VUR diagnosed during follow-up for prenatal hydronephrosis or hydroureter is more common in males [2]. VUR is more common in Caucasian children and typically more severe as compared to African American children [3].

Pediatric patients mostly have a primary VUR, which is due to abnormalities in ureteral implantation into bladder resulting in loss of the normal anti-reflux mechanism at the uretero-vesicular junction. This type of VUR has shown a hereditary nature with clustering in families which implies a genetic role in its pathogenesis, but no single gene has yet been identified. Secondary VUR is less common and results from an increase in bladder pressure caused by conditions such as posterior urethral valves or neurogenic bladder. VUR is associated with recurrent UTI and renal scarring, also called reflux nephropathy (RN). The renal scarring may be congenital in origin, or it occurs as a result of renal parenchymal injury caused by acute pyelonephritis (APN).

Complications Associated with VUR

VUR as a risk factor for UTI has been identified for more than a century. Its association with renal scaring was first demonstrated in early 1960s by Hudson and Edwards [4]. This was followed by further studies in 1970s, particularly by Smellie et al. [5] who reported a significant correlation between VUR (high grade in particular) and renal scaring; 53% of all children with VUR and 79% of those with a high grade VUR. Around the same time, the commonly used term for renal scarring, chronic pyelonephritis, was replaced with the currently used term RN [6].

Urinary Tract Infection

Based on the results of a systematic review from 33 studies that included 4891 children (0–18 years), those with VUR were 1.5 times (95% CI: 1.1–1.9) more likely to have APN, as confirmed by dimercaptosuccinic acid (DMSA) renal scans, as compared to children with no VUR (67 vs 49%; P = 0.004) [7]. A recent 2-year, multi-site prospective cohort study that included 500 children; 305 with VUR in the RIVUR study and 195 with no VUR in the CUTIE (Careful Urinary Tract Infection Evaluation) study, reported that the rates of recurrent febrile UTI were higher in children with VUR (25.4%) as compared to no VUR (17.3%) [8].

In a retrospective study that evaluated risk factors for UTI in children with VUR, recurrent UTI occurred in 120 (16.2%) patients during the follow-up period of 58,856 person-months. UTI incidence rate per 1000 person-months (95% CI) was 9.4 (8.2, 10.8) for severe VUR (Grades IV/V) as compared to 7.8 (6.9, 8.8) for mild to moderate VUR (Grades I–III) (P = 0.03) [9].

High-grade VUR as a risk factor for UTI has also been reported by others. Sjostrom et al. reported a cohort of infants with severe reflux (Grades III–V), 47% had breakthrough UTI during a median follow-up of 39 months [10]. In another study that looked at recurrent UTI in preschool children, VUR was present in 14/34 (34%) of those with recurrent UTI and 69/256 (27%) without recurrence. UTI was significantly associated with bilateral and intrarenal (grade III–V) VUR (OR: 3.5) [11].

Renal Scarring

Renal scarring associated with VUR, also called RN, may be congenital in origin, which is a result of abnormal renal development resulting in focal renal dysplasia, or acquired, which results from pyelonephritis-induced renal injury (Table 1) [12]. However, the differentiation of congenital versus acquired RN on the basis of preceding UTI can be arbitrary because the possibility of a preexisting renal scar before the UTI cannot always be ruled out. Studies have showed a significantly higher likelihood of renal scaring (RR: 2.6 [95% CI: 1.7–3.9]) associated with APN in children with VUR as compared to no VUR [7]. The reported odds ratio of renal scarring with APN in presence of a VUR is 2.8 for patients and 3.7 for the renal units as compared to those with no VUR [13].

Pathogenesis and Risk Factors for Renal Scarring

The exact mechanism for renal scarring following APN is not known. It is believed to be mediated by immunological mechanisms, macromolecular trapping and mesangial dysfunction, vascular alterations, hypertension, and hemodynamic alterations [14]. Renal scarring due to intrarenal reflux occurs mostly at the renal poles because of the presence of extensively fused (compound) renal papillae, which are associated with reflux [15]. The scarring may result from a single episode of pyelonephritis, especially in young children, also called "big bang effect" or the process may take several years [16]. In one study, the mean time from the discovery of VUR to the appearance of renal scarring was 6.1 years [17].

Table 1 Acquired versus congenital reflux nephropathy in children [12]

	Acquired	Congenital
Time of occurrence	Postnatal	Prenatal
History of UTI before diagnosis	Common	Uncommon
Age distribution at diagnosis	All pediatric age groups	Mostly in younger children
Gender distribution	Predominately females	Predominately males
Grade of VUR at the time of diagnosis	Variable, depending on age	Mostly high-grade
Renal histology	Chronic inflammatory changes	Features of renal dysplasia

UTI Urinary tract infection, *VUR* Vesicoureteral reflux

The important risk factors that have been associated with renal scaring after APN are the severity of VUR, recurrent UTI, and delayed treatment of UTI. Other risk factors associated with increased risk of renal scarring with UTI include non-E. coli UTI and genetic susceptibility [8, 18, 19].

Severity of VUR

Renal scarring occurs with APN with or without VUR, but the risk is higher in the presence of VUR, particularly a high-grade VUR. A meta-analysis of the published data revealed that renal damage (per 100 renal units) occurred in 6.2% in those with grades I–III VUR and 47.9% in those with grades IV and V VUR [20]. In the RIVUR study, the proportion of new scars in renal units with grade 4 VUR was significantly higher than in units with no VUR (OR, 24.2; 95% CI, 6.4–91.2) [21]. RIVUR study did not include patients with grade V VUR.

Recurrent UTI

The reported prevalence of renal scarring after febrile UTI is about 15% [22]. It ranges from 3% after the first UTI to 29% after > three febrile UTI [23, 24]. In the RIVUR study, children with a second UTI had significantly more renal scars odds ratio (OR), 2.85; 95% confidence interval (95% CI), 1.38 to 5.92 as compared to those with a single UTI [20]. A post hoc analysis of RIVUR and CUTIE studies revealed that the odds of renal scarring after second febrile UTI was 11.8 (95% CI, 4.1–34.4) times greater than after a single febrile infection, and the odds of renal scarring after three or more febrile infections was 13.7 (95% CI, 3.4–54.4) times greater than after a single febrile infection [25].

Bladder and bowel dysfunction (BBD) is an important risk factor for recurrent UTI. The presence of BBD in patients with primary VUR increases risk of recurrent

UTIs [relative risk (RR): 2.1; 1.7–2.5] [26]. The impact of BBD in children with VUR on renal scaring has been related to; increase in risk of febrile UTI (44% as compared to 13% in those without BBD), delay in VUR resolution at 24 months (31% with BBD and 61% without BBD) and the higher rate of postoperative UTI (22% as compared to 5% without BBD) [27].

Delayed Antibiotic Treatment

A multivariate analysis of 158 children with febrile UTI showed that a delay of greater than 48 h in the initiation of antibiotic treatment was associated with an increased risk of acute lesions on renal scan [28]. The RIVUR study revealed that delayed initiation of antibiotic treatment was associated with an increased risk of new scars; 74% lower in children whose treatment started within 24 h of onset of fever as compared to those whose treatment started after 72 h of fever [25].

Patient Age and Sex

No age is immune from renal scarring due to APN. RIVUR trial reported that the risk for new kidney scarring is higher in older children [21]. Other recent studies have also shown that older children may be at higher risk of kidney scarring [22, 23]. Renal scarring occurs in adult kidneys as well, as is seen in adult transplanted kidneys [29]. Also, adult pig kidneys with VUR and UTI scar as quickly/easily as those of piglets [30].

In some randomized studies, the number of cases reported with renal scarring in children with VUR correlated with patient sex [22, 31]. Studies with more males reported significantly more cases of renal scarring [22]. Another study revealed a strong negative correlation ($r = -0.7$) of acquired RN with the percentage of female patients included in the study (Fig. 1). This was attributed mostly to a higher incidence of congenital RN in male as compared to acquired RN in female patients [21].

Complications of Renal Scarring

The complications of RN are well known but poorly defined because of their insidious onset and slow progression. These include hypertension, proteinuria, tubulopathy, focal segmental glomerular sclerosis and chronic kidney disease (CKD) including end stage kidney disease (ESKD) in some patients (Table 2) [12]. Of these, hypertension and proteinuria are the commonest ones that have a significant bearing on long-term renal outcome, and both are amenable to medical intervention.

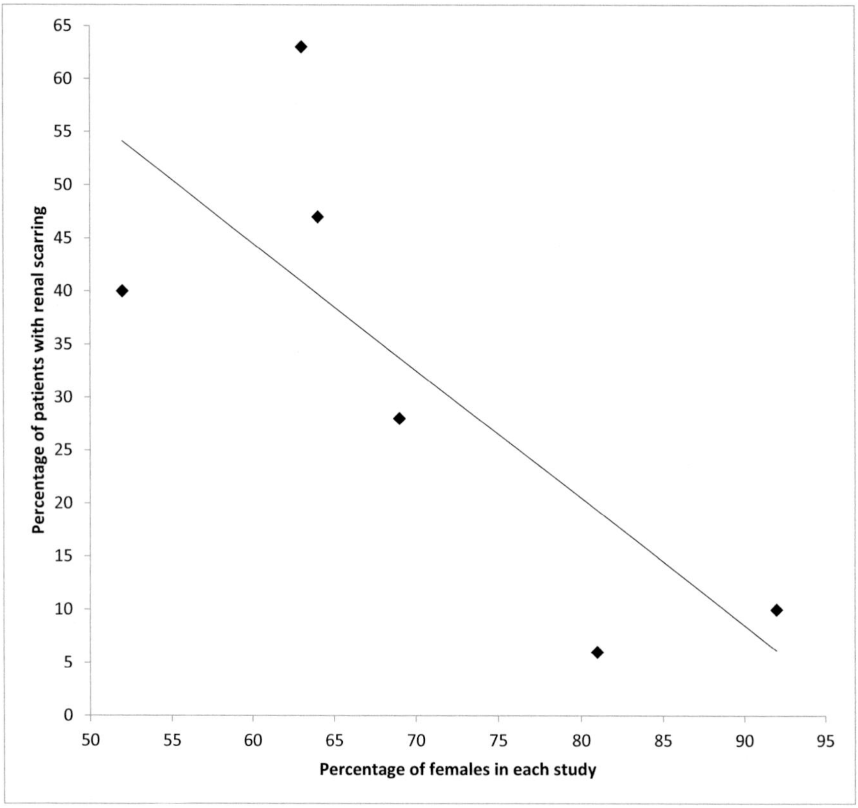

Fig. 1 Correlation of percentage of renal scaring with the percentage of female patients included in various studies ($r = -0.7$) [21]

Table 2 Reported complications of renal scarring [12]

Hypertension
Microalbuminuria/Proteinuria
Focal segmental glomerulosclerosis (FSGS)
Urinary concentration defects
Hyperkalemia and acidosis
Urinary calculi
Growth impairment
Complications during pregnancy
Hypertension, proteinuria, edema, deterioration in renal function, preterm delivery, pre-eclampsia, and fetal loss
Progressive CKD, particularly when scarring is bilateral.

CKD Chronic kidney disease

Hypertension

Hypertension occurs in 10–30% of children and 34–38% of adult patients with renal scarring [32, 33]. In a pediatric study of patients with VUR and renal scarring that were followed for a period of 15 years, about 13% of patients at age 20–31 years were found to be hypertensive [34]. In another study involving 664 VUR patients diagnosed between 1970 and 2004, 3% of patients developed hypertension. The estimated probability of hypertension was 2%, 6%, 15% at 10, 15, and 21 years of age, respectively [35]. In a study that included 159 healthy pediatric patients (median age of 11 years) referred for evaluation of hypertension, 33 (21%) were found to have renal scars by DMSA renal scan [36].

According to a recent study based on the United States Renal Data System (USRDS) data, which reviewed the trends in ESKD attributed to RN from 1996 to 2014, the mean age at the diagnosis of new-onset ESKD secondary to RN was 47 years (IQR 30–65) and this did not change over time 66.8% of all patients with hypertension as a comorbidity [37].

The exact cause for hypertension due to renal scarring is not known but is believed to be due to parenchymal ischemia leading to renin secretion. In a 5-year prospective study of patients with longstanding RN, there was no correlation between blood pressure and plasma renin activity, plasma creatinine concentration, or the degree of scarring. The Degree of renal scaring did not correlate with severity of hypertension [38]. However, a recent study reported a positive correlation between the severity of scarring and hypertension [39].

Proteinuria

Proteinuria due to RN is usually an insidious slowly progressive disease that starts with a mild persistent proteinuria (microalbuminuria). As the disease progresses, overt proteinuria and nephrotic syndrome can develop, which is more commonly seen in adults as compared to pediatric patients. Microalbuminuria has been reported in 51% of pediatric patients (mean age 9.8 + 4.2 years) with RN and overt proteinuria has been reported in 21% of adult patients with RN [40, 41].

The pathogenesis of proteinuria in patients with renal scaring is not well understood and is attributed to immunologic injury, macromolecular trapping and mesangial dysfunction, vascular alterations and hypertension, and glomerular hyperfiltration. The most plausible among these explanations is the hyperfiltration in remaining nephrons. This results in changes in glomerular basement membrane permeability to macromolecules such as albumin and progression of renal disease [42].

In a study of 21 adults (mean age 23.9 years) with history of dilated VUR during infancy, proteinuria was diagnosed in 3 (23%) of the 13 patients with unilateral RN and 2 (50%) of the 4 patients with bilateral RN [43]. In another study of 127 adults (mean age 41 years) with VUR diagnosed during childhood, including 44 (35%) with unilateral and 30 (24%) with bilateral renal scarring, 30 (24%) patients had proteinuria [44].

In patients with RN, the onset of proteinuria predicts progression of renal disease and an overall renal outcome. Studies suggest that the rate of decline in kidney function is proportional to the degree of the proteinuria with the suggested threshold of 0.5 g/24 h as the minimum degree of proteinuria that can affect outcome [45, 46].

Chronic Kidney Disease

RN is a well-known cause of CKD, especially in patients with bilateral severe VUR and proteinuria. According to the North American Pediatric Renal Trials and Collaborative Studies (NAPRTCS) 2008 report, RN was the fourth most common cause of renal failure in children with CKD, on dialysis and post renal transplant [47]. In the Chronic Kidney Disease in Children (CKiD) study, RN was the underlying cause of CKD stage 2 and 3 in 87 (14.8%) of 586 children aged 1–16 years [48]. According to a study by Silva et al., the probability of CKD for patients with bilateral high grade VUR was 15% by 10 years after VUR diagnosis. The three variables that were independently associated with CKD were age at diagnosis >24 months [relative risk (RR) = 4.8, 95% confidence interval (95%CI), VUR grade V (RR = 3.5, 95%CI, 1.5–7.9, P = 0.002), and bilateral renal damage (RR = 2.86, 95%CI, 1.3–6.1, P = 0.007) [49].

Recent literature is indicative of an improving prognosis in patients diagnosed with VUR in childhood. In a study that evaluated the clinical course of 735 children with primary VUR diagnosed between 1970 to 2004, the estimated probability of CKD decreased from 5% to 2% at 10 years after diagnosis in children diagnosed between 1970 to1990 and 1990 to 2004, respectively [50]. Based on the USRDS data, the incidence of patients of any age with ESKD attributed to RN in the US has decreased significantly from 1.9 per million in 1996 to 0.6 per million in 2014 ($p < 0.001$). The respective numbers for children were 0.43 per million and 0.25 per million. The authors attributed this trend to advances in medical and surgical management, change in diagnostic practices from intravenous pyelography to ultrasound and Tc-labelled DMSA scans, and possibly alternative diagnosis such as renal dysplasia in some cases. The study reported that in children, renal dysplasia diagnosis has increased which offsets the decrease in RN incident ESKD cases. The study provided no data on congenital versus acquired RN [37].

The long-term follow-up of patients with ESKD (GFR <15 ml/min/1.73m^2) secondary to RN who have undergone renal transplantation appears to be good. The Australia and New Zealand Dialysis Registry reported on first kidney transplants performed between1985 and 2015 in individuals less than 30 years of age with a diagnosis of CAKUT. The 10-year graft survival in individuals with CAKUT was favorable: patients with RN had a 70% graft survival at 10 years and 49% at 20 years [51].

Table 3 Clinical presentation of reflux nephropathy in adults [12, 31]

	Males	Females
Urinary tract infections	Uncommon	Common
Plasma creatinine	Usually, higher	Usually, normal
End-stage kidney failure	More common	Less common
Proteinuria	Frequent/severe	Infrequent/Less severe
Hypertension	More common	Less common

Reflux Nephropathy in Adults

The diagnosis of RN in adults is mostly a carryover diagnosis from the pediatric age group or is diagnosed because of pregnancy-related complications, recurrent UTI, hypertension, proteinuria, or renal failure. RN in adults shows a more marked differentiation in clinical presentation between the males and the females (Table 3) with adult males presenting mostly with hypertension, proteinuria, and renal failure, whereas the females present mostly with UTI and pregnancy-related complications [12, 31]. The males have a poorer outcome as compared with females, which was previously attributed to a more insidious onset and hence delayed diagnosis in males as compared to earlier diagnosis in females due to recurrent UTI and complications during pregnancy [52]. However, in view of the new knowledge, it is possible that the clinical outcome differences may be because of mostly congenital RN in males as compared to mostly acquired RN in females [31].

In a study that assessed renal function 16–26 years after the first UTI with renal scarring in childhood and compared it with an age-matched cohort, the total glomerular filtration rate (GFR) remained unchanged, but the individual GFR of the scarred kidneys decreased significantly. The decrease in GFR was significant in those with bilateral renal scarring. The median urine albumin/creatinine ratio was 1.2 mg/mmol compared with 0.6 in those with no scarring [53]. In another study on 293 adults (mean age at presentation 31 ± 13.4 years) with RN, females outnumbered males by a ratio of 5:1. The most common presenting complaints for both genders were UTI (65%), hypertension (20%), and proteinuria (6%). However, UTI as a presenting complaint was significantly more common in females as compared with males (72% vs 31%), while proteinuria was significantly more common in males (20% vs 4%). Hypertension was also more common in males (29% vs 18%), but the difference was not significant. VUR was present in 65% females and 75% of males. Of the 147 patients who were followed for a mean period of 6.9 ± 3.6 years, 21 (14%) developed ESKD after a mean follow-up period of 7.0 ± 3.1 years [54].

The complications that have been reported with RN during pregnancy are variable. In a study on 137 women with RN (40% with VUR) with 345 pregnancies, the maternal complications occurred in 39% of the pregnancies. The complications included UTI, hypertension, proteinuria, edema, deterioration in renal function, hematuria, and the renal stones. These complications were significantly more common in those with bilateral renal scarring or impaired renal function (plasma creatinine >0.11 mmol/L) at conception [55]. In another study on 375 pregnancies in 58 women with RN, UTI was the most common complication (22.3%), followed by hypertension (4.3%), preeclampsia (10.4%), fetal loss (10.2%), and preterm delivery (24.2%). The degree of renal function at conception defined the outcome during pregnancy, with compromised fetal prognosis and the progression of maternal disease in those with serum creatinine of >0.22 mmol/L [56].

A more recent study in 87 women with a history of VUR diagnosed during childhood and followed over a median duration of 38 years, maternal complications were detected in 64% and fetal complications in 13% of the cases. Prevalence of UTI (42%), proteinuria (40%), and hypertension (33%) during pregnancy were higher in women with renal scars (48/87) as compared to women with no scarring. The study did not show any increase in the rate of fetal complications or proteinuria due to renal scarring during pregnancy [57].

Conclusion

VUR is a risk factor for recurrent UTI, particularly in those with chronic constipation or BBD. Renal scarring is the most significant complication associated with VUR and the risk factors include high-grade VUR, recurrent UTI, and delayed antibiotic treatment for APN. Hypertension is the commonest complication of renal scarring in children. Recent evidence is indicative of an improving long-term outcome in patients diagnosed with VUR and renal scarring in childhood. Appropriate follow-up of patients with VUR, particularly those with high-grade VUR, is recommended. Patients with renal scarring should be monitored for hypertension and those with significant scarring, particularly bilateral, should be monitored for proteinuria and CKD. Prevention of renal scars and preservation of renal function in those with renal scars remains the most important treatment objective.

References

1. Williams G, Fletcher JT, Alexander SI, Craig JC. Vesicoureteral reflux. J Am Soc Nephrol. 2008;19:847–62.
2. Marra G, Barbieri G, Dell'Agnola CA, Caccamo ML, Castellani MR, Assael BM. Congenital renal damage associated with primary vesicoureteral reflux detected prenatally in male infants. J Pediatr. 1994;124:726–30.
3. Chand DH, Rhoades T, Poe SA, Kraus S, Strife CF. Incidence and severity of vesicoureteral reflux in children related to age, gender, race and diagnosis. J Urol. 2003;170:1548–50.
4. Hodson CJ, Edwards D. Chronic pyelonephritis and vesico-ureteric reflex. Clin Radiol. 1960;11:219–31.
5. Smellie J, Edwards D, Hunter N, Normand IC, Prescod N. Vesico-ureteric reflux and renal scarring. Kidney Int Suppl. 1975;4:S65–72.

6. Bailey RR. The relationship of vesico-ureteric reflux to urinary tract infection and chronic pyelonephritis-reflux nephropathy. Clin Nephrol. 1973;1:132–41.
7. Shaikh N, Ewing AL, Bhatnagar S, Hoberman A. Risk of renal scarring in children with a first urinary tract infection: a systematic review. Pediatrics. 2010;126:1084–91.
8. Keren R, Shaikh N, Pohl H, et al. Risk factors for recurrent urinary tract infection and renal scarring. Pediatrics. 2015;136:e13–21.
9. Dias CS, Silva JMP, Diniz JSS, Lima EM, Marciano RC, Lana LG, Trivelato ALL, Lima MS, Simões e Silva AC, Oliveira EA. Risk factors for recurrent urinary tract infections in a cohort of patients with primary vesicoureteral reflux. Pediatr Infect Dis J. 2010;29:139–44.
10. Sjöström S, Sillén U, Bachelard M, Hansson S, Stokland E. Spontaneous resolution of high grade infantile vesicoureteral reflux. J Urol. 2004;172:694–8. discussion 699.
11. Panaretto K, Craig J, Knight J, Howman-Giles R, Sureshkumar P, Roy L. Risk factors for recurrent urinary tract infection in preschool children. J Paediatr Child Health. 1999;35:454–9.
12. Mattoo TK, Mohammad D. Primary vesicoureteral reflux and renal scarring. Pediatr Clin N Am. 2022;69:1115–29.
13. Peters CA, Skoog SJ, Arant BSJ, et al. Summary of the AUA guideline on management of primary vesicoureteral reflux in children. J Urol. 2010;184:1134–44.
14. Cotran RS. Nephrology forum. Glomerulosclerosis in reflux nephropathy. Kidney Int. 1982;21:528–34.
15. Ransley PG, Risdon RA. Reflux nephropathy: effects of antimicrobial therapy on the evolution of the early pyelonephritic scar. Kidney Int. 1981;20:733–42.
16. Ransley PG, Risdon RA. Renal papillary morphology in infants and young children. Urol Res. 1975;3:111–3.
17. Shindo S, Bernstein J, Arant BSJ. Evolution of renal segmental atrophy (Ask-Upmark kidney) in children with vesicoureteric reflux: radiographic and morphologic studies. J Pediatr. 1983;102:847–54.
18. Ching C, Schwartz L, Spencer JD, Becknell B. Innate immunity and urinary tract infection. Pediatr Nephrol. 2020;35:1183–92.
19. Ragnarsdóttir B, Svanborg C. Susceptibility to acute pyelonephritis or asymptomatic bacteriuria: host-pathogen interaction in urinary tract infections. Pediatr Nephrol. 2012;27:2017–29.
20. Skoog SJ, Peters CA, Arant BSJ, et al. Pediatric vesicoureteral reflux guidelines panel summary report: clinical practice guidelines for screening siblings of children with vesicoureteral reflux and neonates/infants with prenatal hydronephrosis. J Urol. 2010;184:1145–51.
21. Mattoo TK, Chesney RW, Greenfield SP, et al. Renal scarring in the randomized intervention for children with vesicoureteral reflux (RIVUR) trial. Clin J Am Soc Nephrol. 2016;11:54–61.
22. Snodgrass WT, Shah A, Yang M, Kwon J, Villanueva C, Traylor J, Pritzker K, Nakonezny PA, Haley RW, Bush NC. Prevalence and risk factors for renal scars in children with febrile UTI and/or VUR: a cross-sectional observational study of 565 consecutive patients. J Pediatr Urol. 2013;9:856–63.
23. Shaikh N, Craig JC, Rovers MM, et al. Identification of children and adolescents at risk for renal scarring after a first urinary tract infection: a meta-analysis with individual patient data. JAMA Pediatr. 2014;168:893–900.
24. Roberts KB. Urinary tract infections and renal damage: focusing on what matters. JAMA Pediatr. 2014;168:884–5.
25. Shaikh N, Mattoo TK, Keren R, Ivanova A, Cui G, Moxey-Mims M, Majd M, Ziessman HA, Hoberman A. Early antibiotic treatment for pediatric febrile urinary tract infection and renal scarring. JAMA Pediatr. 2016;170:848–54. https://doi.org/10.1001/jamapediatrics.2016.1181.
26. Meena J, Mathew G, Hari P, Sinha A, Bagga A. Prevalence of bladder and bowel dysfunction in toilet-trained children with urinary tract infection and/or primary vesicoureteral reflux: a systematic review and meta-analysis. Front Pediatr. 2020;8:84.
27. Peters CA, Skoog SJ, Arant BS Jr, Copp HL, Elder JS, Hudson RG, et al. Management and screening of primary vesicoureteral reflux in children (2010, amended 2017). American Urological Association. Available at https://www.auanet.org/guidelines/vesicoureteral-reflux-guideline.

28. Fernández-Menéndez JM, Málaga S, Matesanz JL, Solís G, Alonso S, Pérez-Méndez C. Risk factors in the development of early technetium-99m dimercaptosuccinic acid renal scintigraphy lesions during first urinary tract infection in children. Acta Paediatr. 2003;92:21–6.
29. Howie AJ, Buist LJ, Coulthard MG. Reflux nephropathy in transplants. Pediatr Nephrol. 2002;17:485–90.
30. Coulthard MG, Flecknell P, Orr H, Manas D, O'Donnell M. Renal scarring caused by vesicoureteric reflux and urinary infection: a study in pigs. Pediatr Nephrol. 2002;17:481–4.
31. Mattoo TK. Vesicoureteral reflux and reflux nephropathy. Adv Chronic Kidney Dis. 2011;18:348–54.
32. Faust WC, Diaz M, Pohl HG. Incidence of post-pyelonephritic renal scarring: a meta-analysis of the dimercapto-succinic acid literature. J Urol. 2009;181:290–8.
33. Smellie JM, Prescod NP, Shaw PJ, Risdon RA, Bryant TN. Childhood reflux and urinary infection: a follow-up of 10-41 years in 226 adults. Pediatr Nephrol. 1998;12:727–36.
34. Goonasekera CD, Gordon I, Dillon MJ. 15-year follow-up of reflux nephropathy by imaging. Clin Nephrol. 1998;50:224–31.
35. Simoes e Silva AC, JMP S, JSS D, Pinheiro SVB, Lima EM, Vasconcelos MA, Pimenta MR, Oliveira EA. Risk of hypertension in primary vesicoureteral reflux. Pediatr Nephrol. 2007;22:459–62.
36. Ahmed M, Eggleston D, Kapur G, Jain A, Valentini RP, Mattoo TK. Dimercaptosuccinic acid (DMSA) renal scan in the evaluation of hypertension in children. Pediatr Nephrol. 2008;23:435–8.
37. Cornwell LB, Riddell JV, Mason MD. New-onset ESRD secondary to reflux nephropathy has decreased in incidence in the United States. J Pediatr Urol. 2020;16:566.e1–7.
38. Savage JM, Koh CT, Shah V, Barratt TM, Dillon MJ. Five year prospective study of plasma renin activity and blood pressure in patients with longstanding reflux nephropathy. Arch Dis Child. 1987;62:678–82.
39. Gebäck C, Hansson S, Himmelmann A, Sandberg T, Sixt R, Jodal U. Twenty-four-hour ambulatory blood pressure in adult women with urinary tract infection in childhood. J Hypertens. 2014;32:1658–64. discussion 1664
40. Zhang Y, Bailey RR. A long term follow up of adults with reflux nephropathy. N Z Med J. 1995;108:142–4.
41. Karlén J, Linné T, Wikstad I, Aperia A. Incidence of microalbuminuria in children with pyelonephritic scarring. Pediatr Nephrol. 1996;10:705–8.
42. Coppo R, Porcellini MG, Gianoglio B, Alessi D, Peruzzi L, Amore A, Bianchi M, Lace R, Cavalli G, Amprimo MC. Glomerular permselectivity to macromolecules in reflux nephropathy: microalbuminuria during acute hyperfiltration due to aminoacid infusion. Clin Nephrol. 1993;40:299–307.
43. Bailey RR, Lynn KL, Smith AH. Long-term followup of infants with gross vesicoureteral reflux. J Urol. 1992;148:1709–11.
44. Lahdes-Vasama T, Niskanen K, Rönnholm K. Outcome of kidneys in patients treated for vesicoureteral reflux (VUR) during childhood. Nephrol Dial Transplant. 2006;21:2491–7.
45. Neild GH. What do we know about chronic renal failure in young adults? II. Adult outcome of pediatric renal disease. Pediatr Nephrol. 2009;24:1921–8.
46. Neild GH, Thomson G, Nitsch D, Woolfson RG, Connolly JO, Woodhouse CRJ. Renal outcome in adults with renal insufficiency and irregular asymmetric kidneys. BMC Nephrol. 2004;5:12.
47. NAPRTCS. North American Pediatric Renal Transplant Cooperative Study (NAPRTCS); 2008 annual report.
48. Furth SL, Abraham AG, Jerry-Fluker J, Schwartz GJ, Benfield M, Kaskel F, Wong C, Mak RH, Moxey-Mims M, Warady BA. Metabolic abnormalities, cardiovascular disease risk factors, and GFR decline in children with chronic kidney disease. Clin J Am Soc Nephrol. 2011;6:2132–40.

49. Silva JMP, Diniz JSS, Silva ACS, Azevedo MV, Pimenta MR, Oliveira EA. Predictive factors of chronic kidney disease in severe vesicoureteral reflux. Pediatr Nephrol. 2006;21:1285–92.
50. Silva JMP, Diniz JSS, Lima EM, Vergara RM, Oliveira EA. Predictive factors of resolution of primary vesico-ureteric reflux: a multivariate analysis. BJU Int. 2006;97:1063–8.
51. McKay AM, Kim S, Kennedy SE. Long-term outcome of kidney transplantation in patients with congenital anomalies of the kidney and urinary tract. Pediatr Nephrol. 2019;34:2409–15.
52. Williams DG. Reflux nephropathy. Q J Med. 1990;77:1205–7.
53. Wennerström M, Hansson S, Jodal U, Sixt R, Stokland E. Renal function 16 to 26 years after the first urinary tract infection in childhood. Arch Pediatr Adolesc Med. 2000;154:339–45.
54. El-Khatib MT, Becker GJ, Kincaid-Smith PS. Reflux nephropathy and primary vesicoureteric reflux in adults. Q J Med. 1990;77:1241–53.
55. El-Khatib M, Packham DK, Becker GJ, Kincaid-Smith P. Pregnancy-related complications in women with reflux nephropathy. Clin Nephrol. 1994;41:50–5.
56. Jungers P, Houillier P, Chauveau D, Choukroun G, Moynot A, Skhiri H, Labrunie M, Descamps-Latscha B, Grünfeld JP. Pregnancy in women with reflux nephropathy. Kidney Int. 1996;50:593–9.
57. Roihuvuo-Leskinen H-M, Vainio MI, Niskanen KM, Lahdes-Vasama TT. Pregnancies in women with childhood vesicoureteral reflux. Acta Obstet Gynecol Scand. 2015;94:847–51.